PROLOG

Personal Review of Learning in Obstetrics and Gynecology

Gynecologic Oncology and Critical Care

NINTH EDITION

Critique Book

ONLINE ASSESSMENT

See instructions on the inside front cover.

ACOG

American College of Obstetricians & Gynecologists

American College of Obstetricians & Gynecologists

ISBN 978-1-948258-93-7 (trade paperback) | ISBN 978-1-948258-94-4 (ebook)

Printed in the United States of America

1 2 3 4 5 / 0 9 8 7 6

American College of Obstetricians & Gynecologists
409 12th Street SW
Washington, DC 20024-2188

Contributors

PROLOG Editorial Board

PROLOG Task Force for *Gynecologic Oncology and Critical Care,* Ninth Edition

COCHAIRS

Marcela G. del Carmen, MD, MPH
Professor of Obstetrics, Gynecology and Reproductive Biology
Department of Obstetrics, Gynecology and Reproductive Biology
President, Massachusetts General Hospital
Massachusetts General Hospital
Harvard Medical School
Boston, Massachusetts

Michael T. McHale, MD
Clinical Professor
Department of Obstetrics, Gynecology and Reproductive Sciences
Division Director, Gynecologic Oncology
University of California San Diego
Moores Cancer Center
Surgical Director, Perioperative Services
University of California San Diego Health System
San Diego, California

Ryan Spencer, MD, MS
Professor
Division of Gynecologic Oncology
Department of Obstetrics & Gynecology
University of Wisconsin School of Medicine and Public Health
Madison, Wisconsin

Deanna Teoh, MD, MS
Associate Professor
Division of Gynecologic Oncology
Department of Obstetrics, Gynecology and Women's Health
University of Minnesota
Minneapolis, Minnesota

MEMBERS

Dana M. Chase, MD
Professor
David Geffen School of Medicine at UCLA
Los Angeles, California

Leslie H. Clark, MD
Associate Professor of Gynecologic Oncology
Department of Obstetrics and Gynecology
University of North Carolina at Chapel Hill
Chapel Hill, North Carolina

Erica R. Hope, MD
Gynecologic Oncology
Department of Gynecologic Surgery & Obstetrics
Brooke Army Medical Center
Assistant Professor, Uniformed Services University
San Antonio, Texas

Jennifer R. Jorgensen, MD, MPH
Assistant Professor
Department of Obstetrics and Gynecology
Division of Gynecologic Oncology
University of Connecticut School of Medicine
Farmington, Connecticut

Sarah Lindsay, MD, MSc
Assistant Professor
Hartford Healthcare Medical Group
University of Connecticut School of Medicine
Hartford, Connecticut

DISCLOSURE STATEMENT

The Accreditation Council for Continuing Medical Education (ACCME) requires that all faculty and planning committee members disclose any financial interests relative to topics within this edition of PROLOG. This information will be obtained in advance by staff through the American College of Obstetricians & Gynecologists' (ACOG) online disclosure system. There must be ample time for resolution of all potential conflicts of interest. This information (with resolution of any conflicts of interest) should be on file before honoraria are paid.

DISCLOSURE OF FACULTY AND INDUSTRY RELATIONSHIPS

In accordance with ACOG's policy, all faculty and planning committee members have signed a conflict-of-interest statement in which they have disclosed any financial interests or other relationships with industry relative to topics in this edition of PROLOG. Such disclosure allows for better evaluation of the objectivity of the information presented.

CONFLICT OF INTEREST DISCLOSURE

This PROLOG unit was developed under the direction of the PROLOG Editorial Board and Task Force for *Gynecologic Oncology and Critical Care*, Ninth Edition. PROLOG is planned and produced in accordance with the Standards for Commercial Support of the ACCME. Any discussion of unapproved use of products is clearly cited in the appropriate critique.

Current guidelines state that continuing medical education (CME) health care professionals must ensure that CME activities are free from the control of any commercial interest. The task force and advisory committee members declare that neither they nor any business associate nor any member of their immediate families has material interest, financial interest, or other relationships with any company manufacturing commercial products relative to the topics included in this publication or with any provider of commercial services discussed in the volume. All potential conflicts have been resolved through ACOG's mechanism for resolving potential and real conflicts of interest.

Special Acknowledgment

In addition to thanking the advisors, cochairs, and writers for their dedication and many hours of writing, editing, and meeting time, ACOG extends its thanks and gratitude to their institutions and organizations. With their support, task force members were able to devote time and energy to this important volume in the nationally recognized PROLOG series.

Baylor College of Medicine

Brooke Army Medical Center

Case Western Reserve School of Medicine

David Geffen School of Medicine at UCLA

Hartford Health Care

Harvard Medical School

Kaiser Permanente Northern California

Texas Children's Hospital

Tripler Army Medical Center

University of California San Diego Health

University of Connecticut Health Center

University of Connecticut School of Medicine

University of Massachusetts Chan Medical School

University of Michigan

University of Minnesota

University of North Carolina at Chapel Hill

University of Wisconsin School of Medicine and Public Health

Preface

Purpose

PROLOG (Personal Review of Learning in Obstetrics and Gynecology) is a voluntary, strictly confidential self-evaluation program. PROLOG was developed specifically as a personal study resource for the practicing obstetrician–gynecologist. It is presented as a self-assessment mechanism that, with its accompanying performance information, should assist the physician in designing a personal, self-directed, lifelong learning program. It may be used as a valuable study tool, a reference guide, and a means of attaining up-to-date information in the specialty. The content is carefully selected and presented in multiple-choice questions that are clinically oriented. The questions are designed to stimulate and challenge physicians in areas of medical care that they confront in their practices or when they work as consultant obstetrician–gynecologists.

Process

The PROLOG series offers the most current information available in six areas of the specialty: 1) obstetrics; 2) gynecology and surgery; 3) reproductive endocrinology and infertility; 4) urogynecology and reconstructive pelvic surgery; 5) gynecologic oncology and critical care; and 6) patient management in the office. A new PROLOG edition is produced annually, addressing one of these subject areas.

Each unit of PROLOG represents the efforts of a task force of subject matter experts under the supervision of an advisory committee. PROLOG sets forth current information as viewed by recognized authorities in the field of women's health. This educational resource does not define a standard of care, nor is it intended to dictate an exclusive course of management. It presents recognized methods and techniques of clinical practice for consideration by obstetrician–gynecologists to incorporate in their practices. Variations of practice that consider the needs of the individual patient, resources, and the limitations that are special to the institution or type of practice may be appropriate.

Each unit of PROLOG is presented as a two-part book, with performance information and cognate credit available to those who choose to submit their assessment for confidential scoring. The first part of this PROLOG edition is the Critique Book, which contains a discussion or critique of each question. Each critique provides the rationale for correct and incorrect options for each multiple-choice question. Current, accessible references are listed with each critique.

The second part of this PROLOG edition is the Assessment Book, which contains educational objectives for the volume and questions. The questions can be completed by taking an online assessment. Participants can work through the volume at their own pace, choosing to use PROLOG as a closed-book or open-book assessment. Submitting the online assessment is voluntary but encouraged. Participants can earn CME credits only by submitting and passing the online assessment.

Continuing Medical Education Credit

ACCME ACCREDITATION

The American College of Obstetricians & Gynecologists is accredited by the Accreditation Council for Continuing Medical Education (ACCME) to provide continuing medical education for physicians.

AMA PRA CATEGORY 1 CREDIT(S)™

The American College of Obstetricians & Gynecologists designates this enduring material for a maximum of *25 AMA PRA Category 1 Credits*™. Physicians should claim only the credit commensurate with the extent of their participation in the activity.

ACOG COGNATE CREDIT(S)

The American College of Obstetricians & Gynecologists designates this enduring material for a maximum of 25 Category 1 College Cognate Credits. The American College of Obstetricians & Gynecologists has a reciprocity agreement with the American Medical Association that allows *AMA PRA Category 1 Credits*™ to be equivalent to College Cognate Credits.

Participants who submit their assessment for scoring and receive a passing grade of 80% will be credited with 25 CME credits. An individual may request credit only once for each edition. Participants receive CME verification immediately after they pass the online assessment.

Credit for PROLOG: *Gynecologic Oncology and Critical Care*, Ninth Edition, is initially available through December 2028. During that year, the unit will be reevaluated. If the content remains current, credit is extended for an additional 3 years, with credit for the unit automatically withdrawn after December 2031.

Electronic Assessment for CME Credit

To receive the CME credits for this edition, participants must complete an online assessment. Assessment results must be 80% or higher to achieve a passing score and attain CME credit. To access the online assessment, please visit https://prolog.acog.org. Test results and the CME certificate will be available upon completion of the examination.

If you purchased a print book, use the key code located on the inside front cover of the Critique Book and follow the directions provided. If you purchased an eBook, please follow the instructions online through https://prolog.acog.org to purchase and access the assessment.

Conclusion

PROLOG was developed specifically as a personal study resource for the practicing obstetrician–gynecologist. It is presented as a self-assessment mechanism that, with its accompanying performance information, should assist the physician in designing a personal, self-directed learning program. The many quality resources developed by ACOG, as featured in our online store (https://www.acog.org/store), are available to help fulfill the educational interests and needs that have been identified. PROLOG is not intended as a substitute for the certification or recertification programs of the American Board of Obstetrics and Gynecology.

PROLOG CME Schedule

Each volume of PROLOG is accredited for 3 years from its initial publication date. After 3 years, the edition is evaluated for reaccreditation.

Gynecologic Oncology and Critical Care, Eighth Edition	Accredited through 2026
Patient Management in the Office, Eighth Edition	Accredited through 2027
Obstetrics, Ninth Edition	Accredited through 2027
Gynecology and Surgery, Ninth Edition	Accredited through 2027
Reproductive Endocrinology and Infertility, Ninth Edition	Accredited through 2027
Urogynecology and Reconstructive Pelvic Surgery, Second Edition	Accredited through June 2028
Gynecologic Oncology and Critical Care, Ninth Edition	Accredited through 2028

PROLOG Objectives

PROLOG is a voluntary, strictly confidential, personal continuing education resource that is designed to be stimulating and enjoyable. By participating in PROLOG, obstetrician–gynecologists will be able to do the following:

- Review and update clinical knowledge
- Recognize areas of knowledge and practice in which they excel, be stimulated to explore other areas of the specialty, and identify areas requiring further study
- Plan continuing education activities in light of identified strengths and deficiencies
- Compare and relate present knowledge and skills with those of other participants
- Obtain continuing medical education credit, if desired
- Have complete personal control of the setting and of the pace of the experience

The obstetrician–gynecologist who completes *Gynecologic Oncology and Critical Care*, Ninth Edition, will be able to

- identify epidemiologic factors that contribute to the risks of various malignancies and determine appropriate screening tests.
- analyze the pathophysiology and evaluate the histopathology of various malignancies.
- associate symptoms with early onset of specific malignancies, determine appropriate diagnostic tests, and select diagnosis.
- identify physical and surgical findings related to specific stages of malignant disease.
- determine appropriate chemotherapeutic and biological therapy for various types of gynecologic cancer and identify common complications of therapy.
- determine approaches for preoperative assessment, select surgical techniques for gynecologic disorders, and identify common complications of surgery.
- apply knowledge of anatomy, wound management, and appropriate surgical techniques in the surgical therapy of gynecologic disease.
- determine the appropriate treatment of the critical care patient.

Gynecologic Oncology and Critical Care, Ninth Edition, includes the following topics (item numbers appear in parentheses):

Counseling

Bariatric surgery (11)
Familial cancer (24)
Mortality risk factors (17)
Ovarian cancer risk reduction (105)
Ovarian cancer screening (92)
Precision medicine (70)
Recurrent metastatic cancer (55)
Survivorship (152–155)
Vaginal dysplasia (100)

Epidemiology and Biostatistics

Clinical findings and associated hereditary cancer syndromes (93)
Database research (109)
Identifying hereditary cancer syndromes (42)
Kaplan–Meier method (59)
Positive and negative predictive values (90)
Receiver operator characteristic curve (72)
Somatic testing in ovarian cancer (63)
Testing for hereditary cancer syndromes in endometrial cancer (64)
Types of clinical studies (75)

Medical Management

Acupuncture in cancer (51)
Antibody–drug conjugates (31)
Back pain (82)
Cancer diagnosis (91)
Cancer-related electrolyte imbalances (2)
Cervical cancer recurrence (48)
Checkpoint inhibitor toxicity (114–117)
Chemotherapy for recurrent ovarian cancer (50)
Complications of chemotherapy (35)
Deep vein thrombosis (39)
Depression (14)
Diarrhea (47)
Electrolyte abnormalities in advanced cervical cancer (66)
Endometrial cancer evaluation (27)
Endometrial sampling (26)
Evaluation of hematuria (71)
Febrile neutropenia (58)
First-line chemotherapy in ovarian cancer (61)
Geriatric oncology (23)
Hemodynamic monitoring (95)
HER2+ serous endometrial cancer (78)
High-risk gestational trophoblastic neoplasia (140–143)
Hospice (113)
Hypoxia (85)
Initial management of high-risk gestational trophoblastic neoplasia (32)
Low-grade serous ovarian cancer (102)
Maintenance therapy in ovarian cancer (103)
Malignant ovarian germ cell tumor (45)
Management of recurrent malignant ascites (65)
Massive transfusion protocol (5)

Screening and Diagnosis

Surgical Management

A complete subject matter index is included at the end of the Critique Book.

1 Vulvar irritation

A 46-year-old woman presents with new vulvar itching and irritation. Her physical examination is notable for a 2 × 1.5-cm raised gray lesion on the right labium majus. A punch biopsy is performed, and the results are shown in Figure 1-1. The best next step in management is

(A) carbon dioxide laser ablation
(B) cryotherapy ablation
(C) high-potency topical corticosteroid
(D) topical imiquimod
* (E) wide local excision

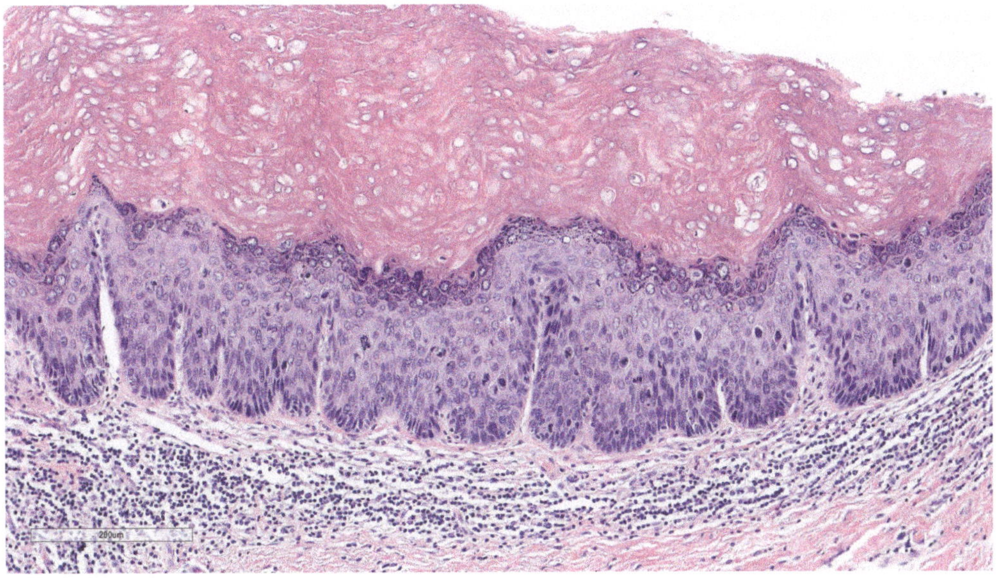

FIGURE 1-1. Vulvar punch biopsy.

Vulvar intraepithelial neoplasia (VIN) rates are on the rise, increasing by 3% per year over 30 years. It can affect any age group, but the incidence is now highest among individuals in their 40s. Vulvar intraepithelial neoplasia is a precancerous lesion with a risk of malignant transformation as well as a risk of concomitant underlying malignancy. It previously was classified into a three-tiered system; however, this was replaced with a single-grade system, in which only high-grade disease is classified as VIN. It is subdivided into usual-type VIN, now termed vulvar high-grade squamous intraepithelial lesion (HSIL), which is strongly associated with human papillomavirus, and differentiated VIN (dVIN, non-HPV associated). Vulvar HSIL is characterized by abnormal cell maturation, enlarged atypical nuclei, and dysplastic features extending above the lower third of the epithelium, as seen in the patient's biopsy; therefore, this patient's diagnosis is HSIL. Differentiated VIN is characterized by more subtle histologic changes, such as basal atypia with premature cell maturation, absence of granular layer, parakeratosis, and enlarged, hyperchromatic nuclei with mitotic figures. It can be difficult to histologically differentiate dVIN and HSIL, and often immunohistochemistry is needed for diagnosis. Differentiated VIN is p53+, and HSIL is p16+. Diagnosis of dVIN often is complicated by the presence of coexisting skin dermatoses, such as lichen sclerosus. Table 1-1 compares and contrasts the features of HSIL and dVIN.

Vulvar HSIL is associated with an underlying invasive squamous cell carcinoma in 20% of patients. This percentage is even higher in patients with dVIN, with some studies reporting the percentage as high as 85%. Due to the high risk of underlying squamous cell carcinoma, wide local excision is recommended as initial management in women with either HSIL (when invasive disease cannot be ruled out) or dVIN. The excision should include a tissue margin of 0.5–1 cm beyond the area of visible disease, although it can be modified to avoid critical structures. Excision specimens should be marked for orientation and sent for pathologic analysis. In this patient with HSIL and possible

*Indicates answer.
Note: See Appendix A for a table of normal values for laboratory tests.

TABLE 1-1. Features of Vulvar High-Grade Squamous Intraepithelial Lesion and Differentiated Vulvar Intraepithelial Neoplasia

VULVAR HIGH-GRADE SQUAMOUS INTRAEPITHELIAL NEOPLASIA	DIFFERENTIATED VIN (dVIN)
Associated with carcinogenic types of HPV	Non-HPV associated
Associated with HPV persistence risk factors, such as smoking and immunocompromise	Associated with vulvar dermatologic conditions, such as lichen sclerosus
Lower association with squamous cell carcinoma and risk of recurrence compared with dVIN	Higher association with squamous cell carcinoma and risk of recurrence
Histologic changes • Abnormal cell maturation • Enlarged atypical nuclei • Dysplastic features extending above the lower third of epithelium	Histologic changes • Basal atypia with premature cell maturation • Absence of granular layer • Parakeratosis • Enlarged, hyperchromatic nuclei with mitotic figures
Immunohistochemical staining: p16+	Immunohistochemical staining: p53+

Abbreviation: HPV, human papillomavirus

Data from Management of vulvar intraepithelial neoplasia. Committee Opinion No. 675. American College of Obstetricians and Gynecologists [published erratum appears in Obstet Gynecol 2017;129:209]. Obstet Gynecol 2016;128:e178–82. doi: 10.1097/AOG.0000000000001713

occult invasive disease, wide local excision is the best initial management option.

Other surgical treatment options, such as carbon dioxide laser ablation and argon beam coagulation, can be considered for individuals with usual-type VIN in whom invasive cancer is not a concern. Multiple representative biopsies should be obtained to exclude invasive disease before beginning treatment. The laser ablation treatment area should include 0.5–1 cm of normal-appearing skin and to a depth of 3 mm into the subcutaneous fat for hair-bearing skin and 2 mm into the dermis for skin with no hair. The large size of this patient's lesion and possible concern for cancer preclude treatment with laser ablation.

Cryotherapy ablation was previously used to treat cervical intraepithelial neoplasia; however, it has largely fallen out of favor as a treatment option due to high rates of recurrence and the availability of more effective treatment options. Cryotherapy should not be used to treat cases of VIN; therefore, it is not the best next step for this patient. Medical treatment options for usual-type VIN are suitable to preserve vulvar anatomy and avoid mutilation in individuals for whom cancer is not a concern. Just as with more conservative surgical treatment, several biopsies are needed to exclude invasive disease. Imiquimod is an immune response modifier that has strong immune infiltration. Response rates with imiquimod treatment range from 35% to 81%, with improved long-lasting results for those with smaller lesions. Topical imiquimod is not an acceptable treatment option for this patient, in whom invasive disease has not been ruled out, and it is less likely to be effective in a larger lesion. Imiquimod may have reduced efficacy in patients who are immunocompromised.

High-potency topical corticosteroids are a highly effective treatment option for skin dermatoses, such as lichen sclerosus, which is associated with vulvar pruritis and irritation. Appropriate treatment of skin dermatoses, particularly lichen sclerosus, can prevent the development of dVIN. In this patient, who has usual-type VIN (vulvar high-grade squamous intraepithelial lesion), topical corticosteroids will not treat the underlying disease.

Cases of usual-type VIN are increasing in the United States. Gynecologists should perform a thorough inspection of the vulva during yearly pelvic examinations, particularly in symptomatic patients. All suspicious vulvar lesions should be biopsied for diagnosis. For individuals in whom occult invasive disease cannot be ruled out, wide local excision is the preferred initial treatment option. Additionally, patients should be counseled on the risk of recurrence and the necessity of long-term follow-up.

Lebreton M, Carton I, Brousse S, Lavoué V, Body G, Levêque J, et al. Vulvar intraepithelial neoplasia: classification, epidemiology, diagnosis, and management. J Gynecol Obstet Hum Reprod 2020;49:101801. doi: 10.1016/j.jogoh.2020.101801

Management of vulvar intraepithelial neoplasia. Committee Opinion No. 675. American College of Obstetricians and Gynecologists [published erratum appears in Obstet Gynecol 2017;129:209]. Obstet Gynecol 2016;128:e178–82. doi: 10.1097/AOG.0000000000001713

Preti M, Joura E, Vieira-Baptista P, Van Beurden M, Bevilacqua F, Bleeker MC, et al. The European Society of Gynaecological Oncology (ESGO), the International Society for the Study of Vulvovaginal Disease (ISSVD), the European College for the Study of Vulval Disease (ECSVD) and the European Federation for Colposcopy (EFC) consensus statements on pre-invasive vulvar lesions. J Low Genit Tract Dis 2022;26:229–44. doi: 10.1097/LGT.0000000000000683

2 Cancer-related electrolyte imbalances

A 58-year-old patient with recurrent platinum-resistant high-grade serous ovarian cancer treated with liposomal doxorubicin and bevacizumab presents to the emergency department. She has experienced worsening oral intake, abdominal pain, and nausea and vomiting during the last week. Her partner reports that she seems confused and disoriented. Her vital signs include a temperature of 37.2 °C (99 °F), a blood pressure of 98/60 mm Hg, a heart rate of 112 bpm, and a respiratory rate of 14, and her oxygen saturation is 99% on room air. On examination, she is oriented to self, but not place or time, and has diffuse abdominal tenderness to palpation without rebound or guarding. Serum electrolytes are notable for concentrations of calcium (14.1 mg/dL) and albumin (3 g/dL). An electrocardiogram demonstrates sinus tachycardia with a shortened QT interval. The best next step in treatment is the administration of

(A) calcitonin
(B) furosemide
* (C) normal saline
(D) prednisone
(E) zoledronic acid

Hypercalcemia occurs in 20–30% of patients with malignancy and is most common in those with advanced-stage disease. Hypercalcemia of malignancy can occur due to tumor secretion of parathyroid hormone, osteolytic metastases, and tumor production of 1,25-dihydroxyvitamin D. Most patients with hypercalcemia of malignancy will have clinical evidence of a malignant diagnosis at the time of increased calcium levels. *Mild hypercalcemia* is defined as serum calcium concentrations of 10.5–12 mg/dL, *moderate* as 12–14 mg/dL, and *severe* as greater than 14 mg/dL. Patients with severe hypercalcemia may experience lethargy, musculoskeletal pain, altered mental status, significant volume depletion, and acute renal insufficiency, and they require prompt treatment regardless of the severity of symptoms.

The patient in this scenario has severe hypercalcemia and should receive prompt interventions to lower calcium levels. Normal saline hydration is the best initial step for patients with severe hypercalcemia because it increases circulating blood volume and renal clearance of calcium. Because patients with severe hypercalcemia have marked intravascular volume depletion, administering isotonic saline for 24–48 hours corrects volume depletion while promoting the excretion of calcium. Care should be taken to avoid fluid overload in patients with impaired renal function or heart failure.

Patients with severe hypercalcemia often will require concurrent treatment with other medications, including bisphosphonates, with or without calcitonin. Calcitonin reduces serum calcium by increasing renal calcium excretion and decreasing bone resorption of calcium. It is considered a weak agent, although it works rapidly within 4–6 hours. Caution should be used because patients can develop tachyphylaxis within 48 hours due to down-regulation of calcitonin receptors. Given the onset of time to action, calcitonin would not be the best next treatment in a patient with severe hypercalcemia.

Furosemide is a diuretic that reduces serum calcium by increasing urinary excretion through prevention of calcium reabsorption in the thick ascending limb of the loop of Henle. Before the development of bisphosphonates, furosemide was a management option among patients with severe hypercalcemia; however, current data do not support routine use in the management of severe hypercalcemia. Furosemide is reserved for the management of fluid overload, and its efficacy in treating hypercalcemia depends on a patient's volume status and fluid balance before administration. It is not the best treatment choice for this patient.

Prednisone is a corticosteroid that can be used to treat hypercalcemia caused by excess extrarenal 1,25-dihydroxyvitamin D. Corticosteroids inhibit osteoclast bone resorption by decreasing tumor production of cytokines, and they also have a direct tumor-lytic effect. Prednisone is typically given over a course of 10 days and is not used as first-line treatment in a patient with severe hypercalcemia in the acute setting; therefore, it is not the correct answer.

Zoledronic acid is a bisphosphonate that induces osteoclast apoptosis. It can also affect the proliferation and differentiation of osteoblasts and neutralize RANKL-mediated stimulation of osteoclasts. Bisphosphonates are part of first-line treatment for hypercalcemia but take approximately 2–4 days to take effect; therefore, starting treatment with intravenous hydration is important to increase calcium excretion and treat symptoms. Zoledronic acid can be started at the time of intravenous hydration to provide long-term treatment of hypercalcemia, but it is not the best initial step due to its delayed effect.

Goldner W. Cancer-related hypercalcemia. J Oncol Pract 2016;12:426–32. doi: 10.1200/JOP.2016.011155

Oueslati I, Kardi A, Yazidi M, Abidi S, Chaker F, Mellassi S, et al. Management of severe hypercalcaemia secondary to primary hyperparathyroidism: the efficacy of saline hydration, furosemide, and zoledronic acid. Endocrinol Diabetes Metab 2022;5:e380. doi: 10.1002/edm2.380

Walker MD, Shane E. Hypercalcemia: a review. JAMA 2022;328:1624–36. doi: 10.1001/jama.2022.18331

3 Laparoscopic complications

A 61-year-old woman with serous endometrial cancer presents for surgical staging. Her history is remarkable for a BMI of 41 and prior colonic resection due to a perforated diverticulitis and subsequent hernia repair with mesh. During laparoscopic entry with an open technique at the umbilicus, the small bowel is encountered during sharp dissection. After additional trocar placement and lysis of adhesions, an 8-mm enterotomy is identified in the ileum. No through and through defect is identified. The best next step is

(A) bowel diversion
(B) omental patch
(C) placement of enteral stent
* (D) primary repair
(E) resection with anastomosis

Bowel injury is a rare but significant complication during abdominal and pelvic surgery. The greatest risk factor for bowel injury is adhesive disease. Immediate identification and appropriate management are critical to optimal patient outcomes.

When feasible, primary repair of a bowel injury is preferred, particularly when approaching a small bowel injury. For the patient in this scenario, who has a less than 1-cm enterotomy, primary repair is the best next step. Primary repair is performed using an interrupted, single-layer closure as shown in Figure 3-1. Some surgeons prefer a second imbricating layer. Primary repair is performed by closing the defect in the longitudinal axis of the bowel to avoid narrowing the bowel lumen. Sutures are initially placed at each apex to elongate the defect perpendicular to the bowel and facilitate the closure. Historically, 3-0 silk suture has been preferred, but many surgeons now choose delayed absorbable suture material, such as polyglactin 910. Sutures are placed approximately 4 mm apart and incorporate 4–5 mm of serosa and the edge of the mucosa in each stitch. Contraindications to primary repair include injury greater than 50% of bowel circumference and bowel ischemia (such as due to mesenteric devascularization or electrosurgery).

Bowel continuity is preferred to diversion, particularly when a small bowel injury is sustained. When primary repair is not feasible due to the extent of injury or devascularization, a bowel resection and anastomosis is the preferred mode of repair. Hand-sewn and stapled anastomoses can be performed. Randomized trials in general surgery have shown the two approaches to be equivalent; however, in some cases, such as severe inflammation or luminal size discrepancy, a hand-sewn anastomosis may be preferred.

If a patient has a high risk of anastomotic leak or a bowel injury that cannot be definitively repaired, diversion of the fecal stream proximal to the injury should be performed. The described patient has a small, sharp injury and is amenable to primary repair; therefore, this is not the best next step. If a bowel resection and diversion are anticipated, a preoperative stomal therapist can help identify an appropriate location for placement of a diverting ostomy that avoids skin folds or the pant waistline. Preoperative marking is best performed with the patient sitting up. If the patient has not undergone preoperative marking, the surgeon should identify an area on the

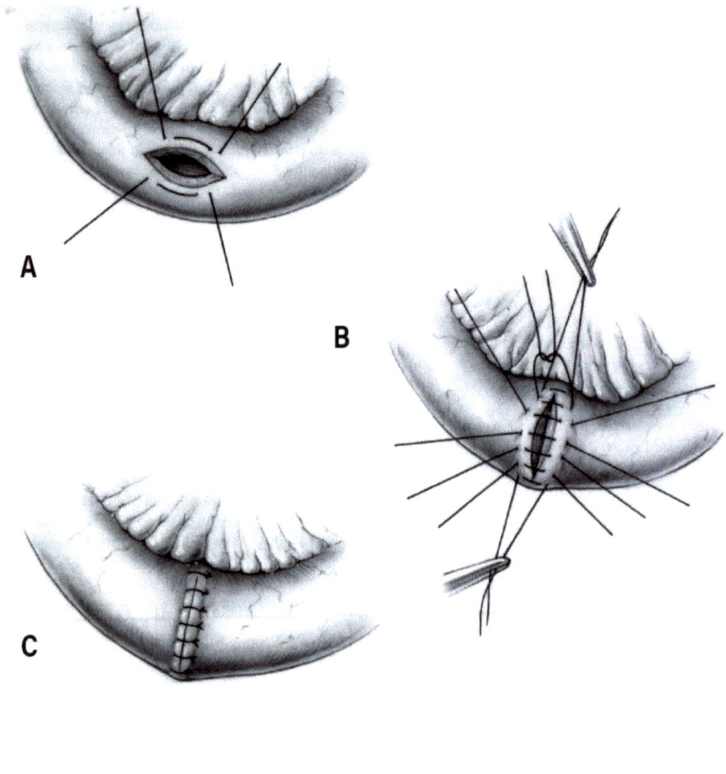

FIGURE 3-1. Image A demonstrates the placement of sutures at the apices of the longitudinal wound to orient the closure of the defect perpendicular to the axis of the bowel. Image B shows the conversion of the longitudinal defect to a transverse defect with interrupted 3-0 imbricating sutures. Image C shows the final closure of the enterotomy. (Reprinted from Urologic and gastrointestinal injuries. In: Yeomans ER, Hoffman BL, Gilstrap III LC, Cunningham F, editors. Cunningham and Gilstrap's operative obstetrics, 3e. McGraw-Hill Education; 2017.)

abdominal wall between the umbilicus and the anterior superior iliac spine or ribs that does not contain a skin fold and allows the bowel to easily traverse the abdominal wall without tension. When a stoma is created for temporary diversion, a loop stoma is preferred because of the ease of reversal and lower morbidity of reversal.

An omental patch, also known as a *Graham patch*, is a technique often used to repair perforated ulcers of the stomach or duodenum. The omentum is sutured with interrupted Lembert sutures to the seromuscular layer of the healthy bowel near the viscus perforation. An omental patch is not an appropriate repair for a primary bowel injury of the ileum. If a patient were undergoing reoperation for delayed recognition of a bowel injury, one might consider an omental patch to address a small defect not amenable to closure due to inflammation or to reinforce the delayed repair or anastomosis.

Endoscopically placed bowel stents for esophageal stricture are being studied in the management of anastomotic leaks after bariatric surgery. The use of an endoscopic stent in the small bowel is experimental and would not be appropriate for primary management of a bowel injury, particularly in the ileum.

Repair of bowel injury is nuanced and requires knowledge of appropriate techniques and challenges. Consultation is appropriate for repair when complex, but gynecologists must understand the basics of bowel repair and perioperative management. Gynecologic surgeons should be facile in identifying injury because delays in diagnosis are associated with significant morbidity and mortality.

Eisner IS, Wadhwa RK, Downing KT, Singhal PK. Prevention and management of bowel injury during gynecologic laparoscopy: an update. Curr Opin Obstet Gynecol 2019;31:245–50. doi: 10.1097/GCO.0000000000000552

Glaser LM, Milad MP. Bowel and bladder injury repair and follow-up after gynecologic surgery. Obstet Gynecol 2019;133:313–22. doi: 10.1097/AOG.0000000000003067

Smyth L, Bendinelli C, Lee N, Reeds MG, Loh EJ, Amico F, et al. WSES guidelines on blunt and penetrating bowel injury: diagnosis, investigations, and treatment. World J Emerg Surg 2022;17:13. doi: 10.1186/s13017-022-00418-y

Stomach. In: Cameron JL, Cameron AM, editors. Current surgical therapy. 14th ed. Elsevier; 2023. p. 81–128.

4 Atypical glandular cells on cervical cytology

A 45-year-old woman presents for evaluation of cervical cytology showing atypical glandular cells (AGCs). She has no concerns at today's visit and no prior history of abnormal cervical cytology. She is not taking hormonal contraception and notes regular menstrual cycles. In addition to colposcopy and endocervical curettage, the best next step is

(A) cervical excisional procedure
* (B) endometrial sampling
(C) human papillomavirus (HPV) testing
(D) pelvic ultrasonography
(E) repeat cervical cytology

Atypical glandular cells on cervical cytology usually originate from the glandular epithelium of the endocervix or endometrium and are found less frequently than squamous abnormalities. Glandular abnormalities are found in less than 1% of abnormal cervical cytology and are most common in patients aged 40 years or older. Patients with a result of AGCs require additional evaluation for premalignant and malignant conditions of the reproductive tract because this cytologic result is associated with cancerous precursors or malignancy in approximately 30% of patients.

In nonpregnant patients with AGCs, colposcopy is recommended regardless of age or HPV result, as noted in the scenario. Endocervical sampling also is recommended at the time of colposcopy due to the endocervical origin of glandular cells. Endometrial sampling is recommended at the time of the colposcopic examination in nonpregnant patients aged 35 years and older (Fig. 4-1). If a patient is younger than 35 years, endometrial sampling is recommended if they are at an increased risk of endometrial neoplasia based on clinical history (eg, abnormal uterine bleeding, obesity, or chronic anovulation).

An excisional procedure would be premature before a complete evaluation for this cytology result. Atypical glandular cells can originate from the cervix, the endometrium, or, less likely, the upper reproductive tract. Additionally, greater than 60% of AGC cytology is due to benign changes, such as reactive or reparative changes, cervical polyps, microglandular hyperplasia, and changes associated with the use of an intrauterine device or tubal metaplasia. Pending results of the testing in this scenario, a cervical excisional procedure may be indicated for a diagnosis of cervical high-grade intraepithelial lesion (cervical intraepithelial neoplasia 2 or 3) or adenocarcinoma in situ, but this is not the best next step for the described patient at this time.

In patients with AGCs, testing for HPV is not reliable for triaging evaluation since 20% of cervical adenocarcinomas are HPV-independent. In addition, AGCs may represent upper

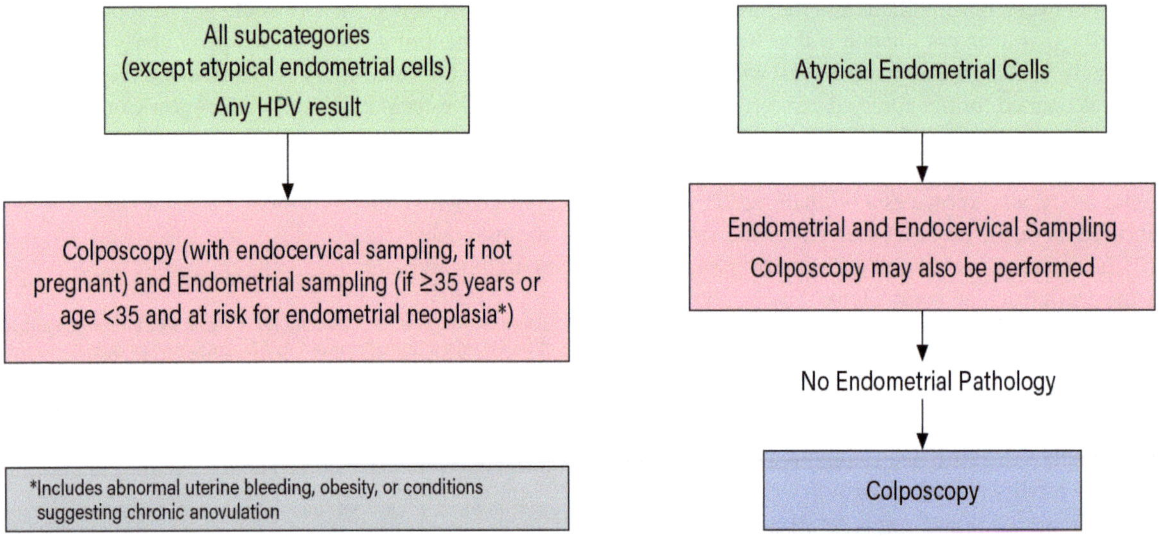

FIGURE 4-1. Management of atypical glandular cells. (Reprinted from Perkins RB, Guido RS, Castle PE, Chelmow D, Einstein MH, Garcia F, et al. 2019 ASCCP risk-based management consensus guidelines for abnormal cervical cancer screening tests and cancer precursors [published erratum appears in J Low Genit Tract Dis 2020;24:427]. J Low Genit Tract Dis 2020;24:102–31. doi: 10.1097/LGT.0000000000000525)

tract pathology. Atypical glandular cells can be associated with cancer of the uterus, fallopian tubes, and ovaries. A systematic review and meta-analysis noted an increased risk of extracervical malignancy (endometrium, fallopian tube, and ovary) among patients with AGC cytology and negative HPV test results. If HPV testing is positive, abnormalities are more likely to be cervical in origin. However, because cervical adenocarcinomas can be present regardless of HPV status, additional AGC cytology evaluation should include cervical evaluation irrespective of HPV test result, evaluation of the uterus based on age and risk factors, and consideration for evaluation of the fallopian tubes and ovaries based on symptoms. Given that HPV testing is not as reliable in patients with AGCs, it is not the appropriate choice in this scenario.

Ovarian cancer has been reported in 0.1–0.6% of individuals with AGCs. Pelvic ultrasonography, although it provides information about uterine and adnexal structures, is not the best method to evaluate premalignant and malignant conditions of the uterus or cervix. Assessing cervical and endometrial pathology with sampling, as previously discussed, is the best next step. If HPV testing is available and negative, this would raise suspicion for an upper genital tract lesion. If the patient undergoes colposcopy and endometrial biopsy with negative results, pelvic ultrasonography should be considered. Pelvic ultrasonography should be included in the baseline evaluation, particularly if patients note other symptoms, such as pelvic pain, bloating, or irregular bleeding, have risk factors for endometrial or ovarian cancer, or both.

Repeating cervical cytology without a diagnostic evaluation is not recommended for AGC cytology because the sensitivity of cytology for adenocarcinoma in situ is lower than that for high-grade squamous intraepithelial lesion (59% compared with 79%). The ASCCP risk-based management guidelines state that patients require repeat screening at more frequent intervals after the initial workup for the AGC result.

Arshi J, Farci F. Atypical glandular cells (AGS). In: StatPearls. StatPearls Publishing; 2025. Accessed March 13, 2025. https://www.ncbi.nlm.nih.gov/books/NBK564318/

Boyraz G, Basaran D, Salman MC, Ibrahimov A, Onder S, Akman O, et al. Histological follow-up in patients with atypical glandular cells on Pap smears. J Cytol 2017;34:203–7. doi: 10.4103/JOC.JOC_209_16

Koutras A, Perros P, Prokopakis I, Ntounis T, Fasoulakis Z, Pittokopitou S, et al. Advantages and limitations of ultrasound as a screening test for ovarian cancer. Diagnostics (Basel) 2023;13:2078. doi: 10.3390/diagnostics13122078

Perkins RB, Guido RS, Castle PE, Chelmow D, Einstein MH, Garcia F, et al. 2019 ASCCP risk-based management consensus guidelines for abnormal cervical cancer screening tests and cancer precursors [published erratum appears in J Low Genit Tract Dis 2020;24:427]. J Low Genit Tract Dis 2020;24:102–31. doi: 10.1097/LGT.0000000000000525

Verdoodt F, Jiang X, Williams M, Schnatz PF, Arbyn M. High-risk HPV testing in the management of atypical glandular cells: a systematic review and meta-analysis. Int J Cancer 2016;138:303–10. doi: 10.1002/ijc.29424

5 Massive transfusion protocol

A patient with a grade 3C placenta accreta spectrum disorder with extension into the parametria has a postcesarean hysterectomy hemorrhage with an estimated blood loss exceeding 5 L. The institutional massive transfusion protocol (MTP) is activated. In an MTP, the best ratio of units of packed red blood cells (PRBCs) to units of fresh frozen plasma (FFP) to six packs of platelets is

(A) 4:2:1
(B) 2:1:1
* (C) 1:1:1
(D) 3:1:2

Optimizing transfusion of blood products is important for reducing morbidity and mortality from rapid, large-volume bleeding. It is estimated that 3–5% of civilian trauma patients receive *massive transfusions*, often defined as exceeding 10 units of PRBCs within the first day after injury. Massive transfusions are seen, with varying frequency, in other populations as well. Gastrointestinal bleeding from esophageal varices, postpartum hemorrhage, and extensive liver and biliary tract operations also are associated with life-threatening blood loss.

In the past, when there was a sudden onset of significant bleeding, the initial resuscitation and support were typically begun by infusing large volumes of crystalloid with transfusion of blood products to follow, based on clinical and laboratory parameters. Several studies have found this approach frequently underestimates transfusion requirements, particularly when there is associated coagulopathy. Excessive administration of crystalloid is associated with worse outcomes compared with transfusion of blood products. Based on these findings, and the experience reported by some trauma centers, the concept of an MTP was developed. Early reports of using MTPs appeared in the literature in the mid-1980s. By 2006, after the publication of several key clinical trials, 85% of trauma centers reported having an MTP in place. By 2016, 98% of trauma centers used an MTP.

A primary advantage of an MTP is the reduction of the risk of coagulopathy. The phenomenon of trauma-induced coagulopathy (TIC) was originally thought to result from infusing large volumes of crystalloid solution along with hypothermia. Subsequent research has shown the mechanism of TIC to be more complex, involving changes in immune function and in the vascular endothelium, as well as the clotting pathways. Trauma-induced coagulopathy has been associated with mortality rates as high as 50% in some series. Early recognition of patients at risk of TIC and avoidance of hemodilution and transfusion of unbalanced volumes of blood components are key contributors to improving outcomes.

Although most of the research on massive transfusion has been conducted in trauma patients in emergency departments, lessons learned apply to patients in other settings, including the operating room. A multidisciplinary team consisting of nurses, anesthesiologists, intensivists, transfusion medicine physicians, and surgeons, in addition to the blood bank and available transport, is charged with the development and implementation of institutional MTPs. Once activated, an MTP requires the blood bank to deliver predetermined packs of blood components (red cells, platelets, and plasma) to the operating room at regular intervals until the bleeding is controlled.

Other definitions have been proposed for the initiation of an MTP, including the critical administration threshold (CAT) and resuscitation intensity (RI) scores. A positive CAT score is determined by the administration of three or more units of PRBCs in a 1-hour time period because of injury. Patients with a positive CAT score have quadruple the mortality compared with those with a negative score.

The RI score accounts for all resuscitation fluids given within 30 minutes of arrival to the emergency department; one point is given for each unit of blood, plasma, or platelets as well as for each liter of crystalloid and each half-liter of colloid. Mortality at 6 hours is tripled for patients who have an RI score of 4 or greater. Regardless of the method used to determine the need to activate the MTP, a formalized, structured protocol avoids delay in initiating transfusion of an appropriate mix of components, reduces overall blood product and crystalloid use, and is more efficient than an individualized approach guided by clinical and laboratory parameters.

Prompt recognition of massive hemorrhage appears to be associated with better outcomes. One study showed that each minute of delay in delivering MTP products was associated with a 5% increase in mortality.

Massive transfusion also is associated with complications. In addition to multiorgan failure that can be associated with hemorrhage and high-volume transfusion, infection, fluid overload, and lung injury have been associated with MTP. The most frequent types of lung injury are transfusion-associated circulatory overload, which is pulmonary edema that results from circulatory overload, and transfusion-related acute injury caused by donor leukocyte antibodies binding to antigens in the pulmonary vessels, which leads to injury and capillary leaks.

For MTP, the preferred ratio of units of PRBCs to units of FFP to platelets is 1:1:1, and this is the best ratio for the described patient. Numerous studies have been conducted to determine the optimal ratio. One of the most influential was the Pragmatic, Randomized Optimal Platelet and Plasma Ratios trial (known as PROPPR). Published in 2015, the PROPPR study randomized 660 patients with severe injuries at 12 North American trauma centers during 2012 and 2013 to transfusion of blood components with ratios of 1:1:1 or 2:1:1 (red blood cells to plasma to platelets). The investigators reported no significant differences in 24-hour (13–17%) or 30-day (22–26%) mortality; however, significantly more patients in the 1:1:1 group achieved hemostasis (86% versus 78%). They found no differences in complication rates between the groups. Modern MTPs typically deliver components in a 1:1:1 ratio, although some centers still may prefer 2:1:1.

Studies have consistently shown that the ratio of PRBCs to platelets should not exceed 3:1. Early mortality is nearly twice as high when the ratio of PRBCs to FFP exceeds 3:1. In one study, patients whose PRBC to platelet ratio was more than 3:1 had an early mortality rate of 50%, compared with 10% for patients whose PRBC to platelet ratio was 1–2:1.

Meneses E, Boneva D, McKenney M, Elkbuli A. Massive transfusion protocol in adult trauma population. Am J Emerg Med 2020;38:2661–6. doi: 10.1016/j.ajem.2020.07.041

Moore, S., Raval,J. Massive transfusion: a review. Ann Blood 2022;7:18. doi: 10.21037/aob-22-3

Young PP, Cotton BA, Goodnough LT. Massive transfusion protocols for patients with substantial hemorrhage. Transfus Med Rev 2011;25:293–303. doi: 10.1016/j.tmrv.2011.04.002

6 Neurologic symptoms

A 68-year-old woman with a history of advanced-stage endometrial cancer presents to the emergency department after a fall. Her history is notable for weakness and headaches during the last several weeks. She also notes nausea and vomiting. A neurologic examination is notable for gait disturbance. Her vital signs are within normal limits, and the laboratory workup is unremarkable. There was no evidence of hemorrhage, hydrocephalus, or mass effect on a noncontrast head computed tomography (CT). The best next step in her evaluation is

(A) contrast-enhanced CT
(B) electroencephalogram (EEG)
(C) lumbar puncture
* (D) MRI
(E) positron emission tomography (PET)

Brain metastases from a gynecologic malignancy are rare, and diagnosis requires retaining a high degree of suspicion in patients presenting with potential neurologic symptoms. Brain metastases can present with a variety of symptoms depending upon the location of the lesion, including headache, vertigo or dizziness, confusion, seizures, impaired vision, falls, or weakness. Brain metastases also should be considered in any patient with persistent nausea and vomiting without an identified etiology. Although still rare, the incidence of brain metastases in ovarian and endometrial cancer seems to be rising. This is likely attributable to improvements in treatment options that allow patients to live longer and thus increase the opportunity for brain metastases to develop. The increased incidence also may be due to improved imaging techniques that identify brain metastases more accurately. Improvements in surgical techniques and radiation therapy, such as stereotactic radiosurgery, also have improved the survival of patients after diagnosis of brain metastases.

The initial workup of neurologic symptoms often includes a non-contrast CT to rule out hemorrhage or mass effect. In many cases, this will lead to a diagnosis of brain metastases; however, non-contrast CT may miss small metastatic lesions. In situations in which suspicion for brain metastases is high, if a CT does not show evidence of a brain metastasis, a brain MRI should be obtained. The addition of contrast to brain CT does increase detection of brain metastases; however, MRI is the most sensitive imaging modality for diagnosis of brain metastases (reported sensitivity nears 100%). Even in patients with a brain metastasis identified on CT, if the number of brain metastases will affect treatment, a brain MRI should be obtained because as many as 20% of patients with solitary brain lesions on CT will have multiple brain metastases on MRI. Use of gadolinium contrast further improves the sensitivity of MRI, particularly for small metastases.

This patient has a history of malignancy and new-onset neurologic symptoms. With an otherwise negative workup, there is a high likelihood that her symptoms could be due to brain metastases. As demonstrated in Figure 6-1, patients with a head CT that is negative for metastasis may still have brain metastases identified on MRI because of the increased sensitivity of MRI. Because there is a high degree of clinical suspicion for brain metastasis, brain MRI is the correct next step in evaluation of the described patient's symptoms.

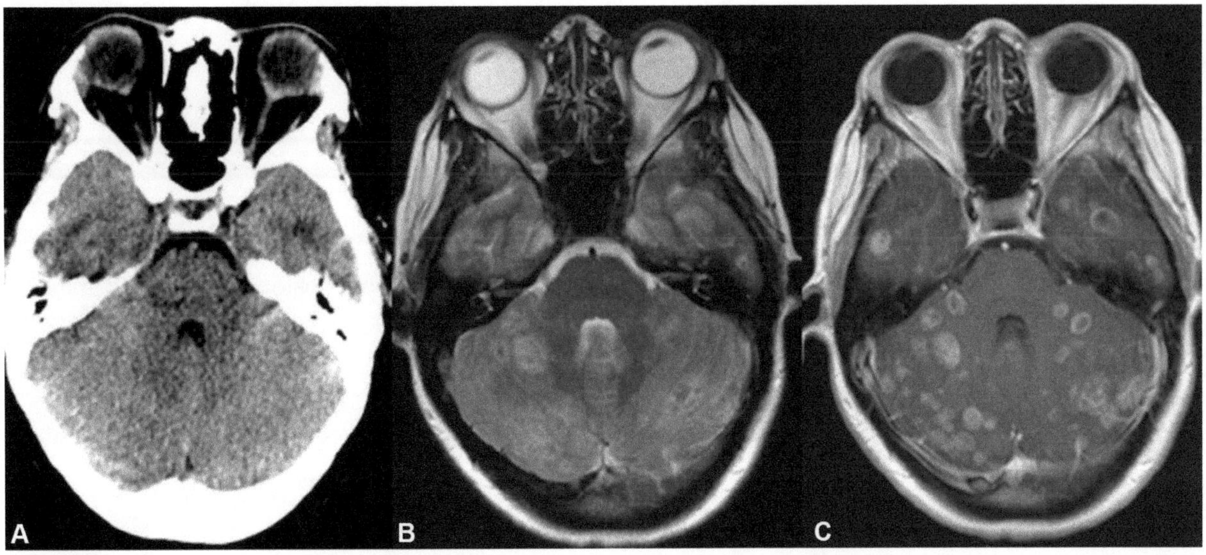

FIGURE 6-1. Noncontrast computed tomography (CT) has low sensitivity for brain metastases. A noncontrast CT image (A) through the posterior fossa is essentially unremarkable. T2-weighted image (B) of the same patient shows extensive abnormality of the cerebellum, with a very large number of metastases most clearly defined by the postcontrast T1-weighted image (C). (Reprinted from Pope WB. Brain metastases: neuroimaging. Handb Clin Neurol 2018;149:89–112. doi: 10.1016/B978-0-12-811161-1.00007-4)

An EEG measures electrical activity of the brain and may be used in the diagnosis of seizure disorders or similar conditions. Although brain tumors may cause changes on EEG, it is not the preferred method for diagnosis due to its lower sensitivity. An EEG may not show changes when tumors are located within the posterior fossa or deep within the cortex, and it is not the best next step for evaluation.

Lumbar puncture is used to evaluate for the presence of cancer in the cerebrospinal fluid or to confirm the presence of leptomeningeal disease. It is less sensitive for brain metastasis than MRI and does not provide information on the location or number of tumors when positive, which may be important for treatment planning. Additionally, lumbar puncture is more invasive than brain imaging. Positron emission tomography is a nuclear medicine imaging technique often used to detect metastatic disease in other areas of the body due to its ability to detect areas of hypermetabolism (as seen in cancer). However, the cerebral cortex is highly metabolic at baseline. When present, brain metastases may actually show up as areas of hypometabolism, making it difficult to distinguish them from other pathology, such as infarction. This limits the usefulness of PET imaging in detecting brain metastases, and it is not the preferred test for diagnosis.

Barajas RF Jr, Cha S. Metastasis in adult brain tumors. Neuroimaging Clin N Am 2016;26:601–20. doi: 10.1016/j.nic.2016.06.008

Lo SS, Gore EM, Bradley JD, Buatti JM, Germano I, Ghafoori AP, et al. ACR Appropriateness Criteria® pre-irradiation evaluation and management of brain metastases. Expert Panel on Radiation Oncology-Brain Metastases. J Palliat Med 2014;17:880–6. doi: 10.1089/jpm.2014.9417

Nasioudis D, Persaud A, Taunk NK, Latif NA. Brain metastases from gynecologic malignancies: prevalence and management. Am J Clin Oncol 2020;43:418–21. doi: 10.1097/COC.0000000000000689

7 Postoperative nutrition

A 51-year-old woman with epithelial ovarian cancer underwent a total abdominal hysterectomy, bilateral salpingo-oophorectomy, omentectomy, peritoneal stripping, extensive lysis of adhesion requiring oversewing of the bowel, and optimal debulking. She is otherwise healthy. In the immediate postoperative period, the best next step for nutrition management is

(A) bowel rest until flatus
(B) clear liquid diet
(C) immunonutrient supplementation
* (D) regular diet
(E) total parenteral nutrition

Optimization of perioperative nutrition is associated with improved outcomes for patients undergoing surgery for gynecologic malignancies. Postoperatively, patients are in a state of catabolism due to inflammatory processes resulting from surgery that can lead to altered organ function and, subsequently, delayed postoperative recovery. Patients with advanced gynecologic malignancies, including advanced ovarian and cervical cancer, commonly present prior to surgery with malnutrition, which contributes to worse outcomes. Optimization of preoperative and postoperative nutrition is associated with improved morbidity and mortality for patients undergoing gynecologic surgery. Researchers have evaluated a variety of preoperative and postoperative interventions to improve perioperative nutrition status (Table 7-1), some of which are included in the Enhanced Recovery After Surgery (ERAS) perioperative pathway.

Early resumption of the patient's regular diet is recommended, typically within the first 24 hours after surgery. This practice is associated with decreased length of stay and faster resumption of bowel function. Although early feeding is associated with an increased risk of nausea without emesis in the immediate postoperative period, studies have otherwise demonstrated no difference in complications compared with delayed feeding. For patients undergoing colorectal surgery, early feeding is associated with improved 5-year survival rates. The optimal postoperative diet is unclear, but ERAS guidelines support a diet with a protein composition of 2 g of protein/kg/d.

Neither bowel rest until flatus nor slow reintroduction of clear liquids is recommended postoperatively. Historically, postoperative feeding after laparotomy was delayed due to concerns for complications related to early feeding. This practice was not evidence-based, and research suggests that delayed or slow resumption of feeding is associated with longer recovery and increased perioperative mortality. These practices are no longer routinely recommended.

Postoperative immunonutrient supplementation is not recommended based on current data. *Immunonutrients* are substances that affect the immune system when used as a supplement and may have a role in decreasing postoperative inflammation. These supplements are the focus of ongoing research on perioperative nutrition. Studies suggest a possible benefit to immunonutrient supplementation for patients undergoing colorectal and urologic surgery, but studies in gynecologic surgery are limited. Preoperative supplementation may provide the most benefit, but the timing of immunonutrient supplementation is unclear. Further research is needed to determine the utility and timing of immunonutrient supplementation in gynecologic surgery.

Nutrition optimization in the postoperative period decreases complications and improves outcomes; however, the universal use of total parenteral nutrition immediately after surgery is not recommended. Total parenteral nutrition is associated with complications, including metabolic disturbances and central line infections, which can impede recovery and increase the length of hospital stay. Parenteral nutrition should be reserved for patients in whom enteral nutrition is not feasible or adequate, such as those with a bowel obstruction, bowel ischemia, or bowel not in continuity, or in those with malnutrition who are unable to meet their nutritional needs with enteral nutrition alone.

Early resumption of enteral nutrition is a safe and effective practice for reducing morbidity and mortality after gynecologic oncology surgery. This practice should be incorporated into postoperative care in addition to screening for malnutrition and the incorporation of other ERAS practices.

TABLE 7-1. Perioperative Nutrition Recommendations

TIME	SUMMARY	REFERENCES
Early pre-op	Preoperative nutritional assessment with validated scoring tool	Kondrup, 2003; Detsky, 1987; Ottery, 1994; Stratton, 2004; Wischmeyer, 2018
	Supplement malnourished patients 10–14 days pre-op	Bozzetti, 2007; Jie, 2012; Weimann, 2017
	Alcohol cessation 4–6 weeks pre-op	Egholm, 2018
Late pre-op	Intake solid foods 6–8 hours pre-op	Brady, 2003; Smith, 2011; Scott, 2014; Merchant, 2016
	Carbohydrate loading drink (50 g maltodextrin) ~3 hours pre-op	Weimann, 2017; Yagci, 2008; Awad, 2013; Gustafsson, 2013; Bilku, 2014; Ljunggren, 2014; Scott, 2014; Smith, 2014; Webster, 2014; Hausel, 2001
	Individualize care in patients with risk of delayed gastric emptying or diabetes	Chen, 1995; Gustafsson, 2008
	Preoperative immunonutrition may be able to alter the immune response to surgery	Moya, 2016; Yeung, 2017; Hamilton-Reeves, 2018; Celik, 2009
Post-op	Nutritional support (ideally enteral feeding) starting within 24 hours postoperatively Consider increased protein and caloric demands of cancer and recent surgery	Schilder, 1997; Pearl, 1998; Cutillo, 1999; Minig, 2009; Charoenkwan, 2014; Bisch, 2018
	Benefits of chewing gum for stimulation of gut motility are controversial	Short, 2015; Atkinson, 2016
	Postoperative immunonutrition may not be as important as preoperative supplementation—further research is needed.	Miyauchi, 2019

Modified from Bisch S, Nelson G, Altman A. Impact of nutrition on enhanced recovery after surgery (ERAS) in gynecologic oncology. Nutrients 2019;11:1088. doi: 10.3390/nu11051088

Berlana D. Parenteral nutrition overview. Nutrients 2022;14:4480. doi: 10.3390/nu14214480

Bisch S, Nelson G, Altman A. Impact of nutrition on enhanced recovery after surgery (ERAS) in gynecologic oncology. Nutrients 2019;11:1088. doi: 10.3390/nu11051088

Boitano TK, Smith HJ, Rushton T, Johnston MC, Lawson P, Leath CA III, et al. Impact of enhanced recovery after surgery (ERAS) protocol on gastrointestinal function in gynecologic oncology patients undergoing laparotomy. Gynecol Oncol 2018;151:282–6. doi: 10.1016/j.ygyno.2018.09.009

Perioperative pathways: enhanced recovery after surgery. ACOG Committee Opinion No. 750. American College of Obstetricians and Gynecologists [published errata appear in Obstet Gynecol 2019;133:1288; Obstet Gynecol 2019;134:1121]. Obstet Gynecol 2018;132:e120–30. doi: 10.1097/AOG.0000000000002818

Scheib SA, Thomassee M, Kenner JL. Enhanced recovery after surgery in gynecology: a review of the literature. J Minim Invasive Gynecol 2019;26:327–43. doi: 10.1016/j.jmig.2018.12.010

Wischmeyer PE, Carli F, Evans DC, Guilbert S, Kozar R, Pryor A, et al. American Society for Enhanced Recovery and Perioperative Quality Initiative joint consensus statement on nutrition screening and therapy within a surgical enhanced recovery pathway. Perioperative Quality Initiative (POQI) 2 Workgroup [published erratum appears in Anesth Analg 2018;127:e95]. Anesth Analg 2018;126:1883–95. doi: 10.1213/ANE.0000000000002743

8 Soft tissue infections

A 54-year-old woman presents to the emergency department with a 2-day history of worsening vulvar swelling and pain. Her medical history is notable for a BMI of 42, hypertension, and type 2 diabetes (her recent outpatient hemoglobin A_{1C} was 10.4). Her vital signs are significant for a temperature of 38.1 °C (100.5 °F), a pulse of 110 bpm, and a blood pressure of 95/60 mm Hg. Her glucose today is 289 mg/dL. On physical examination, there is erythema and edema of the right vulva with central bulla and severe pain with palpation. Blood cultures were obtained, and the emergency department has initiated fluid resuscitation, broad-spectrum antibiotics, and insulin. The best next step in management is

(A) await blood culture results
(B) obtain computed tomography (CT)
(C) perform serial vulvar examinations
* (D) perform surgical debridement
(E) perform vulvar biopsy

This patient is presenting with signs and symptoms of a necrotizing soft tissue infection (NSTI) of the vulva. Necrotizing soft tissue infections are characterized by rapidly progressive infections that cause extensive local tissue destruction and can lead to systemic illness, multisystem organ failure, and even death. Historically referred to as *necrotizing fasciitis*, the condition is increasingly termed *necrotizing soft tissue infection* to encompass infections involving other tissues, such as necrotizing cellulitis or myositis. Treatment is similar regardless of the depth of infection. The true incidence of these infections is unknown due to widely variable reporting practices but is estimated to be as high as 15.5 cases per 100,000 individuals. Early detection and prompt surgical management are critical to decrease morbidity and mortality from these infections.

Necrotizing fasciitis is a deep infection that can lead to destruction of subcutaneous tissues and the fascia. A two-type classification system has been described. Polymicrobial infections are classified as type I, and monomicrobial infections are classified as type II. Type I infections are more common and more likely to develop in patients with risk factors such as diabetes mellitus, obesity, or immunocompromise. Type I infections more frequently develop after instrumentation or surgery or at the site of other wounds, such as diabetic or pressure ulcers. They are more common on the perineum or trunk. Type I infections also can develop at the site of obstetric perineal lacerations or after instrumentation of the uterus. The term *Fournier gangrene* may be used to describe NSTI of the perineum, including the vulva. Type II infections, most commonly caused by group A *Streptococcus*, often present in patients without identifiable risk factors. They are more often seen on the extremities and tend to be more aggressive (mortality rates are greater than 30% in severe cases).

A high degree of clinical suspicion is critical for recognizing NSTIs. Patients presenting with a soft tissue infection who exhibit signs of systemic illness or who show rapid progression or deterioration of their clinical condition should prompt strong consideration of an NSTI.

The diagnosis of NSTI is made clinically. Pain out of proportion to the examination is almost pathognomonic for a necrotizing infection due to the consistency of this finding. Erythema with edema extending beyond the apparent area of infection also is present in more than 50% of patients with an NSTI. When erythema is present, it may progress to reddish-purple tissue and bullae over 24–48 hours, and dark bullae may appear. Findings such as bullae, ecchymosis, and obvious skin necrosis may not be present until later in the disease process because these findings suggest extensive tissue necrosis has already occurred. Laboratory findings can be variable and should not be relied on to make the diagnosis of NSTI. Findings of leukocytosis, increased lactate, and hyponatremia can support the diagnosis of a necrotizing infection, particularly in equivocal cases, but specific laboratory findings are not necessary to make the diagnosis.

The mainstay for the treatment of NSTI is aggressive surgical debridement of necrotic tissue until viable tissue is encountered. Patients often require multiple procedures for serial debridement. Studies have shown that the average number of debridement procedures needed for an affected patient is three to four. Delay in surgical management increases the number and extent of surgical resections and is associated with increased mortality. The patient in this scenario has risk factors for NSTI, including obesity and diabetes with an increased hemoglobin A_{1C}, and is presenting with findings consistent with a vulvar NSTI, including severe pain, erythema, and bullae. The correct management for this patient is prompt surgical debridement of the vulvar infection. Performing serial vulvar examinations would lead to unnecessary delay, resulting in further progression of the necrotizing infection and increased morbidity and mortality for this patient; therefore, this is not the correct answer.

Initial resuscitation and stabilization also are essential, including fluid resuscitation, glucose management, and early initiation of broad-spectrum antibiotics, and these interventions should be performed concomitantly with surgical evaluation and management for best patient outcomes. When possible, blood cultures should be obtained before starting antibiotics, but initiation of broad-spectrum antibiotics and proceeding with surgical debridement should occur while waiting for culture results. For the described patient, waiting for culture results is not the best next step, because it would delay surgical debridement.

When initiating broad-spectrum antibiotics for suspected polymicrobial infections, potential antibiotic choices include piperacillin-tazobactam; a carbapenem plus vancomycin; linezolid; cefotaxime; ceftriaxone plus metronidazole; or clindamycin. Once culture results return, antibiotic coverage should be tailored to culture results. For treatment of type II infections, the recommended therapy is high-dose penicillin and clindamycin. Antibiotics should be continued until no further debridement is needed, and the patient is clinically improved and has been afebrile for 48 hours.

The care of patients with NSTI frequently requires a multidisciplinary approach, and many patients require transfer to a facility with supportive services, such as critical care, expertise in infectious disease and wound care, and availability of plastic surgery. The initial debridement should not be delayed if appropriate critical care and surgical services are available, and postoperative transfer can be performed if needed.

In many patients, imaging will have been obtained during the workup of a patient presenting with a NSTI; however, imaging is not necessary to make or confirm the diagnosis, and gynecologists should not rely on imaging for the diagnosis of NSTI if there is a high degree of clinical suspicion. Obtaining imaging in those patients can cause delays in surgical management, leading to increases in morbidity and mortality. Furthermore, the lack of classic imaging findings should not preclude surgical management of a suspected NSTI when clinical suspicion is high. When obtained, imaging findings of gas within the soft tissues or lack of contrast enhancement of the fascia or affected tissues on CT support the diagnosis of a necrotizing infection. In the described patient, who has several findings of NSTI, obtaining a CT would delay surgical debridement; therefore, this is not the correct answer.

A vulvar biopsy is performed when there is a concern for a malignant or premalignant condition of the vulva. This patient's presentation is more consistent with a necrotizing infection, and a biopsy is not the correct next step. If there is suspicion that the patient's infection represents a superimposed infection of an underlying malignancy, diagnosis can be confirmed by pathologic examination of the debrided tissue rather than by obtaining a vulvar biopsy at presentation.

Bonne SL, Kadri SS. Evaluation and management of necrotizing soft tissue infections. Infect Dis Clin North Am 2017;31:497–511. doi: 10.1016/j.idc.2017.05.011

Courtney-Brooks M, Scalici J, Henretta MS, Modesitt SC, Jazaeri AA, Cantrell LA, et al. Vulvar necrotizing soft tissue infection: a review of a multidisciplinary surgical emergency and management in the modern era. Gynecol Oncol Case Rep 2013;5:6–9. doi: 10.1016/j.gynor.2013.02.002

Stevens DL, Bisno AL, Chambers HF, Dellinger EP, Goldstein EJC, Gorbach SL, et al. Practice guidelines for the diagnosis and management of skin and soft tissue infections: 2014 update by the Infectious Diseases Society of America [published erratum appears in Clin Infect Dis. 2015;60:1448]. Clin Infect Dis 2014;59:e10–52. doi: 10.1093/cid/ciu444

Stevens DL, Bryant AE, Goldstein EJ. Necrotizing soft tissue infections. Infect Dis Clin North Am 2021;35:135–55. doi: 10.1016/j.idc.2020.10.004

9 Nosocomial pneumonia

A 73-year-old patient develops a fever (38.5 °C [101.3 °F]) and shortness of breath 7 days after exploratory laparotomy, total hysterectomy, bilateral salpingo-oophorectomy, and complete cytoreduction for ovarian cancer. Her physical examination is notable for decreased breath sounds on the left and oxygen saturation of 93% on 4 L of O_2 by nasal cannula. Her laboratory test results are notable for a white blood cell count of 16.8×10^3/microliter with 98% neutrophils and a serum creatinine level of 1.74 mg/dL. A chest X-ray demonstrates a left lower lobe infiltrate. The patient has a history of treatment with intravenous antibiotics 4 weeks ago for lower leg cellulitis. In addition to piperacillin-tazobactam, the best antibiotic agent to add to this patient's therapy is

(A) cefazolin
(B) gentamycin
* (C) linezolid
(D) oxacillin
(E) vancomycin

Nosocomial pneumonia (NP), also known as *hospital-acquired pneumonia*, is defined as pneumonia developing in hospitalized patients at least 48 hours after admission. A subset of NP is *ventilator-associated pneumonia*, which is defined as pneumonia developing at least 48 hours after intubation. A survey of 183 U.S. hospitals found that NP accounted for 22% of hospital-acquired infections. Nosocomial pneumonia is a significant contributor to hospital mortality, with reported mortality rates of 20–50%.

Risk factors for NP include older age, high severity of illness, admission to the intensive care unit, and high comorbidity burden. Because aspiration is a common cause of NP, patients with neurologic conditions affecting swallowing are at increased risk, as well as patients on proton-pump inhibitors and histamine-2 receptor blockers, because these drugs lower gastric acid production and allow greater bacterial colonization of the oropharynx. Rigorous preventive oral hygiene regimens and early recognition and treatment of dysphagia have been shown to decrease the risk of NP.

The clinical diagnosis of NP is based on the presence of fever, with evidence of respiratory compromise and productive cough, combined with infiltrates on chest X-ray or chest computed tomography (CT). Chest CT is more sensitive than chest X-ray, particularly for debilitated or bedridden patients, and may demonstrate infiltrate up to 5 days earlier than chest X-ray. Blood and sputum cultures should be obtained to identify the responsible pathogens because bacteremia is present in 25% of patients with NP. To be considered adequate, a sputum sample should demonstrate few or no squamous cells on Gram stain.

Initial empiric antibiotic therapy for NP is recommended in patients who have an identified lung infiltrate and have at least two of three clinical findings: fever, leukocytosis, or cough. In this scenario, the patient has fever and leukocytosis, and it is appropriate to start empiric broad-spectrum coverage with piperacillin-tazobactam. In a study of 17,819 individuals with NP and VAP, the most commonly isolated organisms were, in descending order of frequency, *Staphylococcus aureus*, *Pseudomonas aeruginosa*, *Escherichia coli*, and *Klebsiella pneumoniae*. When available, knowledge of the distribution of pathogens and their sensitivities to antibiotics in the local setting should inform empiric treatment choices to minimize overtreatment and discourage further emergence of antibiotic resistance (Table 9-1).

Coverage for methicillin-resistant *S aureus* (MRSA) is indicated in patients with NP who have specific risk factors for multidrug-resistant organisms, including a history of antibiotic therapy in the last 90 days, such as in the patient described. Empiric coverage also is appropriate in severely ill patients and patients hospitalized in units where more than 20% of *S aureus* isolates are methicillin resistant. A rapid PCR-based test for *S aureus* has a sensitivity of 85% and specificity of 92% among patients with NP, and a negative result can allow safe discontinuation of agents specifically targeting MRSA.

Currently, the two most effective antibiotic agents against MRSA NP are vancomycin and linezolid. A prospective randomized trial comparing the two agents as single-agent therapy in patients with MRSA NP found that compared with vancomycin, linezolid-treated patients had a higher rate of microbiologic success (81.9% versus 60.6%) and a lower rate of nephrotoxicity (8.4% versus 18.2%), although there was no difference in 40-day mortality between groups.

In this scenario, the patient requires additional coverage for MRSA given her recent history of antibiotic treatment. Although vancomycin would otherwise be a reasonable choice, her high creatinine of 1.7 mg/dL increases her risk of vancomycin-associated nephrotoxicity, and the best antibiotic agent to add to her regimen is linezolid.

Gentamicin is an aminoglycoside antibiotic that is used in a wide range of infections and is commonly added to other antibiotics to provide coverage against gram-negative bacteria. Although many staphylococcal species are sensitive to gentamicin, MRSA is typically resistant. Gentamicin also is associated with significant nephrotoxicity; therefore, it is not the best choice for the patient in this scenario.

TABLE 9-1. Recommended Initial Empiric Antibiotic Therapy for Hospital-Acquired Pneumonia (Non-Ventilator-Associated Pneumonia)

NOT AT HIGH RISK OF MORTALITY* AND NO FACTORS INCREASING THE LIKELIHOOD OF MRSA†,‡	NOT AT HIGH RISK OF MORTALITY* BUT WITH FACTORS INCREASING THE LIKELIHOOD OF MRSA†,‡	HIGH RISK OF MORTALITY OR RECEIPT OF INTRAVENOUS ANTIBIOTICS DURING THE PRIOR 90 DAYS*,‡
One of the following:	One of the following:	Two of the following, avoid two β-lactams
Piperacillin-tazobactam§	Piperacillin-tazobactam§	Piperacillin-tazobactam§
OR	OR	OR
Cefepime§	Cefepime§ or ceftazidime§	Cefepime§ or ceftazidime§
OR	OR	OR
Levofloxacin	Levofloxacin Ciprofloxacin	Levofloxacin Ciprofloxacin
	OR	OR
Imipenem§ Meropenem§	Imipenem§ Meropenem§	Imipenem§ Meropenem§
	OR	OR
	Aztreonam	Amikacin Gentamicin Tobramycin
		OR
		Aztreonam‖
	Plus: Vancomycin	Plus: Vancomycin
	OR	OR
	Linezolid	Linezolid
		If MRSA coverage is not going to be used, include coverage for MSSA. Options include: Piperacillin-tazobactam, cefepime, levofloxacin, imipenem, meropenem. Oxacillin, nafcillin, and cefazolin are preferred for the treatment of proven MSSA, but would ordinarily not be used in an empiric regimen for HAP.
If the patient has severe penicillin allergy and aztreonam is going to be used instead of any β-lactam-based antibiotic, include coverage for MSSA.		

Abbreviations: HAP, hospital-acquired pneumonia; IV, intravenous; MRSA, methicillin-resistant *Staphylococcus aureus*; MSSA, methicillin-sensitive *Staphylococcus aureus*.

*Risk factors for mortality include need for ventilatory support due to pneumonia and septic shock.

†Indications for MRSA coverage include intravenous antibiotic treatment during the prior 90 days, and treatment in a unit where the prevalence of MRSA among *S aureus* isolates is not known or is greater than 20%. Prior detection of MRSA by culture or non-culture screening may also increase the risk of MRSA. The 20% threshold was chosen to balance the need for effective initial antibiotic therapy against the risks of excessive antibiotic use; hence, individual units can elect to adjust the threshold in accordance with local values and preferences. If MRSA coverage is omitted, the antibiotic regimen should include coverage for MSSA.

‡If patient has factors increasing the likelihood of gram-negative infection, two antipseudomonal agents are recommended. If patient has structural lung disease increasing the risk of gram-negative infection (ie, bronchiectasis or cystic fibrosis), two antipseudomonal agents are recommended. A high-quality Gram stain from a respiratory specimen with numerous and predominant gram-negative bacilli provides further support for the diagnosis of a gram-negative pneumonia, including fermenting and non-glucose-fermenting microorganisms.

§Extended infusions may be appropriate.

‖In the absence of other options, it is acceptable to use aztreonam as an adjunctive agent with another β-lactam-based agent because it has different targets within the bacterial cell wall.

Modified from Kalil AC, Metersky ML, Klompas M, Muscedere J, Sweeney DA, Palmer LB, et al. Management of adults with hospital-acquired and ventilator-associated pneumonia: 2016 Clinical Practice Guidelines by the Infectious Diseases Society of America and the American Thoracic Society [published errata appear in Clin Infect Dis 2017;64:1298; Clin Infect Dis 2017;65:1435; Clin Infect Dis 2017;65:2161]. Clin Infect Dis. 2016 Sep 1;63(5):e61-111. doi: 10.1093/cid/ciw353

Oxacillin is a penicillinase-resistant β-lactam similar to methicillin. Widespread use of β-lactams to treat staphylococcal infections led to the selection of resistant strains over time, which in turn led to the emergence of MRSA. Because most MRSA is resistant to oxacillin, this is not the correct choice for this patient who requires MRSA coverage.

Cefazolin is a first-generation cephalosporin commonly used for skin infections. It is active against streptococcus species and methicillin-sensitive *S aureus* but typically is not active against MRSA; therefore, cefazolin is not the best antibiotic to add to this patient's regimen.

Kalil AC, Metersky ML, Klompas M, Muscedere J, Sweeney DA, Palmer LB, et al. Management of adults with hospital-acquired and ventilator-associated pneumonia: 2016 clinical practice guidelines by the Infectious Diseases Society of America and the American Thoracic Society [published errata appear in Clin Infect Dis 2017;65:2161; Clin Infect Dis 2017;65:1435; Clin Infect Dis 2017;64:1298]. Clin Infect Dis 2016;63:e61–111. doi: 10.1093/cid/ciw353

Kaneoka A, Pisegna JM, Miloro KV, Lo M, Saito H, Riquelme LF, et al. Prevention of healthcare-associated pneumonia with oral care in individuals without mechanical ventilation: a systematic review and meta-analysis of randomized controlled trials. Infect Control Hosp Epidemiol 2015;36:899–906. doi: 10.1017/ice.2015.77

Kato H, Hagihara M, Asai N, Shibata Y, Koizumi Y, Yamagishi Y, et al. Meta-analysis of vancomycin versus linezolid in pneumonia with proven methicillin-resistant Staphylococcus aureus. J Glob Antimicrob Resist 2021;24:98–105. doi: 10.1016/j.jgar.2020.12.009

Magill SS, Edwards JR, Bamberg W, Beldavs ZG, Dumyati G, Kainer MA, et al. Multistate point-prevalence survey of health care-associated infections [published erratum appears in N Engl J Med 2022;386:2348]. N Engl J Med 2014;370:1198–208. doi: 10.1056/NEJMoa1306801

Zilberberg MD, Nathanson BH, Puzniak LA, Shorr AF. Descriptive epidemiology and outcomes of nonventilated hospital-acquired, ventilated hospital-acquired, and ventilator-associated bacterial pneumonia in the United States, 2012-2019. Crit Care Med 2022;50:460–8. doi: 10.1097/CCM.0000000000005298

10 Placental site trophoblastic tumor

A 39-year-old gravida 1, para 1, had a hysterectomy for a 10-cm myomatous uterus and abnormal uterine bleeding. She had a molar pregnancy 5 years ago. Her preoperative urine test for human chorionic gonadotropin (hCG) was negative. Final pathology showed a vascular myometrial mass invading greater than 50% of the uterine wall. The photomicrographs below show a hematoxylin-eosin–stained section (Fig. 10-1A) and an immunohistochemical stain for Ki-67 (Fig. 10-1B). In this patient, the factor most consistently associated with an unfavorable prognosis is

(A) age less than 40 years
(B) deep myometrial invasion
* (C) long interval from index pregnancy
(D) low hCG
(E) uterine size

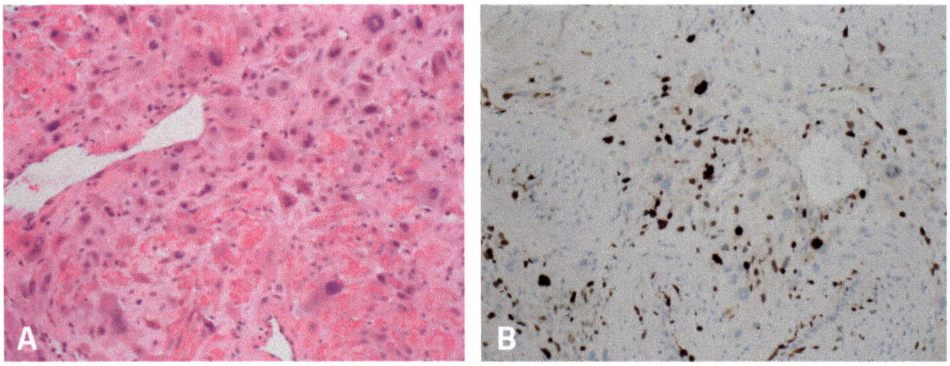

FIGURE 10-1. A. Highly atypical trophoblasts (hematoxylin-eosin). B. Immunohistochemical stain for Ki-67 shows a proliferation index of about 30%, supporting placental site trophoblastic tumor. (Reprinted from Polnaszek B, Mullen M, Bligard K, Raghuraman N, Massad LS. Term pregnancy after complete response of placental site trophoblastic tumor to immunotherapy. Obstet Gynecol 2021;138:115–8. doi: 10.1097/AOG.0000000000004434)

Gestational trophoblastic disease (GTD) is derived from placental tissue and comprises a spectrum of abnormalities, from benign (partial or complete hydatidiform mole and atypical placental site nodule) to malignant (gestational trophoblastic neoplasm [GTN]). Most patients with GTN present after a hydatidiform mole, although any type of gestation can precede the diagnosis. The most common types of GTN are invasive moles and choriocarcinomas. These are usually successfully treated with chemotherapy; however, in certain high-risk circumstances, surgery and radiation also may be required. Epithelioid trophoblastic tumors (ETTs) and placental site trophoblastic tumors (PSTTs) are far less common. They present and are managed quite differently from invasive moles and choriocarcinomas.

Epithelioid trophoblastic tumors primarily originate in chorionic type extravillous (nearly entirely intermediate) trophoblast. There are no villi in the tumor. Epithelioid trophoblastic tumors are relatively resistant to chemotherapy, secrete less hCG, and are usually best treated with hysterectomy.

Placental site trophoblastic tumors also develop from extravillous trophoblast, and villi are not present in these tumors. The incidence of PSTT is approximately 1 in 100,000 pregnancies, and two-thirds are confined to the uterus at the time of diagnosis. Most PSTTs stain strongly for melanoma cell adhesion molecule (Mel-CAM) and human placental lactogen (hPL) and only focally for placental alkaline phosphatase (PLAP). Some cells may stain for p63 and β-hCG. Serum β-hCG levels typically are only mildly increased. A serum hPL level is not helpful for diagnosis or monitoring. Vascular invasion is commonly observed in PSTT, and there is little necrosis and inflammation. Like ETT, because of relative chemotherapy resistance, hysterectomy with lymph node dissection and ovarian conservation is recommended for patients with PSTT. For women who wish to preserve fertility, local excision may be considered.

For patients with metastatic PSTT, a combination of surgery and systemic chemotherapy is recommended. The most effective systemic regimen appears to be EMA-EP (etoposide, methotrexate, actinomycin D/etoposide, cisplatin). Because of the significant toxicity associated with the EMA-EP regimen, there has been interest in developing better-tolerated alternatives. One regimen that appears to be effective and better tolerated is TP/TE (paclitaxel, cisplatin/paclitaxel, etoposide).

Because all trophoblasts express programmed death-ligand 1 (PD-L1), the treatment of patients with chemotherapy-resistant disease using immune checkpoint inhibitors is being explored. Several reports in the literature include relatively modest-sized series of patients with GTN (including a few patients with ETT or PSTT) who have been treated with pembrolizumab and at least one series describing treatment with avelumab. Results have been promising, with complete response rates exceeding 80% for pembrolizumab and nearly 50% for avelumab. Radiation has been reported to provide local control in some cases.

The patient in this scenario has a tumor that consists of intermediate trophoblasts and is consistent with a diagnosis of PSTT. Ki-67 staining shows a proliferation index of approximately 30%.

A long interval from index pregnancy is the most important prognostic factor for the patient. Early diagnosis of PSTT allows prompt initiation of therapy. The probability of successful treatment with combination chemotherapy for patients with metastatic PSTT is highly correlated with time from antecedent pregnancy, highlighting the importance of avoiding delays in diagnosis. In the largest series published to date, which is from the Charing Cross Hospital in London, time from antecedent pregnancy was the most important prognostic factor for overall survival. Advanced International Federation of Gynecology and Obstetrics (FIGO) stage (III or IV) also was significantly associated with worse outcomes; however, time to diagnosis was important, independent of stage. For example, in the Charing Cross experience, all women with stage I PSTT or ETT who received a diagnosis within 4 years of the antecedent pregnancy were long-term survivors, but five out of nine patients with stage I disease who were diagnosed greater than 4 years from antecedent pregnancy died of disease.

Because of resistance to chemotherapy, the World Health Organization (WHO) prognostic scoring is not valid for prognosis or guiding treatment choices in patients with PSTT or ETT. Although high hCG is an adverse prognostic factor for patients with the common forms of GTN, the hCG level does not seem to be associated with outcomes among patients with PSTT. This patient's low hCG will not affect her prognosis.

Whereas the depth of myometrial invasion is prognostic for patients with endometrial carcinoma, it is not an independent factor associated with prognosis for patients with GTN, or any histology, on multivariate analyses. Deep myometrial invasion is not consistently associated with a poor prognosis.

Tumor size, including tumors in the uterus, is a factor in determining the WHO GTN prognostic score; however, it has not been shown to have value in predicting outcomes among women with ETT or PSTT, such as the patient in this scenario with PSTT.

Although age is a factor in the WHO scoring system, data regarding age as a prognostic factor for patients with PSTT are inconsistent. Some series have reported older age as unfavorable, but others have reported worse outcomes among younger patients. In multivariate analysis in the Charing Cross series, age was not independently associated with survival; therefore, the patient's age is not a factor associated with an unfavorable prognosis.

Froeling FE, Ramaswami R, Papanastasopoulos P, Kaur B, Sebire NJ, Short D, et al. Intensified therapies improve survival and identification of novel prognostic factors for placental-site and epithelioid trophoblastic tumours. Br J Cancer 2019;120:587–94. doi: 10.1038/s41416-019-0402-0

Gadducci A, Carinelli S, Guerrieri ME, Aletti GD. Placental site trophoblastic tumor and epithelioid trophoblastic tumor: clinical and pathological features, prognostic variables and treatment strategy. Gynecol Oncol 2019;153:684–93. doi: 10.1016/j.ygyno.2019.03.011

Ngan HY, Seckl MJ, Berkowitz RS, Xiang Y, Golfier F, Sekharan PK, et al. Diagnosis and management of gestational trophoblastic disease: 2021 update. Int J Gynaecol Obstet 2021;155(suppl 1):86–93. doi: 10.1002/ijgo.13877

11 Bariatric surgery

A 32-year-old with a BMI of 45 and type 2 diabetes undergoes a sleeve gastrectomy. Weight loss is likely to most effectively reduce her risk for cancer of the

(A) breast
(B) colon
* (C) endometrium
(D) pancreas
(E) stomach

Bariatric surgery is currently one of the most effective interventions for weight loss and weight maintenance for patients with obesity. Commonly performed procedures are summarized in Table 11-1. Multiple studies have demonstrated an association of obesity and cancer, and bariatric surgery reduces the risk of cancer in multiple cancer types (Table 11-2). This effect is particularly strong for hormonally driven cancer, including breast, ovarian, and endometrial cancer.

Endometrial cancer clearly has been linked to obesity. The protective effect of sustained weight loss after bariatric surgery on the risk of endometrial cancer has been reproduced in multiple studies. After bariatric surgery, patients have a 50–70% reduction in the risk of endometrial cancer. After weight-loss surgery, the patient in this scenario can expect to have the greatest reduction in risk of endometrial cancer.

TABLE 11-1. Bariatric Surgery Types: Benefits and Disadvantages

	ROUX-EN-Y GASTRIC BYPASS	SLEEVE GASTRECTOMY	BILIOPANCREATIC DIVERSION WITH DUODENAL SWITCH	ADJUSTABLE GASTRIC BANDING
Procedure description	Stomach transected to create a 1-ounce pouch with gastrojejunostomy to divert stomach, duodenum, and proximal jejunum	80% of body of stomach is resected	Sleeve gastrectomy is performed with an anastomosis between the proximal duodenum to reduce absorption in addition to gastric changes	Adjustable band is placed proximal to the stomach to constrict the gastric pouch and outlet
Type	Restrictive and malabsorptive	Restrictive	Restrictive and malabsorptive	Restrictive
Benefits	Substantial weight loss with less weight regain	No intestinal anastomosis	Substantial weight loss	Can be adjusted, no intestinal anastomosis
Disadvantages	Higher surgical complications, malabsorption of calcium, iron, and B12	Observational studies show less weight loss and more weight regain than Roux-en-Y	Highest surgical risk	Band erosion, port infection, highest risk of weight regain

TABLE 11-2. Cancer Risk Reduction With Bariatric Surgery in Hormonal Cancer

	RISK REDUCTION	HORMONAL CANCER
Breast cancer	30–50%	Yes
Endometrial cancer	50–70%	Yes
Ovarian cancer	~53%	Yes
Colon cancer	Mixed data	No
Pancreatic cancer	Mixed data	No
Gastric cancer	None	No

Breast cancer also is linked to obesity and is hormonally mediated. The correlation between obesity and premenopausal breast cancer is less significant than that of obesity and postmenopausal breast cancer. Studies of the effects of bariatric surgery on breast cancer in premenopausal patients have shown a 30% reduction in breast cancer risk, whereas studies of postmenopausal patients demonstrate a 50% reduction in risk. The patient in this scenario is 32 years old, and bariatric surgery would result in a greater reduction in endometrial cancer risk than breast cancer risk.

The effect of undergoing bariatric surgery on colorectal cancer risk is mixed, with some studies demonstrating a reduced risk of colon cancer and others suggesting an increased risk of colorectal cancer after bariatric surgery. Multiple population-level cohort studies have indicated that colorectal cancer risk doubles after bariatric surgery. Although the mechanism of increased risk is poorly understood, alterations in the gut microbiome have been proposed as a potential mechanism.

Obesity results in increased activation of the pancreatic beta cells for insulin production, followed by activation of pancreatic stellate cells, resulting in fibrosis and associated increased risk of pancreatic cancer. The effect of bariatric surgery on pancreatic cancer is unclear. Some studies show moderate risk reduction (approximately 25%) for pancreatic cancer, and other studies have not found any benefit.

One historical concern about bariatric surgery was a potential for increased risk of esophageal or gastric cancer due to the increased risk of reflux and metaplasia. To date, studies have not shown a definitive increased risk. Reductions in weight may offset other physiologic changes, but additional research is needed.

Arterburn DE, Telem DA, Kushner RF, Courcoulas AP. Benefits and risks of bariatric surgery in adults: a review. JAMA 2020;324:879–87. doi: 10.1001/jama.2020.12567

Aubrey C, Black K, Campbell S, Pin S. Endometrial cancer and bariatric surgery: a scoping review. Surg Obes Relat Dis 2019;15:497–501. doi: 10.1016/j.soard.2018.12.003

Lim P, Stucky CH, Wasif N, Etzioni DA, Harold KL, Madura JA II, et al. Bariatric surgery and longitudinal cancer risk: a review. JAMA Surg 2024;159:331–8. doi: 10.1001/jamasurg.2023.5809

Schauer DP, Feigelson HS, Koebnick C, Caan B, Weinmann S, Leonard AC, et al. Bariatric surgery and the risk of cancer in a large multisite cohort. Ann Surg 2019;269:95–101. doi: 10.1097/SLA.0000000000002525

12 Surveillance after borderline tumor

A 28-year-old underwent a left oophorectomy for a 12-cm adnexal mass, which was found to be a serous borderline tumor. No other disease was seen at the time of surgery. Her medical history and family history are unremarkable. She has not completed childbearing and asks about surveillance. You inform her that the best test to detect a recurrence is

(A) CA 125 level
(B) computed tomography (CT) of the abdomen and pelvis
(C) human epididymis protein 4 level
(D) MRI
* (E) pelvic ultrasonography

Borderline ovarian tumors are histologically characterized by epithelial proliferation and nuclear atypia in the absence of destructive stromal invasion. The precise incidence of borderline tumors is unknown because only those that undergo surgical removal are reported. Based on data from the California Cancer Registry, the incidence of borderline tumors was 2.5 cases per 100,000 women in 2009, with 61.8% of cases classified as serous and 37.4% as mucinous. Other histologic types of borderline tumors, such as clear cell, endometrioid, and Brenner tumor, make up fewer than 5% of cases.

Borderline tumors are staged using the same staging system as ovarian carcinoma, with 80% of cases being confined to the ovary (stage I) at diagnosis. Compared with primary invasive ovarian carcinoma, the prognosis for patients with borderline tumors is vastly more favorable, with 5-year survival rates for stages I, II, and III disease of 99%, 98%, and 96%, respectively.

Overall recurrence rates range from 4% to 14% across series. Among patients treated with fertility-sparing surgery, the most common sites of recurrence are the involved ovary, with recurrence rates of 25–35% after cystectomy, or the contralateral ovary, with rates of 5–12% after unilateral salpingo-oophorectomy. Although most recurrences are diagnosed within 5 years of the initial surgery, in contrast to high-grade invasive ovarian carcinoma, a higher proportion of borderline recurrences are found more than 5 years after diagnosis and can occur as long as 10–15 years after diagnosis. Although the risk of recurrence after fertility-sparing surgery is higher than after bilateral salpingo-oophorectomy, overall survival rates are unchanged because most tumors recur as borderline tumors, which can be treated easily with re-excision.

The value of active surveillance for patients with a borderline tumor is unclear. Although many recommendations for surveillance exist, currently there are no high-level data demonstrating a benefit. With other diseases, the clinical value of surveillance depends largely on whether asymptomatic recurrences detected by surveillance have a better prognosis than symptomatic recurrences. Because borderline recurrence has no significant effect on survival, any benefit from surveillance to detect a borderline recurrence would have to stem from outcomes other than survival. In patients who have undergone fertility-sparing surgery, surveillance theoretically could enable detection of ovarian recurrence at a smaller tumor size, which may improve the likelihood of ovarian preservation; however, there are no data demonstrating this to be the case.

Whether benefit is derived from surveillance to detect invasive recurrence also is unknown. Based on a systematic review of the literature, the pooled estimate for invasive recurrence risk is 0.5% for patients with early-stage disease and 2% for patients with advanced-stage disease. A 2013 study of 47 reported cases of invasive recurrence found the mean time to progression to carcinoma to be 75 months (range, 11–310) for serous tumors, and 33 months (5–82) for mucinous tumors. Researchers identified two predictors of invasive recurrence: 1) the presence of invasive peritoneal implants and 2) residual disease after surgery. Additionally, the prognostic significance of micropapillary architecture in serous tumors, intraepithelial carcinoma, or stromal microinvasion was questionable due to differences in pathological criteria used in studies and potential bias in how data were collected. Based on these findings, surveillance for invasive recurrence may have the highest yield in patients with residual disease after surgery or with invasive implants; however, data demonstrating improved outcomes among patients whose invasive recurrences were detected through surveillance compared with patients whose recurrences were detected clinically are lacking.

Pelvic ultrasonography is the best strategy for active surveillance because most recurrences occur in the remaining ovarian tissue among patients who had fertility-sparing surgery, such as the described patient. Pelvic ultrasonography is highly sensitive for the detection of adnexal abnormalities, is widely accessible, and is relatively cost-effective, without the risks associated with radiation.

Although CA 125 tumor marker levels are commonly used to monitor for recurrence among patients with high-grade serous ovarian cancer, many borderline tumors do not express high levels of CA 125, and measurement of tumor marker concentrations is not reliable. A study of 164 patients who underwent fertility-sparing treatment for borderline tumor and were monitored with physical examination and ultrasonography every 3 months for 2 years and every 6 months thereafter found that with a median follow-up of 71 months, 24 patients (17%) experienced a recurrence, with pelvic unltrasonography demonstrating an abnormal adnexal mass in 23 patients, whereas CA 125 levels were increased in only eight patients; therefore, CA 125 is recommended for surveillance only in patients whose levels were increased prior to surgery. Given that CA 125 measurement is not a reliable predictor in premenopausal patients due to high false-positive rates, and that the diagnosis of borderline tumor is rarely known preoperatively, many patients who undergo fertility-sparing surgery will not have an assessment of the preoperative CA 125 level.

Among patients with peritoneal implants at diagnosis, data indicate pelvic ultrasonography detects more recurrences than CA 125 concentrations. A study of 45 cases of recurrence among 162 patients with serous borderline tumor with peritoneal implants, approximately one-half of whom had undergone fertility-sparing surgery, found the median time to recurrence was 31 months (range, 4–242 months), with 14 of the 45 recurrences considered invasive. Ultrasonography detected recurrence in 42% of patients, whereas the CA 125 level was increased in 15.6% of all recurrences and in one-half of invasive recurrences. Based on these data, surveillance for invasive recurrence using a combination of ultrasonography and CA 125 testing has been suggested; however, to date there is no evidence this strategy improves outcomes.

Other imaging modalities, such as MRI and CT, are not recommended for use as surveillance tools for recurrent borderline tumor. Particularly for the described patient, whose risk is highest for an adnexal recurrence, MRI and CT offer no significant diagnostic advantage compared with pelvic ultrasonography for the detection of an adnexal mass. They are more costly and, in the case of CT, are associated with potentially harmful cumulative radiation exposure.

Human epididymis protein 4 is a tumor marker approved for monitoring patients with invasive ovarian cancer for relapse. There is no evidence that it is reliable as a diagnostic marker for borderline tumors.

Berrada K, Mariy O, Miara I, Tabakh H, Siwane A, Touil N, et al. Ultrasound imaging of endometriosis. Poster presented at: European Congress of Radiology; March 1–5, 2023; Vienna, Austria. doi: 10.26044/ecr2023/C-22790

Braicu EI, Van Gorp T, Nassir M, Richter R, Chekerov R, Gasimli K, et al. Preoperative HE4 and ROMA values do not improve the CA125 diagnostic value for borderline tumors of the ovary (BOT) a study of the TOC Consortium. J Ovarian Res 2014;7:49. doi: 10.1186/1757-2215-7-49

Daraï E, Fauvet R, Uzan C, Gouy S, Duvillard P, Morice P. Fertility and borderline ovarian tumor: a systematic review of conservative management, risk of recurrence and alternative options. Hum Reprod Update 2013;19:151–66. doi: 10.1093/humupd/dms047

Morris CR, Liu L, Rodriguez AO, Cress RD, Snipes K. Epidemiologic features of borderline ovarian tumors in California: a population-based study. Cancer Causes Control 2013;24:665–74. doi: 10.1007/s10552-013-0145-9

Uzan C, Kane A, Rey A, Gouy S, Pautier P, Lhomme C, et al. How to follow up advanced-stage borderline tumours? Mode of diagnosis of recurrence in a large series stage II-III serous borderline tumours of the ovary. Ann Oncol 2011;22:631–5. doi: 10.1093/annonc/mdq414

13 Bowel preparation

A 65-year-old woman presents with new-onset abdominal pain and bloating. Her past medical history is notable for hypertension, which is well-controlled on medications. The physical examination demonstrates a mobile, 12-cm mass. Computed tomography (CT) demonstrates a 12-cm complex adnexal mass, ascites, and an omental cake without bowel involvement, and the patient is scheduled for an exploratory laparotomy and tumor debulking. Preoperatively, the best gastrointestinal intervention to optimize surgical outcomes is to

(A) avoid oral intake after midnight
(B) begin treatment with oral antibiotics
* (C) have a carbohydrate drink 2 hours before surgery
(D) initiate probiotic therapy immediately
(E) undergo a mechanical bowel preparation

Preoperative preparation is important to minimize surgical and postoperative complications. In patients undergoing debulking surgery for ovarian cancer, additional procedures, such as bowel resection, may be required to achieve optimal cytoreduction. The patient in this scenario is preparing to undergo a debulking procedure. Of the choices listed, drinking a carbohydrate-rich drink up to 2 hours before surgery is the safest recommendation and is a consistent recommendation across many societies.

The Enhanced Recovery After Surgery (ERAS) Society recommends oral carbohydrate loading 2–3 hours before surgery with an isotonic complex carbohydrate solution. Consumption of fluids before surgery is associated with reduced preoperative anxiety, aids in preventing dehydration, and may reduce perioperative insulin resistance. Consumption of 200–250 mL does not appear to increase the risk of aspiration at the time of surgery.

Many recommendations exist regarding ERAS pathways, but there is no consensus regarding the role of bowel preparation, and evidence that preoperative mechanical preparation alone improves surgical outcomes is limited. In gynecologic surgery, data are extrapolated from colorectal literature. A 2011 Cochrane review of 20 randomized controlled trials with 5,805 patients undergoing elective colorectal surgery showed no difference in wound infections or anastomotic leakage rates between those who received a mechanical bowel preparation and those who did not. Mechanical bowel preparation also has been proposed as a way to enhance visualization of the surgical field during laparoscopy; however, a randomized controlled trial of 146 women undergoing laparoscopic hysterectomy with and without bowel preparation showed no differences in surgical outcomes. Mechanical bowel preparation also is time-consuming, expensive, and unpleasant for patients. Given the lack of data demonstrating a benefit of mechanical bowel preparation, it is not the best option for the described patient.

There are data showing reduced rates of infection and anastomotic leakage when oral antibiotics and mechanical bowel preparation are combined. A large-scale study in the United States evaluated the combined use of mechanical bowel preparation and oral antibiotics. It noted that this combination preparation was an independent factor in reducing the incidence of anastomotic leakage, surgical site infections, and postoperative paralytic ileus when compared to oral antibiotics or mechanical bowel preparation alone. A meta-analysis of observational studies evaluated the effectiveness of oral antibiotics with and without a mechanical bowel preparation and surgical site infection risk. Compared to no preparation, surgical site infection risk was significantly reduced when patients received oral antibiotics either alone or combined with a mechanical bowel preparation. The largest study demonstrated no difference between a mechanical preparation with oral antibiotics versus oral antibiotics alone. If a bowel procedure was planned for this patient based on imaging findings, then discussion regarding bowel preparation would be warranted, particularly regarding the use of oral antibiotics. However, mechanical preparation alone would not improve outcomes. As this patient's CT does not raise concerns for bowel involvement, a planned resection is unlikely, and thus, preparation with mechanical preparation or antibiotics is not recommended.

Prebiotics, probiotics, and synbiotics have received attention for their impact on the gut microbiome and systemic anti-inflammatory effects. Literature shows that using probiotics results in little to no difference in perioperative mortality in colorectal surgery but may aid in reducing postoperative infectious complications. Short-term use of probiotics may favorably affect surgical outcomes among patients with planned intestinal surgery; however, their use is not currently endorsed by any societies as part of preoperative preparation.

Fasting starting at midnight is associated with depletion in liver glycogen stores, impaired glucose metabolism, and increased insulin resistance. Data from the anesthesia literature demonstrates that clear fluid intake up to 2 hours before surgery does not increase gastric content or the complication rate. Additionally, patients may ingest solids up to 6 hours before surgery. Given the safety of oral intake with clear liquids up to 2 hours before surgery, fasting starting at midnight is not the best answer in this scenario.

Improving surgical outcomes in a patient undergoing debulking requires a multifaceted approach. Avoiding hypoglycemia and dehydration improves surgical outcomes. Unless bowel resection is anticipated, mechanical bowel preparation should be avoided. If bowel preparation is performed, the surgeon should consider the addition of oral antibiotics and note that this is not a definitive recommendation within gynecologic oncology pathways, particularly as similar surgical site infection outcomes are noted with or without a bowel preparation. Probiotics are not recommended as part of ERAS pathways at this time.

An S, Kim K, Kim MH, Jung JH, Kim Y. Perioperative probiotics application for preventing postoperative complications in patients with colorectal cancer: a systematic review and meta-analysis. Medicina (Kaunas) 2022;58:1644. doi: 10.3390/medicina58111644.

Ju YU, Min BW. A review of bowel preparation before colorectal surgery. Ann Coloproctol 2021;37:75–84. doi: 10.3393/ac.2020.04.01

Kiran RP, Murray AC, Chiuzan C, Estrada D, Forde K. Combined preoperative mechanical bowel preparation with oral antibiotics significantly reduces surgical site infection, anastomotic leak, and ileus after colorectal surgery. Ann Surg 2015;262:416–5. doi: 10.1097/SLA.0000000000001416

National Comprehensive Cancer Network. Palliative care. Version 1.2025 NCCN Clinical Practice Guidelines in Oncology [after login]. NCCN; 2024. Accessed March 13, 2025. https://www.nccn.org/professionals/physician_gls/pdf/palliative.pdf

14 Depression

A 67-year-old presents for a surveillance visit after treatment for stage IIIC serous ovarian carcinoma. She has undergone surgical debulking and completed six cycles of carboplatin-paclitaxel chemotherapy 6 months ago. She is accompanied by her daughter, who expresses concern about the patient's mood, noting increasing irritability, decreased appetite and energy, and insomnia, all of which are interfering with her ability to participate in her daily activities. Her Patient Health Questionnaire 9 (PHQ-9) score is 21. The best next step is to recommend

(A) behavioral activation
(B) cognitive behavioral therapy
(C) electroconvulsive therapy (ECT)
* (D) selective serotonin reuptake inhibitor (SSRI)
(E) tricyclic antidepressant

Major depressive disorder, also known as depression, is a common condition that occurs more frequently in women than men. Screening and treatment for this condition are crucial in the oncology setting. Many screening tools for depression exist with varying sensitivity and specificity. The PHQ-9 is one such tool that has 80% sensitivity and 92% specificity for the diagnosis of depression (Table 14-1). On this assessment, high scores are associated with increasing severity of depression, with thresholds of 5, 10, 15, and 20 correlating to mild, moderate, moderately severe, and severe depression, respectively.

Individuals who have a single episode of major depression are at high risk of recurrence, with 80% experiencing at least one recurrence. This recurrence rate is higher in older individuals due to the increased risk of medical comorbid conditions and higher likelihood of a previous depression diagnosis. Individuals undergoing cancer therapy and those in survivorship are at an increased risk for developing depression. Individuals undergoing cancer treatment who have a comorbid diagnosis of depression have lower survival rates compared with those without depression.

The severity of the depression, in addition to other patient characteristics, affects the recommendations for treatment. Individuals with high-risk characteristics, such as psychotic or bipolar features or an increase in risk of suicide, should be referred to a psychiatrist. Antidepressant therapy is the first-line treatment for individuals with moderate to severe depression or depression persistent for 2 years or longer, and SSRIs are the preferred treatment for most individuals. This class of medication is well tolerated, has few drug interactions, and is relatively safe in the event of an overdose. Selective serotonin and norepinephrine reuptake inhibitors (SNRIs) are an alternative option for first-line therapy for individuals with severe depression. Available data comparing SNRIs to SSRIs suggest similar effectiveness; however, older patients with depression may experience more adverse effects with SNRIs. Given this patient's age and degree of depression, initiation of an SSRI is the best next step.

Behavioral activation is a form of psychotherapy that aims to increase an individual's participation in activities and their positive interactions with their environment. This intervention is not recommended as primary treatment for severe depression but can be considered as an adjunct treatment to pharmacologic therapy. This combination is as effective in treating mild to moderate depression as pharmacotherapy alone and can be considered as an initial approach in patients with less severe depression.

Cognitive behavioral therapy is another form of psychotherapy that aims to modify an individual's thoughts when they interfere with desired behavior and functioning. This intervention is not recommended as primary treatment for severe depression but can be considered as an adjunct treatment to pharmacologic therapy. Cognitive behavioral therapy is as effective in treating mild to moderate depression as

TABLE 14-1. Patient Health Questionnaire 9

NINE-SYMPTOM CHECKLIST				
Name: ______________________		Date: ____________		
Over the last 2 weeks, how often have you been bothered by any of the following problems?	**Not at all**	**Several days**	**More than half the days**	**Nearly every day**
1. Little interest or pleasure in doing things	0	1	2	3
2. Feeling down, depressed, or hopeless	0	1	2	3
3. Trouble falling or staying asleep, or sleeping too much	0	1	2	3
4. Feeling tired or having little energy	0	1	2	3
5. Poor appetite or overeating	0	1	2	3
6. Feeling bad about yourself—or that you are a failure or have let yourself or your family down	0	1	2	3
7. Trouble concentrating on things, such as reading the newspaper or watching television	0	1	2	3
8. Moving or speaking so slowly that other people could have noticed? Or the opposite—being so fidgety or restless that you have been moving around a lot more than usual	0	1	2	3
9. Thoughts that you would be better off dead or of hurting yourself in some way	0	1	2	3
(For office coding: Total Score	________ =	________ +	________ +	________)
If you checked off any problems, how *difficult* have these problems made it for you to do your work, take care of things at home, or get along with other people? ☐ Not difficult at all ☐ Somewhat difficult ☐ Very difficult ☐ Extremely difficult				

Reprinted from Kroenke K, Spitzer RL, Williams JB. The PHQ-9: validity of a brief depression severity measure. J Gen Intern Med 2001;16:606–13. doi: 10.1046/j.1525-1497.2001.016009606.x

pharmacotherapy alone and can be considered as an initial approach in patients with mild or moderate depression. Cognitive behavioral therapy is associated with a decreased risk of relapse after recovery from depression.

Electroconvulsive therapy is not recommended as initial therapy for the described patient. Electroconvulsive therapy can be an appropriate first-line approach for individuals with severe depression with urgent or emergent characteristics or for whom typical treatments are not feasible. These scenarios include individuals with a high risk of suicide, stupor secondary to depression, extreme distress, or inadequate oral intake due to depression. Additionally, ECT can be considered initial therapy for patients who clearly express a preference for this treatment approach. Electroconvulsive therapy leads to rapid improvement in symptoms, but recurrence of symptoms is common. To decrease the risk of recurrence, pharmacotherapy often is indicated after ECT for ongoing treatment.

Although tricyclic antidepressants are approved by the U.S. Food and Drug Administration to treat major depressive disorder and other depressive disorders, these medications are not as effective as SSRIs and are not recommended as first-line treatment of depression. Tricyclic antidepressants may be considered after unsuccessful treatment with SSRIs and other antidepressants. For the patient described, who has severe depression, an SSRI is the first pharmacologic choice.

Assessment of distress symptoms in individuals undergoing cancer therapy is important. Detection of depression during cancer treatment and in survivorship is crucial to adequate treatment and improves outcomes. The severity of depression influences the initial approach to treatment, which may include psychotherapy and medications. Validated screening tools help diagnose depression when patients or family members raise concerns and may help expedite therapy for some patients.

Cuijpers P, van Straten A, Andersson G, van Oppen P. Psychotherapy for depression in adults: a meta-analysis of comparative outcome studies. J Consult Clin Psychol 2008;76:909–22. doi: 10.1037/a0013075

National Comprehensive Cancer Network. Distress management. Version 1.2025. NCCN Clinical Practice Guidelines in Oncology [after login]. NCCN; 2024. Accessed March 13, 2025. https://www.nccn.org/guidelines/guidelines-detail?category=3&id=1431

Unützer J. Clinical practice. Late-life depression. N Engl J Med 2007;357:2269–76. doi: 10.1056/NEJMcp073754

Walker J, Mulick A, Magill N, Symeonides S, Gourley C, Burke K, et al. Major depression and survival in people with cancer. Psychosom Med 2021;83:410–6. doi: 10.1097/PSY.0000000000000942

15 Endometrial cancer

A 31-year-old gravida 1, para 1, with abnormal uterine bleeding receives a diagnosis of grade 1 endometrioid endometrial adenocarcinoma after hysteroscopy with directed sampling. She desires future fertility. You counsel her that imaging is needed to assess her candidacy for fertility-sparing treatment. The best imaging test to assess her fertility status is

(A) computed tomography (CT)
(B) lymphoscintigraphy
* (C) MRI
(D) positron emission tomography (PET)
(E) ultrasonography

Endometrial cancer commonly is found in postmenopausal women, but the incidence of premenopausal endometrial cancer continues to increase because of the obesity epidemic. Currently, as many as 14% of cases of endometrial cancer are diagnosed before menopause, and 4% of patients are aged less than 40 years. The risk of disease spread is directly related to the tumor grade. Low-grade tumors are more likely to be confined to the uterus (80%). Fertility-sparing management with progestins is an option for patients with early-stage disease who meet specific criteria (Box 15-1). Determining which patients are appropriate candidates is the first step after diagnosis.

Magnetic resonance imaging is the best imaging test to assess for myometrial invasion in the described patient. Its sensitivity is superior to that of ultrasonography for myometrial invasion (Fig. 15-1). Magnetic resonance imaging also can help assess the adnexa for metastatic disease and can identify lymphadenopathy with high specificity. Magnetic resonance imaging is the best imaging modality to assess for fertility preservation.

Guidelines from the Society of Gynecologic Oncology state that CT should not be used for diagnosis or to determine the extent of myometrial invasion because its soft tissue contrast resolution is inferior to that of MRI. If symptoms are present or abnormalities found on a physical examination raise concern for metastatic disease, CT is a reasonable step to evaluate for distant spread.

Lymphoscintigraphy is a preoperative procedure that is performed after giving the patient a radioisotope to identify the presence and location of sentinel lymph nodes. Intraoperative injections of methylene blue and indocyanine green are preferred to lymphoscintigraphy use in endometrial cancer due to ease of injection, excellent mapping rates, and shorter operative time. Sentinel lymph node mapping is not part of the evaluation for fertility preservation in endometrial cancer, and it is not the best imaging test in this situation.

BOX 15-1

Recommendations for Fertility Preservation Evaluation in Endometrial Cancer

There is evidence to consider fertility-sparing treatment when the following criteria are met:

- Endometrioid histology, grade 1
- Desire for conservation of uterus with informed consent that data on outcomes are limited
- No myometrial invasion detected preoperatively with MRI or transvaginal ultrasound by a specialized radiologist/sonographer
- No extrauterine disease, confirmed by MRI or CT
- No contraindications to medical management

Evidence for fertility preservation in grade 2 endometrioid endometrial carcinoma is limited but may be considered in some individuals.

Positron emission tomography, usually in conjunction with a CT (PET/CT), has only moderate sensitivity despite its superior utility for assessing lymph node involvement. This test is costly and unnecessary in most cases of endometrial cancer. Additionally, it does not have the soft tissue resolution of MRI and would be an inferior test to diagnose or confirm myometrial invasion.

Ultrasonography performed by an experienced radiologist or sonographer is an alternative if MRI is not available. This can allow evaluation of myometrial invasion as well as adnexal involvement. It would not provide additional information regarding assessment of lymphadenopathy with MRI; consequently, ultrasonography is not the best test for the patient in this scenario.

Fertility-sparing management of endometrial cancer requires a multidisciplinary approach. Modifiable risk factors should be addressed, and a pathologic review of hysteroscopic-guided biopsy is preferred, along with consultation with a fertility specialist.

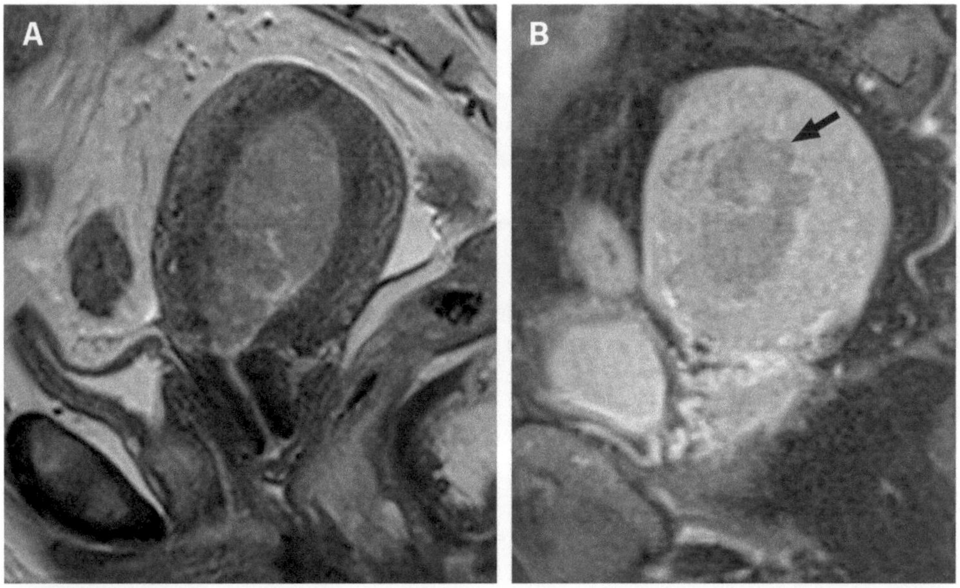

FIGURE 15-1. Post-contrast images of endometrial cancer, International Federation of Gynecology and Obstetrics (FIGO) stage IA. A. Sagittal T2-weighted. B. Parasagittal. There is a large volume of tumor within the endometrial cavity with invasion of the myometrium, extending to less than 50% of the myometrial thickness (arrow). The post-contrast images demonstrate the typical bright enhancement of the myometrium with intermediate enhancement of the tumor. (Reprinted from Patel S, Liyanage SH, Sahdev A, Rockall AG, Reznek RH. Imaging of endometrial and cervical cancer. Insights Imaging 2010;1:309–28. doi: 10.1007/s13244-010-0042-7)

Endometrial cancer. Practice Bulletin No. 149. American College of Obstetricians and Gynecologists. Obstet Gynecol 2015;125:1006–26. doi: 10.1097/01.AOG.0000462977.61229.de

Hamilton CA, Pothuri B, Arend RC, Backes FJ, Gehrig PA, Soliman PT, et al. Endometrial cancer: a Society of Gynecologic Oncology evidence-based review and recommendations, part II. Gynecol Oncol 2021;160:827–34. doi: 10.1016/j.ygyno.2020.12.024

Patel S, Liyanage SH, Sahdev A, Rockall AG, Reznek RH. Imaging of endometrial and cervical cancer. Insights Imaging 2010;1:309–28. doi: 10.1007/s13244-010-0042-7

Rodolakis A, Scambia G, Planchamp F, Acien M, Di Spiezio Sardo A, Farrugia M, et al. ESGO/ESHRE/ESGE guidelines for the fertility-sparing treatment of patients with endometrial carcinoma. Hum Reprod Open 2023;2023:hoac057. doi: 10.1093/hropen/hoac057

16 Minimally invasive surgery for endometrial cancer

A 75-year-old woman with a diagnosis of International Federation of Gynecology and Obstetrics (FIGO) grade 3 endometrial cancer is undergoing surgical staging. A sentinel lymph node (SLN) protocol with indocyanine green tracer injected into the cervix is performed during the operation. A right SLN was detected in the obturator space and was excised. A left SLN was not identified. The best next operative step to evaluate for lymph node metastases is to

(A) inject intrauterine indocyanine green tracer
(B) inject the cervix with isosulfan blue dye
(C) obtain frozen section of the right sentinel node
* (D) perform left-sided lymphadenectomy

Identifying metastatic involvement of regional lymph nodes in endometrial cancer through surgical lymph node assessment has significant diagnostic and prognostic value; however, the extent of lymph node dissection necessary for the management of endometrial cancer is debated. Historically, *complete lymphadenectomy*, defined as the systematic removal of all lymph nodes within the pelvic and para-aortic regions, was undertaken concurrently with hysterectomy in all cases; however, complete lymphadenectomy can result in serious morbidity, and accumulated evidence indicates that the procedure has no intrinsic therapeutic value.

The morbidity associated with retroperitoneal lymphadenectomy increases with the number of lymph nodes removed and the number of retroperitoneal regions involved. Intraoperative complications include increases in bleeding risk, neurologic injury, and anesthesia time. Postoperative complications include increased risk of thromboembolic events, lymphedema, and lymphocyst formation. The occurrence of lymphedema is especially debilitating and is likely underreported in the literature. Reported lymphedema rates vary widely because study findings are influenced by the length of follow-up and the methods used for evaluation. Lymphedema rates may be as high as 40%.

The SLN biopsy technique is an alternative to lymphadenectomy that preserves the diagnostic sensitivity of complete lymphadenectomy while reducing surgical morbidity. The premise is to identify the lymph nodes that are the initial lymphatic drainage site for the primary cancer and therefore most likely to be involved if metastases were present. Candidates for the procedure are patients with apparent uterine-confined disease in which staging information is relevant to adjuvant treatment decisions. Those with abnormal nodes identified on imaging or those with visibly enlarged nodes identified intraoperatively are not candidates for the SLN procedure.

Various factors that influence the diagnostic accuracy of the technique have been identified. These include surgeon experience, tracer type, injection site, pathologic examination technique, and individual patient anatomy. Studies also have consistently demonstrated that strict adherence to an SLN algorithm optimizes the diagnostic accuracy of the technique. The diagnostic performance of this SLN protocol has been evaluated in low- and high-grade endometrial cancer. In the FIRES (Fluorescent Imaging for Robotic Endometrial Cancer Sentinel lymph node biopsy) study, women with clinical stage I endometrial carcinoma of all tumor histologies and grades were included in the cohort, and a sensitivity of 97.2% and a negative predictive value of 99.6% were reported. More recently, the SENTOR study (Sentinel Lymph Node Biopsy Versus Lymphadenectomy for Intermediate- and High-Grade Endometrial Cancer Staging) reported a sensitivity of 96% and a negative predictive value of 99% in higher-grade cancer.

In the SLN algorithm depicted in Figure 16-1, sentinel nodes mapped by tracer must be removed in each hemipelvis. The SLNs removed are assessed by pathology using routine hematoxylin–eosin staining. If negative by hematoxylin–eosin, the diagnostic sensitivity of SLN metastasis is further increased through ultra-staging with serial lymph node sectioning and immunohistochemical staining for cytokeratin. If mapping cannot be

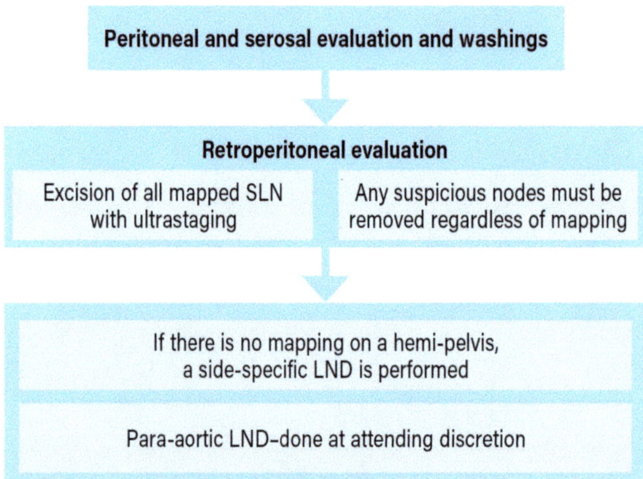

FIGURE 16-1. The sentinel lymph node algorithm for surgical staging of endometrial cancer. Abbreviation: LND, lymph node dissection. (Reprinted from Barlin JN, Khoury-Collado F, Kim CH, Leitao MM Jr, Chi DS, Sonoda Y, et al. The importance of applying a sentinel lymph node mapping algorithm in endometrial cancer staging: beyond removal of blue nodes. Gynecol Oncol 2012;125:531–5. doi: 10.1016/j.ygyno.2012.02.021)

carried out in one or both sides of the pelvis, complete retroperitoneal lymphadenectomy on the non-mapping side must be performed.

In this scenario, surgery is undertaken in a patient with apparent uterine-confined disease who has a grade 3 cancer histology. A right SLN was detected in the obturator space and was excised, but a left SLN was not identified. According to the algorithm, a complete side-specific left pelvic lymphadenectomy should be undertaken, and this is the best next step for the described patient.

Various injection sites and techniques have been evaluated in an effort to improve the diagnostic accuracy of the SLN technique. Sites evaluated include cervical, subserosal/myometrial, and peritumoral (hysteroscopic guided). A cervical injection of tracer into the stroma and submucosa of the cervix has emerged as the recommended technique. It has the advantage of being much quicker, easier, and more reproducible than intrauterine injections. Although cervical injection is theoretically less capable of detecting isolated para-aortic lymph node metastases that may travel through shared adnexal lymphatics, the reported detection rates for cervical injections are comparable to those for intrauterine injections. One additional concern for intrauterine injection is the risk of dispersing malignant cells through the fallopian tubes, and in cases of failed SLN identification, intrauterine tracer injection is not recommended.

Multiple studies also report detection rates when various types of tracers are used. Indocyanine green is a water-soluble compound that emits fluorescence when stimulated under near-infrared light. Compared with blue dye tracer, indocyanine green provides superior visualization and greater ability to remain within the draining lymphatics. Although indocyanine green costs more, it has emerged as the preferred agent due to its higher diagnostic accuracy, safety, and ease of use. Although indocyanine green is the preferred tracer, a repeat injection has not been incorporated into the SLN protocol, but may be considered in individual patients. Re-injection of isosulfan blue is not recommended when an SLN cannot be identified using indocyanine green tracer.

Frozen section is not a routine part of an SLN protocol, and in this case, undertaking frozen section of the excised right SLN will not clarify decision making regarding the status of the left-sided lymph nodes. The right SLN mapped successfully, and this specimen will undergo ultra-staging protocol for pathology assessment as described above. A frozen section may still be undertaken in situations in which it may influence immediate intraoperative decisions, such as characterizing grossly abnormal lymph nodes identified at surgery, but sending a frozen section is not the best next step in this patient's scenario.

In conclusion, SLN mapping has emerged as the standard of care for detecting occult lymphatic metastases in patients diagnosed with apparent uterine-confined endometrial cancer. Although various factors affect the diagnostic accuracy of the technique, strict adherence to the SLN algorithm is crucial. Ongoing research aims to refine the SLN mapping technique and its role in the overall management of endometrial cancer. As medical science progresses toward molecular classification of endometrial cancer for risk stratification, SLN mapping may be further tailored to target more exclusively those at highest risk of nodal involvement of their cancer.

Bodurtha Smith AJ, Fader AN, Tanner EJ. Sentinel lymph node assessment in endometrial cancer: a systematic review and meta-analysis. Am J Obstet Gynecol 2017;216:459–76.e10. doi: 10.1016/j.ajog.2016.11.1033

Cusimano MC, Vicus D, Pulman K, Maganti M, Bernardini MQ, Bouchard-Fortier G, et al. Assessment of sentinel lymph node biopsy vs lymphadenectomy for intermediate- and high-grade endometrial cancer staging. JAMA Surg 2021;156:157–64. doi: 10.1001/jamasurg.2020.5060

Leitao MM Jr, Khoury-Collado F, Gardner G, Sonoda Y, Brown CL, Alektiar KM, et al. Impact of incorporating an algorithm that utilizes sentinel lymph node mapping during minimally invasive procedures on the detection of stage IIIC endometrial cancer. Gynecol Oncol 2013;129:38–41. doi: 10.1016/j.ygyno.2013.01.002

Rossi EC, Kowalski LD, Scalici J, Cantrell L, Schuler K, Hanna RK, et al. A comparison of sentinel lymph node biopsy to lymphadenectomy for endometrial cancer staging (FIRES trial): a multicentre, prospective, cohort study. Lancet Oncol 2017;18:384–92. doi: 10.1016/S1470-2045(17)30068-2

Terada S, Tanaka T, Murakami H, Tsuchihashi H, Toji A, Daimon A, et al. Lymphatic complications following sentinel node biopsy or pelvic lymphadenectomy for endometrial cancer. J Clin Med 2023;12:4540. doi: 10.3390/jcm12134540

17 Mortality risk factors

A 56-year-old woman with a BMI of 45 presents for an annual visit. Five years ago, she underwent a hysterectomy and bilateral salpingo-oophorectomy to treat abnormal uterine bleeding caused by the pathology shown in Figure 17-1. She is concerned about her mortality risk, and you counsel her that her highest risk of mortality is from

* (A) cardiovascular disease
(B) colon cancer
(C) diabetes mellitus
(D) endometrial cancer
(E) fatty liver

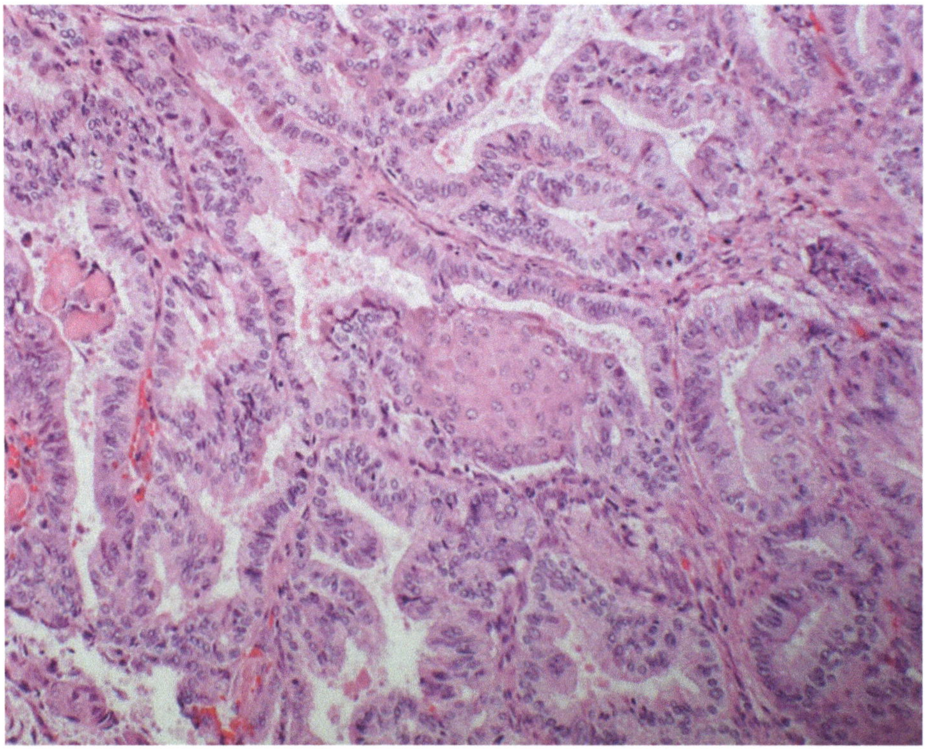

FIGURE 17-1. High-power image with crowded back-to-back glands with nuclear rounding, vesicular nuclei, small nucleoli, and squamous metaplasia. (Courtesy of Dr. Christine Bookhout, Department of Pathology, University of North Carolina.)

The pathology shown in Figure 17-1 is grade 1 endometrial cancer. Endometrial cancer has been highly linked to obesity, which creates hyperinsulinemia, unopposed estrogen, and a proinflammatory state that promotes proliferation of the endometrium. For every 5-point increase in BMI, a person has a 50% increase in lifetime risk of endometrial cancer. It is estimated that more than one half of all endometrial cancer in the United States is directly attributable to obesity.

Because of the association between obesity and metabolic syndrome, women with obesity and endometrial cancer, such as the patient in this scenario, are at an increased risk for many comorbid conditions.

A retrospective review of more than 44,000 patients diagnosed with endometrial cancer found the most common cause of death in this patient population to be cardiovascular disease. Specifically, patients diagnosed with localized, low-grade endometrial cancer were six times more likely to die from cardiovascular disease than endometrial cancer.

The patient in this scenario has presented 5 years after receiving a diagnosis of grade 1 endometrial cancer. After 5 years of surveillance, the risk of recurrent endometrial cancer or death from endometrial cancer is low. Based on the above data, the patient is at highest risk of death from cardiovascular disease. Although endometrial cancer has been associated with diabetes mellitus and fatty liver due to the link between endometrial cancer and obesity, cardiovascular disease remains the most likely cause of death.

Approximately 20% of patients diagnosed with endometrial cancer will die from another malignancy, and 1 in 10 patients with endometrial cancer will harbor a genetic mutation, such as Lynch syndrome, which increases their risk of secondary malignancies (ie, colon cancer). Despite this associated cancer risk, the risk of cardiovascular disease-related mortality is greater than that of colon cancer mortality in this patient population.

Routine health screening, optimization of lifestyle choices, and genetic testing can enhance health and wellness for patients with endometrial cancer and should be incorporated into survivorship plans. Traditional lifestyle interventions often do not affect long-term weight loss; however, bariatric surgery and novel medication options have shown meaningful modification of cardiovascular risk in these patients. Among the bariatric surgery options, gastric-sleeve gastrectomy has been shown to have the highest long-term success. More recently, glucagon-like peptide 1 (GLP-1) agonists, such as semaglutide, have led to sustained weight loss and improved diabetic and cardiovascular outcomes in patients. As science in this space evolves, a multidisciplinary team of specialists can help optimize health and weight in endometrial cancer survivors.

Agnew H, Kitson S, Crosbie EJ. Interventions for weight reduction in obesity to improve survival in women with endometrial cancer. Cochrane Database of Systematic Reviews 2023, Issue 3. Art. No.: CD012513. doi: 10.1002/14651858.CD012513.pub3

Lu KH, Broaddus RR. Endometrial cancer. N Engl J Med 2020;383:2053–64. doi: 10.1056/NEJMra1514010

Popoviciu M, Păduraru L, Yahya G, Metwally K, Cavalu S. Emerging role of GLP-1 agonists in obesity: a comprehensive review of randomised controlled trials. Int J Mol Sci 2023;24:10449. doi: 10.3390/ijms241310449

Ward KK, Shah NR, Saenz CC, McHale MT, Alvarez EA, Plaxe SC. Cardiovascular disease is the leading cause of death among endometrial cancer patients. Gynecol Oncol 2012;126:176–9. doi: 10.1016/j.ygyno.2012.04.013

18 Statistical measures in antibiotic choice

A 52-year-old woman with endometrial adenocarcinoma is scheduled for hysterectomy and surgical staging. Her surgical history includes an appendectomy complicated by a methicillin-resistant *Staphylococcus aureus* wound infection. Considering her potential risk of antibiotic resistance, the most important statistical measure in prophylactic antibiotic selection for this patient is

(A) negative predictive value
* (B) positive predictive value
(C) sensitivity
(D) specificity

Surgical site infections (SSIs) are the most common postoperative complication after gynecologic surgeries in the United States. The estimated rate of SSI after hysterectomy ranges from 1% to 4%, and SSIs are the second most common diagnosis resulting in postoperative admission after hysterectomy. These complications can lead to increased morbidity and higher health care costs. Reducing SSI has become a national initiative to improve surgical outcomes. Surgical site infections are tracked in a national database, and reimbursement by payors may be affected if institutional rates are too high.

Surgical site infection prevention bundles have been instituted at most hospitals to reduce SSI after hysterectomy. Although components of the bundle may vary slightly, all include preoperative antibiotics. Most gynecologic SSIs originate from the endogenous flora of the patient's skin and vagina. These organisms typically include gram-positive cocci from the skin and the aerobes and anaerobes of the vagina but may include enteric flora. Antibiotics administered within 1 hour of incision are meant to provide pharmacologic augmentation to the natural host immunity. Bacterial resistance mechanisms allow evasion of preoperative antibiotics and increase the risk of SSI. This patient has a history of methicillin-resistant infection, which increases her risk of antibiotic resistance in the future. It is imperative to consider this factor when choosing preoperative antibiotics and, specifically, evaluate the likelihood that she would have the same infection at the time of the hysterectomy.

There are four important factors to consider when evaluating a medical or diagnostic test, particularly a screening test: positive predictive value, negative predictive value, sensitivity, and specificity (Appendix B). In this scenario, *positive predictive value* is defined as the probability that the bacteria with an antibiotic-resistant result will be resistant to that antibiotic. Knowing the positive predictive value of antibiotic resistance testing will allow the physician to determine whether the patient is at risk for the same infection at the time of her hysterectomy. The standard choice of a preoperative antibiotic is cephalosporin, but it would not be prudent because cephalosporins are not effective against methicillin-resistant *S aureus*, evidenced by the high positive predictive value of the test that determines that resistance.

Negative predictive value is defined as the probability that the bacteria with an antibiotic-sensitive result will be sensitive to that antibiotic. The negative predictive value of the antibiotic sensitivity testing allows one to determine the proportion of patients with a bacterial infection susceptible to the antibiotic the first time who will continue to show susceptibility at the subsequent infection. The negative predictive value of an antibiotic sensitivity test would allow the determination of future antibiotic sensitivity based on prior sensitivity results with the same bacteria. Negative predictive value in this scenario would not give the information needed regarding the likelihood of antibiotic resistance to cephalosporins in the future; therefore, it is not the most important statistical measure to consider.

Sensitivity is a test's ability to correctly identify an individual with the disease as positive, or, in this scenario, to correctly identify bacteria with the antibiotic resistance as positive (ie, being antibiotic resistant). A highly sensitive test would indicate very few false positives. Conversely, *specificity* is the test's ability to correctly identify an individual without the disease as negative, or, in this scenario, correctly identify bacteria without antibiotic resistance as negative (ie, being antibiotic sensitive). A highly specific test would indicate very few false negatives. Although specificity and sensitivity are useful measures to evaluate the ability of a wound culture to diagnose a patient with an infection, these measurements are less useful when selecting antibiotics and assessing antibiotic resistance. They are less critical statistical measures to consider in this scenario.

Surgical site infections are a major cause of postoperative complications and morbidity. Antibiotic use preoperatively has been shown to reduce the risk of SSIs. When choosing preoperative antibiotics, it is imperative to consider the patient's prior infection history and possible antibiotic resistance.

Andiman SE, Xu X, Boyce JM, Ludwig EM, Rillstone HR, Desai VB, et al. Decreased surgical site infection rate in hysterectomy: effect of a gynecology-specific bundle. Obstet Gynecol 2018;131:991–9. doi: 10.1097/AOG.0000000000002594

Maxim LD, Niebo R, Utell MJ. Screening tests: a review with examples [published erratum appears in Inhal Toxicol 2019;31:298]. Inhal Toxicol 2014;26:811–28. doi: 10.3109/08958378.2014.955932

Prevention of infection after gynecologic procedures. ACOG Practice Bulletin No. 195. American College of Obstetricians and Gynecologists. Obstet Gynecol 2018;131:e172–89. doi: 10.1097/AOG.0000000000002670

19 Surgical site infection prevention

A 54-year-old patient with ovarian cancer undergoes interval debulking surgery with exploratory laparotomy, total abdominal hysterectomy, bilateral salpingo-oophorectomy, and omentectomy. She has a history of diabetes mellitus, and her hemoglobin A_{1C} is 9.5%. Her BMI is 29. She received cefazolin 30 minutes before incision, and her skin and vagina were prepped with chlorhexidine-alcohol skin preparation before surgery. Her midline incision is closed with a series of interrupted subcuticular monocryl sutures. There are no complications during surgery. On postoperative day 5, she develops a wound infection that requires opening the incision and packing. The factor that increased her risk of surgical site infection (SSI) the most is

(A) antibiotic selection
(B) BMI
(C) chlorhexidine-alcohol skin preparation
* (D) diabetes
(E) skin closure method

Surgical site infection remains a troublesome source of high health care costs and postoperative morbidity, affecting up to 30% of patients undergoing gynecologic oncology surgery. Surgical site infections are classified as incisional (eg, vaginal cuff cellulitis) or deep organ/space (eg, vaginal cuff abscess).

Hysterectomy is considered a clean-contaminated wound or an operative wound that encounters bacteria in a controlled condition and without unusual contamination due to vaginal entry. As such, appropriate measures to reduce SSI should be taken. There are several guidelines and toolkits that help reduce the incidence of SSI, including the consensus bundle from The Joint Commission on Surgical Care, Enhanced Recovery After Surgery, the World Health Organization, and the National Healthcare Safety Network. Bundled elements to reduce SSIs typically include antimicrobial prophylaxis, skin preparation, avoidance of hypothermia and surgical drains, and reduction of hyperglycemia.

Preoperative risk assessment should be performed based on patient-specific factors. The WASHING mnemonic was designed as a memory aid for identified surgical risk factors (Box 19-1). Weight is the first independent risk factor, with obesity (BMI greater than 30) being associated with increased risk of infection. Antibiotic-resistant skin flora (eg, methicillin-resistant *Staphylococcus aureus*) should be considered by

BOX 19-1

WASHING Mnemonic for Essential Increased Risk Factors in Surgical Site Infections

- W: Weight
- A: Antibiotic-resistant skin flora, methicillin-resistant *Staphylococcus aureus*
- S: Smoking cessation
- H: Hygiene (skin preparation)
- I: Immune deficiency status
- N: Nutritional status
- G: Glycemic control

Reprinted from Pellegrini JE, Toledo P, Soper DE, Bradford WC, Cruz DA, Levy BS, Lemieux LA. Consensus bundle on prevention of surgical site infections after major gynecologic surgery. Obstet Gynecol 2017;129:50-61. doi: 10.1097/AOG.0000000000001751.

reviewing a patient's medical history and assessing the potential need for repeat screening. Patients who smoke tobacco and are able to abstain for 4 weeks before surgery can reduce their risk of an SSI. Hygiene (skin preparation) should be done with chlorhexidine–alcohol, and patients should shower with chlorhexidine gluconate before surgery when able. Immunodeficiency can increase a patient's risk of infection but may not be modifiable. For patients with immunodeficiency due to chemotherapy, consider the timing of surgery to allow bone marrow recovery time. Nutritional status also should be considered, and surgeons should identify ways to improve a patient's nutritional care before and after surgery. Strict glycemic control during the first 24 hours after gynecologic oncology surgery has been shown to reduce SSIs by 35%.

Hyperglycemia has been specifically identified as an independent risk factor with potential for intervention. Several studies have identified that a glucose level of greater than 200 mg/dL is associated with a higher risk of infection regardless of whether a patient has diabetes. In a cohort study of more than 21,000 patients undergoing gastrointestinal surgery, postoperative hyperglycemia (greater than 250 mg/dL) was found to be associated with a 20% increased risk of readmission. When their preoperative hemoglobin A_{1C} was high, patients had tighter glycemic control and a lower threshold to treat hyperglycemia with insulin. This led to a 17% decreased risk of readmission.

In addition, use of preoperative broad-spectrum antibiotics should be based on the planned procedure. Dosage should be based on weight (increased dosage when weight is greater than 120 kg), with a repeat dose given if extended time of surgery (typically more than 3 hours) or excessive blood loss (greater than 1,500 mL) occurs. Skin preparation should be done with chlorhexidine–alcohol skin preparation rather than povidone–iodine because this decreases SSIs by 40%. Although not approved by the U.S. Food and Drug Administration for vaginal preparation, low concentrations of chlorhexidine gluconate are generally tolerated and can be used. Patients should be normothermic (maintaining their temperature at 36.5 °C [97.7 °F]) throughout surgery because hypothermia has been associated with an increased risk of infection. Drains, such as peritoneal, subcutaneous, and nasogastric types, should be avoided unless absolutely necessary. Hair removal should be done only when it interferes with the incision site, and hair should be clipped rather than shaved (shaving increases the risk of infection).

In this scenario, the factor that increased the patient's risk of an SSI is her uncontrolled diabetes. Appropriate preoperative antibiotics, BMI, skin preparation, and choice of closure do not increase her risk of SSI.

Nelson G, Bakkum-Gamez J, Kalogera E, Glaser G, Altman A, Meyer LA, et al. Guidelines for perioperative care in gynecologic/oncology: Enhanced Recovery After Surgery (ERAS) Society recommendations-2019 update. Int J Gynecol Cancer 2019;29:651–68. doi: 10.1136/ijgc-2019-000356

Pellegrini JE, Toledo P, Soper DE, Bradford WC, Cruz DA, Levy BS, et al. Consensus bundle on prevention of surgical site infections after major gynecologic surgery. AANA J 2017;85:1–12.

Prevention of infection after gynecologic procedures. ACOG Practice Bulletin No. 195. American College of Obstetricians and Gynecologists. Obstet Gynecol 2018;131:e172–89. doi: 10.1097/AOG.0000000000002670

Schmidt PC, Kamdar NS, Erekson E, Swenson CW, Uppal S, Morgan DM. Development of a preoperative clinical risk assessment tool for postoperative complications after hysterectomy. J Minim Invasive Gynecol 2022;29:401–8.e1. doi: 10.1016/j.jmig.2021.10.008

20 Palpable breast mass

A 42-year-old gravida 3, para 3003, presents for her annual well-woman examination. She is currently using a levonorgestrel-releasing intrauterine device for contraception. Her baseline mammogram at age 40 was negative. Her family history includes a grandmother with breast cancer diagnosed when she was 64 years old. On physical examination, the patient is afebrile. She has a 2-cm nontender, firm, mobile mass just lateral to the left nipple with no skin changes. The best next step to evaluate the mass is

(A) core needle biopsy
* (B) diagnostic digital breast tomosynthesis
(C) examination in 2 months
(D) fine needle aspiration
(E) MRI

In 2023, an estimated 300,000 women in the United States received a diagnosis of breast cancer. The lifetime average risk of cancer for a woman is approximately 13%. The most common pre-diagnostic symptom is a palpable breast mass. Most palpable breast masses are benign, and obstetrician–gynecologists may encounter these during well-woman examinations in asymptomatic patients. The evaluation is based on age at diagnosis and clinical suspicion for malignancy.

Masses that are firm and fixed to surrounding tissues with overlying skin findings, such as dimpling or nipple retraction, should raise suspicion for malignancy. Benign masses are more often mobile and rubbery with discrete margins. Fibroadenomas are the most common cause of a breast mass in young women but also may present at later ages. Other benign palpable masses include breast cysts, intraductal papilloma, atypical hyperplasia, tubular adenomas, phyllodes tumor, and lobular carcinoma in situ. At the initial presentation, a physical examination helps identify the location for focused imaging; however, physical examination is not a reliable method of diagnosis, and imaging is necessary to fully evaluate a palpable breast mass. Guidelines from the American College of Radiology specify that imaging for women older than age 40 with a palpable mass starts with diagnostic digital breast tomosynthesis, which allows planar imaging and reconstructions, instead of traditional two-dimensional mammography. This improves lesion detection and characterization, particularly for cancer presenting as a mass, and it is the best next step for the described patient.

The addition of ultrasonography to diagnostic mammography also has been shown to significantly detect cancer and specific benign findings, such as cysts, and it is recommended for patients younger than age 30 years. In these patients, the risk of cancer is significantly lower, and the additional cost and exposure to radiation with mammography are not indicated. On ultrasonography, benign breast findings typically are smooth and well circumscribed, with thin echogenic capsule, ellipsoid shape (wider than tall), and three or fewer gentle lobulations. Ultrasonographic findings indicating malignancy typically are hypoechoic with ill-defined angular margins, taller than wide, with acoustic shadowing and spiculation or microcalcifications. Color Doppler may be helpful when there is significant vascularity with a malignant lesion. For women with a negative mammogram in the prior 6 months, ultrasonography is a reasonable next step for additional imaging of a palpable mass.

Magnetic resonance imaging is a useful screening tool for breast cancer, particularly for women with dense breast tissue and those who may have hereditary breast cancer; however, because of its high cost and limited availability, it is not indicated for the initial workup of a palpable breast mass. Tissue sampling with a core needle biopsy or fine needle aspiration may be performed but would not be done before imaging. During the initial workup, MRI or tissue sampling with core needle biopsy or fine needle aspiration is not the best next step.

For patients younger than 30 years, when clinical suspicion is low for a malignancy or if the mass is unable to be palpated by the patient or physician after initial identification, it is reasonable to monitor the mass for one to two menstrual cycles and reassess with repeat examination in 2 months. The described patient is older than age 30, and repeat examination in 2 months is not the best next step for her. Based on her age and clinical findings, diagnostic mammography with tomosynthesis is the best next step in evaluation.

Diagnosis and management of benign breast disorders. Practice Bulletin No. 164. American College of Obstetricians and Gynecologists [published erratum appears in Obstet Gynecol 2021;137:382]. Obstet Gynecol 2016;127:e141–56. doi: 10.1097/AOG.0000000000001482

Klein KA, Kocher M, Lourenco AP, Niell BL, Bennett DL, Chetlen A, et al. ACR Appropriateness Criteria® palpable breast masses: 2022 update. Expert Panel on Breast Imaging. J Am Coll Radiol 2023;20:S146–63. doi: 10.1016/j.jacr.2023.02.013

National Comprehensive Cancer Network. Breast cancer screening and diagnosis. Version 2.2024. NCCN Clinical Practice Guidelines in Oncology [after login]. NCCN; 2024. Accessed February 24, 2025. https://www.nccn.org/guidelines/guidelines-detail?category=2&id=1421

Siegel RL, Kratzer TB, Giaquinto AN, Sung H, Jemal A. Cancer statistics, 2025. CA Cancer J Clin 2025;75:10–45. doi: 10.3322/caac.21871

21 Vulvar cancer micrometastasis

A 75-year-old patient underwent a partial radical vulvectomy with ipsilateral inguinal sentinel lymph node biopsy for squamous cell carcinoma of the vulva. Final pathology reveals negative surgical margins and a 1-mm metastasis in the sentinel lymph node with no extracapsular spread. The best next step to treat this cancer is

* (A) external beam radiotherapy
(B) full inguinal-femoral lymphadenectomy
(C) immune checkpoint inhibitor
(D) lymph node assessment in 3 months
(E) systemic chemotherapy

Sentinel lymph node biopsy for vulvar cancer is a safe, accurate alternative to full inguinal-femoral lymphadenectomy for select patients. For patients with a tumor sized less than 4 cm without suspicious lymph nodes, it has become the preferred procedure for inguinal-femoral lymph node assessment due to the significant decrease in related morbidity compared with morbidity with full inguinal-femoral lymphadenectomy. However, when metastatic disease is identified in a sentinel lymph node, further treatment of the affected inguinal-femoral groin is indicated. Data from the Groningen International Study on Sentinel Nodes in Vulvar Cancer I (GROINSS-V I) indicate that for any size of sentinel lymph node metastasis, further treatment of the lymph nodes is warranted. Investigators did find that the risk of other involved lymph nodes increased as the size of the sentinel lymph node metastasis increased.

Historically, if cancer was identified within a sentinel lymph node, treatment included performing a subsequent full inguinal-femoral lymphadenectomy, sometimes referred to as a *completion* lymphadenectomy. This was the approach used in the GROINSS-V I observational study. Additionally, if extracapsular extension or more than one positive lymph node was identified after a full inguinal-femoral lymphadenectomy, postoperative external beam radiotherapy to the groin and pelvis was administered. Because this treatment approach resulted in significant morbidity, a subsequent study, GROINSS-V II, sought to evaluate whether radiotherapy without completion inguinal-femoral lymphadenectomy might be a safe and less morbid alternative.

This study used a prospective, observational design whereby the recommended treatment for positive sentinel lymph node was radiotherapy to the inguinal-femoral and the lower external iliac lymph nodes in lieu of completion inguinal-femoral lymphadenectomy. This study found that for patients with a sentinel lymph node micrometastasis (metastases of 2 mm or less without extracapsular extension), the rate of groin recurrence at 2 years was low (1.6%) and was comparable to the rate observed after completion of inguinal-femoral lymphadenectomy (3.6%). Furthermore, toxicity was lower with radiotherapy than with inguinal-femoral lymphadenectomy, including a lower rate of lymphedema. Based on this, the recommended treatment for a micrometastasis within a sentinel lymph node is external beam radiotherapy, and it is the best next step for cancer treatment in the patient described.

Given comparable cancer-related outcomes and a more favorable toxicity profile, radiotherapy is preferred over a full inguinal-femoral lymphadenectomy. This is not the best next step in treatment for this patient.

Although the presented patient has a micrometastasis within an inguinal sentinel lymph node, there is no size of sentinel lymph node metastasis in which the chance of additional lymph node involvement is low enough to forgo any further treatment. Because of this, lymph node assessment in 3 months is not the best option due to the potential risk of untreated cancer within the inguinal-femoral lymph nodes that could lead to a potentially fatal groin recurrence.

Although there is a paucity of trials of systemic therapy in metastatic vulvar cancer, overall response rates to chemotherapy are low, making this an inferior option to radiotherapy for this patient. In general, chemotherapy is reserved for patients with distant metastases or widely metastatic disease.

Because of the rarity of vulvar cancer, there are no prospective trials investigating immune checkpoint inhibition in vulvar cancer treatment. Its value as a vulvar cancer treatment has been extrapolated from trials in other similar cancer of the lower genital tract, such as cervical cancer, with some success. As with chemotherapy, the paucity of data and inconsistency of response, checkpoint inhibition is reserved for patients with distant metastatic disease. There are no data to support its use for the treatment of an isolated sentinel lymph node metastasis, and this is not the best next step for the described patient.

National Comprehensive Cancer Network. Vulvar cancer. Version 4.2024. NCCN Clinical Practice Guidelines in Oncology [after login]. NCCN; 2024. Accessed January 22, 2025. https://www.nccn.org/guidelines/guidelines-detail?category=1&id=1476

Oonk MH, Planchamp F, Baldwin P, Mahner S, Mirza MR, Fischerová D, et al. European Society of Gynaecological Oncology guidelines for the management of patients with vulvar cancer update 2023. Int J Gynecol Cancer 2023;33:1023–43. doi: 10.1136/ijgc-2023-004486

Oonk MH, Slomovitz B, Baldwin PJ, van Doorn HC, van der Velden J, de Hullu JA, et al. Radiotherapy versus inguinofemoral lymphadenectomy as treatment for vulvar cancer patients with micrometastases in the sentinel node: results of GROINSS-V II. J Clin Oncol 2021;39:3623–32. doi: 10.1200/JCO.21.00006

22 Molecular testing

A 60-year-old patient with a history of stage IA, grade 3, endometrioid adenocarcinoma of the uterus presents for routine surveillance. Her cancer was initially managed with surgery and observation. She has been doing well without evidence of disease for 2 years. She now reports new-onset abdominal bloating and early satiety. A physical examination is notable for mild abdominal distension but is otherwise unremarkable. Imaging of the chest, abdomen, and pelvis reveals multifocal peritoneal implants. A biopsy of a peritoneal nodule confirms recurrent endometrioid adenocarcinoma. When considering options for initial systemic therapy, the best initial tumor test is

(A) folate receptor α (FOLR-α)
(B) homologous recombination deficiency (HRD)
(C) human epidermal growth factor receptor 2 (*HER2*)
* (D) mismatch repair (MMR)
(E) phosphatase and tensin analog (*PTEN*)

The treatment of metastatic or recurrent endometrial cancer has evolved in recent years as understanding of the underlying mechanisms in cancer development has progressed. Historically, endometrial cancer was classified by histologic subtype alone; however, the Cancer Genome Atlas offered an evaluation of the genomic and epigenomic landscape of endometrial cancer, which resulted in the delineation of molecular subtypes. This classification of endometrial cancer more accurately reflects the tumor biology and has been correlated with clinical outcomes. It also allows for potential targeted treatment strategies by molecular classification. Based on this, treatment of endometrial cancer has evolved to include components of molecular profiling in addition to histologic subtype (Appendix C).

One such classification involves the DNA repair pathway known as *mismatch repair.* Mismatch repair is a pathway by which a cell can repair errors created during DNA replication. When this pathway does not function properly, a process termed *mismatch repair deficiency* (dMMR/MMRd) can develop. Mismatch repair-deficient cancer can result in a high level of microsatellite instability, and this instability and dMMR often are used to describe the same molecular subtype. Mismatch repair deficiency may be due to sporadic mutations that occur only within the cells that lead to the development of the tumor or inherited germline mutations, such as in Lynch syndrome, in which the mutation is present in cells throughout the body. Tumors that are not dMMR/microsatellite instability-high (MSI-H) are considered MMR proficient (pMMR/MMRp) and microsatellite stable.

Immunotherapy is a type of cancer treatment that recruits the immune system to fight cancer. One such therapy includes immune checkpoint inhibitors. Immune checkpoints are proteins on the surface of immune cells that interact with ligands on nonimmune cells to prevent immune cells from acting on these cells. This limits immune activity that can lead to autoimmune disease. Cancer cells have evolved to use these checkpoints to avoid recognition by the immune system, thereby avoiding destruction. Checkpoint inhibitor drugs, such as pembrolizumab and dostarlimab, work by blocking these checkpoints, specifically the interaction of programmed cell death protein 1 (PD-1) on the immune cell with PD-L1, its ligand, on the tumor cell (Fig. 22-1). This interaction effectively activates the immune cell, allowing it to recognize a cancer cell as foreign and leading to immune-mediated destruction of cancer cells.

Mismatch repair deficiency leads to an increased number of genetic mutations within cancer cells so that they are more recognizable to immune cells and more susceptible to immune destruction when exposed to immune checkpoint inhibitors. The combination of immune checkpoint inhibitors with chemotherapy may further increase recognition of the cancer cells by the immune system because the cytotoxic effects of chemotherapy lead to increased antigen presentation to immune cells, even in MMRp cancer. This has been seen in recent phase 3 studies that demonstrated significant improvements in progression-free survival when checkpoint inhibitors were added to chemotherapy in the treatment of advanced or recurrent endometrial cancer regardless of MMR status. The magnitude of improvement was greater in the dMMR cohorts. In the phase 3 NRG-GY018 trial, the addition of pembrolizumab to carboplatin and paclitaxel followed by pembrolizumab maintenance therapy resulted in a 70% lower risk of disease progression or death than chemotherapy alone in the dMMR cohort, whereas the reduction was 46% in the pMMR cohort. Similar results were seen with the use of the PD-L1 inhibitor dostarlimab in the RUBY trial.

The described patient has a distant recurrence of endometrial cancer. Because she has not yet received systemic therapy, the best initial systemic therapy for this patient is a combination of chemotherapy with carboplatin and paclitaxel and immunotherapy with a checkpoint inhibitor. Although this treatment is approved regardless of MMR status, MMR testing is useful in counseling patients regarding the expected response to checkpoint inhibition. It is the most useful tumor testing to aid in counseling this patient.

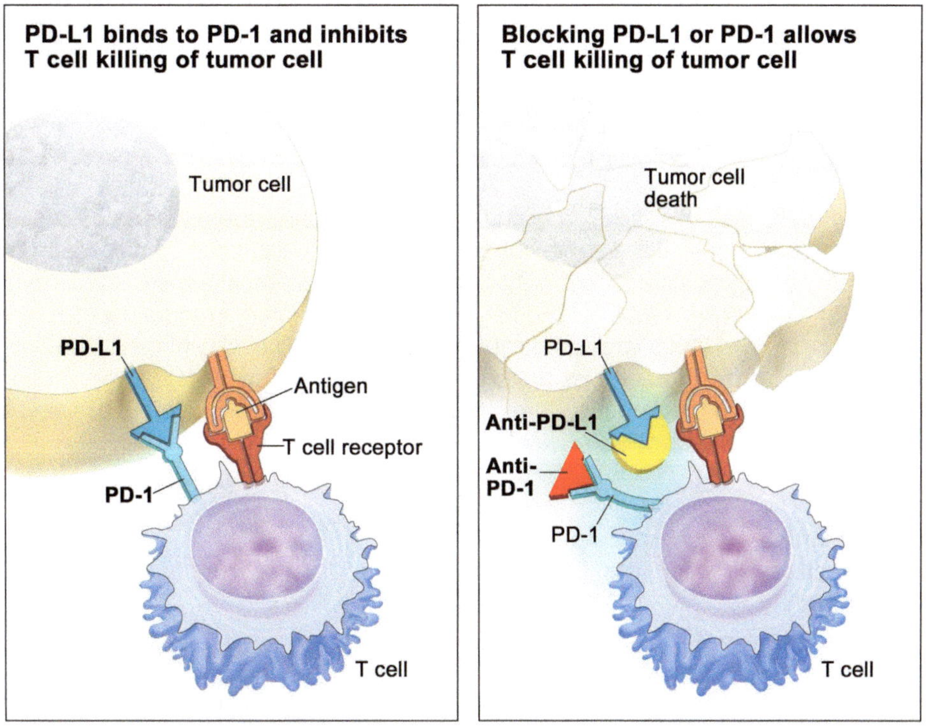

FIGURE 22-1. Checkpoint proteins. Checkpoint proteins, such as PD-L1 on tumor cells and PD-1 on T cells, help keep immune responses in check. The binding of PD-L1 to PD-1 keeps T cells from killing tumor cells in the body (left panel). Blocking the binding of PD-L1 to PD-1 with an immune checkpoint inhibitor allows the T cells to kill tumor cells (right panel). (Reprinted with permission from Terese Winslow.)

The tests for FOLR-α and HRD are options performed in ovarian cancer to inform potential treatment with mirvetuximab sorvavtansine and poly(ADP-ribose) polymerase (PARP) inhibitors, respectively. Mirvetuximab soravtansine is approved for use in recurrent platinum-resistant ovarian cancer with FOLR-α positivity. Patients with ovarian cancer that is homologous recombination deficient may be eligible for PARP inhibitors in either the upfront maintenance setting or at the time of platinum-sensitive recurrence, depending on other patient factors and prior lines of therapy. Because these two tests are not applicable to recurrent endometrial cancer, neither is the best choice in this scenario.

Testing for HER2 on tumor cells is useful in two scenarios. First, if a patient has HER2-positive serous endometrial cancer or carcinosarcoma, trastuzumab can be added to paclitaxel and carboplatin in either the upfront setting (if the patient has advanced-stage disease [II–IV]) or at the time of recurrence, depending on prior lines of therapy. A second scenario in which HER2 testing may be useful is when the U.S. Food and Drug Administration approves treatment with trastuzumab deruxtecan (an antibody–drug conjugate) of any cancer that is HER2 positive in the recurrent setting. However, the use of immunotherapy in patients with MMR deficiency is supported by data from multiple phase III trials showing improvement in overall survival. Although HER2 testing may be important for this patient in the future, chemotherapy with immune checkpoint blockade is the best option at this time, and assessment of her MMR is the best next step.

Finally, *PTEN* is a tumor suppressor gene that is frequently involved in the pathogenesis of endometrioid endometrial cancer. Although it may have been involved in the tumorigenesis of this patient's cancer, it is not useful for determining treatment options.

In patients with advanced or recurrent endometrial cancer, MMR status is important to guide discussion on the expected response to immune checkpoint inhibitors, such as pembrolizumab or dostarlimab. This testing can be performed on a histologic specimen using immunohistochemistry to detect MMR protein expression and is the best test to guide discussion with this patient about the expected response to therapy.

Eskander RN, Sill MW, Beffa L, Moore RG, Hope JM, Musa FB, et al. Pembrolizumab plus chemotherapy in advanced endometrial cancer. N Engl J Med 2023;388:2159–70. doi: 10.1056/NEJMoa2302312

Green AK, Feinberg J, Makker V. A review of immune checkpoint blockade therapy in endometrial cancer. Am Soc Clin Oncol Educ Book 2020;40:1–7. doi: 10.1200/EDBK_280503

Mirza MR, Chase DM, Slomovitz BM, dePont Christensen R, Novák Z, Black D, et al. Dostarlimab for primary advanced or recurrent endometrial cancer. N Engl J Med 2023;388:2145–58. doi: 10.1056/NEJMoa2216334

Olave MC, Graham RP. Mismatch repair deficiency: the what, how and why it is important. Genes Chromosomes Cancer 2022;61:314–21. doi: 10.1002/gcc.23015

23 Geriatric oncology

An 89-year-old patient with newly diagnosed metastatic ovarian cancer presents to the office to discuss treatment recommendations. Her BMI is 24. She has chronic obstructive pulmonary disease, arthritis, and hypertension. On examination, you note a fixed right adnexal mass with impingement on the rectum, a distended abdomen, and decreased breath sounds at the bases. Computed tomography (CT) reveals omental caking, ascites, pleural effusions, and a large adnexal mass. A CT-guided biopsy of the omentum indicates high-grade serous ovarian cancer. You discuss the standard treatment of metastatic ovarian cancer and explain that she may not be able to tolerate systemic therapy due to her age, comorbidities, and cancer burden. The best surrogate to assess her tolerance for chemotherapy is her

(A) BMI calculation
(B) Charlson Comorbidity Index score
* (C) instrumental activities of daily living (IADL) score
(D) nutritional status
(E) performance status assessment

Epithelial ovarian cancer is most often diagnosed in postmenopausal women who are in their early to mid-60s. As the population ages, more cases of ovarian cancer will occur in women aged 80 years and older. Due to comorbidities in older patients, as well as physical limitations and lack of social support, oncologists may be biased against the use of standard therapies, and full-dose chemotherapy or radical surgery may not be considered. Because of the possibility of subjective assessment and discriminating treatment modifications, objective assessment tools have been developed to better assess eligibility for standard therapy and dosing.

Geriatric assessment can include patient-reported measures as well as input from the treatment team regarding the patient's functional abilities, medical conditions, mental health, support at home or in the community, nutrition, and cognitive state. There are several ways to perform a geriatric assessment (Appendix D). Activities of daily living, such as bathing and dressing, are essential for self-care, and the inability to perform these tasks can affect a patient's independence. Instrumental ADLs are similar but include the patient's ability to function within the community.

Instrumental ADLs have been associated with a patient's ability to tolerate and receive chemotherapy for ovarian cancer. In a prospective study of approximately 150 women with ovarian cancer, baseline IADLs were independently associated with completion of four cycles of chemotherapy as well as the experience of toxicity. In this study, baseline IADLs were also associated with survival outcomes, meaning improved functional status correlated with improved outcomes in patients receiving carboplatin and paclitaxel. Instrumental ADLs have been studied in large clinical trials and have been shown to predict toxicities and outcomes such as survival, hospitalizations, and functional decline, and they are the most effective way to predict tolerance to cancer treatment in this patient.

Performance status is an assessment completed by the treatment team. Eastern Cooperative Oncology Group (ECOG) performance status is intended to quantify, with a single number, a patient's functional status; however, it has been shown to poorly correlate with a patient's comorbidities or functional assessment. Performance status is a more subjective assessment, and studies have shown that this assessment does not adequately identify the patients most at risk of intolerable toxicity due to cancer treatment. It is not the best choice for the described patient.

The American Society of Clinical Oncology issued a clinical guideline publication that outlined recommended tools for assessing geriatric patients receiving cancer therapy. One of the recommendations is to assess nutrition. Nutritional status has been associated with mortality in older patients with cancer. A BMI of less than 21 or unintentional weight loss greater than 10% from baseline indicates that nutritional assessment should be undertaken. Neither nutritional assessment nor BMI is consistently associated with tolerance of chemotherapy.

Comorbidities also have been associated with poorer outcomes and toxicity in older patients receiving chemotherapy. The recommendation is to use validated tools, such as the Charlson Comorbidity Index. Some comorbidities that could affect a patient's tolerance of the adverse effects of cancer surgery or treatment and the symptoms associated with metastatic disease include chronic obstructive pulmonary disease, arthritis, poorly controlled diabetes mellitus or hypertension, cardiovascular disease, Parkinson disease, or dementia. Comorbidities have been associated with poor outcomes, such as toxicities, reduced survival, and hospitalizations, and they are less predictive of tolerance than the IADL score.

Although multiple tools can predict outcomes and assess tolerance of chemotherapy in older patients with ovarian cancer, the measurement of IADLs is the most robust and user-friendly tool. Unlike other tools, IADLs can predict functional decline and help to better inform patients about their course with ovarian cancer treatment.

de Arruda FN, Oonk MH, Mourits MJ, de Graeff P, Jalving M, de Bock GH. Determinants of health-related quality of life in elderly ovarian cancer patients: the role of frailty and dependence. Gynecol Oncol 2019;153:610–5. doi: 10.1016/j.ygyno.2019.03.249

Mohile SG, Dale W, Somerfield MR, Schonberg MA, Boyd CM, Burhenn PS, et al. Practical assessment and management of vulnerabilities in older patients receiving chemotherapy: ASCO Guideline for Geriatric Oncology. J Clin Oncol 2018;36:2326–47. doi: 10.1200/JCO.2018.78.8687

Tinquaut F, Freyer G, Chauvin F, Gane N, Pujade-Lauraine E, Falandry C. Prognostic factors for overall survival in elderly patients with advanced ovarian cancer treated with chemotherapy: results of a pooled analysis of three GINECO phase II trials. Gynecol Oncol 2016;143:22–6. doi: 10.1016/j.ygyno.2016.03.018

von Gruenigen VE, Huang HQ, Beumer JH, Lankes HA, Tew W, Herzog T, et al. Chemotherapy completion in elderly women with ovarian, primary peritoneal or fallopian tube cancer an NRG Oncology/Gynecologic Oncology Group study. Gynecol Oncol 2017;144:459–67. doi: 10.1016/j.ygyno.2016.11.033

24 Familial cancer

A 29-year-old gravida 2, para 2, presents for her routine gynecologic examination. Her history is significant for two cesarean deliveries and a tubal ligation. Her family history is notable for epithelial ovarian cancer in her mother (now deceased) at age 54 years. The patient is using combined oral contraceptives (COCs) for cycle control. During your interview, she informs you that her 43-year-old sister received a diagnosis of breast cancer earlier this year and did not have a *BRCA* mutation. Her clinical breast examination is unremarkable. The best next step is to recommend

(A) bilateral salpingo-oophorectomy
(B) cessation of COCs
* (C) genetic testing
(D) pelvic ultrasonography
(E) screening mammography

Hereditary breast and ovarian cancer syndrome is an inherited genetic syndrome that confers an increased risk of these types of cancer in an individual. Families with hereditary breast and ovarian cancer syndrome typically have multiple members with breast cancer, ovarian cancer, or both. The syndrome accounts for 5–10% of all breast cancer and approximately 15% of ovarian cancer. *BRCA1* and *BRCA2* are the most common genetic variants, but as many as 25% are the result of another genetic variant (Table 24-1). Approximately 57% of individuals with *BRCA1* and 49% of individuals with *BRCA2* will develop breast cancer in their lifetime. Approximately 39–46% of individuals with *BRCA1* and 10–27% with *BRCA2* will develop an ovarian type of cancer, such as ovarian, fallopian tube, and primary peritoneal cancer, by age 70 years.

Identification of individuals with hereditary breast and ovarian cancer syndrome allows for additional screening and intervention to prevent or achieve early detection of cancer. This screening process may be limited if the patient does not know their family history (if adopted, for example), has few family members, or has multiple family members with hysterectomy at a young age. Patients at risk for hereditary cancer syndrome can be identified through regular assessment of personal and family history. Family history should include maternal and paternal first- and second-degree relatives, type of cancer, age of onset, and vital status. Gynecologists also should review patients' ancestry because certain ethnic groups are at increased risk of carrying a founder mutation, which is a specific genetic mutation more commonly found in populations that originated from a small ancestral group. Specifically, individuals with Ashkenazi Jewish, French Canadian, and Icelandic ancestry are at increased risk of a founder mutation. Box 24-1 lists the criteria for further genetic evaluation for hereditary breast and ovarian cancer.

This patient's family history is concerning for hereditary breast and ovarian cancer syndrome, and genetic testing is the best next step. Her mother's epithelial ovarian cancer diagnosis warrants additional genetic evaluation in this family, as does her sister's breast cancer diagnosis at age 43 years. Ideally, family members affected by cancer should be tested first because a negative test result indicates the risk of hereditary cancer syndrome is less likely, and unaffected offspring will not need testing. In the event of a positive test result in the proband (the person with a known genetic condition who is the starting point for genetic testing for a family), cascade testing of other family members for the specific gene variant is the most appropriate approach. The described patient has a sister whose testing was negative for *BRCA*, but she may be eligible for expanded panel testing and her current testing may be inadequate. Additionally, despite the sister's prior testing, the described patient is eligible for genetic testing based on her mother's history of ovarian cancer. Because the described patient's mother is deceased, it is appropriate to test the patient. A negative test result does not exclude the possibility of hereditary breast and ovarian cancer syndrome in this family.

Counseling before undergoing genetic testing is crucial to the informed consent process and upholds the ethical principle of autonomy. Genetic testing is a unique scenario in which the results of the testing may affect not only the patient but

TABLE 24-1. Genetic Mutations Associated With Hereditary Breast and Ovarian Cancer Syndrome

GENE	BREAST CANCER RISK	OVARIAN CANCER RISK*	OTHER CANCER RISK
ATM	Increased	No increased risk	Insufficient evidence
BRCA1	Increased	Increased	Prostate
BRCA2	Increased	Increased	Melanoma, pancreas, prostate
BRIP1	No increased risk	Increased	Insufficient evidence
CDH1	Increased	No increased risk	Stomach
CHEK2	Increased	No increased risk	Colon
Lynch syndrome genes: *MSH2*, *MLH1*, *MSH6*, *PMS2*, and *EPCAM*	Insufficient evidence	Increased	Colon, uterine, renal pelvis, small bowel, and others
PALB2	Increased	No increased risk	Unknown
PTEN	Increased	No increased risk	Cowden syndrome†
RAD51C	No increased risk	Increased	Unknown
RAD51D	No increased risk	Increased	Unknown
STK11	Increased risk	Increased risk of sex cord stromal tumors	Peutz–Jeghers syndrome
TP53	Increased	No increased risk	Li–Fraumeni syndrome

*Includes fallopian tube cancer and primary peritoneal cancer.

†Currently referred to as *PTEN hamartoma tumor syndrome.*

Data from National Comprehensive Cancer Network. Genetic/familial high risk assessment: breast and ovarian. Version 2.2017. NCCN Clinical Practice Guidelines in Oncology. Fort Washington (PA): NCCN; 2016. Available at https://www.nccn.org/professionals/physician_gls/pdf/genetics_screening.pdf.

Reprinted from Hereditary breast and ovarian cancer syndrome. Practice Bulletin No. 182. American College of Obstetricians and Gynecologists. Obstet Gynecol 2017;130:e110–26. doi: 10.1097/AOG.0000000000002296

BOX 24-1

Criteria for Further Genetic Evaluation for Hereditary Breast and Ovarian Cancer Syndrome

- Women affected with one or more of the following have an increased likelihood of having an inherited predisposition to breast* and ovarian, tubal, or peritoneal cancer and should receive genetic counseling and be offered genetic testing:
  - Epithelial ovarian, tubal, or peritoneal cancer
  - Breast cancer at age 45 years or less
  - Breast cancer and have a close relative† with breast cancer at age 50 years or less or close relative† with epithelial ovarian, tubal, or peritoneal cancer at any age
  - Breast cancer at age 50 years or less with a limited or unknown family history‡
  - Breast cancer and have two or more close relatives† with breast cancer at any age
  - Breast cancer and have two or more close relatives† with pancreatic cancer or aggressive prostate cancer (Gleason score equal to or greater than 7)
  - Two breast cancer primaries, with the first diagnosed before age 50 years
  - Triple-negative breast cancer at age 60 years or less
  - Breast cancer and Ashkenazi Jewish ancestry at any age
  - Pancreatic cancer and have two or more close relatives† with breast cancer; ovarian, tubal, or peritoneal cancer; pancreatic cancer; or aggressive prostate cancer (Gleason score equal to or greater than 7)
- Women unaffected with cancer, but with one or more of the following have an increased likelihood of having an inherited predisposition to breast and ovarian, tubal, or peritoneal cancer and should receive genetic counseling and be offered genetic testing:
  - A first-degree or several close relatives† that meet one or more of the aforementioned criteria
  - A close relative† carrying a known *BRCA1* or *BRCA2* mutation§
  - A close relative† with male breast cancer

*Invasive and ductal carcinoma in situ breast cancer.

†Close relative is defined as first degree (parent, sibling, offspring), second degree (grandparent, grandchild, uncle, aunt, nephew, niece, half-sibling), or third degree (first cousin, great-grandparent or great-grandchild).

‡Limited family history includes fewer than two first-degree or second-degree female relatives surviving beyond age 45 years.

§Or carrying another known actionable deleterious mutation associated with hereditary breast and ovarian cancer syndrome.

Modified with permission from Lancaster JM, Powell CB, Chen LM, Richardson DL. Society of Gynecologic Oncology statement on risk assessment for inherited gynecologic cancer predispositions. SGO Clinical Practice Committee [published erratum appears in Gynecol Oncol 2015;138:765]. Gynecol Oncol 2015;136:3–7.

Reprinted from Hereditary breast and ovarian cancer syndrome. Practice Bulletin No. 182. American College of Obstetricians and Gynecologists. Obstet Gynecol 2017;130:e110–26. doi: 10.1097/AOG.0000000000002296 also other family members. This counseling should include a discussion of the possible results of the testing and the implications of positive results for her and her family members. The discussion should include the risks, benefits, and other implications of disclosure or nondisclosure to family members. This counseling can be further reinforced upon receipt of genetic testing results but should start before undergoing testing.

Individuals now have access to direct-to-consumer genetic testing for *BRCA*, but their usefulness is limited. This testing is outside of the health care setting, and patients may interpret results themselves and choose not to seek genetic counseling. The consumer test may not evaluate the appropriate breadth of potential genetic mutations. Additionally, testing platforms may have differing technical quality. These features may lead to false-negative or false-positive results. For these reasons, direct-to-consumer testing should be avoided and should not replace formal genetic counseling and testing in the health care setting. Individuals who choose direct-to-consumer testing should confirm the results through clinical testing before acting on the results.

Bilateral salpingo-oophorectomy is not the best next step in this otherwise healthy patient due to the negative effects of surgical menopause and no confirmed increased risk for ovarian cancer. If she undergoes genetic testing and is found to have a *BRCA* mutation, risk-reducing bilateral salpingo-oophorectomy is recommended. Risk-reducing bilateral salpingo-oophorectomy is recommended for individuals with known *BRCA* mutations because this procedure reduces the risk of ovarian cancer by 80%. After risk-reducing salpingo-oophorectomy, there is a residual 3% risk of primary peritoneal carcinoma. Risk-reducing salpingo-oophorectomy is recommended by age 35–40 years for patients with *BRCA1* and age 40–45 years for patients with *BRCA2*. The ultimate timing of the procedure depends on patient factors, including fertility goals. A prospective clinical trial is currently in progress to determine if risk-reducing salpingectomy adequately reduces risk of ovarian cancer without the negative effects of surgical menopause.

Pelvic ultrasonography is not necessary in asymptomatic patients with a family history of breast and ovarian cancer. This approach, along with monitoring the CA 125 level, can be considered in high-risk patients as a short-term screening method before undergoing risk-reducing bilateral salpingo-oophorectomy; however, this screening has not been associated with a decrease in mortality or an increase in survival. It is associated with increased rates of unnecessary surgery and subsequent complications.

The patient in this scenario should not undergo screening mammography at this time. She has a higher-than-average risk of breast cancer based on her family history. Patients with an increased risk of breast cancer should initiate screening mammograms earlier than those of average risk. A breast cancer risk assessment screening tool, such as the modified Gail model or Tyrer–Cuzick risk calculator, can be used to estimate her individual risk of breast cancer. If her lifetime risk of breast cancer is 20% or more, screening mammography is recommended starting at age 30 years. If this patient undergoes genetic testing and is found to have a hereditary breast and ovarian cancer syndrome, additional screening (every 6 months, alternating mammogram and breast MRI) or risk-reducing mastectomy would be recommended. The best next step for this patient is genetic counseling. Genetic testing in this patient will provide better guidance on possible risk-reducing interventions.

Stopping COCs is not indicated in this patient. A family history of breast or ovarian cancer is not a contraindication to hormonal contraception. For patients with *BRCA* mutations, COCs are associated with a decrease in ovarian cancer (reduction after 1 year of use is 33–80% for *BRCA1* and 58–63% for *BRCA2*). Additionally, these individuals also are associated with a decreased risk of endometrial cancer, with no significant increased risk of breast cancer. In patients with a family history of breast and ovarian cancer syndrome, or in those with hereditary cancer syndrome, COCs offer risk reduction of ovarian and endometrial cancer, and their use is appropriate if desired by the patient.

Consumer testing for disease risk. ACOG Committee Opinion No. 816. American College of Obstetricians and Gynecologists. Obstet Gynecol 2021;137:e1–6. doi: 10.1097/AOG.0000000000004200

Counseling about genetic testing and communication of genetic test results. Committee Opinion No. 693. American College of Obstetricians and Gynecologists. Obstet Gynecol 2017;129:e96–101. doi: 10.1097/AOG.0000000000002020

Hereditary Breast and Ovarian Cancer Syndrome. Practice Bulletin 182. American College of Obstetricians and Gynecologists. Obstet Gynecol 2017;130(3):e110-e126. doi: 10.1097/AOG.0000000000002296

Hereditary Cancer Syndromes and Risk Assessment. Committee Opinion 793. American College of Obstetricians and Gynecologists. Obstet Gynecol 2019;134(6):e143-e149. doi:10.1097/AOG.0000000000003563

Monticciolo DL, Newell MS, Moy L, Lee CS, Destounis SV. Breast cancer screening for women at higher-than-average risk: updated recommendations from the ACR. J Am Coll Radiol 2023;20:902–14. doi: 10.1016/j.jacr.2023.04.002

Owens DK, Davidson KW, Krist AH, Barry MJ, Cabana M, Caughey AB, et al. Risk assessment, genetic counseling, and genetic testing for *BRCA*-related cancer: US Preventive Services Task Force Recommendation Statement [published erratum appears in JAMA 2019;322:1830]. JAMA 2019;322:652–65. doi: 10.1001/jama.2019.10987

25 Fertility-sparing management of cervical cancer

A 36-year-old nulligravida who is interested in fertility preservation presents for follow-up after cervical conization for cervical intraepithelial neoplasia 3 (CIN 3). The final pathology from the cone reveals invasive squamous cell carcinoma with a depth of invasion of 6 mm, no lymphovascular space invasion (LVSI), and negative margins. The endocervical curettage also is negative for invasive carcinoma and high-grade dysplasia. Magnetic resonance imaging of the pelvis is normal. The best next step for this patient is

(A) colposcopy and high-risk human papillomavirus (HPV)-based testing at 6 months
* (B) pelvic lymph node sampling
(C) radical hysterectomy
(D) radical trachelectomy
(E) simple hysterectomy

Cervical cancer is diagnosed in more than 13,000 individuals in the United States annually. New diagnoses in the United States are most frequently among women aged 35–44 years. The standard of care for individuals with early-stage disease is hysterectomy with removal of the uterus and cervix, with or without concurrent pelvic lymph node assessment, depending on stage and risk factors. Fertility-sparing treatment is an option and is most validated when the tumor is 2 cm or less in size; however, in some centers, experts will consider fertility-sparing treatment with tumors up to 4 cm. Fertility-sparing treatment is reserved for either squamous cell carcinoma or HPV-related adenocarcinoma and should be avoided in rare histologic subtypes associated with more aggressive behavior.

Negative pelvic lymph node status is a prerequisite for fertility-sparing therapy in all patients, except those with stage IA1 disease (tumor depth less than 3 mm) and no LVSI on cone biopsy, because the presence of positive lymph nodes would necessitate treatment with chemoradiotherapy. Pelvic lymph node assessment, either with sentinel lymph node biopsy or systematic pelvic lymphadenectomy, should be the first step in treating patients seeking to preserve fertility. Accordingly, lymph node assessment is the best next step in the treatment of the patient in this scenario, who has stage IB1 cancer and is interested in fertility-sparing therapy. Individuals choosing fertility-sparing treatment should be counseled that chemoradiation will be recommended in the case of pathologically positive lymph nodes and that alternative fertility options will need to be explored (eg, oocyte cryopreservation with future pregnancy via gestational carrier).

Recent updates to treatment guidelines for early-stage cervical cancer, based on findings from the Prospective Trial of Conservative Surgery for Low-risk Early-stage Cervical Cancer (ConCerv) and Simple Hysterectomy and Pelvic Node Assessment (SHAPE) trial, now provide more conservative surgical approaches for patients regardless of their fertility intentions (Appendix E). Both trials explored conservative surgery for cervical cancer compared with radical surgery. The ConCerv trial was a prospective trial that enrolled women with early-stage, low-risk cervical cancer to evaluate whether conservative surgical options, such as conization or simple hysterectomy, could be considered as alternatives to radical surgery for this patient group. All individuals in the study underwent surgical lymph node assessment. Participants in the study who desired fertility-sparing therapy treated with conization had a 2.4% 2-year recurrence rate. These findings led to significant changes in the fertility-sparing management for patients with early-stage, low-risk disease.

Fertility-sparing management options include conization, simple trachelectomy, radical vaginal trachelectomy, and radical abdominal trachelectomy. Conization alone is sufficient for patients with stage IA1 disease, no LVSI, and negative margins. Patients with stage IA2–IB1 disease meeting low-risk criteria (no LVSI, negative cone margins, squamous cell or usual type adenocarcinoma [grade 1 or 2], depth of invasion of 10 mm or less, and negative imaging) can be treated with cone biopsy and lymph node assessment. In this scenario, the patient has stage IB1 cervical squamous cell carcinoma, expresses a desire for fertility-sparing management, and meets the above criteria. Consequently, she is a suitable candidate for conservative surgery of the cervix and does not need additional uterine surgery. The best next step is to perform pelvic lymph node sampling to assess for potential lymph node metastasis.

Patients who met the criteria for the ConCerv and SHAPE trials (Appendix E), and who did not desire future fertility, underwent laparoscopic simple hysterectomy and pelvic lymph node assessment. In the ConCerv trial, rates of residual disease were 2.5% at the time of hysterectomy, and the recurrence rate was 0% over 2 years. In both trials, the oncologic outcomes were comparable between patients who underwent a simple hysterectomy and those who underwent a radical hysterectomy. Although this patient's disease meets criteria for simple hysterectomy, a simple hysterectomy would not be the best recommendation because she desires future fertility.

Radical trachelectomy, along with pelvic lymph node assessment, can be performed as fertility-sparing therapy for individuals with tumors 2 cm or less in size with LVSI or those with stage IA2–IB1 disease who do not meet the low-risk criteria discussed above. Some surgeons and centers allow radical trachelectomy for tumors as large as 4 cm in size. Radical trachelectomy remains an option for small tumors, although it confers a high risk of surgical complications, and oncologic outcomes are similar with conservative surgery options. Obstetric complications of radical trachelectomy in subsequent pregnancies include preterm labor, ascending infection resulting in preterm premature rupture of membranes, and preterm delivery. Radical trachelectomy would be overtreatment in this patient and is not the best recommendation for her.

Radical hysterectomy with pelvic lymph node assessment is the treatment of choice for individuals with International Federation of Gynecology and Obstetrics (FIGO) stage IA1 disease with LVSI and positive margins for carcinoma on cone biopsy, FIGO stage IA2–IB1 disease not meeting low-risk criteria, and for those with FIGO stage IB2 who do not desire future pregnancy. Radical hysterectomy also is an option for select tumors (sized less than 2 cm) with upper vaginal involvement. The treatment strategy for these individuals aims to avoid combining radical surgery and radiotherapy due to the high morbidity rates with combined therapy. Radical hysterectomy does not align with this patient's wishes for fertility-sparing management; therefore, it is not the best recommendation for this patient.

Repeat colposcopy and HPV-based cotesting in 6 months is a management option for individuals diagnosed with CIN 2 or 3 who are aged less than 25 years, or those aged 25 years and older who are concerned about the effects that treatment may have on future pregnancies. This patient has an occult cancer diagnosis; accordingly, repeat colposcopy and HPV-based cotesting in lieu of lymph node sampling is not an appropriate management strategy.

Conservative surgery with sparing of fertility is an option for some patients with early-stage, low-risk disease who meet specific criteria. In these cases, oncologic outcomes are similar to those of more radical procedures. Patients should be offered and counseled on these options when appropriate.

Bhatla N, Aoki D, Sharma DN, Sankaranarayanan R. Cancer of the cervix uteri [published erratum appears in Int J Gynaecol Obstet 2024;164:1229-30]. Int J Gynaecol Obstet 2018;143(suppl 2):22–36. doi: 10.1002/ijgo.12611

Cibula D, Raspollini MR, Planchamp F, Centeno C, Chargari C, Felix A, et al. ESGO/ESTRO/ESP guidelines for the management of patients with cervical cancer update 2023. Int J Gynecol Cancer 2023;33:649–66. doi: 10.1136/ijgc-2023-004429

Schmeler KM, Pareja R, Lopez Blanco A, Humberto Fregnani J, Lopes A, Perrotta M, et al. ConCerv: a prospective trial of conservative surgery for low-risk early-stage cervical cancer. Int J Gynecol Cancer 2021;31:1317–25. doi: 10.1136/ijgc-2021-002921

Smith ES, Moon AS, O'Hanlon R, Leitao MM Jr, Sonoda Y, Abu-Rustum NR, et al. Radical trachelectomy for the treatment of early-stage cervical cancer: a systematic review. Obstet Gynecol 2020;136:533–42. doi: 10.1097/AOG.0000000000003952

26 Endometrial sampling

A 33-year-old nulligravida presents to your office after hysteroscopy with dilation and curettage. Her biopsy result is shown in Figure 26-1. She desires future fertility. She has a history of polycystic ovary syndrome, a BMI of 38, and factor V Leiden heterozygous status with previous femoral vein thromboembolism. The best next step for the management of this pathology is to

(A) initiate oral contraceptive pills
* (B) insert a levonorgestrel-releasing intrauterine device (LNG-IUD)
(C) perform endometrial ablation
(D) perform a hysterectomy
(E) perform hysteroscopic resection

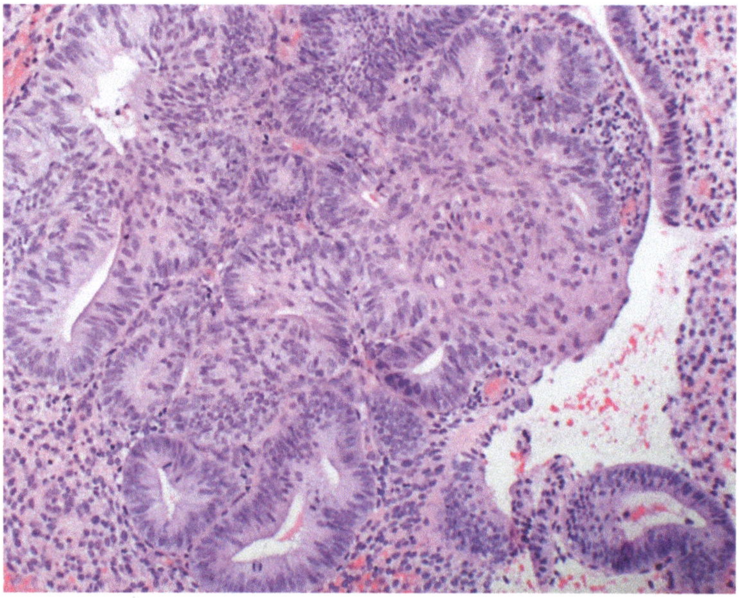

FIGURE 26-1. Glandular crowding and complexity as well as altered cytology characterized by nuclear rounding, vesicular nuclei, small nucleoli, and squamous metaplasia distinct from the surrounding endometrium.

Endometrial intraepithelial neoplasia (EIN), shown in Figure 26-1, is defined by the microscopic presence of glandular crowding and complexity with altered cytology characterized by nuclear rounding, vesicular nuclei, small nucleoli, and squamous metaplasia that is distinct from the surrounding endometrium. Endometrial intraepithelial neoplasia is distinct from endometrial cancer, because the diagnosis of endometrial cancer is reached when back-to-back gland formation measuring more than 2 mm is seen histologically. The categorization of endometrial hyperplasia was changed from the historic simple and complex hyperplasia with or without atypia to the current two-tiered system of non-atypical hyperplasia and EIN.

Endometrial intraepithelial neoplasia is a precursor lesion to endometrial cancer, with approximately 40% of patients harboring concurrent endometrial cancer. The definitive treatment for EIN is extrafascial hysterectomy; however, there are situations in which hysterectomy may not be appropriate. Those desiring fertility, such as the patient in this scenario, or those who are poor surgical candidates due to medical or surgical complexity, may be treated with systemic or local progestin therapy.

For the described patient, who desires future fertility, progestin therapy is the best treatment option. A complete pathologic response of EIN after progestin therapy is reported in 65–100% of patients, with the highest response rates associated with local therapy using IUDs, because issues of compliance are removed. The median time to pathologic response is 6–9 months.

The best next step for the patient in this scenario, who has obesity and is at risk of venous thromboembolism, is local progestin therapy with a LNG-IUD. Levonorgestrel-releasing IUDs deliver 52 micrograms of progesterone locally to the endometrium and are generally used for as long as 5 years in the treatment of EIN or cancer and as long as 8 years for contraception. Localized progestin therapy produces minimal systemic effects and is not associated with weight gain or significantly increased risk of venous thromboembolism. Although systemic progestin therapy, such as megestrol, is an appropriate treatment for patients with EIN, long-term use often causes significant weight gain, which is not advisable in a woman with polycystic ovary syndrome and obesity. Furthermore, systemic progesterone therapy is associated with a risk of venous thromboembolism, and poor adherence may occur. Combined oral contraceptives are generally not favored due to estrogenic stimulation of endometrial proliferation and a progestin dose too low to counteract the proliferation. Additionally, combined oral contraceptives are associated with an increased risk of venous thromboembolism. The LNG-IUD is approved by the U.S. Food and Drug Administration and is an effective treatment for EIN and non-atypical hyperplasia, but there are no evidence-based guidelines for management after placement.

Given that optimal surveillance is not defined, most gynecologic oncologists extrapolate from the National Comprehensive Cancer Network guidelines for fertility-sparing management of low-grade endometrial cancer. These guidelines recommend repeat sampling every 3–6 months until pathologic complete response, followed by continued sampling every 6–12 months. If complete resolution has not occurred by 12 months, hysterectomy strongly should be considered. With complete response, the timing of discontinuation of sampling should be performed on a case-by-case basis. If a patient is actively pursuing pregnancy, it should be encouraged after a complete pathologic response. Because of the risk of cancer recurrence, patients should continue endometrial protection with an LNG-IUD until actively attempting pregnancy. Pregnancy and health optimization with weight loss counseling and referral to a fertility specialist may facilitate improved pregnancy outcomes.

Endometrial ablation should be avoided in all patients with EIN or patients who are at risk for developing EIN or cancer (eg, risk factors for anovulation). Some studies have found endometrial ablation to be associated with challenges in subsequent endometrial sampling. Hormonal treatment of EIN is preferred in patients undergoing conservative management to allow for reversal of EIN and definitive evaluation of resolution as well as future endometrial sampling. Despite some newer ablation techniques reporting lower rates of uterine scarring, these procedures do not adequately treat EIN, which requires progesterone therapy for reversal. The underlying risk of concurrent endometrial cancer in EIN is up to 40%, making tissue ablation of further concern. Finally, pregnancy and fertility are not recommended after ablation due to challenges with implantation and the risk of abnormal placentation.

Hysteroscopic resection, although helpful for more comprehensive evaluation of endometrial pathology, also is not considered a definitive treatment for EIN. A local or systemic LNG-IUD is the best next step for definitive management.

Johns DA, Garza-Leal JG, Diamond MP, Harris M. Post-ablation cavity evaluation: a prospective multicenter observational clinical study to evaluate hysteroscopic access to the uterine cavity 4 years after water vapor endometrial ablation for the treatment of heavy menstrual bleeding. J Minim Invasive Gynecol 2020;27:1273–80. doi: 10.1016/j.jmig.2019.09.775

Management of endometrial intraepithelial neoplasia or atypical endometrial hyperplasia. Clinical Consensus No. 5. American College of Obstetricians and Gynecologists. Obstet Gynecol 2023;142:735–44. doi: 10.1097/AOG.0000000000005297

National Comprehensive Cancer Network. Uterine neoplasms. Version 2.2025. NCCN Clinical Practice Guidelines in Oncology [after login]. NCCN; 2024. Accessed February 26, 2025. https://www.nccn.org/guidelines/guidelines-detail?category=1&id=1473

Ring KL, Mills AM, Modesitt SC. Endometrial hyperplasia. Obstet Gynecol 2022;140:1061–75. doi: 10.1097/AOG.0000000000004989

27 Endometrial cancer evaluation

A 61-year-old receives a diagnosis of grade 2 endometrioid endometrial adenocarcinoma after hysteroscopic biopsy for postmenopausal bleeding. Mismatch repair testing is performed with immunohistochemistry on her tumor specimen with the following results: MSH6 intact, MSH2 intact, PMS2 absent, and MLH1 absent. The best next step in evaluation is to test for

(A) germline mutation
(B) homologous recombination deficiency
(C) microsatellite instability
* (D) promoter methylation

Hereditary causes of endometrial cancer are uncommon and occur in only 3–5% of patients. Lynch syndrome (LS) is the most common heritable cause. It is inherited in an autosomal-dominant fashion and involves deficiencies in mismatch repair genes (*MLH1*, *MSH2*, *MSH6*, *PMS2*, and *EpCAM*). Patients with LS have an increased risk of early-onset endometrial (16–61%) and colon (18–61%) cancer, as well as ovarian cancer (5–10%), but risk varies according to the affected gene. There are several accepted approaches to determining if an endometrial cancer is attributable to LS, including performing mismatch repair or microsatellite instability testing on all patients with endometrial cancer or those with risk factors for hereditary cancer syndromes.

Mismatch repair testing can be performed with immunohistochemistry to detect expression of the four mismatch repair genes. If the genes are functional and all proteins are intact or present, the likelihood of LS is low. If there is a deficiency in MSH2, MSH6, or PMS2 proteins, then the risk of LS increases, and germline testing should be performed.

As in the patient described, when MLH1 is absent (with or without the PMS2 protein, which can exist as a heterodimer), the best next step is to proceed with MLH1 promoter methylation testing (Appendix F). Approximately 20–30% of endometrial cancer will have MLH1 promoter methylation, which is usually a sporadic variant. If testing for promoter methylation is negative, germline testing for LS is indicated; however, if the patient has a significant family history of other LS-related cancer, germline testing is appropriate, regardless of MLH1 promoter methylation status. As such, germline testing is not the most appropriate next step for the patient in the scenario. Endometrial cancer is the most common gynecologic malignancy in the United States, and it is not cost-effective to perform germline testing on all patients when only a small percentage of cases of cancer are hereditary in nature.

Tumor testing for homologous recombination deficiency is performed frequently in ovarian cancer to guide treatment with poly(ADP-ribose) polymerase (PARP) inhibitors, if present. Homologous recombination is an effective mechanism, using the sister chromosome as a template, to perform DNA repair on double-stranded breaks. Deficiency can cause an accumulation of errors in replication, resulting in cell death or use of error-prone repair mechanisms. It is not the next step after mismatch repair protein deficiency if endometrial cancer is identified.

Microsatellite instability is performed on normal and tumor tissue from the same patient to evaluate for changes but would be done instead of immunohistochemical staining for mismatch repair proteins. Microsatellite instability is a factor in this scenario because of the absence of MLH1 and PMS2 proteins. In this patient, deficiencies in mismatch repair proteins have been established, and microsatellite instability is evident. No additional microsatellite instability testing is required.

Lynch syndrome. Practice Bulletin No. 147. American College of Obstetricians and Gynecologists [published erratum appears in Obstet Gynecol 2022;139:696]. Obstet Gynecol 2014;124:1042–54. doi: 10.1097/01.AOG.0000456325.50739.72

National Comprehensive Cancer Network. Uterine neoplasms. Version 2.2025. NCCN Clinical Practice Guidelines in Oncology [after login]. NCCN; 2024. Accessed February 26, 2025. https://www.nccn.org/guidelines/guidelines-detail?category=1&id=1473

Stelloo E, Jansen AM, Osse EM, Nout RA, Creutzberg CL, Ruano D, et al. Practical guidance for mismatch repair-deficiency testing in endometrial cancer. Ann Oncol 2017;28:96–102. doi: 10.1093/annonc/mdw542

28 Treatment of cervical cancer

A 59-year-old woman recently received a diagnosis of cervical cancer. Her pelvic examination reveals a 2-cm cervical lesion. Positron emission tomography/computed tomography (PET/CT) demonstrated a single 3-cm fluorodeoxyglucose-avid right pelvic lymph node. Image-guided biopsy of this node indicates squamous cell carcinoma. The best treatment for her cancer is

(A) pelvic radiotherapy
(B) pelvic radiotherapy with adjuvant chemotherapy
* (C) pelvic radiotherapy with concurrent chemotherapy
(D) radical hysterectomy
(E) radical hysterectomy with pelvic lymphadenectomy

Advanced cervical cancer encompasses a diverse array of clinical presentations. Although the described patient's primary lesion measures only 2 cm, she has a 3-cm metastasis to her right pelvic lymph node. She has International Federation of Gynecology and Obstetrics (FIGO) stage IIIC1 cervical cancer (Appendix G). Although lymph node involvement was not included in earlier FIGO staging criteria, it has always been a major factor in treatment planning. In patients with proven lymphatic involvement, such as the one described in this scenario, the existence of additional microscopic lymphatic involvement within both upstream lymphatic channels and adjacent nodes must be included in treatment planning.

Although it is technically feasible, radical hysterectomy is not appropriate for this patient, irrespective of plans to surgically remove the involved pelvic lymph node or provide subsequent adjuvant radiation after surgery. If radical hysterectomy and pelvic lymphadenectomy were undertaken alone, she would be at high risk of recurrent cancer. Although adding adjuvant external beam radiotherapy after radical hysterectomy is a strategy that can reduce the risk of pelvic recurrence in patients who meet certain criteria, survival outcomes remain poorer with this combined modality strategy in patients with stage III cervical cancer. The incidence of severe toxicity events is significantly higher when combining radical surgery and radiation therapy compared with a strategy of primary chemoradiotherapy alone.

Pelvic radiotherapy with concurrent chemotherapy is the standard of care for the treatment of patients with stage IB3 and higher cervical cancer, and this is the best next step for this patient. Treatment includes external beam radiotherapy with concurrent chemotherapy sensitization and brachytherapy. The external beam radiotherapy targets the cervix and all its draining lymphatics. In this scenario, the larger right pelvic lymph node also may be dosed with additional radiation to sterilize this larger lesion. After completion of external beam radiotherapy, the subsequent application of intracavitary brachytherapy provides additional radiation to the cervix tumor, adjacent parametria, and upper vagina to effectively reach curative doses of radiation while avoiding radiation toxicity.

The standard of care is the addition of weekly cisplatin-based chemotherapy concurrent with external beam radiotherapy. The purpose of additional chemotherapy during external beam radiotherapy is to sensitize the cancer cells to the lethal effects of radiation, thereby improving the overall efficacy of the radiation. This works by several mechanisms, including further potentiating radiation-induced DNA damage, inhibition of DNA repair, synchronization of cells in the radiosensitive G_2/M phase of the cell cycle, and inducing apoptosis. Several trials, as well as a meta-analysis of individual patient data from 13 randomized trials, demonstrate a significant survival benefit of concurrent cisplatin-containing chemoradiation over pelvic radiation alone. Further, the Keynote-18 study demonstrated that the addition of the immunotherapy pembrolizumab to chemoradiotherapy significantly improved progression-free survival in patients with newly diagnosed advanced cervical cancer. Based on recent U.S. Food and Drug Administration approval, National Comprehensive Cancer Network guidelines were updated and now allow the addition of pembrolizumab to chemoradiation in patients with a primary tumor extending to the pelvic sidewall or bladder, or both, or rectal mucosa.

With advances in radiation delivery techniques and the addition of concurrent sensitizing chemotherapy, improvements in pelvic tumor control have positively affected overall survival. As such, recurrences that manifest outside of the prior radiation treatment field now account for a large proportion of deaths due to cervical cancer. Clinical trials have evaluated the efficacy of adding adjuvant systemic chemotherapy after the completion of chemoradiation with the goal of eliminating micrometastases that may exist outside the radiation field; however, findings from the Outback trial, which is the largest phase III, randomized controlled trial to investigate the addition of adjuvant chemotherapy after standard chemoradiation, did not demonstrate a difference in survival rates between those who received additional chemotherapy and those who did not. The trial did demonstrate a significant increase in severe treatment-associated toxicity with the adjuvant chemotherapy after pelvic radiotherapy; therefore, systemic chemotherapy after the completion of chemoradiation is not recommended unless persistent disease or new cancer is identified on completion of initial therapies.

Chemoradiation is the preferred strategy for patients with stage IB3 or higher cervical cancer. Cisplatin is the standard sensitizing chemotherapeutic agent. For patients with stage III to IVA cervical cancer, pembrolizumab also may be added to chemotherapy. In patients with contraindications to cisplatin chemotherapy, such as renal insufficiency, other chemotherapeutic agents, such as paclitaxel, may be substituted.

Chino J, Annunziata CM, Beriwal S, Bradfield L, Erickson BA, Fields EC, et al. The ASTRO clinical practice guidelines in cervical cancer: optimizing radiation therapy for improved outcomes. Gynecol Oncol 2020;159:607–10. doi: 10.1016/j.ygyno.2020.09.015

Franco I, Viswanathan AN. Radiation oncology management of stage III and IVA cervical carcinoma. Int J Gynecol Cancer 2022;32:231–8. doi: 10.1136/ijgc-2021-002491

Guo Q, Wang R, Jin D, Yin Z, Hu B, Li R, et al. Comparison of adjuvant chemoradiotherapy versus radiotherapy in early-stage cervical cancer patients with intermediate-risk factors: a systematic review and meta-analysis. Taiwan J Obstet Gynecol 2022;61:15–23. doi: 10.1016/j.tjog.2021.11.006

Leath CA III, Monk BJ. Twenty-first century cervical cancer management: a historical perspective of the gynecologic oncology group/NRG oncology over the past twenty years. Gynecol Oncol 2018;150:391–7. doi: 10.1016/j.ygyno.2018.06.023

Lorusso D, Xiang Y, Hasegawa K, Scambia G, Leiva M, Ramos-Elias P, et al. Pembrolizumab or placebo with chemoradiotherapy followed by pembrolizumab or placebo for newly diagnosed, high-risk, locally advanced cervical cancer (ENGOT-cx11/GOG-3047/KEYNOTE-A18): a randomised, double-blind, phase 3 clinical trial. Lancet 2024;403:1341–50. doi: 10.1016/S0140-6736(24)00317-9

Reducing uncertainties about the effects of chemoradiotherapy for cervical cancer: individual patient data meta-analysis. Chemoradiotherapy for Cervical Cancer Meta-analysis Collaboration (CCCMAC). Cochrane Database of Systematic Reviews 2010, Issue 1. Art. No.: CD008285. doi: 10.1002/14651858.CD008285

29 Adnexal mass in a pregnant patient

A 37-year-old at 11 2/7 weeks of gestation with an intrauterine spontaneous singleton pregnancy is incidentally found to have a 6-cm unilocular adnexal mass on her first-trimester ultrasound (Fig. 29-1). She is asymptomatic, and her physical examination is normal. Her family history is unremarkable. She has had no previous surgery. The best next step in management is

(A) CA 125 testing
(B) human epididymis protein 4 (HE4)
(C) pelvic MRI
* (D) repeat ultrasonography in 4–6 weeks
(E) surgical resection

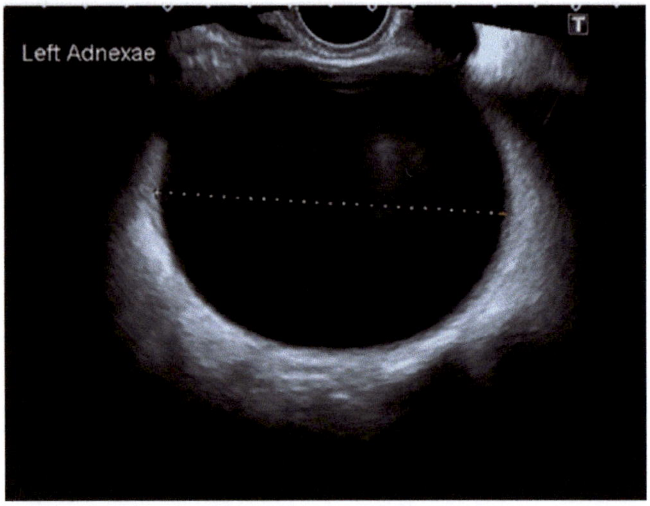

FIGURE 29-1. Ultrasonography showing an adnexal mass. (Reprinted from Puri S. Sonographic assessment of ovarian cysts and masses. In: Jayaprakasan K, Polanski L, Ojha K, editors. Gynaecological ultrasound scanning: tips and tricks. Cambridge University Press; 2020. p. 100–20. Accessed March 17, 2025.)

Adnexal masses are identified in an estimated 0.2–2% of pregnant patients. The incidence of malignant masses in pregnancy is unclear because reported estimates vary widely from less than 1% to 6%. This range reflects differences in study populations, method of identification, and variability in data collection. As with patients who are not pregnant, determining appropriate management and the risks of surgical intervention must be weighed against the potential risk of delayed diagnosis of a malignancy or ovarian torsion.

Ultrasonography is the primary imaging modality for assessing adnexal masses, whether benign or malignant. Pregnant patients display the same characteristics as those who are not pregnant, such as tumor size, solid areas, and vascularity, which are most strongly associated with malignancy. With respect to ovarian cancer types, germ cell tumors account for nearly one-half of the primary ovarian cancer diagnoses during pregnancy, most often related to patient age. Two benign adnexal lesions are specific to pregnancy: 1) luteomas, which can be associated with maternal virilization in 25% of cases, and 2) hyperreactio luteinalis (previously referred to as *theca-lutein cysts*). Both typically present as bilateral solid-appearing masses or ovarian enlargement in the third trimester and spontaneously regress after pregnancy.

In this scenario, the patient is asymptomatic, but ultrasonography shows a 6-cm unilocular or simple cyst. It is well-established that unilocular cysts are associated with a near-zero risk of malignancy in premenopausal and postmenopausal patients. Given the patient's lack of symptoms and the size and benign appearance of the mass, repeat ultrasonography is the best next step. Although the best schedule of repeat imaging has not been established, repeat ultrasound in 4–6 weeks to assess the cyst's stability is reasonable.

Approximately 70% of adnexal masses identified during pregnancy resolve spontaneously, and surgical intervention is rarely required. Surgery is indicated for patients who have symptoms of torsion or whose masses are highly suspicious for malignancy based on ultrasound assessment. Because torsion has been reported to occur most commonly with cysts measuring approximately 10 cm, prophylactic surgery to avoid torsion may be considered for patients with masses this size; however, prospective studies establishing benefit are lacking.

Traditionally, when surgery is indicated, intervention is scheduled between 16 and 20 weeks of gestation when possible, but studies have not shown a significant difference in the rate of adverse outcomes, such as preterm labor or delivery with second-trimester timing, compared with surgery in the first or third trimester. If suspicion for malignancy or torsion is high, surgical intervention should not be delayed. Laparoscopy removal has proven safe in any trimester and is the best surgical approach. In this scenario, given the benign appearance of the cyst, the relatively small size of the mass, and the fact that the patient is asymptomatic, surgical intervention is not indicated and is not the best next step.

Although tumor marker testing can be useful in determining the likelihood of malignancy among patients with adnexal masses, particularly postmenopausal patients, the utility of tumor marker assessment in pregnant individuals is limited. CA 125 levels are generally increased in the first and second trimesters, with levels as high as 2,500 U/mL, and the test is less useful in determining cancer risk in pregnant patients. For this reason, evaluation of CA 125 during pregnancy should be reserved for patients when the suspicion for malignancy is high or there is evidence of metastatic disease. Similarly, although α-fetoprotein, human chorionic gonadotropin, and lactate dehydrogenase proteins are potential markers of germ cell malignancies, levels of these proteins are normally increased in pregnancy. Only extremely high levels or levels clearly discordant with expected levels based on gestational age would be indicative of a potential malignant germ cell tumor and should only be assessed in patients with a highly suspicious ovarian mass.

Human epididymis protein 4, like CA 125, is a surface glycoprotein that can be increased in some cases of ovarian cancer and is approved for use in monitoring for relapse in patients with invasive ovarian cancer. Limited studies suggest that HE4 levels during pregnancy vary widely across individuals, generally increase during pregnancy, and are high in patients with gestational hypertension, gestational diabetes mellitus, preeclampsia, and other pregnancy-related diseases. For these reasons, HE4, like CA 125, is less useful during pregnancy and should only be evaluated when suspicion for cancer is high based on other findings. In the case described, evaluation of CA 125 and HE4 tumor marker levels is not warranted, given the low level of suspicion for cancer based on ultrasound results.

Pelvic MRI is an option that should be reserved for evaluating adnexal masses with highly suspicious characteristics on ultrasonography, or when a nongynecological pelvic process involving structures other than the ovaries is suspected. There is no evidence that MRI without gadolinium causes negative effects in pregnancy. Pelvic MRI is not indicated for this patient, given the simple appearance of her cyst.

Azim SA, Mutz-Dehbalaie I, Wieser V, Berger A, Böttcher B, Fiegl H, et al. Influence of pregnancy-related conditions on human epididymis protein 4 serum levels in comparison to CA 125 a prospective cohort trial. Geburtshilfe Frauenheilkd 2021;81:1047–54. doi: 10.1055/a-1475-4296

Cathcart AM, Nezhat FR, Emerson J, Pejovic T, Nezhat CH, Nezhat CR. Adnexal masses during pregnancy: diagnosis, treatment, and prognosis. Am J Obstet Gynecol 2023;228:601–12. doi: 10.1016/j.ajog.2022.11.1291

Levine D, Patel MD, Suh-Burgmann EJ, Andreotti RF, Benacerraf BR, Benson CB, et al. Simple adnexal cysts: SRU consensus conference update on follow-up and reporting. Radiology 2019;293:359–71. doi: 10.1148/radiol.2019191354

Strachowski LM, Jha P, Phillips CH, Blanchette Porter MM, Froyman W, Glanc P, et al. O-RADS US v2022: an update from the American College of Radiology's Ovarian-Adnexal Reporting and Data System US Committee. Radiology 2023;308:e230685. doi: 10.1148/radiol.230685

30 Treatment planning in cervical cancer

A 42-year-old patient has been experiencing vaginal bleeding for the last 8 months. On examination, her cervix is firm and nodular and measures 7 × 7 cm and extends to the vagina. There is no obvious parametrial involvement on rectovaginal examination. A biopsy of her cervical mass demonstrates invasive squamous cell carcinoma. To determine a treatment plan, the preferred imaging modality is

(A) combined transvaginal and transrectal ultrasonography
(B) intravenous pyelogram
(C) MRI
* (D) positron emission tomography/computed tomography (PET/CT)

Treatment for cervical cancer may range from primary surgical resection to definitive chemoradiation to palliative therapy, depending on factors such as tumor size, local extent, and presence or absence of metastatic disease. Accurately assessing International Federation of Gynecology and Obstetrics (FIGO) stage is essential to determine the best treatment strategy for patients with cervical cancer.

In the current era, staging assessments are done by a detailed physical examination and selected imaging studies. Historically, FIGO staging was based upon clinical examination and supplemented by a narrow range of diagnostic modalities that would be available in low-resource countries, such as cystoscopy, proctoscopy, intravenous pyelogram, and transvaginal and transrectal ultrasonography. Although they provide additional insights into local invasion of the tumor, all these studies are limited in their anatomic focus and are not capable of characterizing the full extent of the disease. The 2018 FIGO staging system was revised to incorporate findings from additional imaging studies, such as CT, MRI, PET, PET/CT, and MRI/PET. These imaging modalities offer more comprehensive characterization of the anatomic disease extent and are the preferred diagnostic modalities for cervical cancer staging. These modalities all differ in their test characteristics and their diagnostic performance, and they have varied roles in the staging of cervical cancer as well as in its subsequent treatment planning, disease response assessment, and post-treatment follow-up.

Positron emission tomography/computed tomography provides higher diagnostic accuracy for assessing retroperitoneal lymph nodes and for detecting metastatic disease compared with stand-alone CT or MRI, and this is the best next step for treatment planning. Due to its greater sensitivity in identifying both regional and distant metastatic disease, whole-body PET/CT is the preferred imaging modality for the initial assessment of patients with stage IB3 and higher cervical cancer. Positron emission tomography/computed tomography combines two imaging techniques to provide simultaneous visualization of both structural and metabolic tumor characteristics. A common radiotracer is F 18 fluorodeoxyglucose, a glucose analogue that localizes to malignant tissue due to its higher metabolic rate and glucose utilization. Positron emission tomography/computed tomography integrates PET and CT components into a single instrument, allowing the simultaneous acquisition of PET and CT data during a single imaging session.

Although stand-alone CT can provide comprehensive anatomic information, it has a lower sensitivity than PET in detecting regional and distant metastatic disease and is not the best next imaging study in this situation. The spatial resolution of contrast-enhanced CT typically is better than that of PET/CT imaging, due to the use of intravenous contrast as well as differences in imaging principles and scanner technologies. Stand-alone contrast-enhanced CT may be useful in certain clinical settings or if PET/CT is not available.

Magnetic resonance imaging typically is not the initial diagnostic modality of choice for staging cervical cancer, particularly in patients whose risk for metastatic disease is increased. The patient in this scenario has a very large cervical mass that extends to her vagina, and her risk of metastatic disease is increased. Identifying the presence of metastatic disease is relevant to her overall staging and subsequent treatment planning. Magnetic resonance imaging is less sensitive for the detection of metastatic disease than PET imaging. Due to the significantly increased length of time necessary for image acquisition, PET typically is applied to more limited anatomic focus. Magnetic resonance imaging is invaluable for subsequent pelvic radiation treatment planning because it provides the most accurate soft tissue and spatial resolution of any imaging modality. Radiation dose and treatment volume are critically informed by the extent of the anatomic disease. Magnetic resonance imaging provides accurate tumor size measurement, assessment of cervical stromal invasion, and identification of local tumor infiltration of pelvic tissues. More accurate assessment of local disease volume facilitates both improved tumor dosing and simultaneous organ sparing. In patients with locally advanced cervical cancer, both PET/CT and MRI often are used.

Serial MRI imaging is increasingly being used for image-guided adaptive brachytherapy, a strategy in which contouring treatment volumes are modified dynamically over time based on follow-up MRI findings while the primary tumor volume recedes with treatment. These techniques improve the therapeutic margin of benefit of radiation and allow for improved cancer outcomes while simultaneously reducing normal organ toxicity. The techniques used when acquiring MRI images are essential to achieving its diagnostic accuracy. The administration of gadolinium-containing contrast agent enhances discrimination between tumor tissue and healthy cervical stroma. Intravenous administration of an antiperistaltic agent reduces interfering bowel activity, and to further improve diagnostic accuracy in assessing organ infiltration, the vagina and rectum can also be filled with contrast gel before the examination.

In summary, the accurate assessment of FIGO stage in cervical cancer is essential for determining the most effective treatment strategy. Positron emission tomography/computed tomography offers the most sensitive and comprehensive initial staging assessment, whereas MRI is invaluable for subsequent treatment planning and response assessment for locally advanced cancer managed by chemoradiation. Ongoing technical advances hold the promise of enhancing current imaging diagnostic capabilities to further optimize treatment planning and outcomes. Potential future directions include the development of molecular imaging probes that better target cancer cells and the integration of artificial intelligence and machine learning to enhance image interpretation.

Bhatla N, Berek JS, Cuello Fredes M, Denny LA, Grenman S, Karunaratne K, et al. Revised FIGO staging for carcinoma of the cervix uteri [published erratum appears in Int J Gynaecol Obstet 2019;147:279-80]. Int J Gynaecol Obstet 2019;145:129–35. doi: 10.1002/ijgo.12749

National Comprehensive Cancer Network. Cervical cancer. Version 3.2025. NCCN Clinical Practice Guidelines in Oncology [after login]. NCCN; 2025. Accessed February 26, 2025. https://www.nccn.org/guidelines/guidelines-detail?category=1&id=1426

Olthof EP, Bergink-Voorthuis BJ, Wenzel HH, Mongula J, van der Velden J, Spijkerboer AM, et al. Diagnostic accuracy of MRI, CT, and [(18)F]FDG-PET-CT in detecting lymph node metastases in clinically early-stage cervical cancer a nationwide Dutch cohort study. Insights Imaging 2024;15:36–1. doi: 10.1186/s13244-023-01589-1

Shakur A, Lee JY, Freeman S. An update on the role of MRI in treatment stratification of patients with cervical cancer. Cancers (Basel) 2023;15:5105. doi: 10.3390/cancers15205105

31 Antibody–drug conjugates

A 32-year-old with stage IVB cervical cancer has completed six cycles of chemotherapy with cisplatin, paclitaxel, bevacizumab, and pembrolizumab, and her fifth cycle of maintenance bevacizumab and pembrolizumab is planned. Today, she presents with new-onset pelvic pain and shortness of breath. Positron emission tomography with computed tomography (PET/CT) shows a progression of the disease. After explaining these results, you recommend discontinuing her current treatment and initiating the antibody–drug conjugate tisotumab vedotin. You discuss the potential adverse events and toxicities of tisotumab vedotin use and recommend pre-infusion management to prevent

(A) alopecia
* (B) blurred vision
(C) fatigue
(D) hypertension
(E) neuropathy

Until the last decade, the treatment of metastatic or recurrent cervical cancer had been limited by low disease response rates and minimal improvements in progression-free and overall survival. The addition of bevacizumab to paclitaxel-based doublet therapy improved overall survival time from 13 to 17 months. A subsequent phase III randomized controlled trial of paclitaxel, cisplatin, and physician's choice bevacizumab with or without the immune checkpoint inhibitor pembrolizumab showed that the addition of pembrolizumab significantly improved overall survival to 2 years. Despite initial responses to therapy, advanced and metastatic cervical cancer often recurs or progresses after triplet or quadruplet therapy, and novel therapies are needed.

Antibody–drug conjugates are a class of therapeutics that target antibodies that are more highly expressed on cancer cells. One of the antibody–drug conjugates enters the cell, and the therapeutic agent, called the *payload*, is cleaved from the antibody, thereby destroying the cancer cell. Neighboring cells also are affected due to a bystander effect. The antibody–drug conjugate tisotumab vedotin has recently gained U.S. Food and Drug Administration approval as a second-line treatment for recurrent cervical cancer. This antibody targets the tissue factor receptor that is highly expressed in cervical cancer and excludes the need to assess for a tissue factor biomarker prior to therapy. The payload is monomethyl auristatin E. Response rates are approximately 20% in patients who have had disease progression after multiagent therapy. Clinical trials have demonstrated a statistically significant improvement in progression-free and overall survival compared with chemotherapy with topotecan, vinorelbine, gemcitabine, irinotecan, or pemetrexed, in recurrent cervical cancer.

Despite the targeted nature of antibody–drug conjugates and the positive effects it has on recurrent cervical cancer, adverse events are common. Tisotumab vedotin has unique toxicities, such as ocular toxicity, that can be particularly challenging (Table 31-1). The most common ocular toxicities include dry eye, conjunctivitis, keratopathy, and blepharitis. Because of these toxicities, patients are required to see an eye care specialist before starting treatment and again before each cycle for the first nine treatments. In addition, there are specific instructions for eye care, such as corticosteroid, vasoconstrictor, and lubricating eye drops administered before, during, and after infusion, as well as application of cold packs to the eyes during infusion. With these strategies, treatment discontinuation due to ocular toxicities is low, and this is the most important adverse event to discuss with the described patient. Because of the need for consultation with an eye specialist and application of eye drops before infusion, pre-infusion management to prevent blurred vision is the correct choice.

TABLE 31-1. Adverse Events With Tisotumab Vedotin

TREATMENT SIDE EFFECT	ALL GRADES, G1–4	GRADE 3 OR GRADE 4 ONLY
Peripheral neuropathy	38%	6%
Ocular toxicities	21–37%	0–1.7%
Epistaxis	26%	0%
Hemorrhage	21%	2%
Gastrointestinal toxicity	18–33%	0–1.6%
Fatigue	28%	6%

In addition to ocular toxicity, this therapy can be associated with peripheral neuropathy and hemorrhage (mostly in the form of nose bleeds). In fact, peripheral neuropathy is common and requires dose reductions for appropriate management. Risk of neuropathy is compounded by the risk of residual neuropathy from previous treatment with paclitaxel and cisplatin. Although counseling regarding this toxicity is important, there are no pre-infusion management recommendations to reduce this risk, and this is not the best choice for the described patient.

Tisotumab vedotin often is associated with fatigue, but no recommended pre-infusion strategies limit this adverse event. Tisotumab vedotin rarely causes alopecia. Although hypertension is a common toxicity seen with bevacizumab, it is not associated with tisotumab vedotin treatment. Tisotumab vedotin provides an effective therapy option for patients whose cervical cancer has progressed during or after multi-agent platinum-based therapy; however, with new therapeutic approaches, awareness and mitigation of unique toxicities are imperative and may require collaboration with other medical specialists.

Coleman RL, Lorusso D, Gennigens C, González-Martín A, Randall L, Cibula D, et al. Efficacy and safety of tisotumab vedotin in previously treated recurrent or metastatic cervical cancer (innovaTV 204/GOG-3023/ENGOT-cx6): a multicentre, open-label, single-arm, phase 2 study. InnovaTV 204/GOG-3023/ENGOT-cx6 Collaborators. Lancet Oncol 2021;22:609–19. doi: 10.1016/S1470-2045(21)00056-5

Crafton SM, Venkat PS, Salani R. A review of the state of cervical cancer: updates from prevention to recurrent disease. Curr Opin Obstet Gynecol 2024;36:28–33. doi: 10.1097/GCO.0000000000000918

Marshall RF, Xu H, Berkenstock M. Ocular toxicities associated with antibody drug conjugates. Curr Opin Ophthalmol 2024;35:494–8. doi: 10.1097/ICU.0000000000001063

Vergote I, González-Martín A, Fujiwara K, Kalbacher E, Bagaméri A, Ghamande S, et al. Tisotumab vedotin as second- or third-line therapy for recurrent cervical cancer. InnovaTV 301/ENGOT-cx12/GOG-3057 Collaborators. N Engl J Med 2024;391:44–55. doi: 10.1056/NEJMoa2313811

32 Initial management of high-risk gestational trophoblastic neoplasia

A 36-year-old gravida 2, para 2, presents with amenorrhea for 2 months followed by irregular vaginal bleeding for the last month. Her most recent pregnancy was a full-term vaginal delivery 2 years ago. Her physical examination is notable for an enlarged 12-week-sized uterus. Her β-human chorionic gonadotropin (β-hCG) concentration is 84,500 mIU/mL, and pelvic ultrasonography shows a 3-cm echogenic mass within the uterine cavity. She undergoes dilation and curettage, and pathology reveals an invasive molar pregnancy. Chest computed tomography (CT) is notable for three lung nodules, and a brain MRI is negative. The best next step is

(A) immunotherapy
(B) single-agent chemotherapy
(C) radiotherapy
* (D) multi-agent chemotherapy
(E) surgical resection

Gestational trophoblastic neoplasia (GTN) is a rare tumor type defined by malignant proliferation of placental trophoblastic cells. Gestational trophoblastic neoplasia comprises invasive molar pregnancy, choriocarcinoma, placental site trophoblastic tumor, and epithelioid trophoblastic tumor. These tumor types are exquisitely chemosensitive, and survival rates are nearly 100% for low-risk disease and 90% for high-risk disease.

Before beginning treatment, it is imperative to determine the International Federation of Gynecology and Obstetrics (FIGO) stage (Appendix H) and calculate the World Health Organization (WHO) prognostic score (Appendix I). *Low-risk disease* is defined as FIGO stages I–II with a WHO prognostic score of less than 7, whereas *high-risk disease* is defined as FIGO stages II–III with a WHO prognostic score of 7 or higher and all FIGO stage IV. The patient in this clinical scenario has FIGO stage III disease (lung metastasis) with a WHO score of 9, indicating high-risk disease. High-risk disease is more likely to develop chemoresistance, and only 36% of patients with high-risk GTN achieve complete response after single-agent chemotherapy.

High-risk disease requires treatment with multi-agent chemotherapy. Although several regimens have been shown to be effective, EMA/CO (etoposide, methotrexate, actinomycin-D, cyclophosphamide, and vincristine) or EMA/EP (etoposide, methotrexate, actinomycin-D, etoposide, and platinum agent [cisplatin]) are the preferred first-line regimens. Both EMA/CO and EMA/EP are associated with significantly higher rates of complete response and significantly lower mortality rates when compared with other multi-agent chemotherapy regimens, and this is the best next step for the patient in this scenario.

Single-agent chemotherapy regimens, such as actinomycin-D (also known as *dactinomycin*) and methotrexate, are very effective for treating low-risk GTN. Response rates for methotrexate and dactinomycin range from 60% to 90%, and all treatment failures can be effectively treated with the single agent that was not initially used. Methotrexate, with its more favorable side effect profile, often is the first-line chemotherapy of choice. Single-agent therapy should not be administered in individuals with high-risk disease, such as the patient in this scenario, due to the risk of developing chemoresistance and treatment failure; therefore, neither dactinomycin nor methotrexate is adequate treatment.

Programmed cell death-ligand 1 (PD-L1) is strongly expressed by GTNs. It is expressed by tumors to suppress the host's anticancer T-cell activity. Pembrolizumab, an immunotherapy, is a monoclonal antibody that blocks this pathway. Pembrolizumab has been shown to be effective in chemoresistant GTN in case reports and is a treatment option in such patients. In this patient, immunotherapy is not the best next step in disease management because it has not failed to respond to multi-agent chemotherapy or recurred after initial multi-agent chemotherapy.

Radiotherapy is rarely used in the treatment of GTN. Radiotherapy can be used to treat brain metastasis, although intrathecal methotrexate may be a more effective option. The described patient does not have metastatic disease to the brain, and radiotherapy is not recommended.

Surgical resection of disease is a treatment option when postmolar GTN is limited to the uterus, when low-risk GTN persists after failure of single-agent chemotherapy, or high-risk GTN persists after failure of chemotherapy. Hysterectomy with salpingectomy is an option for patients whose disease is limited to the uterus. For individuals with extrauterine disease, chemotherapy is the recommended first step in management. This patient has high-risk disease with multiple lung metastases; therefore, surgical resection is not an appropriate initial management option.

High-risk GTN should be treated with multi-agent chemotherapy regimens, preferably EMA/CO or EMA/EP. Gestational trophoblastic neoplasia is highly chemosensitive, with 90% survival rates in patients with high-risk disease.

Albright BB, Ellett T, Knochenhauer HE, Goins EC, Monuszko KA, Kaplan SJ, et al. Treatments and outcomes in high-risk gestational trophoblastic neoplasia: a systematic review and meta-analysis. BJOG 2023;130:443–53. doi: 10.1111/1471-0528.17374

Braga A, Elias KM, Horowitz NS, Berkowitz RS. Treatment of high-risk gestational trophoblastic neoplasia and chemoresistance/relapsed disease. Best Pract Res Clin Obstet Gynaecol 2021;74:81–96. doi: 10.1016/j.bpobgyn.2021.01.005

Ngan HY, Seckl MJ, Berkowitz RS, Xiang Y, Golfier F, Sekharan PK, et al. Diagnosis and management of gestational trophoblastic disease: 2021 update. Int J Gynaecol Obstet 2021;155(suppl 1):86–93. doi: 10.1002/ijgo.13877

33 Basal cell carcinoma of the vulva

A 72-year-old patient presents to your clinic with a 3-month history of increasing vulvar pruritus. On examination, there is a 3-cm papular lesion with central ulceration on the right labium majus that is tender to palpation (Fig. 33-1). A punch biopsy of the lesion reveals nodular-type basal cell carcinoma. The best next step in treatment is

(A) carbon dioxide (CO_2) laser ablation
(B) topical imiquimod
(C) total superficial vulvectomy
(D) vulvar radiotherapy
* (E) wide local excision

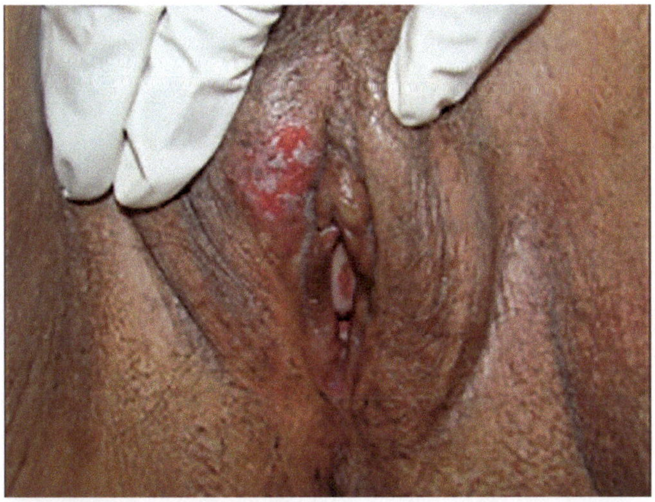

FIGURE 33-1. Vulvar basal cell carcinoma. (Reprinted from Rodríguez VG, De la Fuente García A, Torres MA, Flores MG, Moreno GJ, Candiani JO. Could cryosurgery be an alternative treatment for basal cell carcinoma of the vulva? [published correction appears in Indian Dermatol Online J. 2015 Jul-Aug;6(4):314. doi: 10.4103/2229-5178.160308]. Indian Dermatol Online J. 2014;5(2):160–163. doi:10.4103/2229-5178.131089)

Basal cell carcinoma of the vulva is a rare histologic subtype of vulvar cancer. It accounts for only 5% of cancer affecting the vulva and an even smaller percentage of all diagnosed basal cell carcinoma. Risk factors include basal cell nevus syndrome, a history of radiation therapy, and older age, with a mean age at diagnosis of age 70 years. There have been case reports of basal cell carcinoma developing near lichen and Paget disease of the vulva, but there is not enough information to determine whether these were risk factors for its development.

As with the more common histologic types of vulvar cancer, surgical excision is the mainstay of treatment for vulvar basal cell carcinoma. The primary goal of excision is the complete removal of the tumor with maximal preservation of function. This generally can be accomplished with wide local excision of the full skin thickness with a 1-cm gross margin. Excision of the deeper tissues is not necessary. Due to anatomic and functional constraints, local excision on the vulva can result in narrow excision margins and a resultant higher rate of recurrence. Local recurrence occurs in approximately 10% of patients treated with local excision and may be more common with an inadequate resection margin. A lower recurrence rate has been reported with Mohs microsurgery performed for basal cell carcinoma of the vulva, but the number of reported cases in the literature remains small. This may represent a promising option for decreasing the recurrence rate of vulvar basal cell carcinoma; however, Mohs microsurgery is a specialized surgical procedure. Although its use is increasingly common for skin cancer on other areas of the body, it is not yet widely available for vulvar basal cell carcinoma. Where available, Mohs may be a reasonable option for patients with vulvar basal cell carcinoma; however, traditional wide local excision of the vulva has an excellent 5-year relative survival for individuals with vulvar basal cell carcinoma, and cure rates have been reported to be nearly 100%. Given such high cure rates with local surgical excision, wide local excision of the lesion is the preferred treatment option, and the correct treatment option for this patient.

Carbon dioxide laser ablation and other superficial ablative therapies, such as cryotherapy, often are used to treat vulvar dysplasia, but ablative therapy is not the preferred modality for treatment of cancer due to the higher risk of recurrence or inadequate treatment. Although the use of CO_2 laser ablation to treat basal cell carcinoma has been described, the reported cure rate is lower than the rate for surgical excision. As a result, CO_2 laser ablation is not the best next step in treatment.

Topical imiquimod is a type of medication for skin conditions that works by increasing the immune response in the area of application. It is sometimes used to treat genital condyloma and vulvar dysplasia. There are no reported cases of imiquimod use in vulvar basal cell carcinoma. It has been used in superficial basal cell carcinoma on other areas of the body, and the response rates were inferior to surgical resection. For these reasons, imiquimod is not the best treatment for this patient.

Total superficial vulvectomy, sometimes referred to as *skinning vulvectomy*, involves removing the skin of the entire vulva. This procedure is rarely used in patients with diffuse involvement of the vulvar skin by dermatologic conditions. The described patient has a discrete lesion, and removal of the entirety of the vulvar skin is unnecessary and would lead to increased morbidity. Total superficial vulvectomy is not the best treatment for the described patient.

Radiation therapy may be an effective treatment for vulvar basal cell carcinoma when surgical resection is not feasible; however, radiation therapy requires a protracted course of treatment and comes with significant risks for adverse effects compared with local excision. Thus, for this patient, in whom local excision is feasible, radiotherapy is not the correct choice.

Michalski BM, Pfeifer JD, Mutch D, Council ML. Cancer of the vulva: a review. Dermatol Surg 2021;47:174–83. doi: 10.1097/DSS.0000000000002584

National Comprehensive Cancer Network. Vulvar cancer. Version 4.2024. NCCN Clinical Practice Guidelines in Oncology [after login]. NCCN; 2024. Accessed January 22, 2025. https://www.nccn.org/guidelines/guidelines-detail?category=1&id=1476

Rodríguez VG, De la Fuente García A, Torres MA, Flores MG, Moreno GJ, Candiani JO. Could cryosurgery be an alternative treatment for basal cell carcinoma of the vulva? [published erratum appears in Indian Dermatol Online J 2015;6:314]. Indian Dermatol Online J 2014;5:160–3. doi: 10.4103/2229-5178.131089

Shwe S, Elsensohn AN, Ortiz C, Kraus CN. Mohs micrographic surgery for vulvar malignancies: a systematic review. J Am Acad Dermatol 2022;87:159–62. doi: 10.1016/j.jaad.2021.06.875

34 Molar pregnancy

A 39-year-old gravida 3, para 0020, at 8 weeks of gestation undergoes an ultrasound-guided uterine aspiration and intrauterine device insertion for management of early pregnancy loss. Her preoperative β-human chorionic gonadotropin (β-hCG) concentration is 75,150 mIU/mL. Pathology demonstrates diffusely enlarged hydropic villi without fetal tissue and the presence of cisterns. Genetic testing of the surgical specimen reveals a 46,XX karyotype, and p57 staining is negative. The best next step is to

(A) determine maternal karyotype
* (B) follow β-hCG levels until negative
(C) initiate chemotherapy
(D) remove the intrauterine device

Gestational trophoblastic disease (GTD) is a collection of benign and malignant conditions that occur after a pregnancy. Benign GTD includes molar pregnancy and placental site nodule. Complete molar pregnancy occurs as a result of fertilization of an ovum without maternal DNA, resulting in a diploid karyotype (eg, 46,XX) that is paternal in origin. Complete molar pregnancies lack expression of p57, which is a cyclin-dependent kinase inhibitor that is maternally expressed. Because the genetic makeup of a complete molar pregnancy is paternal in origin, p57 is not present on immunohistochemical staining. Additionally, hydropic villi are typically diffusely seen on histology, and no fetal tissue is present. Partial molar pregnancy often results from two sperm fertilizing a single ovum or from a paternal chromosomal duplication, resulting in a triploid karyotype (eg, 69,XXY). Partial molar pregnancies express p57 because they contain maternal DNA and may have fetal tissue present on histology.

Molar pregnancy is suspected in patients with significant increases in β-hCG levels (frequently more than 100,000 mIU/mL with complete molar pregnancy), those with vesicular appearance of the pregnancy or cystic placental changes on ultrasonography, and those whose uterine size is larger than gestational duration by last menstrual period. In the United States, encountering an enlarged uterus is less common because high-sensitivity pregnancy testing helps diagnose molar pregnancy earlier, and ultrasonography is being performed routinely in first-trimester prenatal care.

Molar pregnancy suspected on preoperative ultrasound or evaluation should be treated surgically, preferably with dilation and curettage, due to the risk of heavy bleeding. The procedure should be done in a setting with the availability of uterotonics and resources to manage heavy bleeding or other complications; however, with earlier diagnosis and intervention, complications are infrequent. Patients at later gestational ages or with more advanced molar pregnancies should undergo dilation and curettage in the hospital setting due to increased risk of hemorrhage or cardiopulmonary complications. Hysterectomy is an option for initial treatment in a patient who has completed childbearing. The diagnosis is then confirmed on pathologic evaluation.

The described patient's pathology is consistent with complete molar pregnancy. After initial treatment with uterine evacuation, serial β-hCG measurement is recommended to assess for postmolar gestational trophoblastic neoplasia (GTN). For this patient with complete molar pregnancy, β-hCG surveillance should be performed every 1–2 weeks until her level has decreased to the lowest level measured by the laboratory, then monthly for 3 months. Patients with partial molar pregnancy should be monitored for 1 month after normalization of β-hCG. A β-hCG concentration that plateaus or increases during surveillance meets criteria for post-molar GTN and should undergo further evaluation (Appendix J). Patients undergoing β-hCG surveillance after GTD is diagnosed should be counseled regarding contraceptive options with a goal of avoiding increased β-hCG due to a new pregnancy or a false-positive result due to luteinizing hormone cross-reactivity during the surveillance phase, which can pose a diagnostic challenge. Systemic hormonal contraception may avoid this cross-reactivity and should be discussed as part of the patient-centered contraception counseling.

Chemotherapy is not recommended for patients with a complete molar pregnancy that resolves after evacuation. Adjuvant chemotherapy in patients with this condition may decrease the risk of developing postmolar GTN. Chemotherapy can be considered in patients with a particularly high risk of postmolar GTN, including those older than 40, those whose initial β-hCG level is greater than 100,000 mIU/mL, those with a significantly enlarged uterus at the time of evacuation, or those with large theca lutein cysts (greater than 6 cm). Complete response to chemotherapy when administered after a confirmed diagnosis of GTN is high enough that adjuvant chemotherapy is generally not recommended. The described patient does not meet these high-risk criteria, and chemotherapy is not the best next step for her.

A maternal karyotype is part of the assessment for recurrent pregnancy loss to evaluate for the presence of a balanced translocation. This test is recommended for patients with three or more early pregnancy losses and can be considered for patients who have experienced two early pregnancy losses. In patients meeting criteria for evaluation, a maternal karyotype should be considered in addition to assessing antiphospholipid antibodies, determining levels of thyroid and prolactin, and evaluating the uterine cavity. Further review of this patient's history is needed to determine her eligibility for recurrent pregnancy loss evaluation.

Intrauterine device removal is not the best next step in the treatment of this patient's complete molar pregnancy. Intrauterine devices are considered category 1 (no restrictions for use) by the Centers for Disease Control and Prevention Medical Eligibility Criteria, and initiation at the time of uterine evacuation is recommended in the setting of suspected GTD.

Patients with molar pregnancy are at high risk of developing GTN, and serial β-hCG measurement to evaluate for postmolar GTN is the most time-sensitive; therefore, it is the best next step for the described patient. Postoperative β-hCG surveillance helps detect and diagnose GTN to allow for prompt treatment if indicated. Approximately 20% of patients with complete molar pregnancies and 4% of patients with incomplete molar pregnancies develop postmolar GTN. Patients with GTN confirmed on β-hCG surveillance should be evaluated with International Federation of Gynecology and Obstetrics (FIGO) criteria for diagnosis of postmolar GTN (Appendix J) and World Health Organization Prognosis Scoring (Appendix I) to determine the appropriate intervention.

Horowitz NS, Eskander RN, Adelman MR, Burke W. Epidemiology, diagnosis, and treatment of gestational trophoblastic disease: a Society of Gynecologic Oncology evidenced-based review and recommendation. Gynecol Oncol 2021;163:605–13. doi: 10.1016/j.ygyno.2021.10.003

National Comprehensive Cancer Network. Gestational trophoblastic neoplasia. Version 2.2025. NCCN Clinical Practice Guidelines in Oncology [after login]. NCCN; 2025. Accessed March 13, 2025. https://www.nccn.org/guidelines/guidelines-detail?category=1&id=1489

Ngan HY, Seckl MJ, Berkowitz RS, Xiang Y, Golfier F, Sekharan PK, et al. Diagnosis and management of gestational trophoblastic disease: 2021 update. Int J Gynaecol Obstet 2021;155(suppl 1):86–93. doi: 10.1002/ijgo.13877

35 Complications of chemotherapy

A 76-year-old patient with metastatic, recurrent ovarian cancer presents to the clinic, reporting weight loss and fatigue. She started her third cycle of weekly paclitaxel with bevacizumab 2 weeks ago. She has nausea but can eat three small meals a day. She had a bowel movement 1 day ago. Her vital signs are unremarkable except for the loss of 2% of her weight since her assessment (before cycle 3). Her BMI today is 17. On examination, her abdomen is distended but nontender. Bimanual examination reveals no palpable pelvic and rectal masses. Computed tomography is ordered, and the results indicate that her pretreatment abdominal tumors have shrunk. The best next step to address her symptoms is to

(A) initiate an appetite stimulant
(B) place an enteral feeding tube
* (C) refer her to a dietitian
(D) start parenteral nutrition

Cancer cachexia is defined as a syndrome associated with loss of skeletal muscle mass that cannot be fully reversed by conventional nutritional support and leads to progressive functional impairment. The diagnosis is based on at least one of two criteria: weight loss greater than 5% over 6 months, or 2–5% weight loss with either a BMI less than 20 or reduced muscle mass. Cancer cachexia is a common condition, affecting over 80% of cancer patients worldwide. It can be associated with poor prognosis, poor quality of life, and death. Due to the negative effects associated with chemotherapy, such as gastrointestinal toxicities and fatigue, cancer treatment can propel the patient into a cachexia-like state. The described patient meets the criteria of cancer cachexia.

Ovarian cancer most often is diagnosed at an advanced stage, and most patients experience multiple recurrences and receive several types of therapy. Patients often present with bloating and ascites, which can make weight loss difficult to appreciate. Early satiety and decreased appetite can be due to tumor burden (ascites and carcinomatosis). Nausea with or without vomiting may be caused by cancer treatment as well as tumor burden. Poor nutritional status and possible cachexia are a concern in these patients.

A patient with cancer can experience three phases of cachexia: precachexia, cachexia, and refractory cachexia. Identifying disease and intervening during each phase are critical to predict the patient's prognosis and improve their experience of cancer treatment. Although *precachexia* has been defined as minimal weight loss (2–5%), with early clinical and metabolic signs predictive of future weight loss, such as anorexia, insulin resistance, inflammation, and hypogonadism, there has yet to be a consensus regarding its definition and early detection. In 2020, the American Society of Clinical Oncology (ASCO) released guidelines for the management of cancer cachexia. Nutritional counseling is associated with improved body weight, and the recommendations endorse referral to a registered dietitian as a practical and harm-free intervention for patients with advanced cancer who experience loss of appetite, weight loss, or both. The best next step for the patient in this scenario is to collaborate with a registered dietitian to establish weight-related goals.

Cancer treatment centers should incorporate nutritional counseling in their treatment protocols. Access to nutritional counseling is associated with improved quality of life and less psychological stress during cancer treatment. Registered dietitians can provide patients and their families with support regarding nutritional status and supplementation. Dietitians working in a cancer center should be trained in using assessments of body composition and physical function. These assessments can help dietitians to counsel patients by offering feeding advice, addressing concerns, providing supplement recommendations, and identifying nutrition-related symptoms.

Overall, enteral tube feeding or total parenteral nutrition to treat or manage cachexia is not recommended. Supplemental nutrition can be considered in certain clinical situations, such as reversible bowel obstruction or short bowel syndrome; however, total parenteral nutrition can be associated with infection and worse survival rates. In the patient described, enteral feeding or parenteral nutrition is not the best next step because she is able to eat and does not have a bowel obstruction.

Oral progesterone agonists have been studied as a treatment for cancer cachexia. Specifically, megestrol acetate has been shown to improve appetite with modest increases in weight; however, in one meta-analysis, this therapy also was associated with an increased risk of death, thromboembolic events, and edema. The ASCO review concludes that a short-term trial of a progesterone agent may be considered, but there is a paucity of evidence to endorse any single pharmacologic agent. There is no U.S. Food and Drug Administration (FDA)-approved medication for cancer cachexia. Anamorelin, a ghrelin receptor agonist, failed to receive FDA approval for cancer-related cachexia. Data supporting the use of other appetite stimulants, such as olanzapine or cannabinoids, are very limited.

Ovarian cancer can present with skeletal muscle loss and cachexia. Muscle loss can be associated with a worse prognosis in this disease. Better interventions are needed to address the nutritional challenges in these patients.

Callaway CS, Mouchantat LM, Bitler BG, Bonetto A. Mechanisms of ovarian cancer-associated cachexia. Endocrinology 2023;165:bqad176. doi: 10.1210/endocr/bqad176

Koshimoto S, Amano K, Mori N, Oyamada S, Arakawa S, Ishiki H, et al. Perspectives of registered dietitians and factors associated with their personal accomplishment in the management of cancer cachexia. Support Care Cancer 2023;31:124. doi: 10.1007/s00520-023-07593-x

Roeland EJ, Bohlke K, Baracos VE, Bruera E, Del Fabbro E, Dixon S, et al. Management of cancer cachexia: ASCO guideline. J Clin Oncol 2020;38:2438–53. doi: 10.1200/JCO.20.00611

Weng C, Huang W, Chang C, Jan Y, Chen T, Lee J. Association of malignant ascites with systemic inflammation and muscle loss after treatment in advanced-stage ovarian cancer. J Cachexia Sarcopenia Muscle 2023;14:2114–25. doi: 10.1002/jcsm.13289

36 Postoperative altered mental status

An 82-year-old woman is evaluated on postoperative day 1 after ovarian cancer debulking surgery. The surgery included extensive pelvic dissection and required 5 hours of operative time. She was given intravenous fluids at a rate of 100 mL/h upon transfer from her post-anesthesia care unit. The next morning, she is lethargic and confused. Her vital signs and laboratory values are noted below in Table 36-1. She weighs 176 lb (80 kg). A physical examination and symptom assessment are otherwise noncontributory. The best next step to evaluate the patient's condition is to obtain

(A) blood cultures
(B) head computed tomography
(C) kidney ultrasound
(D) serial basic metabolic profile
* (E) urine electrolytes

TABLE 36-1. The Described Patient's Vital Signs and Laboratory Study Results

	6 PM	MIDNIGHT	6 AM
Pain Score	8	6	2
Temperature (°C [°F])	37.5 (99.5)	37.1 (98.8)	36.9 (98.4)
Blood pressure	110/75	101/60	98/68
Pulse	101	92	115
Respiratory rate	22	16	18
Oxygen saturation (%)	97	96	98
Urine output (mL/h)	40	16	8
White blood cell count (per mm³)	12,000	—	8,000
Hemoglobin (g/dL)	9	—	9
Creatinine (mg/dL)	0.9	—	2.9
Sodium	137	—	140
Chloride	102	—	101
Bicarbonate	26	—	27
Potassium	4	—	4.1

The most notable abnormality in this clinical scenario is the patient's progressively worsening kidney function. These findings meet the criteria for acute kidney injury (AKI). Her kidney function is acutely decreased, which causes her body to accumulate waste products, such as urea and drug by-products. She will be unable to maintain electrolyte, acid–base, and fluid balance.

Various staging criteria for AKI have been proposed to better characterize the occurrence, severity, and clinical risk that is associated with the clinical syndrome. These are based on serum creatinine, glomerular filtration rate, and urine output. This 176-lb (80-kg) patient has a urine output of 8 mL/h, or 0.1 mL/kg/h, and her serum creatinine is two times her baseline. She is identified to be in the *failure* class by the RIFLE (Risk, Injury, Failure,

Loss of kidney function, and End-stage kidney disease) classification of acute renal injury depicted in Figure 36-1.

Although Enhanced Recovery After Surgery (ERAS) protocols emphasize euvolemia and careful intravenous perioperative fluid management, adequate perfusion of the kidneys is essential for the prevention of insufficient renal perfusion. An older patient undergoing prolonged surgery is at increased risk of AKI. The development of postoperative AKI in patients is associated with significantly higher perioperative morbidity, and it can also facilitate other organ dysfunction that will potentiate further clinical deterioration. Prompt postoperative evaluation of patients who demonstrate evidence of AKI is necessary to identify any potentially reversible factors in a timely manner and prevent progression toward worsening organ dysfunction. Understanding the possible inciting causes for the injury can help identify the most efficient initial diagnostic strategies and clinical interventions. Patients undergoing surgery are exposed to several potential injuries and physiologic stressors that put the kidney at high risk of acute injury, and often it is helpful to organize one's differential diagnosis into 1) prerenal, 2) intrinsic renal, and 3) postrenal etiologies.

Prerenal causes of AKI are due to reduced organ perfusion. The kidneys receive up to 25% of cardiac output, and compromise in the systemic or localized blood flow to the kidney will affect renal function. Patients undergoing ovarian cancer debulking are at a particularly high risk of intravascular volume depletion that affects kidney perfusion. Several factors contribute to intravascular volume loss in this setting. Many patients with advanced ovarian cancer will be intravascularly depleted at their baseline due to malignancy-associated third spacing. These may manifest as ascites, pleural effusion, or interstitial edema. Additionally, gastrointestinal dysfunction is common in patients with advanced ovarian cancer, and third spacing within the intestinal tract can occur with bowel obstruction or in cases of functional ileus due to peritoneal carcinomatosis. Blood loss and insensible losses occurring during a prolonged laparotomy also are potential contributors. Preoperative bowel preparation can also contribute to hypovolemia.

Intrinsic renal factors from AKI cause direct toxicity to the glomeruli, intrinsic vasculature, or renal tubules. Inciting factors in the perioperative setting include acute interstitial nephritis and acute tubular necrosis that may occur as an allergic or toxic reaction to medications and infections.

Postrenal causes of kidney failure include urinary outflow obstruction that secondarily results in increased intratubular pressure and reduction in glomerular filtration. Failure of urine outflow at any level in the urinary tract due to surgical injury to the ureter should be considered in patients undergoing pelvic surgery. Mechanical bladder outlet obstruction or functional failure due to bladder atony may also contribute to AKI.

In this scenario, the patient is 82 years old and has advanced ovarian cancer. She underwent an extensive and prolonged surgical dissection and now has stage II AKI on postoperative day 1. She demonstrates generalized lethargy, but her examination,

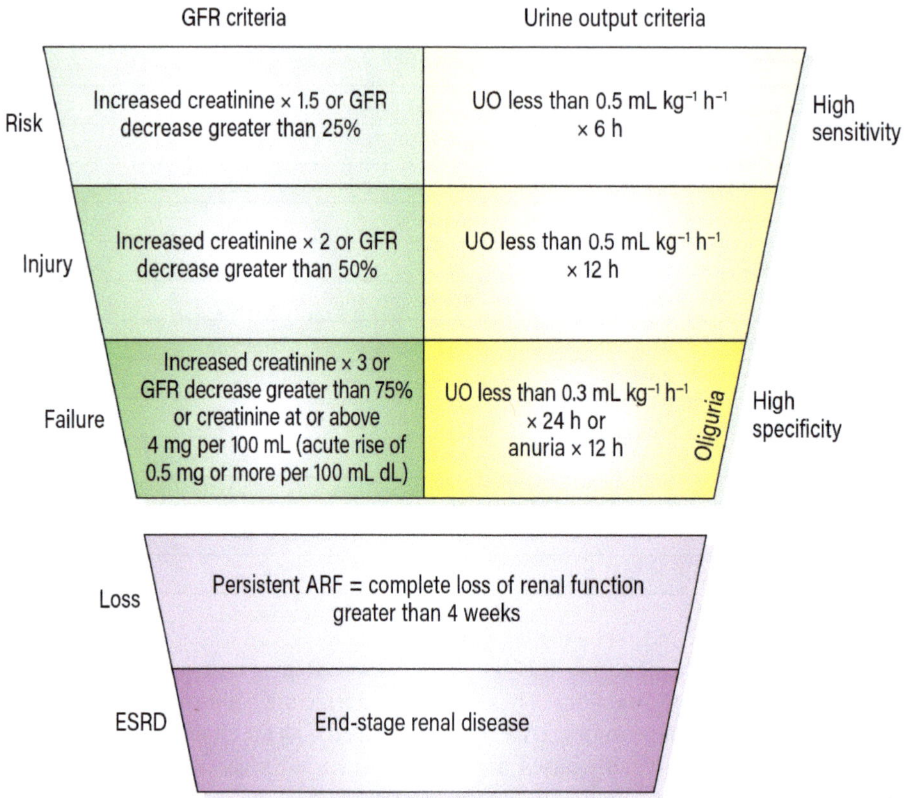

FIGURE 36-1. The RIFLE criteria for defining acute kidney injury. (Reprinted from Ricci Z, Cruz D, Ronco C. The RIFLE criteria and mortality in acute kidney injury: a systematic review. Kidney Int 2008;73:538–46. doi: 10.1038/sj.ki.5002743)

vital signs, and laboratory evaluation are otherwise unremarkable. The differential diagnosis for AKI in her case is very broad and includes prerenal, renal, and postrenal etiologies.

The best next step in evaluation is to obtain urine electrolytes. Urine analysis can aid in distinguishing among AKI etiologies and should be obtained as a priority at this juncture. The urine specific gravity measures urine concentration and can reflect general volume status. Urine electrolytes can be used to calculate the urine fractional excretion of sodium (FENa), a measure of the kidney's handling of sodium. Fractional excretion of sodium is a calculation based on comparing the concentrations of sodium and creatinine in the urine with those of the blood plasma. It is expressed as a percentage (Fig. 36-1). With prerenal causes of AKI, the resorptive capacity of the kidney is preserved and the fraction of sodium excreted will be reduced to less than 1% as an adaptive response to reduced kidney perfusion. On the other hand, the loss of tubular and glomerular function with intrinsic kidney injury can impair the resorptive capacity of the kidney, and sodium preservation will not be reflected in the findings. In such cases, FENa greater than 1% is anticipated.

The other answer options have potential diagnostic value, but because of their relevance or timeliness, they would not be prioritized as the best next step. How these interventions are ultimately prioritized will depend on the results of the FENa and on how one further weighs the entities in the differential diagnosis. A serial basic metabolic profile, for example, will undoubtedly be obtained to monitor trends toward progression or resolution of kidney injury; however, prompt diagnosis is essential to guide her most appropriate immediate intervention and minimize risk for further deterioration. Other diagnostic investigations will be prioritized at this time, rather than adopting a wait-and-see approach.

Acute kidney injury is common in the setting of sepsis, in which endotoxin-induced direct tubular damage and secondary cardiovascular derangements can impair kidney function. This patient does not meet systemic inflammatory response syndrome criteria (Fig. 36-2), and clinical suspicion for sepsis is lower on the differential diagnosis. Moreover, the results of blood cultures will not manifest for some days, and more immediate evaluation tools and interventions are prioritized. In cases of high clinical acuity, if sepsis is on the differential diagnosis, empiric antibiotic treatment can be implemented while waiting for the results of blood cultures.

Kidney ultrasonography can potentially identify surgical injury, leading to hydronephrosis, and also may assess the integrity of the renal vasculature. Based on this clinical scenario, the conditions that kidney ultrasonography could identify, such as bilateral ureteral obstruction or kidney vascular thrombosis, are low on the differential diagnosis. The diagnostic sensitivity of kidney ultrasonography for identifying postoperative ureteral injury varies depending on the type and location of the injury and the timing of the imaging evaluation relative to

FENa

- **FENa < 1% = Prerenal disorder**
- **FENa > 2% = Intrinsic renal disorder**

$$FE_{Na} = 100 \times \frac{\text{sodium}_{urinary} \times \text{creatinine}_{plasma}}{\text{sodium}_{plasma} \times \text{creatinine}_{urinary}}$$

FIGURE 36-2. Fractional excretion of sodium (FENa) calculation.

the injury. Renal ultrasonography has reduced sensitivity in the early postoperative setting. Although kidney ultrasonography is not the best next step for the described patient, it could be considered later in the evaluation if clinical concern for ureteral injury persists.

Assessment of mental status is essential in a bedside evaluation. The patient in this scenario is lethargic without focal findings, making a structural or neurologic event (eg, stroke or hemorrhage) less likely. Given the additional finding of stage II AKI, a metabolic, uremic, or narcotic-induced encephalopathy is favored in the differential diagnosis. Head imaging to evaluate for a structural abnormality is not the best next step but could be obtained if symptoms do not improve with fluid resuscitation and careful medication management.

Acute kidney injury significantly increases the risk of perioperative surgical morbidity and mortality, and patients undergoing ovarian cancer debulking are at a particularly high risk for this complication. Prevention is foundational to minimize AKI occurrence. This includes careful preoperative medical optimization, avoidance of nephrotoxic drugs, and meticulous surgical and anesthesia management to reduce the occurrence of fluid shifts, hypotension, and organ hypoperfusion. If AKI is identified in the postoperative setting, prompt evaluation and intervention are essential to minimize the risk of further deterioration. The FENa is an efficient initial screening tool to discriminate the entities that are highest on the differential diagnosis.

Bell S, Ross VC, Zealley KA, Millar F, Isles C. Management of post-operative acute kidney injury. QJM 2017;110:695–700. doi: 10.1093/qjmed/hcw175

Makris K, Spanou L. Acute kidney injury: definition, pathophysiology and clinical phenotypes. Clin Biochem Rev 2016;37:85–98.

Prowle JR, Forni LG, Bell M, Chew MS, Edwards M, Grams ME, et al. Postoperative acute kidney injury in adult non-cardiac surgery: joint consensus report of the Acute Disease Quality Initiative and PeriOperative Quality Initiative. Nat Rev Nephrol 2021;17:605–18. doi: 10.1038/s41581-021-00418-2

Ricci Z, Cruz D, Ronco C. The RIFLE criteria and mortality in acute kidney injury: a systematic review. Kidney Int 2008;73:538–46. doi: 10.1038/sj.ki.5002743

Ronco C, Bellomo R, Kellum JA. Acute kidney injury. Lancet 2019;394:1949–64. doi: 10.1016/S0140-6736(19)32563-2

37 Early-stage cervical cancer

A 43-year-old gravida 3, para 3, presents with 2 months of postcoital bleeding and dyspareunia. Her surgical history is significant for bilateral tubal ligation. Her physical examination is notable for a 2.5-cm friable mass limited to the posterior lip of the cervix. A biopsy of the mass confirms invasive squamous cell carcinoma. Positron emission tomography with computed tomography is negative for metastatic disease. In addition to pelvic lymph node assessment, the best next step is

(A) cold knife cone
(B) simple trachelectomy
(C) radical trachelectomy
(D) simple hysterectomy
* (E) radical hysterectomy

In the United States, cervical cancer rates have remained stable during the last decade except for individuals in the 30- to 34-year-old age group, in whom incidence has increased by 2.5% per year since 2012. Most of these cases are early-stage disease, allowing for surgical treatment with high cure rates. In this case, the patient has early-stage disease: stage IB2 squamous cell carcinoma of the cervix and a tumor confined to the cervix and measuring between 2 cm to less than 4 cm (Fig. 37-1). Early-stage cervical cancer can be managed with surgery, in which cervical conization, simple hysterectomy, radical trachelectomy, or radical hysterectomy may be performed based on the stage of disease, the extent of spread, and risk factors for more aggressive disease.

Conservative surgery may involve excision of a portion of the cervix (ie, conization), the entire cervix (ie, simple trachelectomy), or the cervix and uterus (ie, simple hysterectomy). In all cases of conservative surgery, surrounding tissues, such as the parametria and the vagina, are left intact. Women with International Federation of Gynecology and Obstetrics (FIGO) stage IA1 disease without lymphovascular space invasion (LVSI) can be treated with cervical conization alone, provided that the cone margins are negative for cancer and high-grade squamous intraepithelial lesion, including cervical intraepithelial neoplasia. Simple extrafascial hysterectomy can be offered to these individuals who do not desire future fertility. Conservative surgery with cervical conization (if fertility-sparing therapy is desired) or simple hysterectomy and pelvic lymph node assessment also can be considered in early-stage, low-risk disease. The Prospective Trial of Conservative Surgery for Low-risk Early-Stage Cervical Cancer (ConCerv) and Simple Hysterectomy and Pelvic Node Assessment (SHAPE) trial investigated conservative surgery in women with early-stage, low-risk cervical cancer. For detailed inclusion criteria defining early-stage, low-risk disease, refer to Appendix E. Participants enrolled in both trials who had more conservative management had similar oncologic outcomes compared to those undergoing more radical procedures. The patient in this scenario has stage IB2 disease, making her ineligible for conservative surgery.

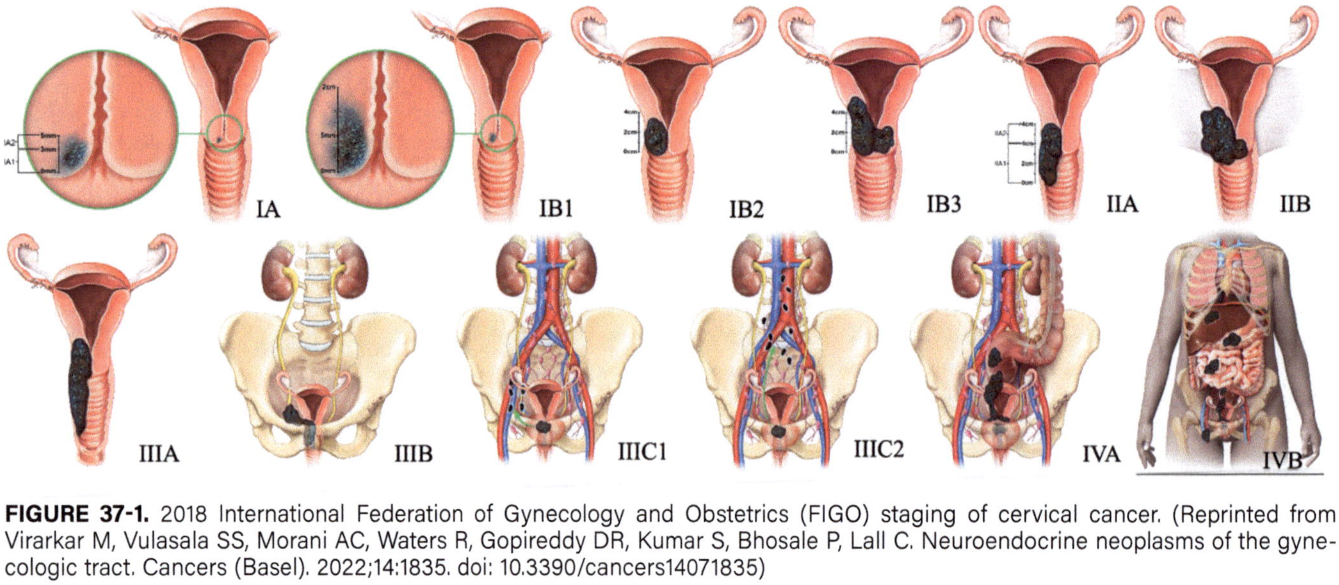

FIGURE 37-1. 2018 International Federation of Gynecology and Obstetrics (FIGO) staging of cervical cancer. (Reprinted from Virarkar M, Vulasala SS, Morani AC, Waters R, Gopireddy DR, Kumar S, Bhosale P, Lall C. Neuroendocrine neoplasms of the gynecologic tract. Cancers (Basel). 2022;14:1835. doi: 10.3390/cancers14071835)

Radical surgery, such as radical trachelectomy and radical hysterectomy, involves removing a wide margin of tissue—typically including the parametria and upper vagina—in addition to en bloc removal of the cervix for a trachelectomy, or cervix and uterus. Radical surgery is the standard of care for FIGO stage IA1 disease with LVSI and positive cone margins for carcinoma, FIGO stage IA2–IB1 disease not meeting low-risk criteria, and FIGO stage IB2. Radical hysterectomy also is an option for select FIGO stage IIA disease. All cases should include pelvic lymph node assessment.

Radical hysterectomy is the treatment of choice for this patient with FIGO stage IB2 disease, given that she has completed childbearing. A radical trachelectomy would be appropriate if she desired fertility-sparing therapy. The criteria for a radical trachelectomy are similar to those of a radical hysterectomy, with a few key exceptions: squamous cell carcinoma, adenocarcinoma or adenosquamous carcinoma, no or minor LVSI, and a tumor size of 4 cm or less (although some centers use a cutoff of 2 cm or less). This patient has completed childbearing, and a radical trachelectomy would not be recommended.

The route of radical hysterectomy, either open or minimally invasive, has come into question in recent years. The Minimally Invasive versus Abdominal Radical Hysterectomy for Cervical Cancer (LACC) trial is a randomized phase 3 controlled trial comparing outcomes for FIGO stages IA1 with LVSI and IA2–IB2 cervical cancer treated with minimally invasive (laparoscopic or robotic) radical hysterectomy with those treated with open abdominal radical hysterectomy. Key findings were significantly lower rates of disease-free survival and overall survival, with a nearly four times increased risk of recurrence with the minimally invasive approach compared to the open approach. Two other epidemiologic studies have shown that minimally invasive radical hysterectomy was associated with lower overall survival compared to open radical hysterectomy. These findings have led to changes in national guidelines both in the United States and Europe. The National Comprehensive Cancer Network and European Society of Gynaecological Oncology guidelines recommend abdominal radical hysterectomy as the standard surgical approach for early-stage cervical cancer. The potential role of minimally invasive surgery for treatment of early-stage cervical cancer with the addition of tumor containment (closure of the upper vagina over the cervix prior to colpotomy) and omission of a transcervical manipulator is currently being explored in the phase III GOG-3043 trial, which randomizes participants to robotic versus open surgery.

Bhatla N, Aoki D, Sharma DN, Sankaranarayanan R. Cancer of the cervix uteri [published erratum appears in Int J Gynaecol Obstet 2024;164:1229-30]. Int J Gynaecol Obstet 2018;143(suppl 2):22–36. doi: 10.1002/ijgo.12611

Cibula D, Raspollini MR, Planchamp F, Centeno C, Chargari C, Felix A, et al. ESGO/ESTRO/ESP guidelines for the management of patients with cervical cancer update 2023. Int J Gynecol Cancer 2023;33:649–66. doi: 10.1136/ijgc-2023-004429

National Comprehensive Cancer Network. Cervical cancer. Version 3.2025. NCCN Clinical Practice Guidelines in Oncology [after login]. NCCN; 2025. Accessed February 26, 2025. https://www.nccn.org/guidelines/guidelines-detail?category=1&id=1426

Plante M, Kwon JS, Ferguson S, Samouëlian V, Ferron G, Maulard A, et al. Simple versus radical hysterectomy in women with low-risk cervical cancer. CX.5 SHAPE investigators. N Engl J Med 2024;390:819–29. doi: 10.1056/NEJMoa2308900

Ramirez PT, Frumovitz M, Pareja R, Lopez A, Vieira M, Ribeiro R, et al. Minimally invasive versus abdominal radical hysterectomy for cervical cancer. N Engl J Med 2018;379:1895–904. doi: 10.1056/NEJMoa1806395

Schmeler KM, Pareja R, Lopez Blanco A, Humberto Fregnani J, Lopes A, Perrotta M, et al. ConCerv: a prospective trial of conservative surgery for low-risk early-stage cervical cancer. Int J Gynecol Cancer 2021;31:1317–25. doi: 10.1136/ijgc-2021-002921

38 Diagnostic tools to evaluate postmenopausal bleeding

A 56-year-old woman presents for follow-up of postmenopausal vaginal bleeding. She experienced menopause when she was 49 years old. Three months ago, she presented to the office with an episode of vaginal spotting. Transvaginal ultrasonography at that time revealed a normal-appearing uterus with an endometrial thickness that measured 1.1 mm. Since that visit, she has had an additional episode of vaginal bleeding. Her pelvic examination reveals vaginal atrophy and is otherwise normal. Her cervical cancer screening is negative from her annual examination 6 months ago. The best next step is

* (A) endometrial sampling
(B) repeat transvaginal ultrasound
(C) systemic hormonal therapy
(D) tranexamic acid
(E) vaginal estrogen

Endometrial cancer is the most common gynecologic cancer in the United States, and 90% of patients with endometrial cancer experience postmenopausal bleeding. Vaginal bleeding in postmenopausal women is most commonly due to vaginal or endometrial atrophy; however, 1–14% of patients are found to have endometrial cancer. Patients with postmenopausal bleeding should be evaluated to rule out endometrial cancer.

One approach to the evaluation of postmenopausal bleeding is to obtain transvaginal ultrasonography to assess endometrial thickness, as was performed in the patient described. This approach is most appropriate in patients without recurrent or persistent bleeding. The measurement of the endometrial thickness is obtained with a sagittal view of the uterus, measuring the endometrium anterior–posteriorly (Fig. 38-1). An endometrial thickness of 4 mm or less has a 99% negative predictive value for endometrial cancer; however, patients who develop recurrent or persistent symptoms should undergo additional evaluation. Repeat transvaginal ultrasonography is not recommended for recurrent postmenopausal bleeding, and this is not the best next step for the patient in this scenario. Even if repeat imaging shows a thin endometrial lining, the recurrent bleeding warrants additional evaluation for an occult cancer and repeat imaging will not provide additional diagnostic information.

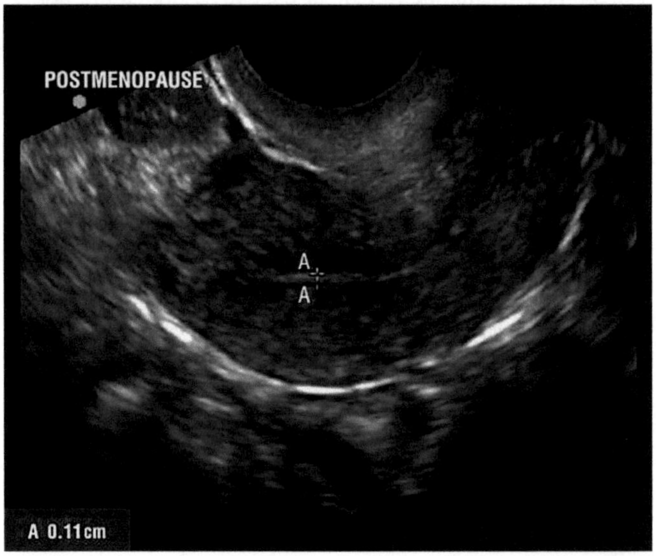

FIGURE 38-1. Assessment of endometrial thickness by ultrasonography. (Reprinted from The role of transvaginal ultrasonography in evaluating the endometrium of women with postmenopausal bleeding. ACOG Committee Opinion No. 734. American College of Obstetricians and Gynecologists. Obstet Gynecol 2018;131:e124–9. doi: 10.1097/AOG.0000000000002631)

The patient in this scenario is presenting with recurrent postmenopausal bleeding, and endometrial sampling is the best next step despite a thin endometrial lining on prior imaging. Although the negative predictive value of a thin endometrial lining is high, this test does not completely exclude cancer and is less effective for excluding non-endometrioid endometrial cancer. Sampling options include endometrial biopsy or dilation and curettage with or without hysteroscopy. Endometrial biopsy is commonly performed due to the ability to obtain pathologic sampling in the clinic and without anesthesia. If this testing also is negative for carcinoma, hysteroscopy with dilation and curettage is recommended to further exclude malignancy due to persistent symptoms.

Although vaginal and endometrial atrophy are the most common causes of postmenopausal bleeding, systemic or vaginal hormonal therapy is not recommended for patients with unexplained vaginal bleeding, such as this patient. Endometrial cancer can be hormonally responsive, and this malignancy should be excluded before prescribing hormone therapy. Once hyperplasia and cancer are excluded, patients can be offered hormone therapy based on their symptoms and findings. For those with evidence of vaginal atrophy, local low-dose estrogen is the preferred initial treatment.

Tranexamic acid is not recommended for the treatment of postmenopausal bleeding. This treatment is used for premenopausal heavy menstrual bleeding or chronic abnormal uterine bleeding to assist with decreasing menstrual blood loss or for management of acute heavy vaginal bleeding, which this patient is not experiencing.

The described patient has recurrent bleeding, and endometrial sampling is the best next step. Sampling also should be considered for patients with an increased risk for cancer or hyperplasia and in those with inconclusive ultrasonography. Inconclusive ultrasonographic findings may occur due to a distorted uterine cavity from fibroids or other structural abnormalities, or technical challenges in obtaining accurate measurements, such as obesity. Gynecologists also should recognize that disparities exist in endometrial cancer outcomes. When compared with White women in the United States, Black women are more likely to receive a diagnosis at a later stage, have more aggressive histology, and have lower 5-year survival rates. Multiple factors are thought to contribute to these disparities, including structural racial inequities in access to care, increased prevalence of leiomyoma among Black women compared with White women (which may distort the endometrial thickness measurement on ultrasonography), and the development of the endometrial thickness thresholds in non-Black populations. Additionally, although transvaginal ultrasonography is effective in excluding endometrioid endometrial cancer when the endometrial thickness is noted to be thin, it is less effective in excluding non-endometrioid subtypes, the latter of which are more common among Black women. Gynecologists should maintain a high index of suspicion for malignancy and evaluate patients with persistent or recurrent postmenopausal bleeding and otherwise normal ultrasonography with endometrial sampling.

Doll KM, Romano SS, Marsh EE, Robinson WR. Estimated performance of transvaginal ultrasonography for evaluation of postmenopausal bleeding in a simulated cohort of Black and White women in the US. JAMA Oncol 2021;7:1158–65. doi: 10.1001/jamaoncol.2021.1700

Long B, Clarke MA, Morillo AD, Wentzensen N, Bakkum-Gamez JN. Ultrasound detection of endometrial cancer in women with postmenopausal bleeding: systematic review and meta-analysis. Gynecol Oncol 2020;157:624–33. doi: 10.1016/j.ygyno.2020.01.032

The role of transvaginal ultrasonography in evaluating the endometrium of women with postmenopausal bleeding. ACOG Committee Opinion No. 734. American College of Obstetricians and Gynecologists. Obstet Gynecol 2018;131:e124–9. doi: 10.1097/AOG.0000000000002631

39 Deep vein thrombosis

A 58-year-old patient with a history of ovarian cancer presents to the clinic for a surveillance visit. She is taking a poly(ADP-ribose) polymerase (PARP) inhibitor after completion of primary taxane and platinum-based chemotherapy. She reports left calf pain that started a few days ago. On examination, her vital signs are within normal limits. Her physical examination is notable for an enlarged left calf that is tender to palpation. Bilateral venous Doppler ultrasonography shows a deep vein thrombosis (DVT). The best next step in treatment is

* (A) direct oral anticoagulant (DOAC)
(B) inferior vena cava filter placement
(C) low-molecular-weight heparin (LMWH)
(D) unfractionated heparin
(E) warfarin

Venous thromboembolism (VTE) is a significant source of morbidity and mortality for patients with cancer, including those with gynecologic malignancies, affecting up to 38% of individuals. In particular, the risk of recurrent VTE and major bleeding events is higher in patients with cancer than in those without cancer. Because of the increased risk of recurrence, longer duration of treatment with an anticoagulant must be considered. The risks of the development of DVT often are not easily modified. Major bleeding due to tumor volume or recent surgery may occur, which necessitates specific selection of anticoagulants for cancer patients.

For many years, the standard of care for a new diagnosis of cancer-associated VTE was admission to the hospital for an unfractionated heparin infusion or injection with transition to LMWH or oral warfarin for long-term outpatient therapy. Although LMWH requires undesirable subcutaneous injections, this class of drugs (enoxaparin) was proven to be superior to oral warfarin in the treatment of cancer-associated VTE in the Comparison of Low-molecular-weight heparin Versus Oral Anticoagulant Therapy for the Prevention of Recurrent Venous Thromboembolism in Patients With Cancer (CLOT) study more than 20 years ago. More recently, DOACs have evolved as an effective treatment for cancer-associated VTE.

Direct oral anticoagulants are a class of drugs that inhibit the ability of factor Xa or thrombin to work directly on the coagulation cascade. They have standard, consistent dosages, leading to more reliable pharmacokinetics. This allows for less variation in therapeutic levels based on underlying medical conditions and fewer food and drug interactions. The benefits of decreased laboratory monitoring and therapeutic range compared with warfarin are significant. In addition, the oral availability of DOACs avoids the burden of injections, leading to increased patient adherence compared to LMWH. Low-molecular-weight heparin is contraindicated in patients with renal disease (creatinine clearance less than 30 mL/min) due to the risk of accumulation of the drug. Direct oral anticoagulants vary in clearance throughout the renal system from 27% (apixaban) to 80% (dabigatran), but several have been shown to be safe in renal dysfunction (apixaban was the preferred choice). Apixaban, edoxaban, and rivaroxaban are acceptable DOAC options.

In 2021, the American College of Chest Physicians published a meta-analysis of randomized controlled trials showing that DOACs are not inferior to LMWH in patients with cancer-associated VTE. Subsequently, they updated their guidelines to recommend DOACs over LMWH except in the setting of luminal gastrointestinal malignancies. National Comprehensive Cancer Network guidelines also recommend DOACs over LMWH for patients without gastric or gastroesophageal lesions. The Society of Gynecologic Oncology has published a clinical practice statement concluding that DOACs are as effective as LMWH for the treatment of VTE and should be offered as initial therapy. Therefore, the correct option for the described patient is treatment with a DOAC.

In the absence of limb-threatening thrombus, hemodynamic instability, or major risk of bleeding, inpatient therapy for VTE is no longer indicated. A 2020 meta-analysis endorsed by the American Society of Hematology, which included seven randomized controlled trials with more than 1,900 patients, reported that outpatient management of uncomplicated VTE was not inferior to inpatient management with respect to outcomes of recurrent VTE and risk of major bleeding. It is more cost-effective to manage patients on an outpatient basis and may contribute to improved quality of life. Individual selection of anticoagulation should be based on renal clearance, ability to tolerate oral medications or do self-injections, and any potential drug–drug interactions. Individuals with intraluminal malignancy are at higher risk of bleeding with DOACs, which should be avoided in these patients.

Inferior vena cava filters placed by interventional radiologists have benefits for patients with DVT who are not candidates for anticoagulant therapy due to the risk of bleeding or anticipated surgical procedures. However, for this patient, who has no contraindications to anticoagulation, placement of an inferior vena cava filter is not the best answer.

The patient in this scenario is a candidate for outpatient anticoagulant therapy, and DOACs are the easiest to administer and do not require laboratory monitoring for therapeutic dosing (as warfarin does); therefore, the best option for the described patient is a DOAC.

Gressel GM, Marcus JZ, Mullen MM, Sinno AK. Direct oral anticoagulant use in gynecologic oncology: a Society of Gynecologic Oncology Clinical Practice Statement. Gynecol Oncol 2021;160:312–21. doi: 10.1016/j.ygyno.2020.11.020

Khatib R, Ross S, Kennedy SA, Florez ID, Ortel TL, Nieuwlaat R, et al. Home vs hospital treatment of low-risk venous thromboembolism: a systematic review and meta-analysis. Blood Adv 2020;4:500–13. doi: 10.1182/bloodadvances.2019001223

National Comprehensive Cancer Network. Cancer-associated venous thromboembolic disease. Version 2.2024. NCCN Clinical Practice Guidelines in Oncology [after login]. NCCN; 2024. Accessed February 24, 2025. https://www.nccn.org/guidelines/guidelines-detail?category=3&id=1423

Ortel TL, Neumann I, Ageno W, Beyth R, Clark NP, Cuker A, et al. American Society of Hematology 2020 guidelines for management of venous thromboembolism: treatment of deep vein thrombosis and pulmonary embolism. Blood Adv 2020;4:4693–738. doi: 10.1182/bloodadvances.2020001830

Stevens SM, Woller SC, Kreuziger LB, Bounameaux H, Doerschug K, Geersing G, et al. Antithrombotic therapy for VTE disease: second update of the CHEST guideline and expert panel report [published erratum appears in Chest 2022;162:269]. Chest 2021;160:e545–608. doi: 10.1016/j.chest.2021.07.055

40 Opioids in cancer-related pain

A 58-year-old patient with platinum-refractory ovarian cancer recently discontinued cancer-directed therapy. She has been seen in the clinic during the last several months with increasing pain due to progressive disease. She is eating and drinking without nausea or vomiting and is having regular bowel movements. For the last several weeks, she has been taking 15 mg of immediate-release oxycodone every 4 hours day and night in addition to over-the-counter pain medications. Her vital signs are normal, and her physical examination is notable for palpable abdominal masses with generalized tenderness but no rebound or guarding. The best next step in this patient's opioid treatment is to

(A) change to a different immediate-release opioid
(B) decrease the oxycodone dosing interval
(C) increase the oxycodone dose
(D) initiate intravenous opioids
* (E) initiate an extended-release opioid

Pain is one of the most common symptoms associated with advanced cancer, particularly at the end of life. *Cancer pain* or *cancer-related pain* are terms used to distinguish pain experienced by patients with cancer from pain experienced by those without malignancy. Treatment of cancer-related pain should be tailored to the individual patient, considering the severity of the pain, patient-specific goals, and the patient's tolerance to opioid therapy.

Although nonpharmacologic interventions may be valuable adjuncts, they rarely are sufficient for the management of cancer-related pain, particularly at the end of life, and pharmacologic analgesics remain the mainstay of cancer pain management. Although optimization of non-opioid medications, such as nonsteroidal anti-inflammatory drugs or acetaminophen, and selective use of other adjunctive agents can be useful for moderate or severe cancer pain, opioid therapy is the most effective option.

Opioid therapy consists of both immediate- and extended-release options. Immediate-release opioid therapy is appropriate for acute pain when quick relief is needed or when pain is expected to be of short duration. Patients with progressive cancer generally experience a persistent baseline level of pain with intermittent fluctuations in intensity. These patients often require higher doses for pain management as they near the end of life. Because of the significant pill burden, increasing dosages of immediate-release opioids can be overwhelming for patients or caregivers. High doses also can result in fluctuations in pain control due to the peaks and troughs created by the pharmacokinetics of immediate-release formulations. For patients with constant, progressive, cancer-related pain, extended-release opioids provide more continuous pain relief over an extended period. The sustained release helps maintain more stable blood levels of pain medication, reducing fluctuations in pain.

Extended-release opioid therapy includes methadone, transdermal fentanyl, and extended-release versions of oxycodone, hydromorphone, hydrocodone, and morphine. Because of the longer half-life and longer duration of potential adverse effects, extended-release opioids should be reserved for severe, continuous pain. They should be considered only for patients who have been receiving consistent, high doses of immediate-release opioids daily for several weeks. A reasonable dose threshold for transitioning patients to extended-release options would be patients using at least 60 morphine milligram equivalents (MME) daily. Changing from an immediate-release to an extended-release formulation requires safe but efficacious prescribing. Equianalgesic tables provide relative potency information about opioids and aid clinicians in calculating dosages when changing medications. This is done by calculating a patient's MME dose of their current medication to allow dose conversions. An MME conversion factor table, such as Table 40-1, can be used for dose conversion by first calculating a patient's daily dose in MME and then multiplying that by the conversion factor for the new medication. For safety, that dose initially is reduced by 30–50% to account for incomplete cross-tolerance and individual variability in opioid pharmacokinetics. Patients on extended-release opioid formulations also should be provided a *rescue dose* of immediate-release opioid to manage breakthrough exacerbations of pain. The rescue dose usually is equivalent to 10–20% of the total opioid daily dose. In many practice environments, access to palliative care providers or other specialists in pain management is available to assist in this transition.

This patient has progressive cancer and has been requiring regular, frequent doses of an immediate-release opioid for the management of her cancer pain. Transitioning to an extended-release opioid would provide more stable, continuous pain relief, and this is the best next step for this patient. Increasing the oxycodone dose or decreasing the interval between dosing would result in increased medication complexity and lead to increased fluctuation in medication levels.

TABLE 40-1. Morphine Milligram Equivalent Doses for Commonly Prescribed Opioids for Pain Management

OPIOID	CONVERSION FACTOR*
Codeine	0.15
Fentanyl transdermal (in micrograms/h)	2.4
Hydrocodone	1.0
Hydromorphone	5.0
Methadone	4.7
Morphine	1.0
Oxycodone	1.5
Oxymorphone	3.0
Tramadol[†]	0.2

*Multiply the dose for each opioid by the conversion factor to determine the dose in MME.

[†]Tramadol is a μ-receptor agonist and norepinephrine and serotonin reuptake inhibitor. MMEs are based on degree of μ-receptor agonist activity; however, it is unknown whether tramadol is associated with overdose in the same dose-dependent manner as observed with medications that are solely μ-receptor agonists.

Modified from Dowell D, Ragan KR, Jones CM, Baldwin GT, Chou R. CDC clinical practice guideline for prescribing opioids for pain United States, 2022. MMWR Recomm Rep 2022;71(No. RR-3):1–95. doi: 10.15585/mmwr.rr7103a1

The use of extended-release opioids simplifies the medication regimen, reducing the burden on patients and caregivers and minimizing disruptions, particularly throughout the night. Intravenous pain medications should be reserved for patients with acute pain crises that cannot be managed in the outpatient setting. Although this patient has worsening pain, she is stable and tolerating oral intake. Her pain can be safely managed with medication adjustments in an outpatient setting, and intravenous medication is not the correct answer choice for her.

Dowell D, Ragan KR, Jones CM, Baldwin GT, Chou R. CDC clinical practice guideline for prescribing opioids for pain United States, 2022. MMWR Recomm Rep 2022;71(No. RR-3):1–95. doi: 10.15585/mmwr.rr7103a1

National Comprehensive Cancer Network. Adult cancer pain. Version 1. 2025 NCCN Clinical Practice Guidelines in Oncology. NCCN; 2025. Accessed March 25, 2025. https://www.nccn.org/professionals/physician_gls/pdf/pain.pdf

41 Risk reduction for recurrent cervical dysplasia

A 31-year-old gravida 1, para 1, presents for follow-up after a loop electrosurgical excision procedure (LEEP) treatment for cervical intraepithelial neoplasia 3 (CIN 3). Her medical history is significant for obesity, with a BMI of 31. A physical examination reveals a well-healed cervical bed with no apparent lesions. Final pathology reveals cervical high-grade squamous intraepithelial lesion (HSIL [CIN 3]) with negative margins and negative endocervical curettings. She has a desire for future fertility but is not actively trying to get pregnant. She does not use tobacco and is in a monogamous, stable relationship. She asks how to decrease her risk of cervical dysplasia in the future. The best next step to reduce her risk of recurrence is

(A) dietary modifications
(B) herbal supplementation
* (C) human papillomavirus (HPV) vaccination
(D) repeat excisional procedure
(E) topical imiquimod

Patients treated for CIN of grade 2 or worse (CIN 2+) are at long-term risk of persistent or recurrent cervical dysplasia after surgical treatment. Although the HPV vaccine is primarily preventive, administering the HPV vaccine series as adjuvant treatment after an excisional procedure for CIN 2 or 3 has been associated with a 65% risk reduction of new or persistent CIN 2 or worse in previously unvaccinated individuals. The risk reduction is attributed to a decreased risk of re-infection or new infection with HPV. Given the safety profile of the vaccine and potential to decrease CIN recurrence risk, adjuvant HPV vaccination should be included as part of shared decision making for age-eligible patients.

Human papillomavirus vaccination is most effective when administered before exposure to HPV. The 9-valent HPV vaccine is the only HPV vaccine available in the United States and is U.S. Food and Drug Administration (FDA) approved for individuals aged 9–45 years. The target age for HPV vaccination is age 9–12 years, with earlier age at initiation associated with a higher likelihood of completing the series on time. The American College of Obstetricians & Gynecologists recommends following current Centers for Disease Control and Prevention recommendations regarding vaccination schedules. Individuals initiating vaccination younger than age 15 years should receive two doses of vaccine, at time 0 and then 6 months after the first dose. Those age 15 years and older should receive three doses, given at times 0, 1–2 months after the first dose, and 4 months after the second dose. Other countries are adopting a single-dose vaccination schedule for the youngest vaccination age groups, and this may be adopted in the United States in the future.

Human papillomavirus vaccination is not recommended during pregnancy. If a series is started and the patient becomes pregnant, completion of the series should be delayed until the pregnancy is complete. Manufacturers of the vaccine have established pregnancy registries to follow outcomes for those women who were mistakenly vaccinated. The vaccine can be given to breastfeeding individuals not previously vaccinated. If the vaccine series is started but subsequent doses are not administered on time, these doses can be administered as the opportunity arises without restarting the vaccination series. Currently, there is no recommendation for individuals who previously received the bivalent or quadrivalent HPV vaccine to be revaccinated with the 9-valent HPV vaccine.

For the described patient, who has already undergone treatment and would like to decrease her future risk of cervical dysplasia, proceeding with HPV immunization is the best next step. The immunization series can be started immediately and completed before the planned pregnancy. Figure 41-1 summarizes age-based recommendations for HPV vaccines.

Dietary changes have been evaluated for prevention of the progression of high-risk HPV infection. A 2018 study performed in Italy investigated dietary patterns and the association with HPV status and risk of CIN 2+. Adherence to a Mediterranean diet was associated with a significantly lower risk of high-risk HPV infection in age-adjusted (odds ratio [OR], 0.76) and multivariate-adjusted models (OR, 0.79). Those who ate a Westernized diet high in plant oils and processed meats had higher odds of high-risk HPV infection (OR, 1.77). The patient in this scenario can be counseled on dietary effects regarding HPV infection and clearance; however, dietary changes alone will not provide the greatest reduction in the recurrence of CIN 2+, and for this reason, this is not the best next treatment.

Herbal medicine has been studied as a supplement to clear HPV infections. Active hexose correlated compound (AHCC) is a proprietary, standardized extract of cultured *Lentinula edodes* mycelia that was developed in Japan in 1992. A randomized, double-blind, placebo-controlled study evaluated the use of AHCC supplements in 50 women older than age 30 years with confirmed persistent high-risk HPV infections. At the time of study completion, a total of 34 patients had received AHCC supplementation, and the overall response rate of cleared persistent HPV infections was 58.8%. This patient has completed treatment for CIN 3 and at this time does not appear to have a persistent HPV infection. Additionally, AHCC is not endorsed as a first-line standard treatment in the management of high-risk HPV infections, and it is not the best next step.

Repeat excisional procedures are acceptable when the first excision has positive margins, although ASCCP's preferred management is HPV-based testing at 6 months, irrespective of margin status, because the risk of HSIL persistence at 6 months is only 17%. Performance of colposcopy with endocervical curettage at the time of the 6-month HPV-based test also is acceptable. Loop electrosurgical excision procedure and cone procedures are associated with similar efficacy in disease control, and clinical judgment is needed when choosing which to use. A LEEP procedure tends to remove less tissue, preserving cervical stroma. For this reason, LEEP has been associated with a decreased risk of cervical insufficiency and obstetric complications when compared with conization. Because cone procedures use a scalpel, the tissue removed has clean edges to evaluate margin status. The surgeon can tailor the size of the cone to focus on known or suspected areas of disease and

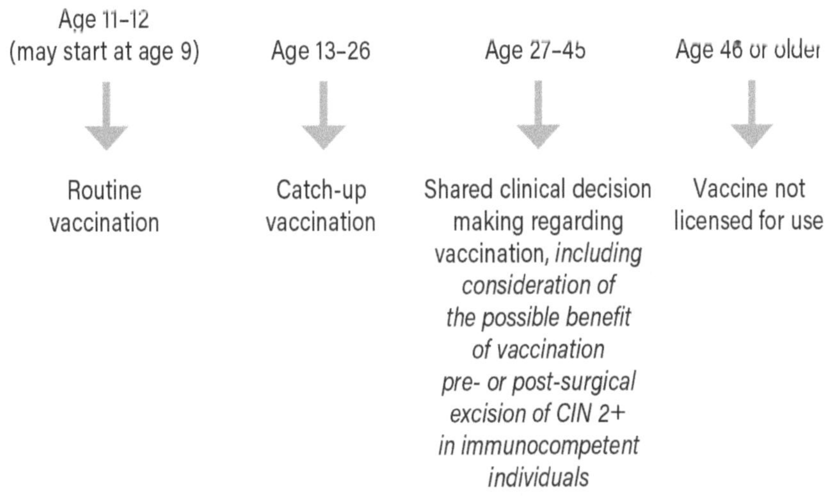

FIGURE 41-1. Recommendations for human papillomavirus vaccination based on age and shared clinical decision making. (Reprinted from Sharpless KE, Marcus JZ, Kuroki LM, Wiser AL, Flowers L. ASCCP committee opinion: adjuvant human papillomavirus vaccine for patients undergoing treatment for cervical intraepithelial neoplasia. J Low Genit Tract Dis 2023;27:93–6. doi: 10.1097/LGT.0000000000000703)

any anatomic variations in the cervical structure, especially after previous excision. Obstetric complications associated with excisional procedures include preterm birth and premature rupture of membranes. A 2022 meta-analysis evaluated 71 studies of local treatment of cervical disease and obstetric outcomes based on cone depth, and techniques that removed more tissue were associated with poorer outcomes. The relative risks for delivery at less than 37 weeks of gestation were 2.70 for conization and 1.56 for large loop excision. Compared with no treatment, the risk of preterm birth was higher in women who required more than one treatment and with increasing cone depth. Factors to consider when recommending a procedure include the ability for follow-up, preexisting anatomy and location of dysplasia, and fertility desires. The described patient desires future fertility and had negative margins; therefore, a repeat excisional procedure is not the correct management.

Topical imiquimod has been studied as a treatment for cervical HSIL compared with excisional procedure, but it has not been studied as an adjuvant treatment to decrease recurrent cervical HSIL. A study conducted among 123 women in the Netherlands noted successful treatment of CIN in 60% of patients in the imiquimod arm and 95% of women in the LEEP arm. Although imiquimod is not FDA approved for this indication and is not considered standard of care, this study provided evidence of the safety of this mode in treating cervical dysplasia. Topical imiquimod may be an alternative for treatment in women who desire to avoid surgical treatment of dysplasia or repeat excisional procedures. Although standardized guidelines are not available for the use of topical imiquimod, studies evaluating this treatment excluded those with prior confirmed CIN 3, concomitant vulvar or vaginal intraepithelial neoplasia, previous cervical malignancy, current malignant disease, immunodeficiency, pregnancy, or lactation. The described patient already has been treated for cervical HSIL, and imiquimod is not the best next step.

Given this patient's diagnosis of cervical HSIL (CIN 3) and desire to decrease the recurrence of dysplasia in the future, proceeding with HPV vaccination is the best option to potentially decrease the risk of recurrent preinvasive disease. Increasing HPV vaccination coverage nationwide will reduce the burden of HPV-associated diseases. A recommendation from a physician for HPV vaccination has the strongest influence on a patient's acceptance of the vaccine. Health care clinics should consider stocking HPV vaccines in their offices to reduce barriers to access.

Hendriks N, Koeneman MM, van de Sande AJ, Penders CG, Piek JM, Kooreman LF, et al. Topical imiquimod treatment of high-grade cervical intraepithelial neoplasia (TOPIC-3): a nonrandomized multicenter study. J Immunother 2022;45:180–6. doi: 10.1097/CJI.0000000000000414

Human papillomavirus vaccination. ACOG Committee Opinion No. 809. American College of Obstetricians and Gynecologists. Obstet Gynecol 2020;136:e15–21. doi: 10.1097/AOG.0000000000004000

Kyrgiou M, Athanasiou A, Paraskevaidi M, Mitra A, Kalliala I, Martin-Hirsch P, et al. Adverse obstetric outcomes after local treatment for cervical preinvasive and early invasive disease according to cone depth: systematic review and meta-analysis. BMJ 2016;354:i3633. doi: 10.1136/bmj.i3633

Perkins RB, Guido RS, Castle PE, Chelmow D, Einstein MH, Garcia F, et al. 2019 ASCCP risk-based management consensus guidelines for abnormal cervical cancer screening tests and cancer precursors [published erratum appears in J Low Genit Tract Dis 2020;24:427]. J Low Genit Tract Dis 2020;24:102–31. doi: 10.1097/LGT.0000000000000525

Sharpless KE, Marcus JZ, Kuroki LM, Wiser AL, Flowers L. ASCCP committee opinion: adjuvant human papillomavirus vaccine for patients undergoing treatment for cervical intraepithelial neoplasia. J Low Genit Tract Dis 2023;27:93–6. doi: 10.1097/LGT.0000000000000703

42 Identifying hereditary cancer syndromes

A 28-year-old woman presents for a well-woman examination. Her family history is significant for endometrial cancer in her mother, breast cancer in her maternal aunt, and colon cancer in her maternal grandfather. Her physical examination is notable for several cutaneous findings (Fig. 42-1). The patient's most likely gene mutation is

(A) *BRIP1*
(B) *MSH6*
* (C) *PTEN*
(D) *STK11*
(E) *TP53*

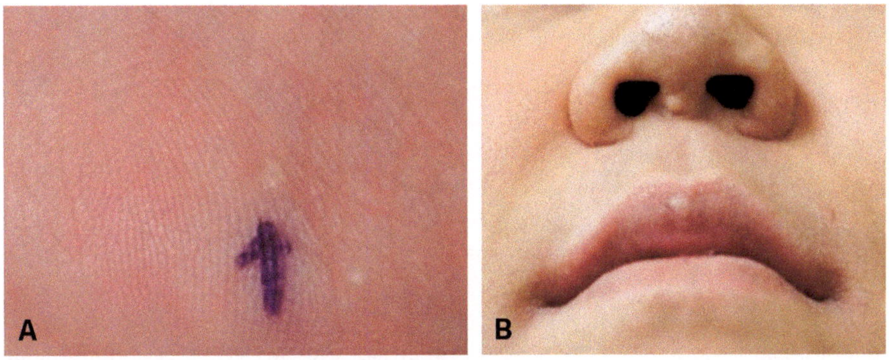

FIGURE 42-1. Patient's palm (A) and face (B). (Reprinted from Lee J, Shin DM, Oh SJ, Park J, Lee D. Ann Dermatol 2023;35:146–50. doi: 10.5021/ad.20.265)

Approximately 5–10% of all cancer can be attributed to a hereditary cancer syndrome. A *hereditary cancer syndrome* is a genetic predisposition to certain types of cancer due to inherited low-penetrance polymorphisms or a single-gene disorder. The most common hereditary cancer syndromes related to gynecologic cancer include hereditary breast and ovarian cancer syndrome, Lynch syndrome, Cowden syndrome, Peutz–Jeghers syndrome, and Li–Fraumeni syndrome (LFS) (Appendix K, Table K-1).

Cowden syndrome is part of the multiple hamartoma syndrome caused by autosomal-dominant mutations in the phosphatase and tensin (*PTEN*) gene, and is now referred to as *PTEN hamartoma tumor syndrome*. It is relatively rare, with a prevalence of 1 in 200,000. Individuals are at risk for breast, endometrial, colon, and thyroid cancer. Individuals typically present with pathognomonic skin lesions, including papules on the face, mucous membranes, and palms. Figure 42-1 illustrates these characteristic lesions. Multiple 1- to 2-mm flat-topped papules are around the patient's mouth and nose, and small whitish papules are on her palms. This patient exhibits these classic mucocutaneous lesions on physical examination and has a family history of the typical cancer associated with Cowden syndrome; therefore, *PTEN* mutation is the most likely gene mutation.

Hereditary breast and ovarian cancer syndromes are most commonly caused by autosomal-dominant mutations in the DNA repair genes *BRCA1* and *BRCA2*. Genes also involved in this pathway include *ATM*, *BRIP1*, *CDH1*, *CHEK2*, *NBN*, *NF1*, *PALB2*, *RAD51C*, and *RAD51D*, which are implicated in a significant number of cases of hereditary cancer, including as much as 25% of hereditary ovarian cancer. *BRIP1* is associated with increased ovarian cancer with an absolute risk of 5–15%; however, it is not associated with increased risk of breast or other cancer. This patient does not have a family history of ovarian cancer; therefore, a *BRIP1* mutation is unlikely to be the cause of her symptoms (Appendix K, Table K-2).

Lynch syndrome is the most common hereditary cause of endometrial cancer and colorectal cancer, accounting for 2–5% of all cases of each. It is the second most common cause of hereditary ovarian cancer. Lynch syndrome is a highly penetrant, autosomal-dominant hereditary cancer syndrome characterized by defects in mismatch repair genes, including *MLH1*, *PMS2*, *MSH2*, *MSH6*, and *EPCAM*. Other cancer associated with Lynch syndrome include cancer of the renal pelvis, small bowel, ureter, pancreas, and stomach. Although this patient does have a family history of endometrial and colon cancer, her physical examination findings and family history of breast cancer make Lynch syndrome less likely.

Peutz–Jeghers syndrome is characterized by gastrointestinal hamartomatous polyposis and mucocutaneous pigmentation in the oral mucosa, lips, nasal flares, fingers, and toes.

It is a rare autosomal-dominant syndrome with an incidence of 1 in 50,000–200,000 live births and is caused by a mutation in the tumor suppressor serine/threonine kinase 11 gene (*STK11*). Individuals with this syndrome are at increased risk of gastrointestinal cancer as well as a predominance of gynecologic malignancies. These malignancies include ovarian sex cord tumors with annular tubules, gastric-type cervical cancer, and breast cancer. This patient's examination is significant for papules but not the mucocutaneous pigmentation seen in more than 95% of individuals with Peutz–Jeghers syndrome.

Li–Fraumeni syndrome is an autosomal-dominant hereditary cancer syndrome caused by germline mutation resulting in the loss of function of the tumor suppressor gene *TP53*. Li–Fraumeni syndrome results in a 50-fold increased risk of developing certain types of cancer. The most common malignancies associated with LFS are colon, brain, osteosarcoma, leukemia, lymphoma, adrenocortical, gastric, and premenopausal breast cancer. The incidence of LFS is approximately 1 in 20,000 people, with more women than men affected. Endometrial cancer is not associated with LFS, and LFS is less likely in this patient.

Several hereditary cancer syndromes increase the risk of gynecologic malignancies. Obstetrician–gynecologists must be well-versed in these syndromes to effectively recognize and diagnose them in their patients. A comprehensive family history should be obtained, and when necessary, patients should be referred for genetic counseling and testing.

Hereditary breast and ovarian cancer syndrome. Practice Bulletin No. 182. American College of Obstetricians and Gynecologists. Obstet Gynecol 2017;130:e110–26. doi: 10.1097/AOG.0000000000002296

Hereditary cancer syndromes and risk assessment. ACOG Committee Opinion No. 793. American College of Obstetricians and Gynecologists. Obstet Gynecol 2019;134:e143–9. doi: 10.1097/AOG.0000000000003562

Kostov S, Watrowski R, Kornovski Y, Dzhenkov D, Slavchev S, Ivanova Y, et al. Hereditary gynecologic cancer syndromes a narrative review. Onco Targets Ther 2022;15:381–405. doi: 10.2147/OTT.S353054

Lee J, Shin DM, Oh SJ, Park J, Lee D. A case of Cowden syndrome presenting with diverse cutaneous manifestations. Ann Dermatol 2023;35:146–50. doi: 10.5021/ad.20.265

43 Abdominal wall hematoma

A 52-year-old patient presents to the emergency department for the abrupt onset of abdominal pain on her left side 3 days after a laparoscopic hysterectomy and bilateral salpingo-oophorectomy. Her medical history is notable for recurrent venous thromboembolism, and she resumed chronic anticoagulation with apixaban 24 hours after her surgery. On examination, the anterior abdominal wall surrounding the left laparoscopic port site is firm. The incision has opened, and there is scant dark red bleeding. She is tachycardic with a heart rate of 115 beats per minute. Her temperature and blood pressure are within normal limits. Her preoperative hemoglobin was 12 mg/dL, and a repeat hemoglobin in the emergency department is 9.5 mg/dL. Computed tomography (CT) with contrast is notable for a hematoma within the left rectus muscle with active extravasation. There is a small amount of complex fluid within the pelvis. She is given intravenous fluid resuscitation with a plan to hold anticoagulation. The best management of the abdominal wall hematoma is

(A) bedside closure of the port site
* (B) endovascular arterial embolization
(C) placement of percutaneous drain
(D) placement of a pressure dressing
(E) surgical exploration and evacuation

This patient has a diagnosis of rectus sheath hematoma secondary to vascular injury from laparoscopic port placement. Lateral laparoscopic ports may cause injury to the inferior epigastric artery or its branches, which can lead to bleeding within the rectus muscle and accumulation of a hematoma within the muscle sheath. Although most of the accumulation remains within the rectus sheath, because of the defect within the posterior rectus fascia from port placement, blood also may enter the peritoneal cavity. Patients on anticoagulation or with coagulation abnormalities are at increased risk for developing an abdominal wall hematoma. The diagnosis of rectus sheath hematoma is confirmed on imaging, and CT is the best imaging modality for verification. Although the diagnosis also can be made with ultrasonography, CT will show additional details about the location, size, and extent of the hematoma. When intravenous contrast is administered, active bleeding can be diagnosed by extravasation or blush of intravenous contrast, which may be important for treatment decisions.

Initial management of a patient with a rectus sheath hematoma should include assessing and stabilizing the patient's condition, including volume replacement and addressing coagulopathies if they exist. Patients on anticoagulation should have their anticoagulation stopped. Whether reversal agents should be administered depends on the degree of coagulopathy (such as the international normalized ratio level in patients on warfarin), degree of bleeding, and patient stability. If patients are unstable or have uncontrolled bleeding, reversal agents should be administered. The specific reversal agent will depend on the anticoagulant.

If no extravasation is noted on imaging, the patient is stable, and the hematoma is not growing, observation is a reasonable option because the pressure within the rectus sheath may impede further bleeding. However, if there is active extravasation on imaging, the hematoma is enlarging, or the patient is experiencing significant blood loss, intervention should be undertaken to stop the bleeding. Interventional radiology localization and arterial embolization is preferred to a surgical approach because open surgical localization of the bleeding vessel can be challenging and can lead to injury of additional vessels.

Additionally, endovascular embolization allows retention of the confined space within the rectus sheath, which can further tamponade the bleeding vessels. Interventional radiology embolization generally is accomplished by common femoral artery puncture with angiography to identify the area of bleeding with subsequent arterial embolization. If no visible extravasation is identified, empiric embolization of the proximal inferior epigastric artery generally is performed. The overall success rate of embolization is reported to be 90%, with most failures occurring in patients with severe underlying systemic disease leading to profound coagulopathy.

Once the bleeding stops and the patient is stable, treatment is directed at symptom management. Most hematomas reabsorb spontaneously, avoiding further intervention. If necessary, large hematomas can be drained percutaneously or, rarely, with surgical exploration. The most common complication after treatment of a hematoma is infection with development of an abscess, which requires drainage. For patients who were anticoagulated at the time of hematoma formation, resumption of anticoagulation will depend on the reason for anticoagulation, patient stability, and the patient's underlying disease, such as active malignancy. For most patients, anticoagulation can be resumed once bleeding has stopped and hemoglobin levels have stabilized. Patients on anticoagulation are at an increased risk for recurrent bleeding, particularly when managed conservatively.

The described patient is on therapeutic anticoagulation, and her imaging shows active bleeding into a rectus sheath hematoma. The patient is presenting to a tertiary care emergency department where interventional radiology services should be available, and the most appropriate treatment for this hematoma is endovascular arterial embolization. As discussed above, this has many advantages over open surgical exploration and evacuation, making that an incorrect answer in this situation. If this patient were presenting to a facility without the ability to perform endovascular embolization, stabilization, reversal of anticoagulation with andexanet alpha, and open surgical exploration and evacuation may be the correct approach.

Although there is some drainage of the hematoma through the port site, closure of the port site will not address the bleeding from the deeper abdominal wall vasculature, and this is not the best management. Likewise, pressure dressing often is used for superficial bleeding at an incision site, such as from the skin edge or subcutaneous tissues. Although it may be used as an adjunct in the case of rectus hematoma, bleeding within the abdominal wall is not sufficiently managed with pressure alone, and this is not the best management for this patient.

Shikhman A, Tuma F. Abdominal hematoma. In: StatPearls. StatPearls Publishing; 2025. Accessed March 13, 2025. https://www.ncbi.nlm.nih.gov/books/NBK519551/

Sobkin PR, Bloom AI, Wilson MW, LaBerge JM, Hastings GS, Gordon RL, et al. Massive abdominal wall hemorrhage from injury to the inferior epigastric artery: a retrospective review. J Vasc Interv Radiol 2008;19:327–32. doi: 10.1016/j.jvir.2007.11.004

44 Recurrent vulvar pruritus

An 88-year-old woman presents with vulvar pruritus. She has multiple medical comorbidities, including congestive heart failure and chronic obstructive pulmonary disease (COPD). Her examination findings are shown in Figure 44-1A and -1B. Five years ago, she underwent an excision of a similar right vulvar lesion. Vulvar and perineal biopsies are obtained at her current visit (Fig. 44-2A and -2B) and are consistent with pathology from her previous excision 5 years ago. The best next step is

* (A) topical imiquimod
(B) Mohs micrographic surgical excision
(C) simple vulvectomy
(D) radical vulvectomy
(E) external beam radiotherapy

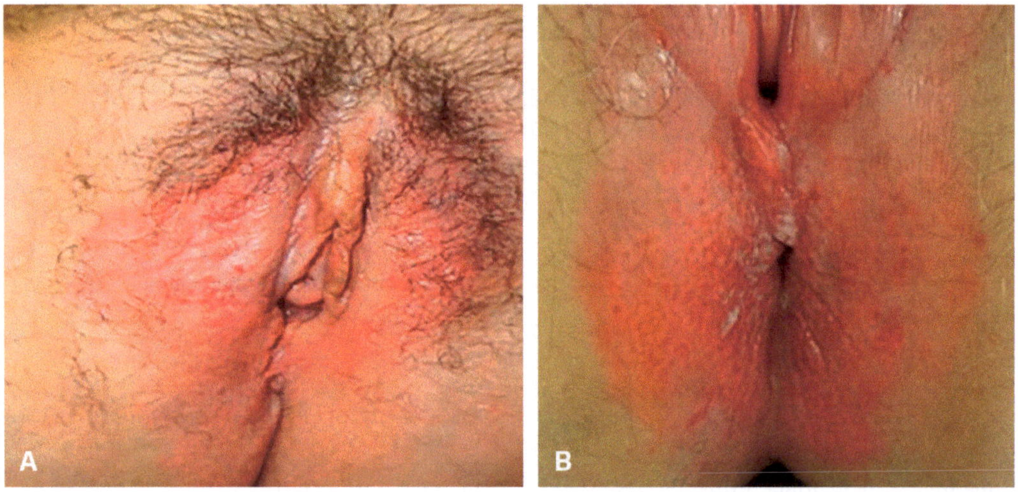

FIGURE 44-1. A. Vulvar examination findings. (Reprinted from Mayo-Martínez F, Moro R, Millán-Esteban D, Ríos-Viñuela E, Bautista IJ, Nagore E, et al. Topical imiquimod in primary cutaneous extramammary Paget's disease: a systematic review. Cancers (Basel) 2023;15:5665. doi: 10.3390/cancers15235665). B. Perineal and perianal examination findings. (Reprinted from Santos MD, Soares F, Presa-Fernandes JM, Silva DS. Perianal Paget disease: different entities with the same name. Cureus 2021;13:e15161. doi: 10.7759/cureus.15161)

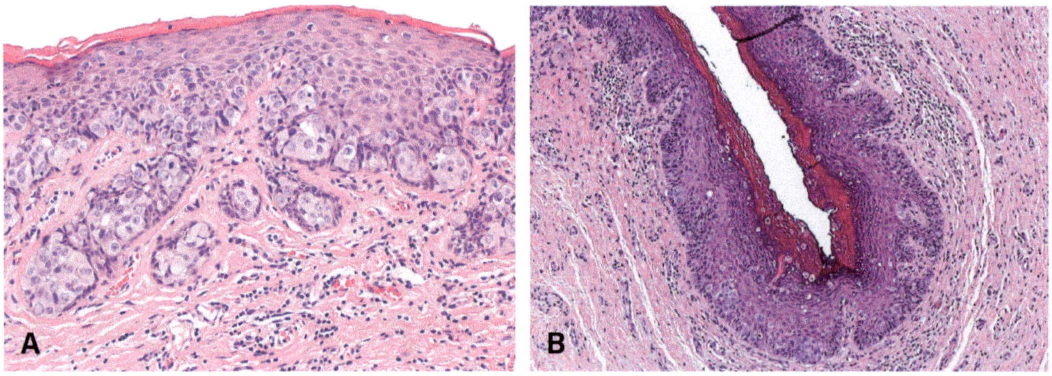

FIGURE 44-2. A. Representative vulvar biopsy: low-power magnification. (Reprinted from Mayo-Martínez F, Moro R, Millán-Esteban D, Ríos-Viñuela E, Bautista IJ, Nagore E, et al. Topical imiquimod a primary cutaneous extramammary Paget's disease: a systematic review. Cancers (Basel) 2023;15:5665. doi: 10.3390/cancers15235665). B. Representative vulvar biopsy with high-power magnification. (Reprinted from Salari E, Ma L. Vulva and vagina: other carcinomas, Paget disease. Pathology Outlines; 2024. Accessed March 17, 2025. https://www.pathologyoutlines.com/topic/vulvapagetsdisease.html. Courtesy of PathologyOutlines.com, contributed by Priya Nagarajan, MD, PhD)

The patient in this scenario has a recurrence of primary, noninvasive extramammary Paget disease (EMPD) of the vulva. Figure 44-1A and -1B depicts typical physical examination findings of erythematous, eczematous, and thickened epidermis. The visibly involved epithelium in this case appears extensive and includes the bilateral vulva as well as the perineum and perianus. On biopsy, an in situ adenocarcinoma is seen. Large, pale, vacuolated cells originating within the lower layers of the epidermis are scattered widely and extend upward toward the surface. There is no evidence for invasion of the Paget cells into the underlying tissue on the biopsy depicted. In practice, immunohistochemical stains also can be used to confirm the diagnosis of recurrent Paget disease and distinguish it from other entities on the differential.

Vulvar EMPD is a rare entity that can present significant diagnostic ambiguity due to its varied pathogenesis. Additional misperceptions may exist regarding the potential natural history of this disease, which can lead to some uncertainty in determining the best management practices. This is particularly evident in the setting of vulvar EMPD. The etiologic distinctions in Box 44-1 are helpful to understand this disease.

The most common form of EMPD that gynecologists diagnose is primary to the vulva (cutaneous) and is noninvasive, and this is the diagnosis of the described patient. Several classification systems for EMPD have been proposed (for one example, see Box 44-2).

Primary vulvar EMPD is an intraepithelial adenocarcinoma that often is associated with pruritus and burning vulvar pain of varying degrees. It has a relatively indolent biology and remains confined to the epidermis in most cases. Progression to underlying invasive EMPD is uncommon, occurring in fewer than 10% of cases of primary vulvar EMPD. Before initiating treatment for vulvar EMPD, a survey to screen for adenocarcinoma is warranted. This may include mammogram, colonoscopy, gynecologic screening, urine cytology, and cystoscopy.

Wide local excision (simple vulvectomy) is the cornerstone of therapy for primary vulvar EMPD. The goal is excision of the lesion with negative margins at pathology. Only the epidermis, dermis, and the superficial aspect of the underlying subcutaneous tissue are removed in wide local excision; however, the disease often is multifocal and typically extends microscopically beyond the visibly abnormal area seen on physical examination. The persistence and recurrence of noninvasive vulvar EMPD after surgical excision are common. True recurrence risks are difficult to define accurately, ranging from 20% to 75% in the literature, with published reports being influenced by both the length and the intensity of surveillance methods used in their follow-up.

The management of recurrent vulvar EMPD requires careful consideration and counseling. Given the frequency of recurrence, patients are vulnerable to repeated operations that can have significant physical, functional, sexual, and psychological consequences. Alternative therapies exist for patients when surgery is not advised. Decisions about therapeutic interventions for recurrence should be individualized. Treatment decisions in these situations must simultaneously manage the patient's vulvar symptoms and the risk for progression to invasive cancer

BOX 44-1

Etiologic Distinctions of Extramammary Paget Disease

1. Etiologic distinction of extramammary Paget disease (EMPD) is histologically similar to mammary Paget disease, but with key differences in the location of the skin manifestations as well as in its association with underlying malignancy. In mammary Paget disease, the rash occurs around the areolar skin and nipple area and is almost always associated with an underlying breast carcinoma. In EMPD, rashes most commonly affect the vulva, but also can affect the perianus, axilla, penis, and scrotum. Moreover, although more than 90% of mammary Paget disease is associated with an underlying carcinoma, EMPD is far less commonly associated with an underlying malignancy.
2. In vulvar EMPD, the cells typically originate from the pluripotent intraepidermal stem cells. Alternatively, they can migrate directly from the underlying glandular cells of the skin and appendages. More rarely, it can emerge as a metastatic event to the vulva. Thus, an initial distinction in vulvar EMPD is whether the condition is 1) primary to the vulva (cutaneous origin) or 2) secondarily involving the vulva (non-cutaneous origin, most commonly gastrointestinal or genitourinary). Primary cutaneous Paget disease is far more common, representing more than 95% of cases diagnosed.
3. Primary vulvar Paget disease typically occurs spontaneously. Less commonly, it develops as a paraneoplastic phenomenon manifesting as an abnormal response to an underlying neoplasm that exists elsewhere at a distant site. The potential of vulvar EMPD to be either a metastatic event or a paraneoplastic phenomenon compels clinicians to investigate for a malignant process outside of the vulva. Often this includes additional screening at initial diagnosis to exclude underlying malignancy outside the vulva.
4. Cases of vulvar EMPD that are of primary cutaneous origin can have either in situ (noninvasive) or invasive forms. The noninvasive forms represent more than 90% of primary vulvar EMPD.

BOX 44-2

Proposed Wilkinson Classification System

Type I: Paget disease of primary cutaneous origin

- **Ia:** as a primary intraepithelial neoplasm
- **Ib:** as an intraepithelial neoplasm with subsequent invasion
- **Ic:** as a manifestation of underlying adenocarcinoma of skin appendage or vulval glandular origin

Type II: Paget disease of noncutaneous origin

- **IIa:** secondary to anorectal carcinoma
- **IIb:** secondary to urothelial neoplasia
- **IIc:** as a manifestation of another noncutaneous carcinoma: endocervical, endometrial or ovarian adenocarcinoma, etc.

Reprinted from Wilkinson EJ, Brown HM. Vulvar Paget disease of urothelial origin: a report of three cases and a proposed classification of vulvar Paget disease. Hum Pathol 2002;33:549–54. doi: 10.1053/hupa.2002.124788 and must consider the balance between treatment efficacy and treatment-related morbidity. Patient age and medical fitness also will influence best-care decisions.

There is increasing evidence supporting the safety and efficacy of topical 5% imiquimod for the management of recurrent vulvar EMPD, and it is the most appropriate next step in this patient's treatment, given her age, medical comorbid conditions, and the extent of the lesion that needs to be treated. Imiquimod is an immune response modifier that activates Toll-like receptor 7 on immune cells within the skin, prompting these cells to produce cytokines that initiate an immune response against abnormal cells within the epithelium. It is approved by the U.S. Food and Drug Administration for the treatment of anogenital warts, actinic keratosis, and superficial basal cell carcinomas. Gynecologic oncologists often use it as a therapy for additional conditions, such as vulvar, vaginal, and cervical intraepithelial neoplasia and vulvar EMPD. Efficacy data shows response rates that range from 50% to 65%. The duration of the responses is not well understood. The frequency of application and the length of use vary greatly in the studies. In practice, dosage depends on the severity of the lesions, the findings at interval of response assessment, and the tolerance of the treatment. Typically, topical imiquimod is self-administered to affected skin one to three times per week, with reassessment examinations recommended at 3- to 4-month intervals.

Although it is generally well tolerated, topical imiquimod may cause local skin reactions at the application site (redness, itching, burning, swelling, flaking). These adverse effects are usually mild to moderate and usually are resolved by modifying the frequency of application. Topical imiquimod provides the ideal balance of efficacy and treatment-associated toxicity in the patient described in this scenario, and it is the best next step in her treatment.

Because this patient is 88 years old with congestive heart failure and extensive involvement of EMPD on the vulva and perianus, surgery carries a higher risk of morbidity. Excising the entire diseased area with a simple vulvectomy to obtain adequate surgical margins would require removing extensive portions of the bilateral vulva as well as the epithelium of the perineum and perianus. An extensive surgery of this kind for a relatively indolent in situ lesion would not be the best next step for this frail patient.

A radical vulvectomy typically would be appropriate for a diagnosis of invasive cancer. In this procedure, the affected vulvar area is excised with additional care to achieve both wider and deeper surgical margins. A radical vulvectomy often is combined with the removal of inguinal lymph nodes to evaluate for regional cancer metastasis. The patient in this scenario does not have invasive vulvar EMPD; therefore, neither the deeper margin of a radical vulvectomy nor lymphadenectomy is necessary, and this is not the best next step for this patient.

Mohs surgery is a specialized surgical technique used primarily for the treatment of skin cancer, often for lesions in a cosmetically sensitive area. Mohs surgery is an iterative process of tissue removal, mapping, processing, microscopic examination, and subsequent additional tissue removal when positive margins are encountered. Although Mohs surgery offers real-time margin assessment during surgery to optimize the success of achieving negative margins, it is time-consuming and unrealistic for large and geographically extensive lesions of the kind in this patient's scenario. Given the perianal involvement of the disease, negative surgical margins would be difficult to achieve, and an attempt would risk anal scarring and permanent stricture. For these reasons, Mohs surgery is not the best next step.

Radiation therapy is a valuable adjunct to the management of typical invasive squamous cell carcinoma of the vulva. It is used for a variety of clinical situations as primary therapy, adjuvant therapy, or for disease recurrence. Radiation, however, is typically not used as a primary treatment for in situ or preinvasive vulvar diseases, and there are no aggregated data on its efficacy in recurrent in situ Paget disease.

Vulvar Paget disease is a challenging entity from a diagnostic and a treatment standpoint. Primary management often is surgical, but recurrence rates are high and repetitive surgical interventions have consequences. Nonsurgical options for recurrent vulvar Paget disease are evolving and increasingly being used as an alternative to surgery, but additional therapeutic options are needed. Ongoing research is investigating new topical therapies that could be added to our current limited armamentarium.

Caruso G, Barcellini A, Mazzeo R, Gallo R, Vitale MG, Passarelli A, et al. Vulvar Paget's disease: a systematic review of the MITO Rare Cancer Group. Cancers (Basel) 2023;15:1803. doi: 10.3390/cancers.15061803

Kibbi N, Owen JL, Worley B, Wang JX, Harikumar V, Downing MB, et al. Evidence-based clinical practice guidelines for extramammary Paget disease. JAMA Oncol 2022;8:618–28. doi: 10.1001/jamaoncol.2021.7148

Snast I, Sharon E, Kaftory R, Noyman Y, Oren-Shabtai M, Lapidoth M, et al. Nonsurgical treatments for extramammary Paget disease: a systematic review and meta-analysis. Dermatology 2020;236:493–9. doi: 10.1159/000506832

Wilkinson EJ, Brown HM. Vulvar Paget disease of urothelial origin: a report of three cases and a proposed classification of vulvar Paget disease. Hum Pathol 2002;33:549–54. doi: 10.1053/hupa.2002.124788

45 Malignant ovarian germ cell tumor

A 33-year-old gravida 2, para 2, presents with a 4-month history of right lower quadrant pain, bloating, and constipation. She has no medical comorbidities and has completed childbearing. Her physical examination is significant for an enlarged right ovary, and ultrasonography reveals a 12-cm complex cyst with a hyperechoic solid nodule. She undergoes a laparoscopic right salpingo-oophorectomy, and an intraoperative frozen section reveals an immature teratoma. A total hysterectomy, left salpingo-oophorectomy, lymphadenectomy, and peritoneal biopsies are performed for surgical staging. The final pathology confirms an immature teratoma with high-grade neural elements confined to the right ovary. The best treatment to prevent disease recurrence is

* (A) bleomycin, etoposide, and cisplatin (BEP)
(B) carboplatin and paclitaxel
(C) external beam radiotherapy
(D) megestrol acetate
(E) pembrolizumab

Malignant ovarian germ cell tumors (GCTs) account for 2–5% of all ovarian malignancies. Sixty percent are confined to the ovary at the time of surgery, and the 5-year survival exceeds 95%. Germ cell tumors are divided into three main categories: 1) primitive GCTs, 2) teratomas, and 3) monodermal and somatic-type tumors associated with dermoid cysts (Box 45-1). Teratomas include benign mature teratomas and malignant immature teratomas.

Most immature teratomas, similar to other GCTs, are unilateral and often present with stage I disease. Immature teratomas are graded on a scale from 1 to 3 based on the amount of immature neuroepithelium. Like other types of ovarian cancer, immature teratomas appear to be confined to the ovary (ie, stage I disease), and patients should undergo surgical staging. The extent of staging will depend on the intraoperative findings and the fertility desires of the patient. For patients who have completed childbearing, total hysterectomy, bilateral salpingo-oophorectomy, lymphadenectomy, peritoneal biopsies, and pelvic washings should be performed. Fertility preservation is a viable option given that most cases are unilateral, diagnosed at an early stage (stage I), and respond well to adjuvant chemotherapy. Fertility-sparing surgical staging should include unilateral salpingo-oophorectomy, lymphadenectomy, peritoneal biopsies, and pelvic washings. In the pediatric population, lymphadenectomy often is omitted if not pathologically enlarged on imaging and at the time of surgery. In all fertility-sparing cases, the contralateral ovary should be carefully inspected, and if it appears normal, biopsy is not recommended. Every attempt should be made to preserve the contralateral ovary and uterus.

Recurrence risk of immature teratomas is associated with tumor grade, and reoccurance rates are as high as 70% in those with high-grade tumors. Adjuvant chemotherapy is recommended for adult patients with high-grade immature teratomas regardless of stage, given the high recurrence rates. Studies in adult patients have shown decreased risk of recurrence for patients who received adjuvant chemotherapy compared with those who underwent surveillance alone.

In contrast, children and adolescents with immature teratomas are treated with postoperative surveillance regardless of grade or stage. Studies in the pediatric population show that surgical excision alone is effective for most patients. Those with recurrences often are cured with surgery, chemotherapy, or both. There is an ongoing prospective randomized trial exploring the role of chemotherapy in immature teratomas in both pediatric and adult patients, and the results of this trial could lead to a shift in treatment paradigms for all age groups.

For immature teratomas, platinum-based adjuvant chemotherapy is associated with a 5-year overall survival rate of

BOX 45-1

Classification of Germ Cell Tumors of the Ovary

Benign
- Dermoid tumors (mature tissues derived from one germ cell layer)
- Mature teratomas (mature tissues derived from two or three germ cell layers)

Malignant
- Primitive germ cell tumors
  - Dysgerminoma
  - Yolk sac tumor
  - Embryonal carcinoma
  - Nongestational choriocarcinoma
- Immature teratoma

Data from Veneris JT, Mahajan P, Frazier AL. Contemporary management of ovarian germ cell tumors and remaining controversies. Gynecol Oncol 2020;158:467–75. doi: 10.1016/j.ygyno.2020.05.007

100%. Bleomycin, etoposide, and cisplatin is the preferred combined chemotherapy regimen. Etoposide and cisplatin is an option for patients in whom bleomycin should be avoided, such as those with significant smoking history, reduced renal function, or pre-existing lung disease. This patient does not have any of the above; therefore, BEP is the treatment of choice to reduce her risk of recurrence.

Although carboplatin and paclitaxel are commonly used in other gynecologic malignancies, this regimen has not been studied in individuals with GCTs, including immature teratomas, and it is not the first-line adjuvant treatment for this patient.

Radiotherapy often was used as adjuvant treatment for patients with GCTs in the past, particularly in dysgerminomas. Recent advances with combination chemotherapy have led to a decline in radiation use for this patient population. Radiation therapy carries a higher risk of premature ovarian failure compared with chemotherapy and also is associated with an increased risk of secondary malignancies. For these reasons, it is a less favorable option in the first-line management of ovarian GCTs and is not the best next step to reduce the risk of recurrence in this patient with a high-grade, immature teratoma.

Adjuvant hormonal therapy, such as megestrol acetate, is an effective treatment option in tumors with high levels of hormonal receptor expression, as seen in endometrioid tumors for example. Germ cell tumors do not frequently express hormonal receptors and are not used as adjuvant therapy for malignant GCTs like immature teratomas.

Immunotherapy agents, such as pembrolizumab, are increasingly used in the treatment for advanced, metastatic gynecologic cancer. Pembrolizumab has been studied in advanced and metastatic GCTs. It has been found to have limited antitumor activity likely secondary to the low tumor mutational burden found in GCTs. Pembrolizumab is not the treatment of choice to reduce recurrence risk in the adjuvant setting.

Germ cell tumors, including immature teratoma, typically are diagnosed at stage I, and many patients have excellent prognoses. Recurrence risk is considerable in individuals with high-grade immature teratomas, and adjuvant treatment with BEP is recommended by the National Comprehensive Cancer Network to reduce this risk.

El Helali A, Kwok GS, Tse KY. Adjuvant and post-surgical treatment in non-epithelial ovarian cancer. Best Pract Res Clin Obstet Gynaecol 2022;78:74–85. doi: 10.1016/j.bpobgyn.2021.06.001

Salani R, Khanna N, Frimer M, Bristow RE, Chen L. An update on post-treatment surveillance and diagnosis of recurrence in women with gynecologic malignancies: Society of Gynecologic Oncology (SGO) recommendations. Gynecol Oncol 2017;146:3–10. doi: 10.1016/j.ygyno.2017.03.022

Veneris JT, Mahajan P, Frazier AL. Contemporary management of ovarian germ cell tumors and remaining controversies. Gynecol Oncol 2020;158:467–75. doi: 10.1016/j.ygyno.2020.05.007

46 Surgical management of borderline tumor

A 37-year-old underwent a right ovarian cystectomy for a 12-cm complex left adnexal mass. The contralateral ovary was normal appearing, and no extraovarian disease was noted. Intraoperative rupture of the mass occurred. Pathology demonstrated a serous borderline tumor with micropapillary features. Her risk of recurrence is increased most by

(A) her age
(B) intraoperative rupture
(C) micropapillary architecture
* (D) ovarian cystectomy
(E) size of mass

Borderline tumors are atypical proliferative ovarian tumors differentiated histologically from ovarian carcinoma by the absence of stromal invasion. Compared with the prognosis for patients with invasive ovarian carcinoma, the prognosis for patients with borderline tumors is excellent, with survival rates of 100% at 5 years and 96% at 10 years for patients with stage I disease, and 98% at 5 years and 88% at 10 years for patients with stage III disease.

Serous tumors comprise most borderline tumors, although mucinous tumors are more common in Asian populations. The tumors are bilateral in 15–40% of patients and associated with extraovarian disease in 15–35% of patients. Among patients with borderline tumors with peritoneal implants, the implants are noninvasive in 85% of patients. In contrast, peritoneal implants associated with primary ovarian mucinous borderline tumors are rare, and the European Society for Medical Oncology and European Society of Gynaecological Oncology state that extraovarian disease associated with a mucinous borderline tumor is likely a metastasis from either an undetected focus of carcinoma within the ovary or a mucinous carcinoma in another organ.

Surgical treatment involves complete removal of visible disease but otherwise is largely determined by patient age and fertility plans. Given a median age at diagnosis of 46 years, borderline tumors frequently occur in patients of childbearing age, and many patients undergo fertility-sparing surgery with ovarian cystectomy or unilateral salpingo-oophorectomy, both of which are considered adequate treatment for apparent early-stage disease. Cystectomy often is done to preserve the ovary, although hormone levels and fertility potential typically remain the same after unilateral salpingo-oophorectomy, provided the contralateral ovary is normal. Cystectomy is associated with a 30% recurrence risk, compared with a 5–10% recurrence risk after unilateral salpingo-oophorectomy. The diagnosis of borderline tumor often is not established until after surgery when final pathology results become available. Reoperation for removal of the involved ovary after cystectomy may be appropriate for some patients, depending on their age and fertility wishes. Among patients with mucinous tumors, evidence of microinvasion (invasion of less than 5 mm) has been associated with a higher risk of malignant recurrence. Because recurrence with mucinous carcinoma often is fatal due to its resistance to treatment, completion oophorectomy is recommended for mucinous borderline tumors with microinvasion treated by cystectomy.

Among patients who do not desire fertility, surgical removal is achieved by unilateral or bilateral salpingo-oophorectomy with or without elective hysterectomy, depending on laterality of disease, patient age, and preferences. Historically, removal of remaining ovarian tissue on completion of childbearing has been recommended for patients with a history of borderline tumor, but there are no data demonstrating benefit from this practice. For a patient who underwent a unilateral salpingo-oophorectomy but does not desire future childbearing, it is questionable whether the potential benefit of reoperation to remove remaining ovarian tissue outweighs the known risks of surgery and potential increased risks of other morbidities, including cardiovascular disease and dementia, which have been associated with bilateral salpingo-oophorectomy.

Reoperation for the purpose of staging in patients with apparent early-stage disease is difficult to justify because the only finding that would significantly change management is the discovery of invasive implants. In patients with advanced disease and extraovarian disease incompletely resected at primary surgery, reoperation to remove residual disease is appropriate to reduce the risk of recurrence and assess for invasive implants. Surgical removal is especially important for invasive implants because they tend to respond poorly to chemotherapy. Gross residual noninvasive disease also has been associated with an increased risk of invasive recurrence.

The described patient has an apparent stage I serous borderline tumor. Her tumor was removed by cystectomy, which confers a risk of recurrence of approximately 30%, and this is the factor that has the greatest influence on her risk of recurrence.

Intraoperative rupture has been reported to be associated with recurrence among patients with early-stage invasive epithelial ovarian cancer in some studies, but other studies have not found it to predict recurrence independent of other prognostic factors. Because of the distinctly different biology of borderline tumors, extrapolation of data from invasive ovarian cancer to borderline cancer is highly questionable. There is little direct evidence demonstrating that intraoperative rupture of borderline tumors influences recurrence risk.

The size of an adnexal mass does not predict the recurrence of a borderline tumor. Mucinous tumors are on average larger at presentation than serous tumors, but mucinous tumors are rarely associated with extraovarian disease. Because they are more often bilateral and associated with extraovarian disease, recurrence is more common among serous tumors.

Older age is not a predictor of recurrence independent of other prognostic factors. In a retrospective analysis of 950 patients, age of less than 40 years was a risk factor for recurrence, but this was attributable to a higher proportion of women undergoing fertility-sparing surgery. Although the risk of recurrence was higher among younger patients, when the disease recurred in older patients, it was more likely to be extraovarian and invasive. For the described patient, who is 47 years old, the fact that she had a cystectomy, not her age, is the most significant risk factor for recurrence overall.

Micropapillary architecture is found in a subset of serous borderline tumors. Tumors displaying a micropapillary pattern more often are associated with advanced stage, bilateral disease, residual disease, microinvasion, and invasive implants compared with serous tumors without micropapillary architecture. Although controversy persists over whether micropapillary architecture is an independent prognostic factor for recurrence, recent analyses suggest that it does not predict recurrence in the absence of invasive implants.

Chevrot A, Héquet D, Fauconnier A, Huchon C. Impact of surgical restaging on recurrence in patients with borderline ovarian tumors: a meta-analysis. Eur J Obstet Gynecol Reprod Biol 2020;248:227–32. doi: 10.1016/j.ejogrb.2020.03.023

Colombo N, Sessa C, du Bois A, Ledermann J, McCluggage WG, McNeish I, et al. ESMO-ESGO consensus conference recommendations on ovarian cancer: pathology and molecular biology, early and advanced stages, borderline tumours and recurrent disease. Int J Gynecol Cancer 2019;29:728–60. doi: 10.1136/ijgc-2019-000308

Morice P, Uzan C, Fauvet R, Gouy S, Duvillard P, Darai E. Borderline ovarian tumour: pathological diagnostic dilemma and risk factors for invasive or lethal recurrence. Lancet Oncol 2012;13:e103-15. doi: 10.1016/S1470-2045(11)70288-1

Trillsch F, Mahner S, Woelber L, Vettorazzi E, Reuss A, Ewald-Riegler N, et al. Age-dependent differences in borderline ovarian tumours (BOT) regarding clinical characteristics and outcome: results from a sub-analysis of the Arbeitsgemeinschaft Gynaekologische Onkologie (AGO) ROBOT study. Ann Oncol 2014;25:1320–7. doi: 10.1093/annonc/mdu119

47 Diarrhea

A 67-year-old patient with ovarian cancer presents with worsening diarrhea 14 days after cytoreductive surgery. She reports 2 days of watery diarrhea with associated abdominal cramping. In the office, she has normal vital signs with mild abdominal tenderness and no rebound or guarding. Her serum laboratory values are within normal limits, her computed tomography result is unremarkable, and her stool cultures reveal a gram-positive, spore-forming anaerobic bacterium. The best management for this condition is to administer

(A) bezlotoxumab
* (B) fidaxomicin
(C) metronidazole
(D) tigecycline
(E) vancomycin

Clostridioides difficile (formerly known as *Clostridium difficile*) is a gram-positive, spore-forming anaerobic bacterium and is the most common cause of health care-associated diarrhea in the developed world. Infection with *C difficile* is associated with significant morbidity and mortality, particularly in older adults and those who are immunocompromised. Appropriate diagnosis and management of *C difficile* colitis are important.

Upon diagnosis of *C difficile* colitis, all concomitant antibiotics should be discontinued, and appropriate antibiotic treatment initiated. The antibiotic of choice for treatment of an initial episode of *C difficile* colitis is oral fidaxomicin, and this is the best next step in the management of this patient's condition. Fidaxomicin is a narrow-spectrum macrocyclic antibiotic with excellent efficacy and tolerability in the treatment of *C difficile* colitis. Multiple phase III randomized controlled trials comparing fidaxomicin to vancomycin have found similar short-term cure rates (approximately 90%), but fidaxomicin also has a lower risk of recurrence than vancomycin (4–15% recurrence with fidaxomicin versus 18–25% for vancomycin). Experts believe this reduced recurrence risk occurs because of fewer alterations in the gut microbiota relative to vancomycin.

Recurrence after initial treatment is another key clinical consideration in the management of *C difficile* colitis. The initial choice of antibiotic treatment can reduce the risk of recurrent infection. Treatment of *C difficile* infection with oral metronidazole or oral vancomycin has been associated with approximately 25% recurrence. These antibiotics should not be considered as first-line therapy, and neither is the best next step for the patient in this scenario. If fidaxomicin is not available, oral vancomycin is considered a second-line alternative.

Bezlotoxumab is a monoclonal antibody that targets the *C difficile* toxin B. The addition of bezlotoxumab to standard-of-care antibiotics, such as vancomycin, resulted in similar cure rates but a 10% reduced risk of recurrence in two phase III, placebo-controlled trials. In these trials, most patients received oral vancomycin as standard of care, and the benefit of adding bezlotoxumab to fidaxomicin for the initial episode of *C difficile* diarrhea is currently unclear. Caution should be exercised in prescribing bezlotoxumab to patients with a history of congestive heart failure because heart failure was more commonly reported in the bezlotoxumab arm (12.7%) compared with placebo (4.8%).

Fecal microbiota transplantation (FMT) is another therapy with increasingly positive evidence for the treatment of recurrent and refractory *C difficile* colitis. Fecal microbiota transplantation should be considered after a second or subsequent recurrence or in cases of severe, complicated *C difficile* infection. Some studies have shown FMT to be a potential alternative to surgical resection in severe, refractory cases. Although single FMT may be successful in some cases, multiple infusions may be required. A multidisciplinary team approach is critical to provide the best care in severe, refractory infection.

Tigecycline also has shown in vitro activity against *C difficile*. Intravenous tigecycline has been studied in observational cohort studies but not in randomized trials, and existing data do not support its use. Intravenous tigecycline can be considered in cases of severe or refractory *C difficile* infection in conjunction with infectious disease consultation.

Guery B, Menichetti F, Anttila V, Adomakoh N, Aguado JM, Bisnauthsing K, et al. Extended-pulsed fidaxomicin versus vancomycin for Clostridium difficile infection in patients 60 years and older (EXTEND): a randomised, controlled, open-label, phase 3b/4 trial. EXTEND Clinical Study Group. Lancet Infect Dis 2018;18:296–307. doi: 10.1016/S1473-3099(17)30751-X

Louie TJ, Miller MA, Mullane KM, Weiss K, Lentnek A, Golan Y, et al. Fidaxomicin versus vancomycin for Clostridium difficile infection. OPT-80-003 Clinical Study Group. N Engl J Med 2011;364:422–31. doi: 10.1056/NEJMoa0910812

Ray J, LaBundy J. Lower gastrointestinal tract disorders. Clin Updates Womens Health Care 2022;XX(5):1–74.

van Prehn J, Reigadas E, Vogelzang EH, Bouza E, Hristea A, Guery B, et al. European Society of Clinical Microbiology and Infectious Diseases: 2021 update on the treatment guidance document for Clostridioides difficile infection in adults. Guideline Committee of the European Study Group on Clostridioides difficile. Clin Microbiol Infect 2021;27(suppl 2):S1–21. doi: 10.1016/j.cmi.2021.09.038

Wilcox MH, Gerding DN, Poxton IR, Kelly C, Nathan R, Birch T, et al. Bezlotoxumab for prevention of recurrent Clostridium difficile infection. MODIFY I and MODIFY II Investigators. N Engl J Med 2017;376:305–17. doi: 10.1056/NEJMoa1602615

48 Cervical cancer recurrence

A 42-year-old patient with a history of stage IB2 squamous cell carcinoma of the cervix who underwent chemoradiation therapy with cisplatin 4 years ago presents for a follow-up visit. She reports an unintentional 30-lb weight loss and new left leg swelling. Positron emission tomography shows a new fluorodeoxyglucose F 18 (FDG)-avid pelvic mass concerning for rectal invasion and multiple FDG-avid liver lesions. Tumor testing is positive for programmed death-ligand 1 (PD-L1). The best next step in treatment is chemotherapy combined with

(A) bevacizumab
(B) gemcitabine
* (C) pembrolizumab
(D) tisotumab vedotin
(E) topotecan

Recurrent cervical cancer is a challenging clinical situation. Historically, the best option for treatment of recurrent cervical cancer was a combination of platinum and taxane chemotherapy; however, molecular and biologic understanding of cancer continues to evolve, and significant advances in cancer therapeutics have been made. Newer clinical trials have shown improvements in survival with the addition of novel therapeutics to the chemotherapy backbone. Evolving options for treatment are shown in Table 48-1.

Programmed death-ligand 1 binds with the T-cell receptor programmed cell death protein 1 (PD-1) to prevent an immune response against those cells. Malignant cells often overexpress proteins involved in preventing immune response, such as PD-L1, to evade a T-cell-mediated tumor response and subsequent cell death. Immune checkpoint inhibitors are therapeutics designed to activate the immune system by blocking the tumor surveillance interaction between PD-L1-positive cells and the PD-1 receptors on T cells to activate the immune

TABLE 48-1. Evolving Therapeutics in Cervical Cancer Treatment

	MECHANISM OF ACTION	DRUGS IN CLASS	ADVERSE EVENTS
Antiangiogenics	Monoclonal antibody against vascular endothelial growth factor, platelet-derived growth factor, and other targets	Bevacizumab* Cetuximab Trastuzumab Sorafenib Sunitinib Imatinib Pazopanib Lenvatinib Everolimus	· Hypertension · Venous thromboembolism · Gastrointestinal fistula or perforation
Immune checkpoint inhibitors	Monoclonal antibody against programmed cell death protein 1 and programmed death-ligand 1 or cytotoxic T-lymphocyte-associated antigen 4	Pembrolizumab* Dostarlimab Avelumab Cemiplimab Nivolumab Ipilimumab Durvalumab Atezolizumab	· Colitis · Dermatitis · Thyroid dysfunction · Pneumonitis
Antibody-drug conjugate	Antibody delivers payload directly to tumor	Tisotumab vedotin* Trastuzumab deruxtecan†	· Ocular toxicity · Vary by agent

*U.S. Food and Drug Administration approved in cervical cancer.

†U.S. Food and Drug Administration approved for 3+ HER2 IHC expression.

response against those tumor cells. Current immune checkpoint inhibitors include monoclonal antibodies against PD-1 (pembrolizumab, nivolumab, cemiplimab, and dostarlimab), PD-L1 (atezolizumab, durvalumab, avelumab), or cytotoxic T-lymphocyte-associated antigen 4 (CTLA-4) (ipilimumab).

Pembrolizumab is an anti-PD-L1 monoclonal antibody. The Keynote 826 trial, a phase III randomized trial of 548 patients with recurrent or metastatic cervical cancer, studied pembrolizumab in combination with chemotherapy. The trial evaluated the addition of pembrolizumab to chemotherapy with or without bevacizumab. Similar adverse effect profiles were seen in both arms of this trial. Patients with PD-L1+ tumors who were randomized to pembrolizumab had improved overall survival with a 36% reduced risk of death at 24 months. There was an 8-month improvement in overall survival with the addition of pembrolizumab. As a result, the addition of pembrolizumab to chemotherapy in recurrent cervical cancer has been approved by the U.S. Food and Drug Administration as the new standard of care for patients with tumors expressing PD-L1, and adding pembrolizumab is the best next step in treatment for the patient in this scenario.

Before the advent of immune therapy, bevacizumab had shown added benefit to cytotoxic chemotherapy in the treatment of recurrent or metastatic cervical cancer. Bevacizumab is a monoclonal antibody against vascular endothelial growth factor (VEGF). In a randomized phase III trial of 452 patients receiving chemotherapy with cisplatin and paclitaxel with or without bevacizumab, receipt of bevacizumab was associated with a 3.7-month improvement in median overall survival. Notable adverse effects of adding bevacizumab to chemotherapy included increased risk of hypertension (25% versus 2%), blood clots (8% versus 1%), and gastrointestinal fistulas (3% versus 0%). Follow-up data from this trial indicate fistula rates of 15%. Although bevacizumab should be considered in patients with recurrent cervical cancer—with or without immune therapy, based on the results of Keynote 826 discussed above—this patient's suspected rectal invasion is at increased risk of gastrointestinal fistula, and chemotherapy/immunotherapy without bevacizumab is recommended.

Antibody–drug conjugates are another novel strategy for cancer treatment. These drugs are designed with an antibody linked to a drug that targets novel or upregulated antigens on tumor cells. The antibody binds to the antigen on the cancer cell, and the drug then enters the target cell. Tisotumab vedotin is an antibody–drug conjugate against tissue factor, which is upregulated in cervical cancer. Although data supporting the efficacy of single-agent tisotumab vedotin in cervical cancer are promising, clinical trials are ongoing to evaluate the safety and efficacy of this therapeutic with cytotoxic chemotherapy. This is not the best next step for the patient in this scenario.

Gemcitabine and topotecan are agents used to treat recurrent cervical cancer. A phase III trial comparing multiple platinum-containing doublets for recurrent cervical cancer did not show a benefit with the addition of gemcitabine or topotecan to cisplatin therapy, and the use of one of these agents is not the best next step to treat the described patient's recurrent cervical cancer.

Colombo N, Dubot C, Lorusso D, Caceres MV, Hasegawa K, Shapira-Frommer R, et al. Pembrolizumab for persistent, recurrent, or metastatic cervical cancer. KEYNOTE-826 Investigators. N Engl J Med 2021;385:1856–67. doi: 10.1056/NEJMoa2112435

Karpel HC, Powell SS, Pothuri B. Antibody-drug conjugates in gynecologic cancer [published erratum appears in Am Soc Clin Oncol Educ Book 2023;43:e390772CX1]. Am Soc Clin Oncol Educ Book 2023;43:e390772. doi: 10.1200/EDBK_390772

Monk BJ, Sill MW, McMeekin DS, Cohn DE, Ramondetta LM, Boardman CH, et al. Phase III trial of four cisplatin-containing doublet combinations in stage IVB, recurrent, or persistent cervical carcinoma: a Gynecologic Oncology Group study. J Clin Oncol 2009;27:4649–55. doi: 10.1200/JCO.2009.21.8909

Peng H, He X, Wang Q. Immune checkpoint blockades in gynecological cancer: a review of clinical trials. Acta Obstet Gynecol Scand 2022;101:941–51. doi: 10.1111/aogs.14412

Tewari KS, Sill MW, Long HJ III, Penson RT, Huang H, Ramondetta LM, et al. Improved survival with bevacizumab in advanced cervical cancer [published erratum appears in N Engl J Med 2017;377:702]. N Engl J Med 2014;370:734–43. doi: 10.1056/NEJMoa1309748

49 Complications of an epidural after surgery

Recent literature has suggested that epidural anesthesia for postoperative pain relief may not be the best option for patients undergoing gynecologic surgery. In addition to the risks of urinary retention and difficulty ambulating, the main reason for the decrease in the use of epidural anesthesia is

* (A) anesthesia failure
(B) cardiac arrest
(C) epidural abscess
(D) neuraxial hematoma

In theory, epidural anesthesia after major abdominal operations offers meaningful advantages compared with alternative methods. For more than 20 years, epidurals have been used to reduce the use of opioids, to achieve quicker return of gastrointestinal function, and to provide excellent pain relief, leading to faster recovery. In practice, it is not clear that these advantages have been realized. Because epidural anesthetics are invasive, labor intensive, and expensive, studies now are weighing their effectiveness against that of other approaches. A substantial body of literature calls the widespread use of postoperative epidural anesthesia into question and, consequently, epidurals are being used less frequently than they were in the past.

One of the factors that has dampened the enthusiasm for postoperative epidurals is the development of Early Recovery After Surgery (ERAS) protocols, which appear effective in achieving many of the same goals, without the risks and inconvenience of an epidural. Although there is no universally accepted definition of an ERAS protocol, most protocols have several features in common. With the intent to maintain, as much as is possible, normal physiology during the postoperative period, most protocols involve preoperative education and counseling, optimization of nutritional status, avoidance of prolonged fasting, maximization of nonopioid pain management strategies, maintenance of normal fluid balance and body temperature, administration of nerve blocks, early ambulation, and appropriate antibiotic and venous thromboembolism prophylaxis.

Beyond the increasing deployment of ERAS bundles, epidurals are being used less often because many alternatives to postoperative epidural anesthesia now are available, such as nerve blocks, paravertebral blocks, and direct infiltration of the incision with local anesthetic in the operating room. In addition, local anesthetics can be delivered through a catheter placed in the surgical incision and can remain in place for some time after surgery.

Reports have not consistently demonstrated that postoperative epidurals are associated with lower mortality rates or fewer complications, and there is concern that they may impair mobilization in certain groups. With the growing awareness of the importance of reducing the risk of postoperative thromboembolic events, increasing numbers of patients receive pharmacologic prophylaxis with an anticoagulant, which can complicate epidural catheter placement and removal. Patients with postoperative epidurals require closer monitoring than do those without epidurals, leading to increased cost of care. There is some evidence that postoperative epidurals, when used as a component of ERAS protocols, are associated with higher probabilities of infection, cardiac and pulmonary complications, and longer length of hospital stay.

The most frequent complication of postoperative epidural is failure to provide adequate analgesia. A number of studies have reported failure rates, and the frequency ranges from 16% to nearly 50%. Four studies have found that failures occur more than 40% of the time. Reasons for inadequate pain relief include leaking of infusate around the catheter, catheters becoming dislodged or displaced, blockage, and one-sided, or incomplete, blocks.

Cardiac arrest is an uncommon complication of epidural use and is not a causal factor. A Canadian study of more than 35,000 patients found that the risk of cardiac arrest was 1 in 5,000 for patients who had a postoperative epidural. A study of patients at increased risk of cardiovascular events undergoing noncardiac operations found higher frequencies of cardiovascular death and nonfatal myocardial infarction and cardiac arrest among patients who had epidurals, but this incidence is much lower than the risk of inadequate analgesia. There is no evidence that postoperative epidurals reduce the risk of cardiac complications.

Neuraxial hematoma is a relatively rare, but potentially devastating, complication that may require emergent decompression to preserve spinal cord function and avoid permanent injury. It is estimated that the risk of neuraxial hematoma with an epidural is 1 in 26,400. Because of its rarity, neuraxial hematoma treatment does not affect the frequency of epidural use. Likewise, epidural abscess is a rare but serious complication that does not affect the incidence of epidural use. One estimate of the frequency of abscess after an epidural is 1 in 27,000. Treatment typically requires surgical drainage, periodic irrigation, and antibiotics.

Dhondt LA, Vereen MS, van de Laar RL, Stolker R, Dirckx M, van Beekhuizen HJ. Efficacy of locoregional analgesic techniques after laparotomy for gynecologic cancer: a systematic review. Int J Gynecol Cancer 2024;34:1423–30. doi: 10.1136/ijgc-2024-005404

Rawal N. Epidural analgesia for postoperative pain: Improving outcomes or adding risks? Best Pract Res Clin Anaesthesiol 2021;35:53–65. doi: 10.1016/j.bpa.2020.12.001

Rawal N. Epidural technique for postoperative pain: gold standard no more? Reg Anesth Pain Med 2012;37:310–7. doi: 10.1097/AAP.0b013e31825735c6

Wagemans MF, Scholten WK, Hollmann MW, Kuipers AH. Epidural anesthesia is no longer the standard of care in abdominal surgery with ERAS. What are the alternatives? Minerva Anestesiol 2020;86:1079–88. doi: 10.23736/S0375-9393.20.14324-4

50 Chemotherapy for recurrent ovarian cancer

A 62-year-old patient presents to the emergency department reporting shortness of breath, nausea and vomiting, and a swollen abdomen. She finished six cycles of chemotherapy for stage IIIC ovarian cancer 3 months ago. Tumor testing is notable for homologous recombination proficiency and low folate receptor α expression. She has persistent neuropathy from her previous treatments, which limits her daily activities. On examination, her blood pressure is 110/60 mm Hg. Her lungs have decreased breath sounds at the bases bilaterally, and her abdomen is distended. Her white blood cell count is 10×10^9/L, and her creatinine level is 0.9 mg/dL. Computed tomography results show bilateral pleural effusions and peritoneal carcinomatosis. Computed tomography-guided peritoneal biopsy confirms recurrent ovarian cancer. The best next step is chemotherapy with

(A) carboplatin, paclitaxel, and bevacizumab
(B) mirvetuximab soravtansine
* (C) pegylated liposomal doxorubicin with bevacizumab
(D) topotecan

More than 80% of patients with ovarian cancer will have complete resolution of disease after surgical debulking and first-line platinum-based chemotherapy, but eventually most patients develop recurrent disease. *Platinum-resistant ovarian cancer* is routinely defined as disease recurrence within 6 months after completing platinum-based chemotherapy. Platinum-resistant disease is challenging to treat, and response rates are less than 40%, with overall survival less than 2 years. The standard approach to the treatment of platinum-resistant ovarian cancer has been non-platinum chemotherapy with or without anti-vascular endothelial growth factor (VEGF) therapy with bevacizumab, and clinical trial enrollment should be considered when available (Table 50-1).

In 2014, the AURELIA trial (bevacizumab combined with chemotherapy for platinum-resistant recurrent ovarian cancer: The AURELIA Open-Label Randomized Phase III Trial) established a new standard of care for platinum-resistant ovarian cancer. In this phase III randomized controlled trial, patients received physician's choice chemotherapy with paclitaxel, pegylated liposomal doxorubicin, or topotecan with or without bevacizumab. Chemotherapy with bevacizumab resulted in statistically significant improvements in progression-free survival

TABLE 50-1. Preferred Intravenous Cytotoxic Chemotherapies for Epithelial Ovarian Cancer

OPTIONS FOR FIRST-LINE METASTATIC OVARIAN CANCER	OPTIONS FOR PLATINUM-RESISTANT OVARIAN CANCER	OPTIONS FOR PLATINUM-SENSITIVE OVARIAN CANCER
• Carboplatin/paclitaxel with or without bevacizumab every 3 weeks followed by bevacizumab surveillance (if used during six cycles of chemotherapy)	• Docetaxel • Gemcitabine • Liposomal doxorubicin/bevacizumab* • Paclitaxel (weekly)/bevacizumab* • Topotecan/bevacizumab* • Mirvetuximab soravtansine-gynx (75% or more positive FRα-expressing tumor cells) • Trastuzumab deruxtecan (HER3+ tumors)	• Carboplatin/gemcitabine/bevacizumab* • Carboplatin/liposomal doxorubicin/bevacizumab* • Carboplatin/paclitaxel/bevacizumab* • Cisplatin/gemcitabine

*Bevacizumab demonstrated superiority in outcomes but is contraindicated in certain clinical situations.

Data from National Comprehensive Cancer Network. Ovarian cancer: continue including fallopian tube cancer and primary peritoneal cancer. Version 2.2025. NCCN Clinical Practice Guidelines in Oncology [after login]. NCCN; 2025. Accessed June 10, 2025. https://www.nccn.org/professionals/physician_gls/pdf/ovarian.pdf

and improvements in quality of life. The combination therapy led to improvements in quality of life, an important endpoint for this morbid, life-threatening disease. Despite the superior response rates, many oncologists are reluctant to use paclitaxel in this clinical setting due to the risk of neuropathy and alopecia. Based on these data, for this patient with platinum-resistant disease, the non-platinum agent pegylated liposomal doxorubicin in combination with bevacizumab is the best treatment option.

Platinum-sensitive recurrence is defined as progression after 6 months from last platinum-based treatment. It is likely that a patient with platinum-sensitive disease will be retreated with a platinum-based therapy with or without bevacizumab. Prior studies have demonstrated activity of carboplatin with paclitaxel, pegylated liposomal doxorubicin, or gemcitabine with or without bevacizumab. This patient has platinum-resistant disease with progression 3 months after completion of platinum-based therapy, and the platinum-based options (single-agent carboplatin; cisplatin and paclitaxel; carboplatin, paclitaxel, and bevacizumab) are not the best treatment options. Despite the term *platinum-resistant*, platinum can be used in some patients with platinum-resistant disease. Literature has suggested that cisplatin with gemcitabine is an active regimen and could be a reasonable recommendation, but this doublet therapy has not been considered the control arm for trials in this resistant population.

Based on the AURELIA trial, the National Comprehensive Cancer Network recommended topotecan for the treatment of platinum-resistant disease; however, in subgroup analyses of the AURELIA trial, single-agent topotecan resulted in no partial or complete responses; therefore, single-agent topotecan is not the best next treatment for the described patient's disease.

Mirvetuximab soravtansine is an antibody–drug conjugate directed at folate receptor α. It is currently U.S. Food and Drug Administration-approved for platinum-resistant ovarian cancer treatment in tumors that have high expression of folate receptor α. It has shown improvements in both progression-free and overall survival. It is not appropriate to use in this patient because she has low folate receptor α expression.

The therapeutic options for platinum-resistant ovarian cancer are limited in both efficacy and tolerability. With the introduction of antibody–drug conjugates into the gynecologic cancer treatment space, new options recently have been approved for these patients. To use these new medications, the patient's tumor must be biomarker positive, which limits the utility of these drugs in all patients. Clinical trials continue to be an important and necessary option for these patients.

Coleman RL, Brady MF, Herzog TJ, Sabbatini P, Armstrong DK, Walker JL, et al. Bevacizumab and paclitaxel-carboplatin chemotherapy and secondary cytoreduction in recurrent, platinum-sensitive ovarian cancer (NRG Oncology/Gynecologic Oncology Group study GOG-0213): a multicentre, open-label, randomised, phase 3 trial. Lancet Oncol 2017;18:779–91. doi: 10.1016/S1470-2045(17)30279-6

National Comprehensive Cancer Network. Ovarian cancer/fallopian tube cancer/primary peritoneal cancer. Version 3.2024. NCCN Clinical Practice Guidelines in Oncology [after login]. NCCN; 2024. Accessed January 22, 2025. https://www.nccn.org/guidelines/guidelines-detail?category=1&id=1453

Pujade-Lauraine E, Hilpert F, Weber B, Reuss A, Poveda A, Kristensen G, et al. Bevacizumab combined with chemotherapy for platinum-resistant recurrent ovarian cancer: the AURELIA open-label randomized phase III trial [published erratum appears in J Clin Oncol 2014;32:4025]. J Clin Oncol 2014;32:1302–8. doi: 10.1200/JCO.2013.51.4489

Richardson DL, Eskander RN, O'Malley DM. Advances in ovarian cancer care and unmet treatment needs for patients with platinum resistance: a narrative review. JAMA Oncol 2023;9:851–9. doi: 10.1001/jamaoncol.2023.0197

51 Acupuncture in cancer

A 76-year-old patient is undergoing chemotherapy for the treatment of advanced ovarian cancer. She is experiencing many bothersome symptoms related to her treatment and is interested in pursuing acupuncture. The best use of acupuncture in cancer patients is to

(A) decrease symptoms of depression
* (B) enhance pain management
(C) improve chemotherapy effectiveness
(D) increase the immune response
(E) prevent nausea

Acupuncture is an ancient medicinal practice that involves the placement of thin needles into the skin at specific points by trained practitioners. The use of acupuncture has been studied in relation to several adverse effects caused by cancer and cancer therapy with varying results. These studies have shown benefit from the inclusion of acupuncture as a complementary treatment modality in cancer patients with symptoms including pain, nausea, and neuropathy, but many of these studies are small, retrospective, low quality, and lacking a control group.

Acupuncture has been shown to be associated with a significant decrease in pain intensity in patients with cancer. Recently, acupuncture has been studied in more robust prospective studies, including those with sham controls, increasing the quality of evidence supporting its use. One such area of study includes the use of acupuncture in the treatment of cancer-related pain. When used in addition to traditional methods of pain management, such as opioid therapy, acupuncture has been shown to lead to a further reduction in pain compared with traditional pain management therapies alone. A similar study showed that there was a more significant reduction in cancer-related pain with the use of acupuncture than with sham controls. These and other studies support the efficacy of acupuncture in reducing the intensity and amount of pain experienced by patients with cancer-related pain. Other complementary therapies that may improve cancer pain include yoga, music therapy, and meditation, including mindfulness-based practice, although the data supporting the use of these therapies is of variable quality.

Although there is some support for the idea that acupuncture may have immunomodulatory effects, the immune effects of acupuncture have not been specifically studied in cancer patients, and increasing the immune response is not supported by available data. Likewise, no studies have shown that acupuncture increases the effectiveness of chemotherapy.

Acupuncture has been more extensively investigated in chemotherapy-induced nausea and vomiting and has been shown to provide benefit in some studies. These studies are of limited use because they are challenging to interpret or broadly apply due to a lack of standardization of the chemotherapy regimen for participants. The risk of chemotherapy-induced nausea and vomiting varies widely by specific chemotherapeutic medication, and this can significantly confound these results. Additionally, several older studies that showed a reduction in chemotherapy-induced nausea and vomiting with acupuncture may not be applicable to current chemotherapy protocols due to the increased effectiveness of modern antiemetic medications that were not available at the time of the older studies. Because of these concerns, the data supporting the use of acupuncture for chemotherapy-induced nausea and vomiting is of lower quality than that supporting its role in pain management. Similarly, the data regarding the potential mental health benefits of acupuncture to improve depression and anxiety are of limited size and quality and do not reach the level of the data supporting the use of acupuncture for the management of cancer-related pain.

He Y, Guo X, May BH, Zhang AL, Liu Y, Lu C, et al. Clinical evidence for association of acupuncture and acupressure with improved cancer pain: a systematic review and meta-analysis. JAMA Oncol 2020;6:271–8. doi: 10.1001/jamaoncol.2019.5233

Li H, Schlaeger JM, Jang MK, Lin Y, Park C, Liu T, et al. Acupuncture improves multiple treatment-related symptoms in breast cancer survivors: a systematic review and meta-analysis. J Altern Complement Med 2021;27:1084–97. doi: 10.1089/acm.2021.0133

Yang J, Wahner-Roedler DL, Zhou X, Johnson LA, Do A, Pachman DR, et al. Acupuncture for palliative cancer pain management: systematic review. BMJ Support Palliat Care 2021;11:264–70. doi: 10.1136/bmjspcare-2020-002638

52 Cervical cancer screening in a low-resource setting

A 41-year-old woman presents to a health clinic where you often volunteer in Uganda. Her sister was recently treated for cervical cancer, which prompted the patient to seek cervical cancer screening. The patient's community clinic does not have the resources to provide this screening, and because she does not have reliable transportation, she has never been screened. No laboratory services are available to you in the location. On examination during her clinic visit today, her cervix is grossly normal. She wants to know if anything can be done at this visit. You inform her that the best next step is

(A) cryotherapy
(B) excisional procedure
(C) random cervical biopsy
* (D) visual inspection with acetic acid

Improvements in cervical cancer prevention, such as human papillomavirus (HPV) vaccination, early detection, and treatment of precancerous lesions, have contributed to decreased mortality in many high-resource countries; nevertheless, countries and communities with inadequate health care resources continue to experience significant mortality due to cervical cancer. Approximately 90% of cervical cancer-related mortality occurs in these locations. This disparity is due to differences in HPV vaccination coverage, access to screening and treatment of precancerous lesions, and availability of cervical cancer treatment. Screening and treatment in these areas may differ from the standard of care because of barriers to access.

Cervical cancer screening is transitioning to HPV-based testing because it informs decisions about current and future risk of disease. In the United States, options include primary HPV testing or co-testing (cytology and HPV testing simultaneously). The World Health Organization recommends HPV-based testing but without additional guidance on how it should be implemented or managed. Implementation of HPV-based testing can be limited in high- and low-resource settings, including in the United States. In high-resource settings, barriers to implementation include limited availability of the test and the need for new laboratory infrastructure to accommodate the increased demand for screening. The same barriers are more pronounced in low-resource settings where existing health care resources are strained. In addition, patients experience delays that result in a loss to follow-up.

The World Health Organization has developed worldwide goals aimed at eliminating cervical cancer as a public health problem and reducing disparities by 2030. This strategy includes expanding HPV vaccination coverage to more than 90% of girls before they are 15 years old, increasing screening with high-performance testing to 70% of adolescents and women by the age of 35 years and again at 45 years, and increasing access to treatment of precancerous and cancerous lesions to more than 90% (Box 52-1). Human papillomavirus vaccination is most effective when administered to younger individuals. These three approaches are crucial to address current disparities at different stages in the disease course.

BOX 52-1

The 2030 Targets Toward Elimination of Cervical Cancer

Meeting the following 90–70–90 targets by 2030 will put all countries on the path to elimination:

- **90%** of girls fully vaccinated with HPV vaccine by 15 years of age
- **70%** of women screened using a high-performance test by 35 years of age and again by 45 years of age
- **90%** of women identified with cervical disease are treated
  - **90%** of women with precancer treated
  - **90%** of women with invasive cancer managed.

Reprinted from WHO Global strategy to accelerate the elimination of cervical cancer as a public health problem. Geneva: World Health Organization; 2020.

Worldwide, HPV vaccination uptake is overall low. Efforts to improve HPV vaccination uptake are ongoing globally in an effort to reduce mortality due to cervical cancer. Human papillomavirus vaccination is effective in low-resource settings and will assist in overcoming challenges in screening and treatment through primary prevention. Resolving barriers to HPV vaccination is paramount to addressing the global disparities of this disease.

The patient in this scenario does not have access to testing in her community clinic, and she does not have reliable transportation. The health clinic in which she is being seen today also has limited resources, and the approach to screening is influenced by these factors. Although primary HPV testing is preferred, referral for testing would not address the barriers she faces and would not be possible at this visit today. In this scenario, visual inspection with 5% acetic acid is the best available modality for her screening. This screening method involves applying dilute acetic acid to the patient's cervix and examining the cervix with a light source. The appearance of an acetowhite lesion at or adjacent to the squamocolumnar junction is a positive result (Fig. 52-1). This screening method requires minimal resources

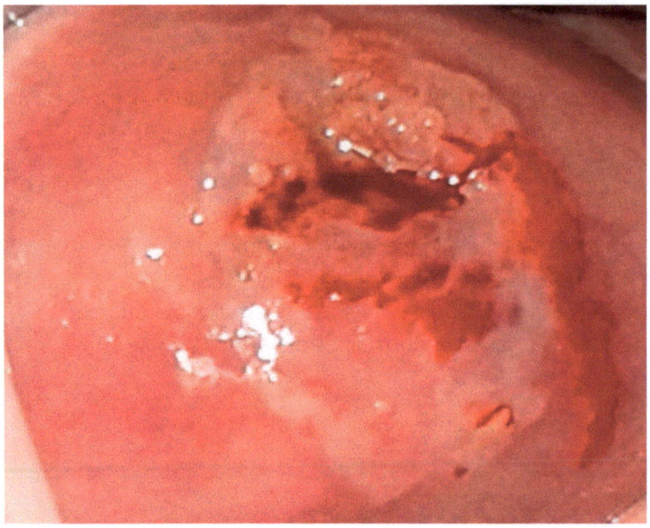

FIGURE 52-1. Positive visual inspection with acetic acid with an acetowhite area on the posterior aspect of the cervix. (Reprinted from World Health Organization. Training of health staff in VIA, HPV detection test and cryotherapy. Trainees' handbook. WHO; 2017. Accessed March 13, 2025. https://www.who.int/publications/i/item/9789290225553)

and has sensitivity similar to that of cervical cytology. Patients with a positive visual inspection with 5% acetic acid may then undergo same-day treatment if available, such as cryotherapy, thermal ablation, or loop electrosurgical excision procedure.

Cryotherapy is not the best next step for the described patient. It is an appropriate treatment for cervical intraepithelial neoplasia, but it requires an evaluation for a lesion first. Patients with a fully visualized squamocolumnar junction are candidates for cryotherapy when an acetowhite lesion involves less than 75% of the cervix and does not extend into the endocervical canal. If visual inspection with acetic acid shows a lesion that meets these criteria, cryotherapy is a good option for same-day treatment. If invasive cervical cancer is suspected, an excisional procedure, not cryotherapy, would be the treatment of choice. The patient in this scenario should be evaluated first with visual inspection with acetic acid, and if appropriate, an excisional procedure could follow. Excision is indicated if cervical high-grade squamous intraepithelial lesion is suspected or confirmed, or for diagnosis if invasive cervical cancer is suspected on initial cytology or inspection.

Obtaining a random cervical biopsy is not the best next step for this patient. Visual inspection with acetic acid is preferred because it provides a systematic visual evaluation of the cervix to detect abnormalities to appropriately triage and direct further treatment. This further treatment can occur the same day if available. Furthermore, this health care setting does not have access to a laboratory, and pathologic evaluation may not be feasible.

Patients in low-resource settings experience unique barriers to cervical cancer screening. Visual inspection with acetic acid is an effective cervical cancer screening option that requires few resources and allows for same-day treatment when available. Notably, visual inspection with acetic acid has not been associated with decreased mortality from cervical cancer compared with primary HPV screening; and further efforts should address increasing access to primary HPV screening, including HPV screening with self-swab, to mitigate disparities throughout the world.

Cervical cancer screening in low-resource settings. Committee Opinion No. 624. American College of Obstetricians and Gynecologists. Obstet Gynecol 2015;125:526–8. doi: 10.1097/01.AOG.0000460763.59152.9e

Kundrod KA, Smith CA, Hunt B, Schwarz RA, Schmeler K, Richards-Kortum R. Advances in technologies for cervical cancer detection in low-resource settings. Expert Rev Mol Diagn 2019;19:695–714. doi: 10.1080/14737159.2019.1648213

Marcus JZ, Cason P, Downs LSJ, Einstein MH, Flowers L. The ASCCP Cervical Cancer Screening Task Force endorsement and opinion on the American Cancer Society updated cervical cancer screening guidelines. J Low Genit Tract Dis 2021;25:187–91. doi: 10.1097/LGT.0000000000000614

Perkins RB, Guido RS, Castle PE, Chelmow D, Einstein MH, Garcia F, et al. 2019 ASCCP risk-based management consensus guidelines for abnormal cervical cancer screening tests and cancer precursors. 2019 ASCCP Risk-Based Management Consensus Guidelines Committee [published erratum appears in J Low Genit Tract Dis 2020;24:427]. J Low Genit Tract Dis 2020;24:102–31. doi: 10.1097/LGT.0000000000000525

World Health Organization. Global strategy to accelerate the elimination of cervical cancer as a public health problem. WHO; 2020. Accessed March 13, 2025. https://www.who.int/publications/i/item/9789240014107

World Health Organization. Training of health staff in VIA, HPV detection test and cryotherapy. Trainees' handbook. WHO; 2017. Accessed March 13, 2025. https://www.who.int/publications/i/item/9789290225553

53 Endometrial intraepithelial neoplasia

A 35-year-old, otherwise healthy woman receives a diagnosis of endometrial intraepithelial neoplasia (EIN) on dilation and curettage. The most appropriate surgical procedure to manage EIN is

(A) hysteroscopic endometrial resection
(B) radiofrequency endometrial ablation
(C) supracervical hysterectomy
* (D) total hysterectomy

Endometrial intraepithelial neoplasia is a precancerous condition. The risk of progression to invasive endometrial carcinoma has been estimated at approximately 30%. Most cases of EIN are attributable to excess exposure of the endometrium to estrogen. The incidence rate of endometrial cancer in patients with untreated EIN is approximately 8% per year. Approximately 40% of patients with a preoperative diagnosis of complex endometrial hyperplasia will have an invasive cancer diagnosed at the time of hysterectomy. Most cancer that occurs in conjunction with EIN is well-differentiated (grade 1) and superficially invasive or confined to the endometrium with good prognosis.

Total hysterectomy is the best procedure to prevent the development of invasive cancer over time and to fully evaluate for concurrent cancer if present. The disease cure rate for EIN by total hysterectomy is essentially 100%. The management of the ovaries is an individualized decision and involves consideration of age, comorbidities, suitability for postmenopausal hormone therapy, family and personal history, and patient preference. If the ovaries are retained, it is reasonable to perform salpingectomy, which may reduce the risk of serous ovarian cancer in the future. Hysterectomy is the best procedure for the patient in this scenario, who has a diagnosis of EIN.

Because residual endometrium may be present, supracervical hysterectomy should not be performed in patients with EIN. If hyperplastic endometrium is present below the margin of resection, malignancy could be present or develop in the stump. Residual malignancy exposes the patient to a risk of local spread and necessitates additional treatment, including a second operation with possibly increased morbidity.

Endometrial intraepithelial neoplasia is an absolute contraindication to ablation regardless of technique. Hysteroscopic endometrial resection and radiofrequency ablation (along with all other ablative techniques) are not appropriate. These procedures have been demonstrated to leave a substantial proportion of the endometrium untreated. Most patients do not become amenorrheic after ablation, and any residual endometrium, if hyperplastic, could progress to invasive malignancy. Prior ablation is likely to increase the difficulty of evaluating bleeding episodes that could occur in the future.

Management of endometrial intraepithelial neoplasia or atypical endometrial hyperplasia. Clinical Consensus No. 5. American College of Obstetricians and Gynecologists. Obstet Gynecol 2023;142:735–44. doi: 10.1097/AOG.0000000000005297

Trimble CL, Kauderer J, Zaino R, Silverberg S, Lim PC, Burke JJ II, et al. Concurrent endometrial carcinoma in women with a biopsy diagnosis of atypical endometrial hyperplasia: a Gynecologic Oncology Group study. Cancer 2006;106:812–9. doi: 10.1002/cncr.21650

54 Rare ovarian tumors

A 53-year-old woman underwent surgical exploration for an 8-cm complex adnexal mass with corpuscular fluid and vascular solid components. The result from intraoperative frozen section is shown in Figure 54-1. You perform comprehensive surgical staging that ultimately reveals stage IC2 cancer. You recommend primary chemotherapy followed by

- (A) endocrine therapy
- * (B) evaluation in 3 months
- (C) poly(ADP-ribose) polymerase (PARP) inhibitor
- (D) programmed cell death protein 1 (PD-1) inhibitor
- (E) vascular endothelial growth factor inhibitor

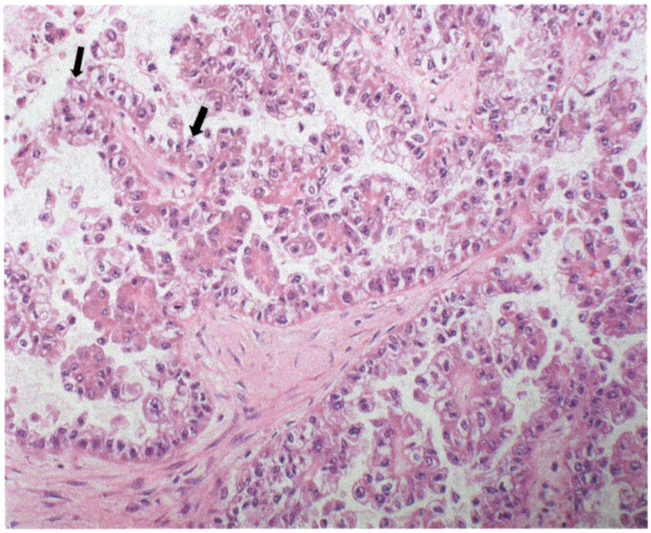

FIGURE 54-1. High-grade nuclei with prominent nucleoli, nuclear hobnailing (arrows), and distinct clear to eosinophilic cytoplasm with hyalinized core. (Courtesy of Dr. Christine Bookhout, Department of Pathology, University of North Carolina.)

The histology in Figure 54-1 demonstrates clear cell carcinoma of the ovary. Clear cell carcinoma of the ovary is a rare subtype of epithelial ovarian cancer that occurs in approximately 10% of cases of ovarian cancer. Relative to serous cancer, clear cell cancer tends to present at a younger age and earlier stage. Endometriosis is a well-established risk factor for clear cell carcinoma of the ovary. Clear cell carcinoma of the ovary is biologically distinct from other epithelial cancer and often associated with alterations in the AT-rich interaction domain 1A (ARID1A) and phosphatidylinositol-4,5-bisphosphate 3-kinase (PIK3) catalytic subunit alpha (PIK3CA). Clear cell carcinomas display high-grade nuclei with prominent nucleoli, nuclear hobnailing, and distinctive clear to eosinophilic cytoplasm, which leads to the formation of glandular and papillary structures with hyalinized cores (Fig. 54-1).

Determination of the ideal management of clear cell carcinomas is challenging because the rarity of these tumors limits large prospective trials. There are mixed data on the benefit of adjuvant chemotherapy in surgically staged, stage I clear cell carcinoma. In a patient with stage IC2 cancer, National Comprehensive Cancer Network guidelines recommend adjuvant chemotherapy based on data from large prospective trials in ovarian cancer that included patients with clear cell histology. In early-stage clear cell ovarian cancer, administration of three cycles of combination platinum and taxane chemotherapy, rather than six cycles, may be adequate based on a secondary analysis of Gynecologic Oncology Group (GOG) 157 and a multicenter cohort study showing no difference in survival for three versus six cycles of chemotherapy. Given these data, active surveillance is the best next step for the described patient, and a surveillance visit with evaluation can be performed in 3 months.

Patients with hormonally responsive malignancies may benefit from ongoing endocrine therapy after chemotherapy. Clear cell carcinoma generally is not hormonally driven and usually does not express estrogen receptors, and maintenance endocrine therapies are not the best next step in the treatment of the described patient.

In certain patients with stage II to IV ovarian cancer, a maintenance treatment strategy using PARP inhibitors can be effective. These agents work by blocking PARP inhibitors from repairing DNA damage, which leads to tumor cell death. Clinical application of PARP inhibitors in high-grade serous and endometrioid ovarian cancer treatment has been studied in multiple prospective trials. They are most effective in patients whose tumors are deficient in homologous recombination repair, including those with *BRCA* germline or somatic mutations; however, no participants with clear cell carcinoma were included in these trials. Patients with stage I cancer are not eligible to receive PARP inhibitors, and this is not the best next step for the patient described.

The role of immunotherapy, such as anti-cell death protein 1 antibodies, continues to expand. Although 15% of clear cell carcinomas will have mismatch repair deficiency or high tumor mutational burden, suggesting a potential role for immunotherapy, there are no data to support the routine use of immune checkpoint inhibitors in the maintenance of stage I clear cell carcinoma. The role of immunotherapy in treating clear cell carcinoma is an area of active research but is not the best next step for the described patient at this time.

The first U.S. Food and Drug Administration-approved maintenance therapy in ovarian cancer was bevacizumab. Bevacizumab is a monoclonal antibody against vascular endothelial growth factor. Gynecologic Oncology Group 218, which primarily evaluated serous malignancies, showed a modest 4-month benefit in progression-free survival in patients with stage III and IV ovarian cancer, but only 3% of participants had clear cell histology. Available data do not support the use of anti-vascular endothelial growth factor therapy in stage I ovarian cancer.

Burger RA, Brady MF, Bookman MA, Fleming GF, Monk BJ, Huang H, et al. Incorporation of bevacizumab in the primary treatment of ovarian cancer. Gynecologic Oncology Group. N Engl J Med 2011;365:2473–83. doi: 10.1056/NEJMoa1104390

Gadducci A, Multinu F, Cosio S, Carinelli S, Ghioni M, Aletti GD. Clear cell carcinoma of the ovary: epidemiology, pathological and biological features, treatment options and clinical outcomes. Gynecol Oncol 2021;162:741–50. doi: 10.1016/j.ygyno.2021.06.033

National Comprehensive Cancer Network. Ovarian cancer/fallopian tube cancer/primary peritoneal cancer. Version 3.2024. NCCN Clinical Practice Guidelines in Oncology [after login]. NCCN; 2024. Accessed January 22, 2025. https://www.nccn.org/guidelines/guidelines-detail?category=1&id=1453

Prendergast EN, Holzapfel M, Mueller JJ, Leitao MM Jr, Gunderson CC, Moore KN, et al. Three versus six cycles of adjuvant platinum-based chemotherapy in early stage clear cell ovarian carcinoma a multi-institutional cohort. Gynecol Oncol 2017;144:274–8. doi: 10.1016/j.ygyno.2016.12.004

55 Recurrent metastatic cancer

A 73-year-old patient with recurrent platinum-resistant metastatic ovarian cancer, who was previously treated with three lines of chemotherapy, is brought to the emergency department by her family due to abdominal pain, bloating, nausea, and vomiting. She is currently enrolled in a clinical trial. On evaluation in the emergency department, her vital signs reveal a temperature of 36.3 °C (97.3 °F), blood pressure of 90/60 mm Hg, heart rate of 120 beats per minute, a respiratory rate of 20 breaths per minute, and oxygen saturation of 90% on room air. Her examination is notable for abdominal bloating with a palpable fluid wave, and computed tomography (CT) reveals progressive disease with moderate volume ascites and metastatic implants of the liver and spleen. Her family reports she has had increasing difficulty with activities of daily living and now spends most of her days in bed. In addition to hospital admission, the best next step for her cancer care is to

(A) change the chemotherapy regimen
(B) consult hospice for enrollment
(C) continue clinical trial treatment
* (D) perform a goals-of-care assessment

Epithelial ovarian cancer is a chemotherapy-responsive disease, with approximately 70–80% of cancer responding to initial chemotherapy. Despite high initial response rates, recurrent disease occurs in more than 50% of patients within the first 2 years of completion of first-line therapy. Given the high recurrence rate, many patients are exposed to multiple treatment regimens. Clinical trial enrollment, when available, is a mainstay of treatment among patients with ovarian cancer, particularly in a recurrent setting.

To evaluate patients in a consistent manner while on clinical trial, standard criteria are used for measuring how the disease affects a patient's daily living abilities. This is referred to as a *performance* or *functional* status. The Eastern Cooperative Oncology Group (ECOG) Performance Status Scale is one measurement that is used, and it describes a patient's level of functioning as it pertains to their ability to care for themselves, participate in daily activities, and have physical abilities (Table 55-1). This scale allows clinicians to assess changes in a patient's level of functioning as a result of a treatment regimen or disease status.

TABLE 55-1. Eastern Cooperative Oncology Group Performance Status Scale

GRADE	ECOG PERFORMANCE STATUS
0	Fully active, able to carry on all pre-disease performance without restriction
1	Restricted in physically strenuous activity but ambulatory and able to carry out work of a light or sedentary nature, eg, light house work, office work
2	Ambulatory and capable of all self-care but unable to carry out any work activities; up and about more than 50% of waking hours
3	Capable of only limited self-care; confined to bed or chair more than 50% of waking hours
4	Completely disabled; cannot carry on any self-care; totally confined to bed or chair
5	Dead

Reprinted from Oken MM, Creech RH, Tormey DC, Horton J, Davis TE, McFadden ET, et al. Toxicity and response criteria of the Eastern Cooperative Oncology Group. Am J Clin Oncol 1982;5:649–55.

This patient is presenting with metastatic recurrent disease and prior lines of treatment with worsening functional status. On the ECOG Performance Status Scale, this patient would now be classified as having a performance status of 3, given that she is now in bed for more than 50% of waking hours and is capable of limited self-care. The American Society of Clinical Oncology recommends clinicians reassess a patient's goals, priorities, and desires for information whenever a significant change in a patient's care is being considered. Given the change in this patient's status and the prior treatments she has received, a goals-of-care meeting with the patient, her family, and other caregivers is the best next step to discern the patient's wishes and provide care in line with her goals.

A new chemotherapy regimen may be an option for patients with recurrent or progressive disease. Patients with years to months to live and a good performance status (less than 2) are likely to be interested in continuing anticancer therapy. Chemotherapy can be used to provide symptom palliation, maintain stable disease, and provide an opportunity to use newer agents with possibly fewer toxicities; however, repetitive administration of chemotherapy may be harmful to a patient's quality of life. Regarding this patient, proceeding immediately to a new chemotherapy regimen without assessing her overall health status and goals of care would be premature; therefore, it is not the best next step for her cancer care at this time.

Clinical trial enrollment is encouraged among patients with advanced and recurrent ovarian cancer. If progressive disease or excessive toxicity from the chemotherapy treatment is noted during trial monitoring, patients should be assessed for a change in treatment or discussion about palliation pending the degree of disease, symptoms, and functional status. After the patient's current symptoms are under control, she may be able to resume care on the clinical trial. However, if progressive disease is noted or unmanageable toxicity is encountered, a change in management, including other potential therapy options if available, and discussion of best supportive care/hospice care are warranted. This is best decided through a goals-of-care meeting. The clinician should not assume the patient can continue on the clinical trial until her overall status and goals are evaluated. For this reason, continuation on the trial is not the best next step.

As the functional status of a patient worsens, the options of discontinuing treatment and initiating goal-directed supportive care should be discussed, including referral to palliative care or hospice. The National Comprehensive Cancer Network recommends that patients be referred to palliative care if there is evidence of worsening prognosis, which includes a decline in performance status to 3 or worse, uncontrolled symptoms, or distress despite anticancer therapy. This recommendation stems from studies that show positive effects on early use of referrals to palliative care and fewer emergency department visits, hospitalizations, and intensive care unit admissions. Palliative care can be administered while a patient is still receiving cancer treatment. Hospice care, generally reserved for patients who are not receiving treatment for the underlying disease, may be appropriate for this patient. Hospice focuses on comfort and quality of life for a person who is approaching the end of life and is provided for a patient with a terminal illness with an anticipated survival of 6 months or less if the illness runs its natural course. Making an assumption that the patient desires to enroll in hospice without a goals-of-care discussion would not be appropriate. It would defy the right to autonomy and participation in health care decisions and is not the appropriate next step for the described patient.

Discussions regarding prognosis and end-of-life care can be challenging. Recommendations exist regarding strategies for communication of change in prognosis. Published frameworks such as GUIDE can be used to aid in relaying information. GUIDE stands for Get ready, Understand, Inform, Demonstrate empathy, and Equip (Table 55-2). If using GUIDE to discuss serious news with a patient, the clinician should take time to prepare and ensure all appropriate information, as well as people, are available for a meeting. This includes ensuring a private place to have the discussion. Once in an appropriate setting, the clinician can assess the patient's understanding of the situation, for example, by asking, "What is your understanding of your illness at this time?" Once the clinician understands what the patient knows, news should be delivered clearly using a one-sentence headline, such as "The computed tomography shows that the cancer has gotten worse." Although additional information will need to be discussed, patients and family members are likely to experience emotional responses to hearing difficult news; therefore, before moving on to the next steps, it is important to acknowledge any emotions explicitly. After this, the clinician can equip the patient and family for the next steps in treatment or discussion about options in care. This allows the patient to participate in their health care decisions and ensures that recommendations regarding treatment and associated risks are discussed in accordance with the patient's wishes.

TABLE 55-2. GUIDE Tool for Breaking Bad News

STEP	WHAT YOU SAY OR DO
Get Ready—Info, People, Place	"Let me take a minute to make sure I've got what I need." • Make sure you have all the information you need at hand. • Make sure you have all the right people in the room. • Find a place with some privacy.
Understand what the patient knows	Question examples: "What thoughts have you had since the biopsy?" "What have you taken away from other doctors so far?"
Inform starting with a headline	"The CT shows that the cancer has gotten worse." • Give the information clearly and to the point with a one-sentence headline of the most important piece of information you want them to take away. • Avoid jargon. • After the headline, you will need to give more information, but after giving the headline, STOP.
Demonstrate empathy—respond directly to emotion	"I can see this news is not what you were hoping for." • Expect the patient's first response to be emotion. • Acknowledge the emotion explicitly.
Equip the patient for the next step	"Is there anything I could do to make this a little easier?" "I want you to be prepared for the next step. Can I explain..." • Don't dismiss concerns or say that everything will be fine.

Reprinted from VitalTalk. Serious news: breaking bad news using the GUIDE tool. VitalTalk; 2019. Accessed March 13, 2025. https://www.vitaltalk.org/guides/serious-news/

Baile WF, Buckman R, Lenzi R, Glober G, Beale EA, Kudelka AP. SPIKES-a six-step protocol for delivering bad news: application to the patient with cancer. Oncologist 2000;5:302–11. doi: 10.1634/theoncologist.5-4-302

Gilligan T, Coyle N, Frankel RM, Berry DL, Bohlke K, Epstein RM, et al. Patient-clinician communication: American Society of Clinical Oncology consensus guideline. J Clin Oncol 2017;35:3618–32. doi: 10.1200/JCO.2017.75.2311

Mori M, Morita T, Bruera E, Hui D. Prognostication of the last days of life. Cancer Res Treat 2022;54:631–43. doi: 10.4143/crt.2021.1573

National Comprehensive Cancer Network. Palliative care. Version 1.2025 NCCN Clinical Practice Guidelines in Oncology [after login]. NCCN; 2024. Accessed March 13, 2025. https://www.nccn.org/professionals/physician_gls/pdf/palliative.pdf

Oken MM, Creech RH, Tormey DC, Horton J, Davis TE, McFadden ET, et al. Toxicity and response criteria of the Eastern Cooperative Oncology Group. Am J Clin Oncol 1982;5:649–55.

Seol A, Yim GW, Chung JY, Kim SI, Lee M, Kim HS, et al. Identification of patients with recurrent epithelial ovarian cancer who will benefit from more than three lines of chemotherapy. Cancer Res Treat 2022;54:1219–29. doi: 10.4143/crt.2021.1010

56 Radiation proctitis

A 48-year-old patient with stage IIIA squamous cell carcinoma of the cervix presents for routine surveillance. She completed chemoradiation 12 months ago. Her medical history is notable for hypertension and a 10-pack-year smoking history. She reports recent-onset fecal urgency, bloody diarrhea, and periodic stool incontinence. On physical examination, there is no evidence of recurrent disease; however, a rectal examination is painful and blood is noted. She undergoes a diagnostic sigmoidoscopy, which confirms the diagnosis of radiation proctitis. Subsequent management with sucralfate retention enemas does not relieve her symptoms. The best next treatment to address her symptoms is

(A) corticosteroid suppositories
(B) mesalamine
(C) ozone therapy
(D) pentoxifylline and vitamin E
* (E) rectal formalin application

Radiation therapy is the mainstay of treatment for locally advanced cervical cancer, and pelvic radiation therapy is used to treat other types of gynecologic cancer as well. Radiation therapy uses high-energy rays to generate ionizing radiation, which impairs or halts the division of the rapidly dividing tumor cells. Although advances in technology have allowed more precise delivery of radiation therapy to the target tissues, proximal organs, such as the rectum, are within the field of radiation due to their proximity to gynecologic tumors. As such, radiation proctitis is one of the most common complications of radiation therapy to the pelvis.

Radiation proctitis is characterized by damage to the rectal epithelium caused by secondary exposure to ionizing radiation. It can be classified as acute or chronic based on the timing of symptoms relative to radiation. Acute radiation proctitis occurs during or immediately after radiation therapy and is characterized by superficial mucosal injury. Chronic radiation proctitis involves full-thickness mucosal injury and has a delayed onset relative to radiation therapy. Chronic radiation proctitis most commonly presents within 14 months of radiation exposure, but it can present several years after radiation therapy. Risk factors for its development include hypertension, diabetes mellitus, smoking, and inflammatory bowel disease.

The diagnosis of radiation proctitis is suspected clinically and confirmed by direct visualization of the rectum with sigmoidoscopy (Fig. 56-1). This procedure should be performed by an experienced endoscopist due to the increased friability of the tissues leading to an increased risk of perforation. Treatment is based on the severity of symptoms but generally progresses in a stepwise fashion from medical treatments, such as mesalamine enemas or rectal formalin application; to interventional treatments, such as endoscopic argon beam plasma coagulation; to hyperbaric oxygen therapy; and to surgery, such as diversion of the bowel.

Medical treatment options include sucralfate enemas or formalin application to the rectum. Formalin treatment for radiation-induced proctitis works by acting as a chemical cautery, directly targeting and sealing fragile, newly formed blood vessels or telangiectasia in the damaged rectal mucosa, effectively stopping bleeding by inducing localized tissue necrosis through protein coagulation when applied topically; essentially, it "scleroses" the bleeding vessels, preventing further hemorrhage. Sucralfate forms a protective layer over the bowel walls and protects the fragile blood vessels from breaking. Sucralfate enemas are self-administered by the patient at home, whereas formalin application is performed by an endoscopic provider in an outpatient clinic setting or in a minor procedure room with intravenous sedation. Although the quality of evidence supporting formalin application is of slightly higher quality than that supporting sucralfate retention enemas, the ability to render enema treatments at home makes sucralfate enemas a reasonable choice as an initial therapy as was used in this

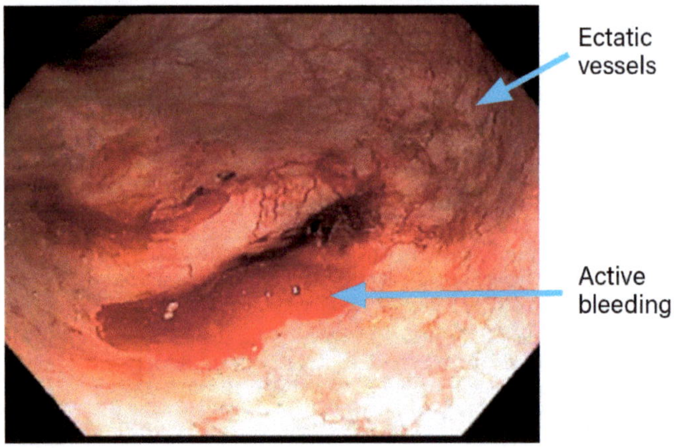

FIGURE 56-1. Sigmoidoscopy showing chronic radiation proctitis, telangiectasia, and an area of active bleeding. (Reprinted from Patel A, Pathak R, Deshpande V, Patel SH, Wickremesinghe PC, Vadada D. Radiofrequency ablation using BarRx for the endoscopic treatment of radiation proctopathy: a series of three cases. Clin Exp Gastroenterol 2014;7:453–60. doi: 10.2147/CEG.S66534)

patient. If sucralfate enemas are not effective, the best next alternative is medical management with formalin application to the rectal mucosa, and this is the best next option for the patient in the scenario.

Other medical treatments, such as mesalamine, ozone therapy, and corticosteroid suppositories, have not proved to be effective and are no longer recommended as first-line therapy for radiation proctitis, and these suppositories are not the best next treatment of this patient's symptoms. Pentoxifylline and vitamin E have shown some promise in the treatment of necrosis resulting from radiation therapy and in the prevention of fibrosis; however, neither has been shown to be effective for radiation proctitis.

Dahiya DS, Kichloo A, Tuma F, Albosta M, Wani F. Radiation proctitis and management strategies. Clin Endosc 2022;55:22–32. doi: 10.5946/ce.2020.288

Paquette IM, Vogel JD, Abbas MA, Feingold DL, Steele SR. The American Society of Colon and Rectal Surgeons clinical practice guidelines for the treatment of chronic radiation proctitis. Dis Colon Rectum 2018;61:1135–40. doi: 10.1097/DCR.0000000000001209

Sauvage L, Bentahila R, Tran Y, Guénégou-Arnoux A, Fabiano E, Bats A, et al. Radiation proctitis in patients with locally advanced cervical cancer treated by chemoradiation: analysis and predictive factors from a retrospective cohort. Am J Clin Oncol 2024;47:311–6. doi: 10.1097/COC.0000000000001092

57 Endometrial cancer surveillance

A 64-year-old patient presents for a surveillance visit 3 months after robot-assisted laparoscopic hysterectomy, bilateral salpingo-oophorectomy, and pelvic lymph node dissection for a stage IA, grade 2, endometrioid endometrial adenocarcinoma. She reports no changes to her health, no new bladder or bowel symptoms, and no bleeding. The best way to assess for cancer recurrence is to perform

(A) CA 125 tumor marker testing
(B) computed tomography (CT) of the abdomen and pelvis
* (C) pelvic examination
(D) positron emission tomography combined with computed tomography (PET/CT)
(E) vaginal cytology

The number of endometrial cancer survivors in the United States is estimated to be 600,000. This number is expected to increase given the aging population and increasing endometrial cancer incidence. General gynecologists frequently are part of a team that provides surveillance to endometrial cancer survivors. The clinical value of surveillance depends on several factors (Box 57-1). The Society of Gynecologic Oncology surveillance recommendations and the National Comprehensive Cancer Network (NCCN) guidelines for surveillance of patients with a history of endometrial cancer recommend a physical examination (including speculum, pelvic, and rectovaginal examinations) combined with symptom review every 3–6 months for the first 2 years and every 6–12 months for the next 3 years. A pelvic examination is the best surveillance strategy for the patient in this scenario. The guidelines emphasize the importance of patient education regarding symptoms and symptom recognition, given that most recurrences are symptomatic. Vaginal bleeding is the most common symptom of local recurrence, whereas distant recurrence can be associated with a variety of symptoms, including weight loss, pain, cough, and lethargy.

BOX 57-1

Factors That Affect the Clinical Value of Surveillance

- accuracy of surveillance methods
- availability of effective treatment for recurrent disease
- likelihood of recurrence
- whether asymptomatic recurrences (detected by surveillance) have a better prognosis than symptomatic recurrences

Historically, surveillance strategies for endometrial cancer have included routine vaginal cytology, but several recent studies have found that vaginal cytology rarely detects endometrial cancer recurrence that is not otherwise associated with vaginal bleeding or other abnormal findings on pelvic examination. Study results indicated that vaginal cytology is subject to false-positive results, particularly among patients who have received vaginal radiation therapy. As a result, the use of routine vaginal cytology for endometrial cancer surveillance is no longer recommended.

Patients with advanced disease or high-risk histology are more likely to experience a distant recurrence. Although CT can detect distant disease, most patients with distant recurrence are symptomatic, and many studies have found that the prognosis among symptomatic patients is not significantly worse than that of asymptomatic patients. Because of the potential harms of repeated imaging, including cumulative radiation exposure and the risk of incidental findings, routine imaging with CT in the absence of clinical indication is not recommended. By the same rationale, PET/CT also is not recommended. Although PET/CT is more sensitive than CT, it is less specific and associated with approximately three to five times higher radiation exposure compared with CT of the abdomen and pelvis.

Until recently, prospective data were not available, and surveillance guidelines have been informed almost entirely by retrospective, observational data; however, a large pragmatic trial evaluating surveillance after treatment for endometrial cancer, the TOTEM (temozolonide and topotecan) study, was published in 2022. In this prospective study, 1,866 patients in remission after treatment for endometrial cancer, stratified by risk of recurrence, were randomized to a minimal or intensive surveillance strategy (Table 57-1). After a median follow-up of 69 months, there was no significant difference in 5-year survival between the minimal and intensive groups (91.9% versus 90.6%, respectively), leading the authors to conclude that routine vaginal cytology and laboratory or imaging tests should not be included in surveillance, even for high-risk patients.

In this study, nearly all (171/175) cancer recurrences occurred within 5 years, and 75% occurred in the first 2 years, confirming the potential value of more intense surveillance during the first 2 years. No recurrences were detected by cytology alone, confirming that cytology offers little additional value. Approximately 50% of patients with recurrent disease were symptomatic at the time of detection, and annual CT did not improve survival. However, distant recurrence has generally been associated with poor prognosis, potentially making CT monitoring more valuable in this subset of individuals. Although routine use of CT is not recommended, there may be a role for its use in select patients. The described patient has low-risk disease and routine surveillance imaging with CT or PET/CT would not be justified.

In the TOTEM study, no benefit was found from CA 125 monitoring; however, the study included relatively few patients with serous histology, in whom CA 125 is more frequently increased. The NCCN recommends CA 125 monitoring be considered for patients whose CA 125 level was high at the time of diagnosis; however, this is not the case for the patient described.

Because both arms of the TOTEM trial included frequent physical examinations, its results do not indicate the optimal frequency of scheduled visits. Because only 10.1% of recurrences were detected by examination alone, it may be that a less frequent visit schedule would be equally effective. Trials evaluating the frequency of visits and comparing scheduled versus patient-initiated visits are currently underway.

Most patients with endometrial cancer (85%) have early-stage disease, which is associated with a risk of recurrence ranging from 1% to 15% depending on other pathologic factors. A significant proportion of recurrences are local recurrences in the vaginal vault or pelvis, which are usually detected on physical examination and often are salvageable; therefore, pelvic examination is the highest value procedure for detecting recurrence and is the best strategy for continued surveillance for the patient in this scenario.

TABLE 57-1. Minimal and Intensive Surveillance Regimens for Low- and High-Risk Patients

	LOW RISK OF RECURRENCE		HIGH RISK OF RECURRENCE	
Surveillance Method	**Minimal Surveillance Strategy**	**Intensive Surveillance Strategy**	**Minimal Surveillance Strategy**	**Intensive Surveillance Strategy**
Physical and pelvic examination	Every 6 mo (total 11 visits/5 y)	Every 4 mo for 2 y, then every 6 mo (total 13 visits/5 y)	Every 4 mo for 2 y, then every 6 mo (total 13 visits/5 y)	Every 4 mo (total 14 visits/5 y)
Vaginal cytology	No	Annually	No	Annually
CT of chest, abdomen, pelvis	No	Annually for 2 y	Annually for 2 y	Annually
CA 125	No	No	No	Every visit
Abdominal and pelvic ultrasound	No	No	No	Twice a year for 3 y, then annually

American Cancer Society. Key statistics for endometrial cancer. ACS; 2025. Accessed March 17, 2025. https://www.cancer.org/cancer/endometrial-cancer/about/key-statistics.html

Ezendam NP, de Rooij BH, Kruitwagen RF, Creutzberg CL, van Loon I, Boll D, et al. ENdometrial cancer SURvivors' follow-up carE (ENSURE): less is more? Evaluating patient satisfaction and cost-effectiveness of a reduced follow-up schedule: study protocol of a randomized controlled trial. Trials 2018;19:227. doi: 10.1186/s13063-018-2611-x

Salani R, Khanna N, Frimer M, Bristow RE, Chen L. An update on post-treatment surveillance and diagnosis of recurrence in women with gynecologic malignancies: Society of Gynecologic Oncology (SGO) recommendations. Gynecol Oncol 2017;146:3–10. doi: 10.1016/j.ygyno.2017.03.022

Zola P, Ciccone G, Piovano E, Fuso L, Di Cuonzo D, Castiglione A, et al. Effectiveness of intensive versus minimalist follow-up regimen on survival in patients with endometrial cancer (TOTEM Study): a randomized, pragmatic, parallel group, multicenter trial. J Clin Oncol 2022;40:3817–27. doi: 10.1200/JCO.22.00471

58 Febrile neutropenia

A 55-year-old patient with recurrent, metastatic cervical cancer is receiving chemotherapy with cisplatin, paclitaxel, bevacizumab, and pembrolizumab. She presents during cycle 1, day 7, with an at-home temperature of 38.2 °C (100.8 °F) and poor intake. Her vital signs on arrival are blood pressure of 88/50 mm Hg, heart rate of 110 beats per minute, temperature of 38 °C (100.4 °F), a respiratory rate of 18 breaths per minute, and oxygen saturation of 94% on room air. Her physical examination is notable for abdominal pain to palpation without rebound or guarding. Her white blood cell count is 1.2×10^3/L with an absolute neutrophil count of 400 per microliter, and her serum creatinine concentration is 1.3 mg/dL. Computed tomography is negative (no bowel wall thickening and no radiographic source of infection). Intravenous hydration is started, and urine and blood cultures are pending. She has a prior documented allergic reaction to penicillin and cephalosporins. The best initial antibiotic regimen is

(A) ciprofloxacin
(B) levofloxacin
* (C) meropenem
(D) vancomycin

Neutropenia is a major risk factor for the development of infections among patients undergoing treatment for malignancy. Signs and symptoms of infection may be muted among patients with low neutrophil counts, but fever remains an early sign. *Febrile neutropenia* is defined as a single temperature greater than 38.3 °C (100.9 °F) or a sustained temperature of greater than 38 °C (100.4 °F) for 1 hour or longer in a patient with an absolute neutrophil count (ANC) of less than 500 cells/microliter or an ANC expected to decrease to less than 500 cells/microliter within 48 hours. Patients presenting with neutropenic fever require urgent empiric antibiotic treatment.

The patient in this scenario presents with a sustained fever and has an ANC of less than 500. In addition to searching for a source of infection, prompt administration of antibiotics is important for decreasing morbidity. The Multinational Association of Supportive Care in Cancer (MASCC) risk index score aids in identifying patients with febrile neutropenia who are at low risk for mortality. The factors included in this scoring system are noted in Table 58-1. Patients who score 21 or higher are considered to be at low risk for complications and may be considered for outpatient management. This patient has a score of 12 (moderate symptoms comprising diarrhea and abdominal pain, solid tumor, outpatient at time of symptom onset, and age less than 60 years) and is classified as high risk.

Patients considered high risk should be admitted to the hospital for evaluation and treatment and immediately receive broad-spectrum intravenous antibiotics that provide antipseudomonal activity. Although gram-positive bacteria are the most frequent pathogens identified during neutropenic fever, broad coverage against aerobic gram-negative pathogens is important, given their virulence and association with severe sepsis. Single-agent therapy is preferred, but combination treatment should be considered if antimicrobial resistance is suspected (eg, history of methicillin-resistant

TABLE 58-1. The Multinational Association for Supportive Care in Cancer Score

CHARACTERISTIC	WEIGHT
Burden of febrile neutropenia	
No or mild symptoms	5
Moderate symptoms	3
No hypotension (SBP greater than 90 mm Hg)	5
No active COPD	4
Solid tumor or no previous fungal infection	4
No dehydration requiring parenteral fluids	3
Outpatient status	3
Age less than 60 y	2

Abbreviations: COPD, chronic obstructive pulmonary disease; SBP, systolic blood pressure.

NOTE. Applicable points are added to create a cumulative score. The maximum score is 26, and a score greater than 20 has a predicted low risk (less than 10%) for serious medical complications during the course of the febrile neutropenia.

Reprinted from Zimmer AJ, Freifeld AG. Optimal management of neutropenic fever in patients with cancer. J Oncol Pract 2019;15:19–24. doi: 10.1200/JOP.18.00269

Staphylococcus aureus). Of the choices listed, meropenem is the only broad-spectrum agent. Meropenem provides activity against most gram-positive, gram-negative, and anaerobic organisms and is a Category 1 recommendation by the National Comprehensive Cancer Network in the treatment of neutropenic fever. Additionally, among patients with renal failure or renal disease, meropenem is preferred as it is associated with lower rates of seizures compared with imipenem combined with cisplatin.

Patients who meet low-risk criteria during neutropenic fever can receive antibiotics as an outpatient. Patients with febrile neutropenia may be eligible for discharge if they meet certain criteria, including a residence 1 hour or less or 30 miles or less from the clinic or hospital, ability to comply with frequent follow-up, availability of a family member or caregiver 24 hours a day, access to a phone and transportation 24 hours a day, and no history of non-adherence to treatment protocols. Amoxicillin and clavulanate is an oral antibiotic that can be used in low-risk patients who are not suspected to be colonized by extended-spectrum β-lactamase-producing gram-negative bacilli. Because the patient in this scenario falls into a high-risk category based on her MASCC score, she should be admitted for intravenous antibiotics. In addition, the patient is allergic to penicillin.

Ciprofloxacin has activity against gram-negative and atypical organisms, such as *Legionella*, and less activity against gram-positive organisms. It has no activity against anaerobes, and gram-negative resistance is increasing in many hospital centers. Given its more limited coverage profile, ciprofloxacin would not be an appropriate first-line agent in this patient's care.

Levofloxacin also provides coverage against gram-negative and atypical organisms. It has improved activity against gram-positive bacteria when compared with ciprofloxacin but has no activity against anaerobic organisms and would not be appropriate in the initial management of febrile neutropenia.

Vancomycin has gram-positive activity only and would not be an appropriate initial treatment in a patient with neutropenic fever because coverage against gram-negative organisms is needed due to concerns of virulence and potential for sepsis. It can be added to empiric therapy if there is concern for methicillin-resistant *S aureus* due to history or current results.

Febrile neutropenia is a medical emergency. The MASCC score triages patients to high or low risk and appropriate inpatient or outpatient management. Among patients who are high risk, empiric broad-spectrum intravenous antibiotics should be initiated after blood cultures have been obtained.

Klastersky J, de Naurois J, Rolston K, Rapoport B, Maschmeyer G, Aapro M, et al. Management of febrile neutropaenia: ESMO Clinical Practice Guidelines. Ann Oncol 2016;27:v111–8. doi: 10.1093/annonc/mdw325

National Comprehensive Cancer Network. Prevention and treatment of cancer-related infections. Version 3. 2024 NCCN Clinical Practice Guidelines in Oncology. NCCN; 2024. Accessed March 25, 2025. https://www.nccn.org/professionals/physician_gls/pdf/infections.pdf

Taplitz RA, Kennedy EB, Bow EJ, Crews J, Gleason C, Hawley DK, et al. Outpatient management of fever and neutropenia in adults treated for malignancy: American Society of Clinical Oncology and Infectious Diseases Society of America clinical practice guideline update. J Clin Oncol 2018;36:1443–53. doi: 10.1200/JCO.2017.77.6211

Zimmer AJ, Freifeld AG. Optimal management of neutropenic fever in patients with cancer. J Oncol Pract 2019;15:19–24. doi: 10.1200/JOP.18.00269

59 Kaplan-Meier method

A study of a new treatment is underway. The primary outcome is overall survival, and you want to analyze the study's data with the Kaplan–Meier method. The probability calculation for Kaplan–Meier at each time interval is represented by

(A) change in percent death/change in time
(B) number of deaths/patients enrolled
(C) number of disease-free survivors/number of patients at risk
* (D) number of survivors/number of patients at risk

Survival analysis extends our ability to understand outcomes beyond simply occurrence or non-occurrence by accounting for the time from a certain point to the event of interest. Fundamental assumptions in survival analyses are that all subjects have been followed from the same point (t0) to the time of the event, and that they are followed and evaluated in the same manner. A typical choice for t0 is the date of randomization on a randomized trial, treatment on a nonrandomized therapeutic trial, or diagnosis on an observational study.

Survival data are analyzed to calculate hazard rates (probabilities of the event happening during a very short time interval). This is called the *hazard ratio*, and it is a commonly reported statistic for comparing outcomes between two groups of study participants.

There are several approaches to survival analysis. The most commonly used are the Life Table method, the Kaplan–Meier method, and the Cox proportional hazards method.

The Life Table method is the simplest and involves creating an actuarial table (life table) consisting of a number of fixed duration time periods, and the frequency of events occurring during each interval is calculated. Events are assumed to take place at the midportion of each interval. A cumulative event rate, by a certain time, is calculated by multiplying the rate of events occurring during each interval up to that time. The cumulative event rate (eg, death, progression, or survival) is plotted on the y axis, and the intervals are plotted on the x axis, generating a graphic representation.

The Kaplan–Meier Product Limit method also is relatively simple to use and interpret, and it is nonparametric (ie, it can be used independent of assumptions made about the shape of the survival function). The Kaplan–Meier method is similar to the Life Table method, except that it is more precise. With Kaplan–Meier, the intervals are not of fixed length; rather, exact survival times are used instead of assuming that events occur at the midpoint of a fixed duration interval. In effect, the duration of each interval is determined by the time between events. Cumulative survival probability is calculated in the same manner as in a Life Table analysis.

The underlying concept is that the Kaplan–Meier method permits calculation of the chance that an individual will have survived to a particular time. The total time of observation is divided into a series of consecutive intervals. Intervals may be of different lengths, as above, and each patient's first interval begins at time of their enrollment (t0). For the entire population, the probability of surviving a specific interval is calculated as follows: (number of patients who were known to be alive at the end of the interval)/(number of patients who were known to be alive at the start of the interval). All patients included in the calculation of the probability of surviving the interval must have been monitored throughout the interval (status must be known at both the start and the end). The cumulative probability of surviving from enrollment to the completion of the nth interval is the product of the probabilities of surviving all the intervals up to and including the nth.

Figure 59-1 shows two Kaplan–Meier curves representing the persistence (survival) of unilocular cysts compared with septated ovarian cysts. Cumulative survival is plotted on the y axis and time on the x axis. Each discrete point represents a persistent cyst. A limitation of the Kaplan–Meier analysis is that it is not straightforward to adjust for multiple covariates.

The Cox proportional hazards method is similar to a logistic regression model and is particularly well suited to analysis of multiple covariates. As in the Kaplan–Meier method, assumptions about the shape of the survival curve are unnecessary; however, the hazard ratio is assumed to be equal throughout the entire time of the study (the hazard rates must be proportional). If the proportional hazards assumption is violated, the Cox model must be modified.

The probability that is calculated in each time interval of a Kaplan–Meier analysis is (number of survivors)/(number of patients at risk). This calculation is made in each interval when conducting a Kaplan–Meier analysis. Plotting the product of all interval probabilities of survival up to a certain point will yield a survival curve.

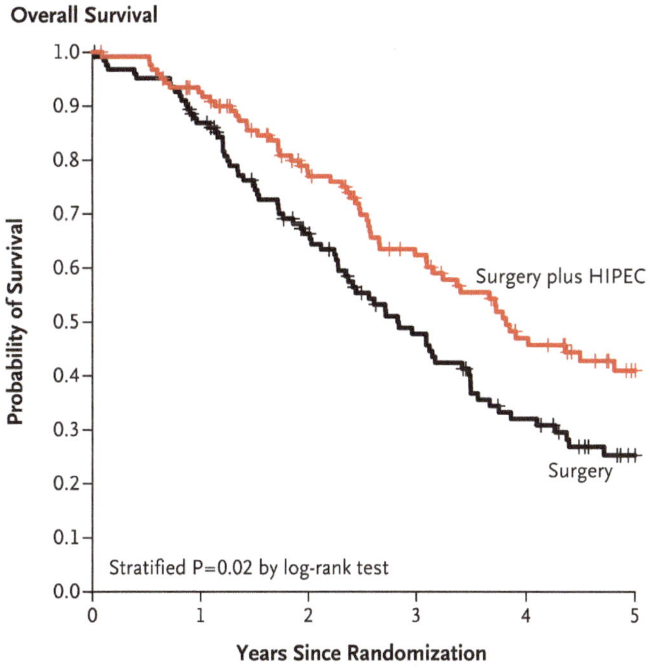

FIGURE 59-1. Kaplan–Meier curve of overall survival comparing patients with stage III epithelial ovarian cancer treated with surgery with or without hyperthermic intraperitoneal chemotherapy (HIPEC). (Reprinted from van Driel WJ, Koole SN, Sikorska K, Schagen van Leeuwen JH, Schreuder HW, Hermans RH, et al. Hyperthermic intraperitoneal chemotherapy in ovarian cancer. N Engl J Med 2018;378:230–40. doi: 10.1056/NEJMoa1708618)

This calculation of (change in percent death)/(change in time) approximates the tangent to the mortality curve, which is the hazard rate of death at a specific time. The calculation of (deaths)/(patients enrolled) illustrates the mortality rate and does not account for time to death; likewise, calculating (disease-free survivors)/(number of patients treated) in this scenario is not the best choice. If the outcome were progression-free survival, this would be appropriate.

Barraclough H, Simms L, Govindan R. Biostatistics primer: what a clinician ought to know: hazard ratios [published erratum appears in J Thorac Oncol 2011;6:1454]. J Thorac Oncol 2011;6:978–82. doi: 10.1097/JTO.0b013e31821b10ab

Bewick V, Cheek L, Ball J. Statistics review 12: survival analysis. Crit Care 2004;8:389–94. doi: 10.1186/cc2955

Bland JM, Altman DG. Survival probabilities (the Kaplan-Meier method). BMJ 1998;317:1572–80. doi: 10.1136/bmj.317.7172.1572

Efron B. Logistic regression, survival analysis, and the Kaplan-Meier curve. Journal of the American Statistical Association 1988;83:414–25. doi: 10.1080/01621459.1988.10478612

Rich JT, Neely JG, Paniello RC, Voelker CC, Nussenbaum B, Wang EW. A practical guide to understanding Kaplan-Meier curves. Otolaryngol Head Neck Surg 2010;143:331–6. doi: 10.1016/j.otohns.2010.05.007

60 Initial management of ovarian cancer

A 57-year-old woman is referred to you after reporting 6 months of pelvic pain, bloating, and early satiety. Her past medical history is notable for hypertension and poorly controlled diabetes mellitus, with a hemoglobin A_{1C} (Hb A_{1C}) of 9.2 mg/dL. The physical examination is notable for a moderately distended abdomen and palpable masses to the level of the umbilicus with fluid wave. Her CA 125 is 432 U/mL. Computed tomography (CT) of her chest, abdomen, and pelvis reveals bilateral adnexal masses, moderate ascites, omental nodularity to the greater curvature of the stomach, mesenteric lymphadenopathy, and a 4-cm liver mass near the portal vein. A CT-guided biopsy of the omentum shows high-grade serous carcinoma of müllerian origin. The best next step in treatment is

(A) chemoradiation
(B) hospice referral
* (C) neoadjuvant chemotherapy
(D) primary cytoreductive surgery

Surgical management with comprehensive staging and optimal tumor debulking plays an important role in survival outcomes among patients with ovarian cancer. For patients with newly diagnosed ovarian cancer, assessment of disease distribution and medical comorbidities is important in treatment planning. If patients demonstrate limited disease, such that all disease can be removed during surgery, primary debulking surgery should be considered. The patient in the scenario has apparent stage IIIC disease (disease outside of the pelvis and upper abdominal disease) and has poorly controlled diabetes. The disease distribution described is unlikely to lead to optimal debulking to less than 1 cm of residual disease. Given this, she will benefit from neoadjuvant chemotherapy before having an interval debulking surgery.

Optimal tumor debulking is defined as less than 1 cm of residual disease, but the ultimate goal of surgery is to have no residual disease. The amount of residual disease has the greatest prognostic effect on overall and progression-free survival. A retrospective study evaluated the effect of residual disease on survival and noted that patients with no gross residual disease had the longest overall survival at 86 months compared with 46 months for patients with 0.1–1 cm of disease and remaining disease greater than 1 cm at 37 months. In a separate meta-analysis, the median progression-free survival for patients with no residual disease was 25.6 months compared with 17.2 months for patients with remaining disease of greater than 0–1 cm and 12.2 months for residual disease greater than 1 cm.

Computed tomography can aid feasibility assessment and surgical planning. Triage laparoscopy has been used as a tool to aid in the identification of disease suitable for optimal cytoreduction. The laparoscopic-based Fagotti scoring model assesses the presence or absence of seven criteria (Table 60-1). Each item on the scoring model receives a score of 0 (not present) or 2 (present). A score of more than 8 is associated with a low likelihood of achieving optimal cytoreduction. In these cases, neoadjuvant chemotherapy followed by interval surgical cytoreduction and adjuvant chemotherapy is recommended. In patients in whom CT may not clearly demonstrate upper abdominal disease distribution, a triage laparoscopy for scoring and proceeding to debulking surgery can be performed. The patient in this scenario has evidence of disease at the omentum with extension to the stomach, liver, and bowel mesentery, all of which make the likelihood of optimal debulking low.

In patients who are not surgical candidates based on age, fragility, poor performance status, or comorbidities, or those who have a disease burden that is unlikely to be optimally cytoreduced, neoadjuvant chemotherapy is given with the intent to allow for medical improvement or clinical response, or both, that would increase the likelihood of optimal cytoreduction at time of interval surgery. Several trials have compared neoadjuvant chemotherapy followed by interval debulking surgery and adjuvant chemotherapy to primary debulking surgery followed by chemotherapy. Results across trials demonstrated that patients treated with neoadjuvant chemotherapy had improved surgical outcomes with shorter operative time, less blood loss, fewer surgical complications, and shorter hospital stays. Patients who received neoadjuvant chemotherapy also had fewer extensive and complicated surgeries to achieve optimal cytoreduction and had a lower risk of death. Randomized trials outside of the United States have found noninferior survival for patients receiving neoadjuvant chemotherapy versus primary debulking surgery; however, these trials reported lower overall survival and lower rates of optimal debulking compared with U.S. studies. This raises questions about generalizability to U.S. practice where aggressive debulking is more common. Because this patient does not appear to have disease amenable to optimal cytoreduction, proceeding with neoadjuvant chemotherapy is the best next step in treatment.

Hospice care focuses on the care, comfort, and quality of life of a person with a serious illness who is approaching the end of life. Hospice referrals can be provided when a doctor believes the patient has 6 months or less left to live if the illness is allowed to progress naturally. In contrast, palliative care is specialized medical care for patients living with serious illnesses. Patients enrolled in palliative care may receive medical

TABLE 60-1. Fagotti Scoring Algorithm

TUMOR CHARACTERISTIC	SCORE
Peritoneal carcinomatosis: Massive peritoneal involvement and/or miliary pattern of distribution	0 (not present) or 2 (present)
Diaphragmatic surface involvement: Widespread infiltrating carcinomatosis and/or confluent nodules to most of diaphragm surface	0 (not present) or 2 (present)
Mesenteric involvement: Large infiltrating nodules and/or involvement of the root of the mesentery based on limited movement of intestinal segments	0 (not present) or 2 (present)
Omental involvement: Tumor diffusion of the omentum up to the greater curvature of the stomach	0 (not present) or 2 (present)
Bowel involvement: Tumor infiltration of large or small bowel requiring intestinal resection, sigmoid, and/or	0 (not present) or 2 (present)
Stomach involvement: Obvious tumor infiltration into gastric wall	0 (not present) or 2 (present)
Liver involvement: Liver surface lesions greater than 2 cm in size	0 (not present) or 2 (present)

Reprinted from Fleming ND, Nick AM, Coleman RL, Westin SN, Ramirez PT, Soliman PT, et al. Laparoscopic surgical algorithm to triage the timing of tumor reductive surgery in advanced ovarian cancer. Obstet Gynecol 2018;132:545–54. doi: 10.1097/AOG.0000000000002796

care for their symptoms while also receiving treatment for their disease. Early hospice referrals can lead to improved quality of life, but in a patient with newly diagnosed ovarian cancer that has a high likelihood of response to primary therapy, a hospice referral would be premature. If she is able to undergo chemotherapy and eventually have surgery followed by chemotherapy, her estimated progression-free survival is around 2 years. Therefore, hospice is not the best answer in this scenario. If this patient declined all medical and surgical interventions, or if she were too medically ill to receive therapy, then it would be appropriate to discuss hospice care.

Chemoradiation therapy is not the primary treatment for epithelial ovarian cancer and is a treatment most commonly used for vulvar and cervical cancer. Although ovarian cancer is a radiosensitive malignancy, transperitoneal spread is the most common route. Historically, whole abdominal radiotherapy was evaluated for sterilization of large volumes of micrometastatic intraperitoneal disease; however, the dose limitations needed to minimize organ toxicities were ineffective in eradicating the tumor burden. Currently, improved radiation techniques that allow for focal radiation may be used for palliation of isolated and particularly bothersome metastatic disease (eg, spinal metastases) but is not considered the primary modality of therapy for patients with metastatic ovarian cancer.

Broekman KE, van der Aa MA, Nijman HW, Jalving M, Reyners AK. End-of-life care for patients with advanced ovarian cancer in the Netherlands: a retrospective registry-based analysis. Gynecol Oncol 2022;166:148–53. doi: 10.1016/j.ygyno.2022.04.017

Cummings M, Nicolais O, Shahin M. Surgery in advanced ovary cancer: primary versus interval cytoreduction. Diagnostics (Basel) 2022;12:988. doi: 10.3390/diagnostics12040988

Fleming ND, Nick AM, Coleman RL, Westin SN, Ramirez PT, Soliman PT, et al. Laparoscopic surgical algorithm to triage the timing of tumor reductive surgery in advanced ovarian cancer. Obstet Gynecol 2018;132:545–54. doi: 10.1097/AOG.0000000000002796

61 First-line chemotherapy in ovarian cancer

A 56-year-old patient with stage IVA ovarian cancer with preoperative pleural effusions presents for postoperative follow-up 2 weeks after an exploratory laparotomy, total abdominal hysterectomy, omentectomy, and tumor debulking. She had unresectable disease in the lesser sac and small bowel mesentery. She has no other medical problems. On examination, her midline incision is well healed. In addition to carboplatin, the best chemotherapy regimen for this patient is

(A) gemcitabine and bevacizumab
(B) paclitaxel alone
* (C) paclitaxel and bevacizumab
(D) pegylated liposomal doxorubicin

Most patients with ovarian cancer present with stage III or IV disease because they often are asymptomatic in the early stages. In addition, the symptoms of ovarian cancer can be vague, such as abdominal bloating or pain, urinary frequency, and early satiety. The initial approach to treatment includes consideration for primary debulking surgery or neoadjuvant chemotherapy. The decision to proceed with surgery is based on several factors, including the ability to resect all visible disease, the patient's performance status, and the presence of comorbidities that might prevent an immediate surgical intervention (eg, clinically significant pulmonary emboli). A review of preoperative images with or without assessment with diagnostic laparoscopy can help guide this decision.

Stage IVA ovarian cancer is defined by the presence of malignant pleural effusions. This is not necessarily a contraindication for primary debulking surgery consideration, but it has been demonstrated that *suboptimal debulking*, defined as gross residual disease greater than 1 cm, is associated with a poorer prognosis compared with optimal or complete cytoreduction. Progression-free and overall survival are inferior in patients when complete resection is not achieved.

In patients with advanced-stage epithelial ovarian cancer (stage III and IV), the standard-of-care chemotherapy is carboplatin and paclitaxel. Multiple phase III clinical trials have demonstrated the benefit of the addition of anti-angiogenesis therapy, such as bevacizumab, to the standard treatment, especially in patients with stage IV or suboptimally debulked disease. In addition, the use of anti-angiogenesis therapy has been shown to reduce pleural effusions and ascites. In patients with high-risk disease, the addition of anti-angiogenesis therapy outweighs the potential risks (hypertension, proteinuria, impaired wound healing, bowel perforation). For the described patient, the addition of bevacizumab to paclitaxel is recommended for the treatment of stage IV disease or in suboptimally debulked patients, especially with ascites or pleural effusions, or both. The addition of bevacizumab to carboplatin and paclitaxel was associated with a 30% reduction in the risk of progression or death in a subset of patients with stage IV disease. There was a 39% reduction in the risk of progression or death in the subset of patients with suboptimally debulked stage III disease.

There are some situations in which the addition of paclitaxel to the treatment regimen is not recommended. First, due to the potential for the development or worsening of peripheral neuropathy with paclitaxel, the oncologist may choose to avoid this agent in patients who present with severe peripheral neuropathy before treatment. Second, if neuropathy presents and progresses during treatment, the oncologist may choose to substitute gemcitabine or pegylated liposomal doxorubicin for paclitaxel. Second-line or later-line, platinum-sensitive recurrent disease can be treated with other platinum doublets. In many cases, platinum combined with non-taxane agents is used to limit toxicities, such as alopecia and peripheral neuropathy. Neither gemcitabine and bevacizumab nor pegylated liposomal doxorubicin is the appropriate treatment choice for this patient in the first-line setting.

This patient has no contraindications to paclitaxel, and platinum–taxane doublet is the standard treatment for her disease. She does not have preexisting neuropathy, and she has suboptimally debulked disease, large-volume ascites, and pleural effusion. The addition of bevacizumab to platinum–taxane chemotherapy is the best choice for her treatment.

Aghajanian C, Blank SV, Goff BA, Judson PL, Teneriello MG, Husain A, et al. OCEANS: a randomized, double-blind, placebo-controlled phase III trial of chemotherapy with or without bevacizumab in patients with platinum-sensitive recurrent epithelial ovarian, primary peritoneal, or fallopian tube cancer. J Clin Oncol 2012;30:2039–45. doi: 10.1200/JCO.2012.42.0505

Coleridge SL, Bryant A, Kehoe S, Morrison J. Neoadjuvant chemotherapy before surgery versus surgery followed by chemotherapy for initial treatment in advanced ovarian epithelial cancer. Cochrane Database of Systematic Reviews 2021, Issue 7. Art. No.: CD005343. doi: 10.1002/14651858.CD005343.pub6

Karam A, Ledermann JA, Kim J, Sehouli J, Lu K, Gourley C, et al. Fifth Ovarian Cancer Consensus Conference of the Gynecologic Cancer InterGroup: first-line interventions. Ann Oncol 2017;28:711–7. doi: 10.1093/annonc/mdx011

Oza AM, Cook AD, Pfisterer J, Embleton A, Ledermann JA, Pujade-Lauraine E, et al. Standard chemotherapy with or without bevacizumab for women with newly diagnosed ovarian cancer (ICON7): overall survival results of a phase 3 randomised trial. ICON7 trial investigators. Lancet Oncol 2015;16:928–36. doi: 10.1016/S1470-2045(15)00086-8

Pujade-Lauraine E, Wagner U, Aavall-Lundqvist E, Gebski V, Heywood M, Vasey PA, et al. Pegylated liposomal doxorubicin and carboplatin compared with paclitaxel and carboplatin for patients with platinum-sensitive ovarian cancer in late relapse. J Clin Oncol 2010;28:3323–9. doi: 10.1200/JCO.2009.25.7519

62 Fertility-sparing treatment of endometrial cancer

A 38-year-old nulligravida with a history of polycystic ovary syndrome undergoes hysteroscopy with dilation and curettage for abnormal uterine bleeding. The pathology demonstrates grade 1 endometrioid endometrial adenocarcinoma that is ERPR+. Magnetic resonance imaging of the pelvis shows normal-appearing ovaries, no evidence of residual endometrial mass or myometrial invasion, and no pelvic lymphadenopathy. She strongly desires fertility-sparing treatment. The factor that best predicts this patient's response to treatment is

(A) absence of lymphadenopathy
(B) absence of myometrial invasion
(C) absence of ovarian involvement
(D) her age
* (E) progesterone receptor status

Endometrial cancer is the most prevalent gynecologic cancer in the United States. Although most patients are diagnosed after menopause at an average age of 60 years, approximately 14% of patients are premenopausal. Patients younger than age 40 years with endometrial cancer are more likely to have early-stage, low-grade disease; however, up to 20% may have extrauterine spread at diagnosis. This risk increases to 50% with higher-grade tumors. Because the standard treatment for endometrial cancer involves total hysterectomy, younger patients may desire fertility preservation, and identifying appropriate candidates for conservative management with progestins is of utmost importance (Box 62-1).

BOX 62-1

Fertility-Sparing Treatment Recommendations for Endometrial Cancer

Recommendations

Review of initial pathology by an experienced histopathologist

- A request for a second opinion by an experienced histopathologist is recommended if fertility-sparing treatment is considered (Level of evidence III, Grade A).
- The G1, G2, G3 grading system is recommended. The binary grading system for endometrial carcinoma should not be used for these patients (Level of evidence III, Grade A).
- The use of immunohistochemistry (PTEN, ARID1A, etc) for the evaluation of several biomarkers is not recommended for diagnostic purposes (Level of evidence IV, Grade D).

Differentiation of the tumor

- Fertility-sparing treatment is considered for endometrioid patients with endometrial carcinoma with Grade 1, Stage IA without myometrial invasion and without risk factors (Level of evidence V, Grade A).
- Evidence for Grade 2 endometrioid endometrial carcinoma is limited. Therefore, fertility-sparing treatment should be discussed on a case-by-case basis (Level of evidence IV, Grade C).

Establishing a reliable histopathology

- Hysteroscopic-guided endometrial biopsy is preferred over blind biopsy for confirming the diagnosis of endometrial carcinoma (Level of evidence III, Grade A).

Myometrial invasion

- Preoperative assessment of myometrial invasion in patients with endometrial carcinoma should be performed using MRI or transvaginal US by a specialized radiologist/sonographer. Standardized high-quality protocols for MRI should be used to reach the highest possible accuracy (Level of evidence III, Grade A).
- Computed tomography should not be used for preoperative assessment of myometrial invasion in patients with endometrial carcinoma (Level of evidence III, Grade A).

Exclude extrauterine disease/ synchronous or metastatic

- Magnetic resonance imaging or CT is recommended for detecting pelvic or para-aortic lymph nodes and distant metastases (Level of evidence II, Grade B).
- Adnexal involvement should be ruled out by pelvic MRI or transvaginal US (Level of evidence II, B).

Reprinted from Rodolakis A, Scambia G, Planchamp F, Acien M, Di Spiezio Sardo A, Farrugia M, et al. ESGO/ESHRE/ESGE guidelines for the fertility-sparing treatment of patients with endometrial carcinoma. Hum Reprod Open 2023;2023:hoac057. doi: 10.1093/hropen/hoac057

BOX 62-2

Recommendations for Medical Treatment of Endometrial Cancer

Recommendations

Selection of medication

- A combined approach consisting of hysteroscopic tumor resection, followed by oral progestins and/or levonorgestrel intrauterine device, is the most effective fertility-sparing treatment both for complete response rate and live birth rate compared with other treatment options (Level of evidence II, Grade B).
- Gonadotropin-releasing hormone analogues should not be considered as a first-line treatment (Level of evidence II, Grade B).

The role of hysteroscopic resection

- If an early and focal myometrial invasion (1–2 mm) is suspected from the resection material, a fertility-sparing approach may be discussed on a case-by-case basis. In this circumstance, complete hysteroscopic lesion resection, followed by oral progestins and/or levonorgestrel intrauterine device, can be proposed as fertility-sparing treatment (Level of evidence IV, Grade C).

Dose of progestins

- Orally administered megestrol acetate at a dose of 160–320 mg/d or medroxyprogesterone acetate at a dose of 400–600 mg/d is recommended (Level of evidence III, Grade B).
- A levonorgestrel intrauterine device at a dose of 52 mg, alone or in combination with oral progestins, is a safe and effective approach (Level of evidence III, Grade B).

Duration of treatment

- The recommended duration of therapy is 6–12 months, within which a complete response should be achieved (Level of evidence III, Grade B).
- The maximum time to achieve complete response should not exceed 15 months (Level of evidence IV, Grade C).
- In the absence of any kind of response at 6 months, multidisciplinary counselling is recommended for adapting the management on a case-by-case basis (Level of evidence IV, Grade B).

Response (partial vs complete vs no response)

- Hysteroscopic resection followed by progestins either by oral and/or intrauterine device administration is recommended to achieve both the highest complete response rate and the highest live birth rate (Level of evidence II, Grade B).
- Weight control during fertility-sparing treatment is highly recommended to increase the chance of response (Level of evidence II, Grade A).

Follow-up with maintenance treatment for patients willing or not willing to conceive immediately

- Two consecutive endometrial biopsies showing complete response with a minimal interval of 3 months are necessary to consider the success of the fertility-sparing treatment (Level of evidence IV, Grade C).
- The complete response is mandatory to consider follow-up with maintenance treatment until pregnancy is planned (Level of evidence II, Grade A).
- Clinical pelvic examination and US scan are recommended at every 3-month follow-up visit (Level of evidence IV, Grade B).
- Endometrial histological assessment should be performed every 3–6 months by hysteroscopy according to the results of imaging (Level of evidence IV, Grade B).
- MRI could be considered on a case-by-case basis (Level of evidence IV, Grade C).

Pregnancy

- Women undergoing fertility-sparing treatment for endometrial hyperplasia or endometrial carcinoma should be encouraged to actively aim to conceive as soon as the complete response is achieved (Level of evidence V, Grade B).
- ART should be considered in order to improve success rate and reduce the interval to conception without a higher risk of recurrence (Level of evidence III, Grade B). However, natural conception may be considered in women with good reproductive potential within a defined time (6–9 months) (Level of evidence V, Grade C).
- Close surveillance by a multidisciplinary team should be continued and maintenance therapy with a levonorgestrel intrauterine device should be recommended to women who decline surgery after delivery and who do not plan their second pregnancy immediately after the first one (Level of evidence III, Grade B).

Recurrence rate after fertility-sparing treatment

- The risk of recurrence after fertility-sparing treatment for endometrial carcinoma may be equal for progestins or a levonorgestrel intrauterine device (Level of evidence II, Grade B).

Definitive and completion surgeries

- Definitive surgery is recommended in cases of non-responders, inability to conceive, recurrence or disease progression (Level of evidence II, Grade A).
- For patients with a strong desire to preserve fertility, a second conservative approach can be considered on a case-by-case basis (Level of evidence IV, Grade B).
- Completion surgery is recommended after completing childbearing (Level of evidence II, Grade A).
- Removal of ovaries should be considered on a case-by-case basis (Level of evidence III, Grade B).

Reprinted from Rodolakis A, Scambia G, Planchamp F, Acien M, Di Spiezio Sardo A, Farrugia M, et al. ESGO/ESHRE/ESGE guidelines for the fertility-sparing treatment of patients with endometrial carcinoma. Hum Reprod Open 2023;2023:hoac057. doi: 10.1093/hropen/hoac057

The most important predictor of response to medical treatment with progestins is progesterone receptor status. Hormone receptor-positive tumors, particularly those that are progesterone receptor-positive, are more common in grade 1 endometrioid endometrial cancer and have a higher response rate to progestin therapy (up to 72%).

Medical therapy in lieu of hysterectomy should be reserved for those who want to maintain fertility, and they should be referred to a fertility specialist for evaluation and counseling. A hysterectomy is recommended after childbearing. Young age at diagnosis should increase suspicion of a hereditary syndrome, such as Lynch syndrome, which might increase the risk of other malignancies, such as colorectal and ovarian cancer. In this setting, it is appropriate to offer enhanced surveillance or risk-reducing surgery.

Typically, only patients with tumors limited to the endometrium are considered candidates for fertility preservation, and the degree of myometrial invasion is not the most important predictor of response to medical therapy (Box 62-2). The presence or degree of myometrial invasion increases the risk of extrauterine disease. It does not predict response better than tumor grade. Whereas pelvic ultrasonography or MRI can be used to assess depth of invasion, MRI has the higher sensitivity (sensitivity: pelvic ultrasonography, 75%, versus MRI, 83%). In addition, MRI allows for assessment of other pelvic organs and for the presence of pelvic lymphadenopathy or extrauterine cancer spread.

The presence of lymphadenopathy, regardless of how it is identified, raises concern for at least stage III disease. These patients are not eligible for fertility-sparing therapy; rather, a hysterectomy with lymphadenectomy is recommended. Concern for stage III endometrial cancer also may include a recommendation for adjuvant treatment. Lymphadenopathy, if identified, is an exclusionary criterion for fertility-sparing medical therapy and is not a predictor of response. Fertility preservation would not be considered for patients suspected to have ovarian metastatic cancer or evidence of ovarian metastatic disease. Similarly, because ovarian involvement is a contraindication for fertility-sparing medical therapy, it would not be an appropriate predictor of response to conservative treatment.

Patients with grade 1 endometrioid histology without myometrial invasion or evidence of extrauterine disease who want to preserve future fertility may defer a hysterectomy and undergo hysteroscopic tumor resection. Additionally, these patients should be candidates for treatment with progestins (Box 62-2). Mismatch repair testing should be performed on tumor specimens for Lynch syndrome testing, especially in younger patients because they have a lower response rate to medical therapy, have an increased recurrence risk, and are at risk for other types of cancer.

Hamilton CA, Pothuri B, Arend RC, Backes FJ, Gehrig PA, Soliman PT, et al. Endometrial cancer: a Society of Gynecologic Oncology evidence-based review and recommendations, part II. Gynecol Oncol 2021;160:827–34. doi: 10.1016/j.ygyno.2020.12.024

Rodolakis A, Scambia G, Planchamp F, Acien M, Di Spiezio Sardo A, Farrugia M, et al. ESGO/ESHRE/ESGE guidelines for the fertility-sparing treatment of patients with endometrial carcinoma. Hum Reprod Open 2023;2023:hoac057. doi: 10.1093/hropen/hoac057

63 Somatic testing in ovarian cancer

A 46-year-old patient received a new diagnosis of stage IIIC ovarian cancer and presented for follow-up after cycle 3 of adjuvant therapy with carboplatin and paclitaxel. Her germline genetic testing showed a *BRCA* wild type with a variant of unknown significance in *BRIP1*. She is curious about what maintenance therapy may be advised after her sixth cycle of chemotherapy. You inform her that, in addition to germline testing, the best next step to determine her maintenance plan is to test the tumor for

(A) *BRIP1* mutation
* (B) homologous recombination deficiency (HRD)
(C) programmed death-ligand 1 (PD-L1) immunohistochemistry
(D) vascular endothelial growth factor immunohistochemistry

Approximately 50% of patients with epithelial ovarian cancer have somatic alterations or mutations in the homologous recombination repair (HRR) pathway. A somatic mutation or alteration is present in the tumor and does not always indicate that the patient carries a germline or inherited mutation. Germline mutation tests are performed on patients' blood or saliva, but the tumor is required to test for somatic mutations (Fig. 63-1). It is now standard of care to test a patient with ovarian cancer for other inherited, germline mutations as well as somatic, tumor alterations or mutations. The HRR pathway repairs double-stranded DNA breaks. If this pathway is not intact, mutations can accumulate and lead to carcinogenesis. The BRCA protein is a component of this HRR pathway, as are other proteins, such as ATM, BRIP1, and RAD51C. Roughly one-half of epithelial ovarian cancer is homologous repair deficient, of which 15% are due to germline *BRCA* mutations, 5–10% due to somatic *BRCA* mutations, and 25% due to mutations or epigenetic abnormalities in other genes involved in the HRR pathway (Fig. 63-1). Currently, except in patients with *BRCA* mutations, testing individual proteins or gene mutations is not recommended because testing for the characteristic homologous repair deficiency is more effective.

Testing patients with ovarian cancer for *BRCA* mutations (somatic and germline) and HRD is now considered standard of care because these results can direct treatment management. After carboplatin and paclitaxel chemotherapy is completed in first-line ovarian cancer, maintenance therapy should be considered because it can improve progression-free and overall survival to varying degrees by biomarker subtype in patients with advanced ovarian cancer. Several clinical trials have explored biomarker-directed and non-biomarker-directed maintenance therapies for treating advanced ovarian cancer (Table 63-1). Consideration for maintenance treatment should take into account *BRCA* mutation status (somatic or germline),

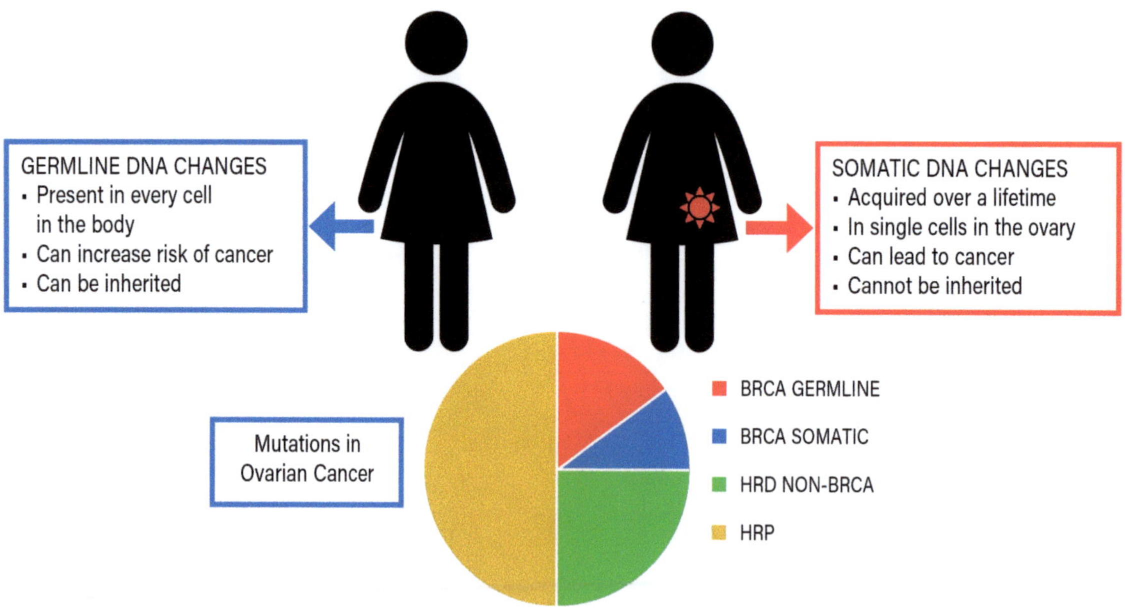

FIGURE 63-1. Somatic versus germline testing.

TABLE 63-1. Use of Maintenance Therapy by Tumor Characteristic

TUMOR CHARACTERISTIC	CHEMOTHERAPY BACKBONE	BEVACIZUMAB	POLY(ADP-RIBOSE) POLYMERASE (PARP) INHIBITOR
BRCA mutated (somatic or germline)	Platinum + taxane	Physician's choice	At completion of chemotherapy +/− bevacizumab
HRD	Platinum + taxane	Physician's choice	At completion of chemotherapy +/− bevacizumab
HR proficient (HRD negative)	Platinum + taxane	Physician's choice	Physician's choice +/− bevacizumab

Abbreviations: HRD, homologous repair deficient; PARP, poly(ADP-ribose) polymerase.

HRD, stage of disease, and whether the patient has received bevacizumab with the first round of chemotherapy.

Patients with mutated *BRCA* should receive first-line maintenance therapy with a poly(ADP-ribose) polymerase (PARP) inhibitor, which is associated with improved progression-free and overall survival in several randomized clinical trials. If the platinum-based chemotherapy was used and a response to treatment occurs, the PARP inhibitor olaparib can be added to bevacizumab for maintenance in patients with HRD in the tumor. This approach has shown benefit in progression-free and overall survival. Niraparib is an option irrespective of homologous repair status, although the benefit in terms of progression-free survival is more modest for homologous repair-proficient tumors. Although benefit with niraparib has been demonstrated in terms of progression-free survival, it has not improved overall survival in any patient cohort. The best next step in management is tumor testing for HRD to guide decision making regarding maintenance PARP inhibitor therapy.

Programmed death-ligand 1 status is not currently tested to determine therapy, such as immunotherapy, in ovarian cancer. Although adding a checkpoint inhibitor or immunotherapy to the treatment of metastatic ovarian cancer has been explored, results to date have not shown significant improvements in progression-free survival.

In the management of advanced ovarian cancer at diagnosis, the addition of targeted therapies, such as anti-angiogenesis and PARP inhibitor maintenance, relies on tumor testing results. This tumor testing can predict response to therapy and prognosis. The choice to use these therapies alone or in combination partially depends on physician and patient preference, but in *BRCA*-mutated and HRD tumors, improvements in outcomes have been demonstrated when these therapies are added. Testing for HRD is the best next step for the described patient because it will inform decision making about proceeding with a maintenance PARP inhibitor alone, in combination with bevacizumab, or bevacizumab alone.

Goh JC, Gourley C, Tan DS, Nogueira-Rodrigues A, Elghazaly H, Edy Pierre M, et al. Optimizing treatment selection and sequencing decisions for first-line maintenance therapy of newly diagnosed advanced ovarian cancer. Gynecol Oncol Rep 2022;42:101028. doi: 10.1016/j.gore.2022.101028

Moore KN, du Bois A. Homologous recombination deficiency testing in first-line ovarian cancer. Ann Oncol 2022;33:231–3. doi: 10.1016/j.annonc.2021.12.013

O'Malley DM, Krivak TC, Kabil N, Munley J, Moore KN. PARP inhibitors in ovarian cancer: a review. Target Oncol 2023;18:471–503. doi: 10.1007/s11523-023-00970-w

Vergote I, González-Martín A, Ray-Coquard I, Harter P, Colombo N, Pujol P, et al. European experts consensus: BRCA/homologous recombination deficiency testing in first-line ovarian cancer. European experts' consensus group. Ann Oncol 2022;33:276–87. doi: 10.1016/j.annonc.2021.11.013

64 Testing for hereditary cancer syndromes in endometrial cancer

A 57-year-old gravida 4, para 4, receives a diagnosis of stage IA, grade 1, endometrioid endometrial adenocarcinoma after hysterectomy and surgical staging. There is no myometrial invasion or lymphovascular space invasion, and pelvic washings are negative. Her brother has a history of colon cancer at age 55 years. The best next somatic test to assess her risk of genetic cancer is

(A) CpG island hypermethylation
(B) homologous recombination deficiency
* (C) mismatch repair (MMR) protein expression
(D) *p53* overexpression

More than 67,000 new cases of uterine cancer were estimated to be diagnosed in 2024. Of these cases of cancer, approximately 3–5% will have a hereditary origin. Lynch syndrome is an autosomal-dominant genetic mutation in MMR genes affecting 1 in 600 to 1 in 3,000 individuals. This genetic syndrome accounts for most hereditary endometrial cancer. The risk of endometrial cancer in Lynch syndrome is 18–61%, at times exceeding that of colorectal cancer.

Immunohistochemistry testing for the presence of MMR protein expression in the tumor specimen is the best next test to perform for the patient in this scenario. Deficiencies in MMR protein expression raise the concern for Lynch syndrome and may indicate the need for germline testing. The MMR proteins include MLH1, MSH2, MSH6, and PMS2. If the proteins are reported as intact, they are present and functional. If there is absent MLH1, or a loss of both MLH1 and PMS2, testing should be performed to determine whether this is due to a somatic mutation from MLH1 promoter hypermethylation. If hypermethylation is present, the absence of proteins is due to somatic mutations, and the patient is unlikely to have Lynch syndrome. If hypermethylation is absent, referral to a genetic counselor for Lynch syndrome germline testing is indicated; moreover, if there is any other pattern of absent MMR protein expression, the patient should be immediately referred to a genetic counselor for Lynch syndrome germline testing as well. The MMR somatic testing algorithm is shown in Appendix F.

Although epigenetic changes that cause CpG island hypermethylation are important in the testing algorithm for Lynch syndrome as noted above, CpG island hypermethylation is not the best initial test to elucidate a possible inherited cancer syndrome from a germline mutation.

Homologous recombination deficiency is tested routinely in patients with ovarian cancer because they are especially susceptible to treatment with poly(ADP-ribose) polymerase (PARP) inhibitors. The process of homologous recombination is a key mechanism for DNA repair, particularly double-stranded breaks. This deficiency can be exploited in patients with homologous recombination deficiency (*BRCA*, among others) by inhibiting PARP (single-strand break repair). This dual blockade can lead to lethal damage or facilitate a more error-prone repair and cause cell death. This therapy is not approved for use in endometrial cancer, and it is not the best next step for this patient.

Abnormalities in protein expression of the tumor suppressor gene *p53* are common in many types of cancer. Its loss of function, which may be observed as underexpression or overexpression, contributes to carcinogenesis through unregulated cell cycle proliferation. Its overexpression is a poor prognostic factor in endometrial cancer and is more often associated with type II histologies (as much as 90%). Although this information may provide additional prognostic data, *TP53* germline mutations (Li–Fraumeni syndrome) are estimated to be present in only 0.2% of all adult patients with cancer, and this is not the best next step.

Despite the presence or absence of abnormalities in MMR proteins, a significant family history of cancer that includes cancer associated with Lynch syndrome (eg, colorectal, endometrial, ovarian, gastric, urinary tract, or biliary tract) should prompt further evaluation according to national guidelines for germline testing.

Lynch syndrome. Practice Bulletin No. 147. American College of Obstetricians and Gynecologists [published erratum appears in Obstet Gynecol 2022;139:696]. Obstet Gynecol 2014;124:1042–54. doi: 10.1097/01.AOG.0000456325.50739.72

Mamat Yusof MN, Chew KT, Kampan NC, Shafiee MN. Expression of PD-1 and PD-L1 in endometrial cancer: molecular and clinical significance. Int J Mol Sci 2023;24:15233. doi: 10.3390/ijms242015233

Nakamura M, Obata T, Daikoku T, Fujiwara H. The association and significance of p53 in gynecologic cancers: the potential of targeted therapy. Int J Mol Sci 2019;20:5482. doi: 10.3390/ijms20215482

Tao MH, Freudenheim JL. DNA methylation in endometrial cancer. Epigenetics 2010;5:491–8. doi: 10.4161/epi.5.6.12431

65 Management of recurrent malignant ascites

A 68-year-old patient presents with abdominal distension, shortness of breath, and unintentional weight loss. She is being treated for recurrent platinum-resistant ovarian cancer and started chemotherapy 2 weeks ago. She has had four recent paracenteses for ascites, most recently 1 week ago, and she desires more long-term relief of her symptoms. On examination, she has a distended abdomen with a notable fluid wave. Computed tomography demonstrates large ascites, peritoneal carcinomatosis, and enlarged pelvic and periaortic lymph nodes. Her CA 125 concentration is 1,258 U/mL, and her creatinine level is 1.4 mg/dL. The best next step to achieve long-term relief for her symptoms is to

(A) administer albumin
(B) administer a diuretic
(C) perform cytoreductive surgery
(D) perform an ultrasound-guided paracentesis
* (E) place an indwelling peritoneal catheter

In the setting of advanced or metastatic cancer, fluid can accumulate in the peritoneal cavity. This fluid, termed *malignant ascites*, is caused by inflammation of the peritoneal surfaces and capillary leak syndrome within malignant tumors. Ascites is most common in ovarian cancer and also can be seen in advanced endometrial or cervical cancer. Ascites in the setting of cancer is exudative, and it is transudative in the setting of cirrhosis, heart failure, or kidney disease. The serum-ascites albumin gradient (SAAG) is used to differentiate the two. A SAAG of less than 1.1 g/dL in the setting of malignant ascites is considered low. The presence of ascites is associated with increased morbidity and mortality due to malnutrition, shortness of breath, renal insufficiency, and bowel obstruction. Reducing the distension and discomfort caused by ascites can improve a patient's functional and physical status. Medications and procedures can be used to reduce the amount of ascites. Paracentesis will temporarily reduce the volume of peritoneal fluid and improve symptoms. If the cancer responds to anticancer therapies, the volume of ascites will decrease and may even resolve; however, several weeks or cycles of treatment may be required for clinical response, and the disease response often is limited in recurrent disease settings, especially in platinum-resistant disease.

Paracentesis, usually image-guided, is the most commonly used acute management approach for malignant ascites. It provides immediate relief for the patient, and the risk of complications, such as peritonitis, hypotension, hypoproteinemia, bowel perforation, and intraabdominal bleeding, is rare. Repeated paracentesis can result in loculated ascites, which results in difficulty evacuating the ascites, and it requires several visits for the patient. More than one visit can be challenging for the patient, their support system, and the health care system. Given the desire for long-term symptomatic improvement, ultrasound-guided paracentesis is not the best next step for this patient.

Indwelling peritoneal catheters are an alternative to repetitive paracentesis. An interventional radiologist places the catheter, and once placed, the patient and their support people can drain the fluid at home. These catheters have been shown to decrease hospital visits and provide relief similar to that of repetitive paracentesis. This intervention is associated with a low risk of peritonitis, sepsis, or hypotension. Because the relief of ascites accumulation can take several treatment cycles to achieve, patients need a longer-lasting intervention. Paracentesis alone provides symptomatic relief for 10 days on average, whereas an indwelling catheter provides immediate relief at any time for the patient, even while at home, and therefore, it is a more appropriate intervention for patients requiring frequent paracenteses. An indwelling peritoneal catheter is the best next step for this patient with platinum-resistant ovarian cancer who is starting a new treatment.

Medical management of malignant ascites with diuretics is ineffective. Although diuretics may be helpful for patients with hepatic metastasis and ascites due to portal hypertension (transudative), this approach has been less successful in patients with malignant ascites due to carcinomatosis and an inability for intravascular volume to affect intraperitoneal fluid production from a tumor; moreover, diuretics can lead to hypotension, hypovolemia, renal failure, and electrolyte imbalance.

Intravenous administration of albumin is used to prevent negative sequelae of removing a large volume of ascites (more than 500 cc) but does not decrease the amount of ascites. When a large volume of ascites is removed by paracentesis, circulatory dysfunction can result. This can be partially prevented by infusing intravenous albumin after paracentesis. Intravenous albumin can decrease electrolyte imbalances from large-volume paracentesis secondary to large shifts of intravascular volume, but this is not the best next step.

Whereas cytoreductive surgery is used commonly at the time of diagnosis of ovarian cancer, secondary cytoreduction in the setting of recurrent disease is only beneficial for carefully selected patients. Clinical trial results suggest that patients with platinum-sensitive ovarian cancer who have a strong performance status, ascites volume less than 500 cc, and no residual tumor at the time of primary cytoreduction are most likely to benefit from secondary cytoreduction. In addition, the recurrent disease must be in area(s) that can be completely resected at the time of secondary debulking. This patient has large-volume and persistent ascites as well as carcinomatosis and platinum-resistant cancer, and secondary cytoreduction is not the best option.

The management of malignant ascites remains challenging. Procedures, such as paracentesis, provide immediate relief, but long-term relief requires effective cancer therapy. In the setting of disease resistant to therapy and frequent paracenteses, indwelling peritoneal catheters are an option for ascites relief while avoiding frequent hospital visits. More research is needed to establish better therapies for platinum-resistant or platinum-refractory disease.

Conte C, Fagotti A, Avesani G, Trombadori C, Federico A, D'Indinosante M, et al. Update on the secondary cytoreduction in platinum-sensitive recurrent ovarian cancer: a narrative review. Ann Transl Med 2021;9:510. doi: 10.21037/atm-20-4690

Hou W, Sanyal AJ. Ascites: diagnosis and management. Med Clin North Am 2009;93:801–17, vii. doi: 10.1016/j.mcna.2009.03.007

Kietpeerakool C, Rattanakanokchai S, Jampathong N, Srisomboon J, Lumbiganon P. Management of drainage for malignant ascites in gynaecological cancer. Cochrane Database of Systematic Reviews 2019, Issue 12. Art. No.: CD007794. doi: 10.1002/14651858.CD007794.pub3

Meyer L, Suidan R, Sun C, Westin S, Coleman RL, Mills GB. The management of malignant ascites and impact on quality of life outcomes in women with ovarian cancer. Expert Rev Qual Life Cancer Care 2016;1:231–8. doi: 10.1080/23809000.2016.1185369

Narayanan G, Pezeshkmehr A, Venkat S, Guerrero G, Barbery K. Safety and efficacy of the PleurX catheter for the treatment of malignant ascites. J Palliat Med 2014;17:906–12. doi: 10.1089/jpm.2013.0427

66 Electrolyte abnormalities in advanced cervical cancer

A 49-year-old woman presents to the emergency department with vaginal bleeding and pelvic and low back pain. Vital signs include a temperature of 37.1 °C (98.7 °F), blood pressure of 112/70 mm Hg, heart rate of 95 beats per minute, respiratory rate of 16 breaths per minute, and oxygen saturation of 98% on room air. She has tenderness to palpation in the bilateral lower abdominal quadrants without rebound or guarding. Speculum examination reveals a fungating cervical mass encompassing the cervix and extending into the upper vagina. On bimanual examination, an 8-cm mass is palpable, and bilateral parametrial invasion is suspected. Computed tomography (CT) confirms the presence of a tumor, with bilateral hydronephrosis noted. Serum testing is notable for potassium of 6.45 mEq/L. Her electrocardiogram (ECG) result is shown in Figure 66-1. The best next treatment is to initiate

* (A) calcium gluconate
(B) dialysis
(C) furosemide
(D) insulin
(E) patiromer

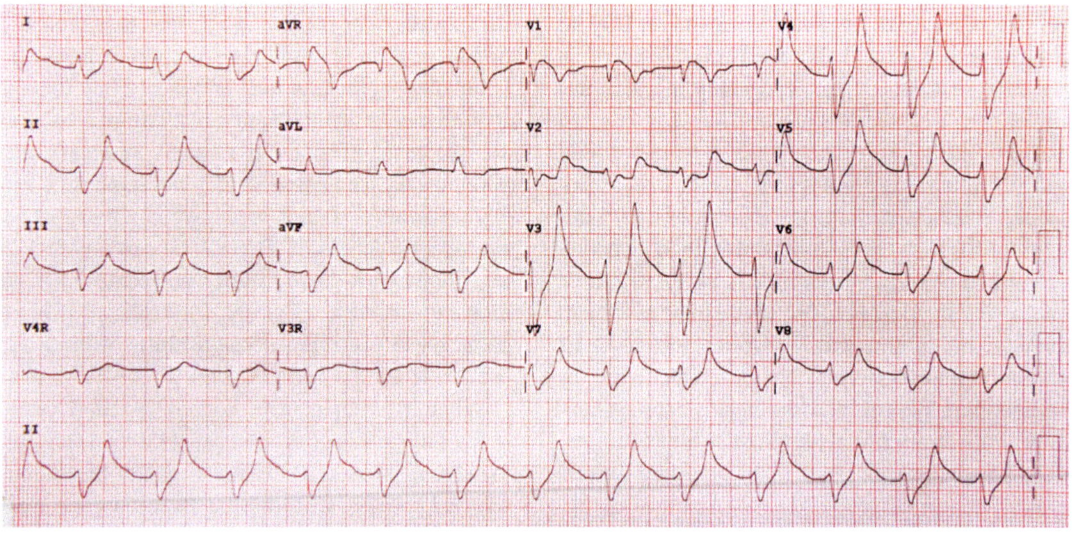

FIGURE 66-1. Normal electrocardiogram. (Reprinted from Hicks B. Hyperkalemia on ECG. J Educ Teach Emerg Med 2016;1:V7-8.)

Electrolyte abnormalities are a common laboratory finding in patients presenting with advanced cervical cancer. Determining the urgency of hyperkalemia is dependent on the signs and symptoms of the patient, the severity of the potassium elevation, and the underlying cause of hyperkalemia. Signs and symptoms associated with hyperkalemia include muscle weakness or paralysis, cardiac conduction abnormalities, and cardiac arrhythmias, including sinus bradycardia, sinus arrest, ventricular tachycardia, fibrillation, and asystole. Cardiac abnormalities usually occur with a potassium concentration of 7 mEq/L or higher but may occur at lower levels in patients with an acute increase in serum potassium or underlying cardiac conditions.

There are several ECG changes associated with hyperkalemia. A peaked T wave (Fig. 66-2) with a shortened QT interval is the earliest change, followed by progressive lengthening of the PR interval and QRS duration. Over time, the P wave may disappear and the QRS complex will widen to a sine wave pattern. Without treatment, this can progress to asystole.

The patient in this scenario presents with an increased potassium concentration and peaked T waves on ECG. The ECG changes meet the criteria for a hyperkalemic emergency, and thus treatment to stabilize the myocardium is the most urgent intervention and should precede treatments to reverse the hyperkalemia (Fig. 66-3). Treatment for hyperkalemic emergency is intravenous calcium to stabilize the myocardium and antagonize the membrane actions of the potassium. Calcium can be administered as calcium gluconate or calcium chloride, but calcium gluconate generally is preferred because it is less irritating when compared with calcium chloride. Calcium gluconate should be infused over 2–3 minutes with constant cardiac monitoring and can be repeated after 5 minutes if ECG changes persist or recur. After stabilization of the myocardium, additional therapies should be administered to lower potassium as noted in Box 66-1.

The remaining treatment options decrease potassium levels and should be considered after stabilization of the myocardium. Dialysis is indicated in patients with hyperkalemia and severe kidney impairment (estimated glomerular filtration rate [GFR] less than 15–29 mL/min). Patients who have moderate hyperkalemia (K 6.5–7.5 mmol/L) and normal kidney function or mild (GFR greater than 60 mL/min) to moderate (GFR greater than 30 mL/min) impairment can usually be managed without dialysis.

Furosemide, a loop diuretic, increases potassium loss in the urine by increasing distal sodium delivery in the ascending limb of Henle, which stimulates potassium excretion. The expected drop in potassium after administration is variable. Effects of this medication are slow and can take up to an hour. Adding furosemide to this patient's regimen is an appropriate second step in lowering potassium levels after stabilization of the myocardium with intravenous calcium.

Insulin lowers serum potassium by driving potassium into cells through the enzyme Na^{+}-K^{+}-ATPase (also known as the sodium pump or sodium-potassium pump) in skeletal muscle and will only transiently lower the potassium concentration,

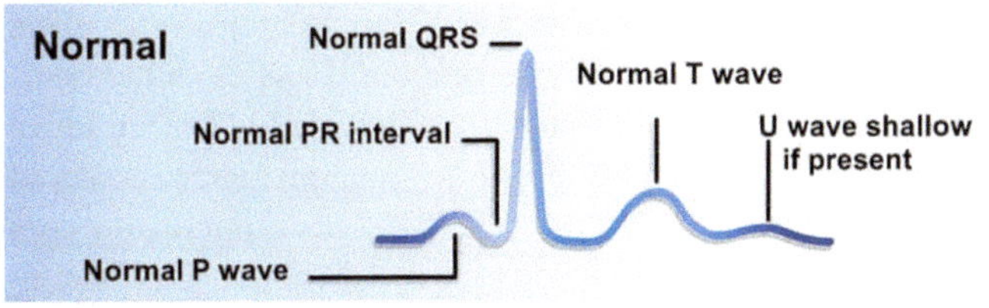

FIGURE 66-2. Normal electrocardiogram result. (Reprinted from Teymouri N, Mesbah S, Navabian SMH, Shekouh D, Najafabadi MM, Norouzkhani N, Poudineh M, Qadirifard MS, Mehrtabar S, Deravi N. ECG frequency changes in potassium disorders: a narrative review. Am J Cardiovasc Dis. 2022 Jun 15;12(3):112-124)

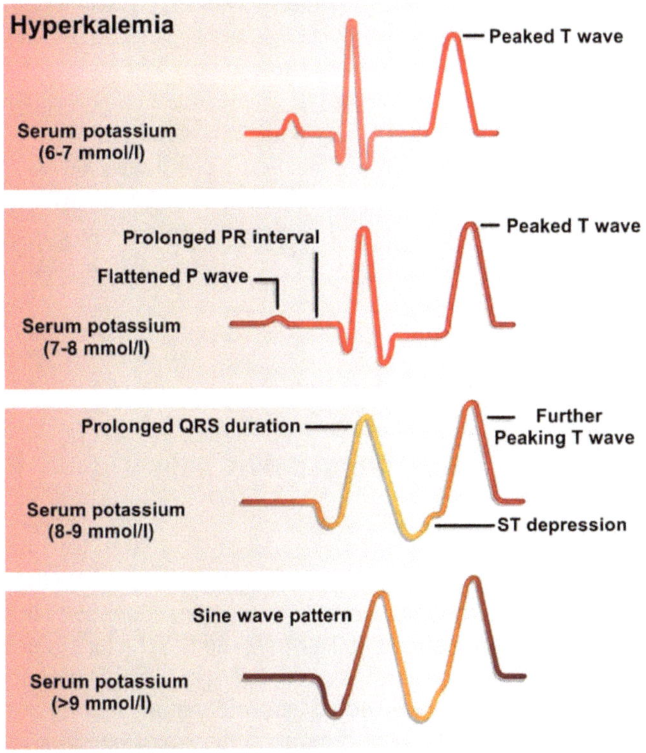

FIGURE 66-3. Electrocardiogram changes. (Reprinted from Teymouri N, Mesbah S, Navabian SMH, Shekouh D, Najafabadi MM, Norouzkhani N, Poudineh M, Qadirifard MS, Mehrtabar S, Deravi N. ECG frequency changes in potassium disorders: a narrative review. Am J Cardiovasc Dis. 2022 Jun 15;12(3):112-124)

BOX 66-1

Treatment of Hyperkalemia

1. Antagonize membrane actions of potassium
   - Calcium gluconate or calcium chloride
2. Drive potassium intracellularly
   - Insulin +/− glucose pending glucose level
   - Beta-2-adrenergic agonist
3. Remove potassium from the body
   - Loop or thiazide diuretic
   - Cation exchange resin
   - Dialysis (if severe hyperkalemia or renally compromised)

so this is not the correct answer. Glucose typically is given with insulin to prevent hypoglycemia. If serum glucose is 250 mg/dL or higher, insulin should be held. The effect of insulin begins 10–20 minutes after administration, peaks at 30–60 minutes, and lasts 4–6 hours. Serum potassium concentration is expected to drop by 0.5–1.2 mEq/L after administration. Although the patient in this scenario could receive insulin as part of the treatment for hyperkalemia, the timing for insulin to take effect is too great in the setting of cardiac changes on ECG.

Patiromer is an oral gastrointestinal cation exchanger that will bind potassium in the colon in exchange for calcium. It has been available on the U.S. market since 2015 and can be used in chronic hyperkalemic states. A study among emergency departments noted a single dose of oral patiromer at 25.2 g reduced serum potassium within 2 hours of administration. Although this medication will also aid with potassium excretion, the time to effect would limit its use acutely in the setting of ECG changes, and therefore this is not the best answer.

Urgent treatment of hyperkalemia varies depending on symptoms, degree of increased potassium, and presence of cardiac changes on ECG. Among patients with potassium of 6.5 mEq/L or higher or ECG changes, or both, the myocardium must first be stabilized. Patients without clinical manifestations of hyperkalemia, absence of cardiac abnormalities, and no evidence of ongoing potassium absorption can benefit from having their potassium levels lowered more slowly.

Colbert GB, Patel D, Lerma EV. Patiromer for the treatment of hyperkalemia. Expert Rev Clin Pharmacol 2020;13:563–70. doi: 10.1080/17512433.2020.1774363

Littmann L, Gibbs MA. Electrocardiographic manifestations of severe hyperkalemia. J Electrocardiol 2018;51:814–7. doi: 10.1016/j.jelectrocard.2018.06.018

Mushiyakh Y, Dangaria H, Qavi S, Ali N, Pannone J, Tompkins D. Treatment and pathogenesis of acute hyperkalemia. J Community Hosp Intern Med Perspect 2012;1(4). doi: 10.3402/jchimp.v1i4.7372

Sterns RH, Grieff M, Bernstein PL. Treatment of hyperkalemia: something old, something new. Kidney Int 2016;89:546–54. doi: 10.1016/j.kint.2015.11.018

Weiss JN, Qu Z, Shivkumar K. Electrophysiology of hypokalemia and hyperkalemia. Circ Arrhythm Electrophysiol 2017;10:e004667. doi: 10.1161/CIRCEP.116.004667

67 Worsening pelvic pain

A 65-year-old woman presents to the emergency department with pelvic pain that has been present for 2 months and has worsened to a pain score of 10 out of 10 today. Oxycodone has previously been prescribed for pain management. Her past medical history is notable for hypertension, depression managed with cognitive behavioral therapy, liver cirrhosis, and endometrial cancer. She has a firm, immobile pelvic mass on examination. Selected laboratory study results are shown in Table 67-1. The factor that puts this patient at greatest risk for opioid-induced respiratory depression is

* (A) altered kidney function
(B) depression
(C) endometrial cancer
(D) hypertension
(E) liver cirrhosis

TABLE 67-1. The Described Patient's Laboratory Study Results

LABORATORY STUDY	VALUE
Alanine aminotransferase	17 units/L
Aspartate aminotransferase	16 units/L
Creatinine	2.1 mg/dL

Obstetrician–gynecologists manage various types of pain, ranging from postoperative pain and endometriosis-related discomfort to pain associated with cancer. Opioids often are a necessary element in multimodal pain regimens; however, they are associated with significant risks to patients and society due to opioid use disorders and opioid overdose-related deaths. Although the true prevalence of opioid use disorder in the United States is difficult to determine, it is estimated to be 2.04–2.77% of the population—approximately 6.7–7.6 million people. Individuals with cancer have high rates of pain (30–50%), and opioid use disorder is increasingly recognized in this population.

The incidence of opioid-related adverse events, including opioid-induced respiratory depression, overdose, and overdose-related death, is increasing. Risk factors for these conditions include young age, medical and psychological comorbidities, history of substance use disorder, and stress. Strong predictors of opioid-induced respiratory depression, which can lead to death, include substance use disorder within the last 6 months, bipolar disorder, schizophrenia, cerebrovascular disease, renal disease, heart failure, benign pancreatic disease, and concurrent benzodiazepine or antidepressant use.

Opioids are primarily metabolized within the liver, and metabolites are excreted by the kidneys. These metabolites can be inactive or active, and some active metabolites may be more potent than the parent drug. Individuals with chronic renal disease are at increased risk of adverse events due to reduced elimination and increased accumulation of the parent drug, the active metabolites, or both. Various opioid agents undergo different mechanisms of metabolism. For instance, oxycodone is primarily metabolized by the CYP450 system in the liver to active metabolites cleared by the kidney, resulting in a high risk for drug–drug interactions and an increased risk of toxicity. Other opioids, such as hydromorphone, do not undergo metabolism by the CYP450 system and, therefore, have much less potential for drug–drug interactions and toxicity in patients with renal failure. The patient in this scenario has altered kidney function (creatinine 2.1) and was prescribed oxycodone. She is at increased risk of adverse events, including opioid-induced respiratory depression.

Although hypertension often leads to altered kidney function and chronic kidney disease, hypertension alone does not increase the risk of opioid-related adverse events. Hypertension can lead to stress, which puts an individual at risk. Similarly, endometrial cancer may increase the risk of opioid use disorder due to cancer-related pain and emotional and psychosocial stress caused by the diagnosis. The possible sequelae of these diagnoses rather than the diagnoses themselves put individuals at increased risk of opioid-related adverse events.

Although this patient does have liver cirrhosis, she is not in liver failure as evidenced by normal results on liver function tests. Although liver failure could increase the risk of opioid-related adverse events due to decreased metabolism, it is not a strong predictor for opioid-induced respiratory depression.

Depression and other psychiatric comorbidities increase the risk of developing opioid use disorder as well as opioid-related adverse events. Before beginning opioid therapy, it is imperative to obtain a full history, including psychiatric conditions and use of antidepressants, antipsychotics, and anxiolytics. Use of antidepressants is a strong predictor for opioid-induced respiratory depression. Although this patient has a diagnosis of depression, which puts her at risk for opioid-related adverse events, she is not currently taking antidepressants, so this is not the greatest risk factor for her.

Rates of opioid use adverse events are on the rise. It is imperative for the prescribing physician to consider the patient's psychological, social, and medical comorbidities when choosing to initiate opioids and opioid selection. When prescribing opioids, clinicians also should consider providing naloxone to address potential opioid-related adverse events, especially opioid-induced respiratory depression. Numerous studies highlight the effectiveness of making naloxone readily available within the community to mitigate opioid-related emergencies.

Clark AK, Wilder CM, Winstanley EL. A systematic review of community opioid overdose prevention and naloxone distribution programs. J Addict Med 2014;8:153–63. doi: 10.1097/ADM.0000000000000034

Davison SN. Clinical pharmacology considerations in pain management in patients with advanced kidney failure. Clin J Am Soc Nephrol 2019;14:917–31. doi: 10.2215/CJN.05180418

Ganguly A, Michael M, Goschin S, Harris K, McFarland DC. Cancer pain and opioid use disorder. Oncology (Williston Park) 2022;36:535–41. doi: 10.46883/2022.25920973

Keyes KM, Rutherford C, Hamilton A, Barocas JA, Gelberg KH, Mueller PP, et al. What is the prevalence of and trend in opioid use disorder in the United States from 2010 to 2019? Using multiplier approaches to estimate prevalence for an unknown population size. Drug Alcohol Depend Rep. Published online April 8, 2022. doi: 10.1016/j.dadr.2022.100052

Webster LR. Risk factors for opioid-use disorder and overdose. Anesth Analg 2017;125:1741–8. doi: 10.1213/ANE.0000000000002496

68 Postoperative complications in an unstable patient

A 63-year-old woman presents to the emergency department with abdominal pain 12 days after a debulking procedure with hysterectomy, bilateral salpingo-oophorectomy, rectosigmoid resection with anastomosis, and omentectomy. Vital signs include a temperature of 38.1 °C (100.5 °F) and a heart rate of 120 beats per minute. Intravenous fluids and broad-spectrum antibiotics are started, and laboratory values are pending. Computed tomography (CT) results are shown in Figures 68-1 and 68-2. The best next step in management is

(A) serial abdominal examinations
(B) Gastrografin study
(C) nasogastric decompression
(D) interventional radiology consultation
* (E) surgical exploration

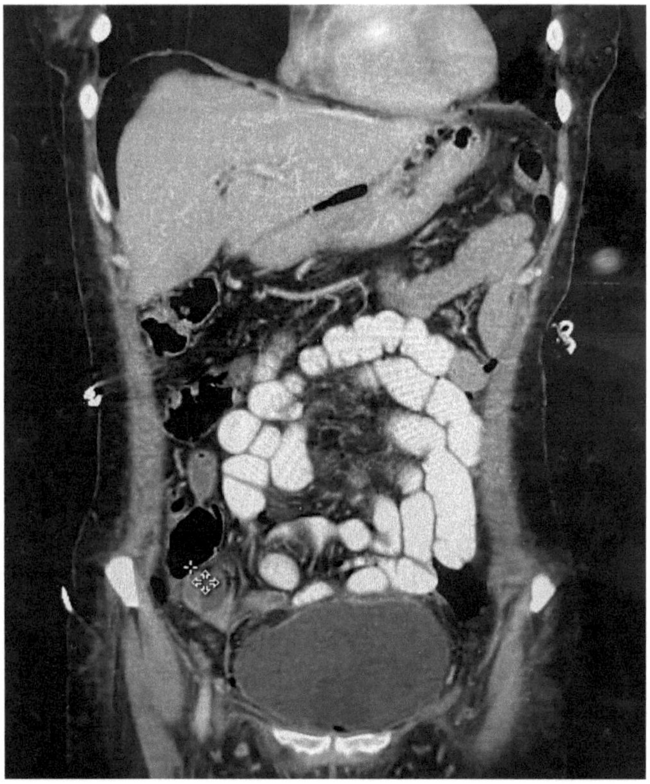

FIGURE 68-1. Computed tomography of the described patient, coronal view.

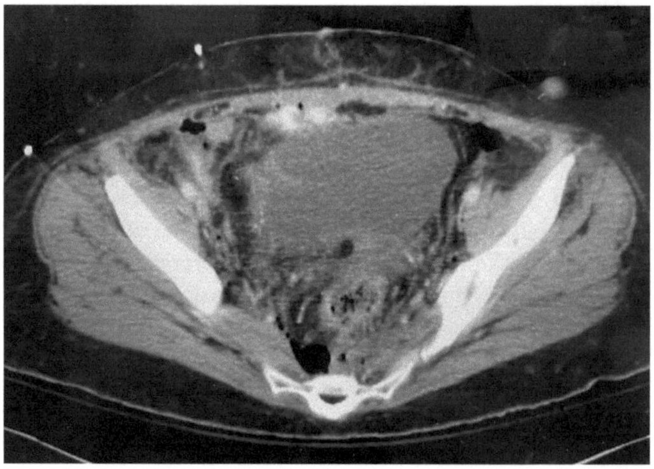

FIGURE 68-2. Computed tomography of the described patient, axial view of the pelvis.

The described patient's computed tomography results show a large volume of free air in the abdomen (Fig. 68-1) and scattered extraluminal free air in the pelvis (Fig. 68-2), which raises concern for viscus perforation. Peritonitis in the setting of free air is a surgical emergency that requires immediate exploration. Given the described patient's recent bowel resection, an anastomotic leak or other delayed bowel perforation should be highly suspected.

Patients with suspected perforation, hemodynamic instability, or both, require immediate surgical exploration to prevent clinical decline and either repair of the viscus perforation or diversion proximal to the perforation. Because the patient in this scenario has signs of hemodynamic instability and free air on imaging, immediate surgical exploration with laparotomy is the best next step in her treatment. At the time of exploration, the primary goal is to wash out the abdomen, repair or resect the perforation if feasible, and likely divert the fecal stream.

Anastomotic leakage is a challenging postoperative complication. Clinical management has evolved over the last several decades, and multiple nonsurgical options are available, depending on patient presentation and clinical stability. In patients with anastomotic leak without peritonitis who are hemodynamically stable, conservative management with percutaneous drainage with or without fecal diversion may be feasible. If a patient is hemodynamically stable with a contained pelvic leak, treatment options include diverting ileostomy combined with transanal or percutaneous drainage. More recently developed endoscopic procedures, including stent or clip placement or endoluminal vacuum-assisted therapy may also be feasible. Some surgeons favor protective diversion at the time of initial anastomosis formation. Data on this practice are mixed, but protective stomas may reduce the risk of reoperation for anastomotic leak.

Additional studies and procedures should not delay immediate treatment for a patient with hemodynamic instability and suspected bowel perforation. Serial abdominal examinations are not the best next step as they would delay the appropriate definitive evaluation and treatment of the patient's condition. In a patient with stable clinical presentation and unclear source of small volume free air postoperatively, serial examinations may help guide treatment and the role of surgical exploration.

Gastrografin is a water-soluble contrast media that is safe for use in the setting of possible bowel perforation. It can be administered orally or rectally in combination with X-rays or computed tomography to assess for obstruction or bowel perforation. Delaying surgical exploration with a Gastrografin study in the described patient with sepsis and high suspicion for bowel perforation based on surgical history, symptoms, and computed tomography findings, would not be appropriate and therefore is not the best next step. However, in a clinically stable patient with an indeterminate presentation of bowel perforation, a Gastrografin study may assist in the diagnosis and treatment planning.

Nasogastric decompression is a helpful tool in the management of postoperative small bowel obstruction, but it is not appropriate for anastomotic leak or bowel perforation. Small bowel obstruction does not present with free air; rather, it presents with dilated loops of small bowel with a transition point on CT imaging. In stable patients with bowel obstruction, initial conservative management with bowel decompression and nasogastric tube is appropriate. Bowel obstructions associated with peritonitis, mesenteric edema, or concern for bowel ischemia require surgical intervention. In the setting of free air, nasogastric tube placement is not appropriate medical management.

A consultation with an interventional radiologist can help determine if a percutaneous drainage catheter is an option for stable patients with contained bowel perforation and no peritoneal signs on examination. Success rates of conservative drainage vary, and reoperation or proximal surgical diversion may be required. Given the high morbidity and mortality of gastrointestinal leakage, this strategy should be undertaken only in well-selected patients. The patient described in this scenario is not stable, and delaying surgical intervention for consultation with interventional radiology would not be appropriate.

Chiarello MM, Fransvea P, Cariati M, Adams NJ, Bianchi V, Brisinda G. Anastomotic leakage in colorectal cancer surgery. Surg Oncol 2022;40:101708. doi: 10.1016/j.suronc.2022.101708

Clifford RE, Fowler H, Govindarajah N, Vimalachandran D, Sutton PA. Early anastomotic complications in colorectal surgery: a systematic review of techniques for endoscopic salvage. Surg Endosc 2019;33:1049–65. doi: 10.1007/s00464-019-06670-9

Scotté M, Mauvais F, Bubenheim M, Cossé C, Suaud L, Savoye-Collet C, et al. Use of water-soluble contrast medium (gastrografin) does not decrease the need for operative intervention nor the duration of hospital stay in uncomplicated acute adhesive small bowel obstruction? A multicenter, randomized, clinical trial (Adhesive Small Bowel Obstruction Study) and systematic review. Surgery 2017;161:1315–25. doi: 10.1016/j.surg.2016.11.026

Shalaby M, Emile S, Elfeki H, Sakr A, Wexner SD, Sileri P. Systematic review of endoluminal vacuum-assisted therapy as salvage treatment for rectal anastomotic leakage. BJS Open 2018;3:153–60. doi: 10.1002/bjs5.50124

69 Pain management for laparotomy

A 43-year-old patient presents for a preoperative evaluation before total abdominal hysterectomy for chronic pelvic pain and abnormal uterine bleeding due to multiple uterine leiomyomas. Her uterine size is approximately 28 weeks on physical examination, and you plan to perform a midline vertical incision. She expresses concern regarding anticipated pain after surgery and would like to minimize her need for opioid medications. You discuss a multimodal pain regimen with her, including acetaminophen, gabapentin, and celecoxib, to decrease opioid use. The best time to initiate this regimen is

(A) the day before surgery
* (B) preoperatively on the day of surgery
(C) in the post-anesthesia care unit
(D) at discharge from the hospital

Pain management after hysterectomy is an important component of perioperative care. Adequate pain management shortens recovery and improves patient experience. Different routes of hysterectomy confer different amounts of postoperative pain, with minimally invasive approaches (vaginal and laparoscopic) typically causing less pain than open surgery. Hysterectomy using laparotomy is indicated in certain clinical scenarios. Although the approach to pain management after hysterectomy may be tailored based on the route of hysterectomy and patient characteristics, a standardized multimodal approach can effectively minimize opioid requirements.

Historically, pain after hysterectomy has been treated with liberal use of opioid analgesics. Opioid analgesics have secondary effects that can negatively affect a patient's postoperative recovery by causing nausea and vomiting, slowed bowel function, and decreased postoperative mobility. These limitations, and the growing opioid epidemic, have called for an evidence-based approach to perioperative pain management. Research has focused on the utilization of a multimodal pain management strategy to treat postoperative pain. This multimodal strategy is associated with decreased opioid use, decreased pain scores, and improved patient experience, particularly with open approaches. This strategy is part of the Enhanced Recovery after Surgery (ERAS) program to promote healing and recovery in the perioperative state.

The multimodal pain management approach supported by ERAS includes scheduled nonsteroidal anti-inflammatory drugs (NSAIDs), such as ketorolac or ibuprofen, or cyclooxygenase-2 (COX2) inhibitors, acetaminophen, gabapentin, and oral opioids if necessary.

The best time to initiate this multimodal pain regimen is preoperatively on the day of surgery, and this is the best next step for the patient described above. Administration begins in the preoperative area. Preemptive administration decreases opioid use postoperatively, promotes recovery, and minimizes pain. The strategy also is appropriate after surgery; however, effectiveness is maximized if it is initiated preoperatively. An intravenous route for opioids or a patient-controlled analgesia pump can be added if needed.

Preemptive treatment with a multimodal pain regimen earlier than the day of surgery is not supported by current research and is not recommended as a standardized approach to perioperative pain management. Initiation of the regimen the day before surgery is not the best next step. Continuing the multimodal regimen postoperatively is appropriate; however, the improvement in outcomes is seen most significantly when administration begins preoperatively. Initiation of the regimen in the post-anesthesia care unit or on discharge from the hospital after surgery are not appropriate next steps.

Enhanced Recovery After Surgery also supports the use of other pain management strategies, such as epidural analgesia, transverse abdominus plane block, and incisional infiltration of bupivacaine, when appropriate. These modalities are associated with decreased opioid use in the immediate postoperative period—particularly for gynecologic surgery performed with laparotomy. Reducing pain perioperatively is thought to decrease stress response and shorten recovery time. Epidural analgesia may affect mobility postoperatively, may cause hypotension, and is associated with longer length of stay compared with transverse abdominus plane block. Infiltration of bupivacaine is effective in reducing opioid use perioperatively and is easily accessible. Gynecologists should weigh the risks and benefits of these adjunct analgesia options based on individual patient characteristics. It is unclear if epidural analgesia and transverse abdominal plane block result in decreased opioid use and stress response after minimally invasive gynecologic surgery.

Madsen AM, Martin JM, Linder BJ, Gebhart JB. Perioperative opioid management for minimally invasive hysterectomy. Best Pract Res Clin Obstet Gynaecol 2022;85:68–80. doi: 10.1016/j.bpobgyn.2022.05.006

Nelson G, Bakkum-Gamez J, Kalogera E, Glaser G, Altman A, Meyer LA, et al. Guidelines for perioperative care in gynecologic/oncology: Enhanced Recovery After Surgery (ERAS) Society recommendations-2019 update. Int J Gynecol Cancer 2019;29:651–68. doi: 10.1136/ijgc-2019-000356

Perioperative pathways: enhanced recovery after surgery. ACOG Committee Opinion No. 750. American College of Obstetricians and Gynecologists [published errata appear in Obstet Gynecol 2019;133:1288; Obstet Gynecol 2019;134:1121]. Obstet Gynecol 2018;132:e120–30. doi: 10.1097/AOG.0000000000002818

Scheib SA, Thomassee M, Kenner JL. Enhanced recovery after surgery in gynecology: a review of the literature. J Minim Invasive Gynecol 2019;26:327–43. doi: 10.1016/j.jmig.2018.12.010

Tseng JH, Cowan RA, Afonso AM, Zhou Q, Iasonos A, Ali N, et al. Perioperative epidural use and survival outcomes in patients undergoing primary debulking surgery for advanced ovarian cancer. Gynecol Oncol 2018;151:287–93. doi: 10.1016/j.ygyno.2018.08.024

70 Precision medicine

A 55-year-old patient with stage IIIC high-grade serous ovarian cancer undergoes adjuvant chemotherapy after primary debulking surgery. She has no evidence of disease after platinum-based chemotherapy. Her germline testing for heritable genetic syndromes was negative for known mutations. The best biomarker to determine the efficacy of maintenance therapy is

(A) folate receptor α (FOLR1)
* (B) homologous recombination deficiency (HRD)
(C) human epidermal growth factor receptor-2 (HER2)
(D) programmed death-ligand 1 (PD-L1)
(E) tumor mutational burden (TMB)

Precision medicine in the form of targeted therapy continues to evolve in gynecologic oncology. During the last decade, multiple new therapies received indications for treatment based on molecular markers for cervical, endometrial, and ovarian cancer. This is a paradigm that has long been used in other solid tumors, including lung and breast cancer. Therapies targeting actionable mutations have been shown to improve survival outcomes and quality of life. Some of the more commonly used molecular targets for gynecologic oncology are shown in Appendix C.

In ovarian cancer, *BRCA* mutations are associated with improved progression-free survival (PFS), overall survival (OS), platinum sensitivity, and ability to achieve optimal cytoreduction at the time of debulking surgery. The presence of a *BRCA* mutation or an HRD predicts tumor response to therapy with a poly(ADP-ribose) polymerase (PARP) inhibitor. Several studies have proven this benefit, either as a single agent or in combination with bevacizumab as a maintenance strategy for patients after platinum-based frontline chemotherapy.

The SOLO-1 trial showed that patients with a BRCA-mutated tumor (germline or somatic) who received olaparib as maintenance therapy had an OS of 67.0% versus 46.5% in patients receiving placebo. Data from results at 41 months showing a 70% reduction in progression or death led to U.S. Food and Drug Administration (FDA) approval of olaparib as monotherapy maintenance in patients with BRCA-mutated tumors. PAOLA-1 added olaparib maintenance to frontline therapy with carboplatin, paclitaxel, and bevacizumab followed by bevacizumab maintenance for patients with BRCA-mutated or HRD tumors. This showed an improvement in PFS with a hazard ratio of 0.59 with the addition of olaparib, and led to FDA approval for patients with *BRCA 1/2*-mutated tumors (germline or somatic) or tumors with genomic instability (a proxy measure for the presence of homologous recombination deficiency). In the PRIMA trial, niraparib maintenance was compared to placebo in patients receiving frontline chemotherapy regardless of tumor *BRCA* or HRD status. The trial showed improved PFS in all patients receiving niraparib maintenance, with marked improvement in PFS for patients with *BRCA*-mutated and HRD tumors. The FDA recommends niraparib for all patients as a single agent after complete or partial response to platinum-based first-line therapy. However, given the less than 3-month improvement in PFS in patients with homologous repair-proficient tumors, shared decision-making regarding risks and benefits of maintenance niraparib therapy is recommended for this group of patients. For the described patient, who has no evidence of disease after primary therapy, tumor testing for homologous repair deficiency for consideration of maintenance PARP-inhibitor therapy is the best next step.

At this time, other genomic and molecular testing is primarily used to guide treatment in the recurrent setting. Folate receptor α is a cell surface receptor that mediates the transportation of folate into the cell. It is upregulated in cancer cells, including up to 80% of ovarian cancer cells. *High expression* of folate receptor α is defined as greater than 75% tumor cells staining with 2+/3+ intensity, and it predicts response to mirvetuximab, an antibody–drug conjugate used for treatment of platinum-resistant ovarian cancer. The phase 3 MIRASOL trial showed significant PFS and OS benefits for patients with platinum-resistant ovarian cancer when compared with the investigator's choice of chemotherapy. Testing for FOLR1 is important for determining treatment options in the recurrent setting but is not the best next step for this patient at this time.

Checkpoint inhibitors, a form of immunotherapy, include PD-1 inhibitors and PD-L1 inhibitors. For some tumors, including cervical cancer, PD-L1 tumor expression as measured by immunohistochemistry is used as a biomarker for the use of a checkpoint inhibitor, such as pembrolizumab (a PD-1 inhibitor). PD-L1 has not been found to be a biomarker for checkpoint inhibitor response in ovarian cancer, and this is not the best option for the described patient.

Tumor mutational burden also is used as a biomarker for use of PD-L1 inhibitors. Tumor mutational burden is broadly defined as the number of somatic mutations per megabase of genomic sequence and can be a useful biomarker in metastatic or unresectable solid tumors. A *high* TMB is defined as more than 10 mutations per megabase. In the phase II Keynote-158 study, high TMB in a variety of metastatic or unresectable solid tumors was associated with a durable response to checkpoint inhibition and led to tumor-agnostic FDA approval of pembrolizumab for TMB-high disease. Although its efficacy as a biomarker for checkpoint inhibitor response is more uncertain in ovarian cancer, pembrolizumab remains a therapy option for TMB-high ovarian cancer without other good options for therapy. Use of TMB would not be appropriate in this setting because the patient has just completed frontline therapy and has other effective options for the treatment of recurrent disease in the future.

Human epidermal growth factor receptor-2 has long been a biomarker for breast cancer in predicting response to trastuzumab. Patients with HER2-positive uterine cancer also have been shown to have improved PFS with the addition of trastuzumab to primary chemotherapy. Recently, trastuzumab deruxtecan (T-Dxd) has been approved for HER2+ (IHC3+) in metastatic solid tumors in patients who have received prior treatment and are not candidates for any other therapy. Trastuzumab deruxtecan is an antibody–drug conjugate consisting of trastuzumab linked to topoisomerase 1 inhibitor (deruxtecan). This could potentially be an option for patients in the recurrent setting, but not the maintenance setting, and it is not the best option for the patient in this scenario.

Molecular testing and its prognostic and therapeutic implications are rapidly evolving. At this time, for this patient with ovarian cancer and no evidence of disease after primary therapy, the most important biomarker for maintenance therapy is HRD status, which makes homologous recombination deficiency the correct answer. FOLR1, TMB, and HER2 status may be useful for treatment planning in the recurrent setting but would not guide immediate therapy. PD-L1 has not been shown to be a good biomarker for checkpoint inhibitor response in ovarian cancer.

Arend RC, Jackson-Fisher A, Jacobs IA, Chou J, Monk BJ. Ovarian cancer: new strategies and emerging targets for the treatment of patients with advanced disease. Cancer Biol Ther 2021;22:89–105. doi: 10.1080/15384047.2020.1868937

Hill BL, Graf RP, Shah K, Danziger N, Lin DI, Quintanilha J, et al. Mismatch repair deficiency, next-generation sequencing-based microsatellite instability, and tumor mutational burden as predictive biomarkers for immune checkpoint inhibitor effectiveness in frontline treatment of advanced stage endometrial cancer. Int J Gynecol Cancer 2023;33:504–13. doi: 10.1136/ijgc-2022-004026

Hinchcliff EM, Westin SN. Next generation sequencing for gynecologic malignancy: promise and potential pitfalls. Gynecol Oncol 2021;163:217–9. doi: 10.1016/j.ygyno.2021.10.005

Wolford JE, Ferrigni E, Margul D, Herzog TJ. Integrating precision medicine into the contemporary management of gynecologic cancer. Curr Oncol Rep 2022;24:889–904. doi: 10.1007/s11912-021-01163-2

71 Evaluation of hematuria

A 64-year-old gravida 5, para 5, completed chemoradiation for stage IIA2 squamous cell carcinoma of the cervix 7 years ago. She has a 60-pack-year smoking history and past medical history of chronic obstructive pulmonary disease and coronary artery disease. She now presents to the emergency department with intermittent severe pelvic pain. She also reports worsening urinary incontinence, urinary frequency, and intermittent hematuria over the past 2 years. Her pelvic examination demonstrates vaginal agglutination, and the apex of the vagina and cervix cannot be evaluated. A urine sample demonstrates gross hematuria with associated small clots. Computed tomography demonstrates diffuse bladder wall hypertrophy, with muscosal irregularity and intraluminal debris. The best next step in evaluation is

* (A) cystoscopy
(B) positron emission tomography (PET)
(C) tampon test
(D) urine cytology
(E) urodynamic testing

Gynecologic cancer and its treatment can significantly affect the anatomy and function of pelvic organs. Bladder dysfunction is particularly common after treatment with chemoradiation for locally advanced cervical cancer. Urinary incontinence and frequency are reported in 50% and 70% of patients after treatment, respectively. Severe urinary dysfunction also is reported, with 9% of women experiencing constant urinary leakage after chemoradiation.

Radiation-induced bladder toxicity can be suspected in any person with bladder symptoms and a history of pelvic radiation. A prominent feature of late radiation damage is the obliteration of tissue microvasculature, also known as *obliterative endarteritis*. Ischemia leads to further necrosis of the mucosa and detrusor muscle and stimulates progressive fibrosis and contracture of the bladder wall. Hematuria or frank blood, reduction of bladder compliance and capacity, loss of detrusor function, and stricture and fistula are all potential consequences. Radiation-induced ischemia and fibrosis are not static and can progress, leading to worsening bladder dysfunction over time.

This patient has severe bladder dysfunction that is consistent with chronic radiation cystitis. This patient's urinary incontinence, urinary frequency, and hematuria are chronic and progressive. Severe pain that is described as contraction-like can be due to bladder spasms. A pelvic examination demonstrates vaginal agglutination that is almost certain to be associated with radiation-induced vaginal mucosal desquamation. The computed tomography (CT) in this scenario demonstrates diffuse bladder wall hypertrophy, with mucosal irregularity and intraluminal debris likely representing blood clots. Such findings are highly consistent with the progressive fibrotic changes in bladder contracture that can occur after high-dose radiation. This patient's history of smoking and cardiovascular disease further increases her risk for bladder ischemia, which amplifies the possibility of late radiation toxicity. The differential diagnosis for this clinical presentation includes urinary tract infection, fistula, and recurrent or secondary malignancy.

Cystoscopy is the best next step to evaluate this patient's condition. It effectively addresses many entities on the differential diagnosis and can be used for therapeutic intervention for her severe hematuria. Telangiectasia, bleeding vessels, ulcers, and malignancy can be identified by direct visualization. Clot evacuation, biopsy, and cauterization of bleeding vessels can be performed. Bladder capacity, fistula, and ureteral integrity can then be identified with a retrograde pyelogram at the time of cystoscopy. It is important to note that urinary tract infection is on the differential diagnosis. Although cystoscopy is generally not recommended in patients with active urinary tract infection, the acuity of this clinical presentation renders the benefits of the procedure greater than this theoretical risk. Using appropriate antibiotic prophylaxis can minimize the risk of infectious complications in patients undergoing cystoscopy.

A tampon test is a simple and cost-effective method for detecting vesicovaginal fistula. To perform this test, a tampon is placed in the vagina. The bladder is then filled with a dilute solution of indigo carmine or methylene blue or other liquid with detectable color that is safe for bladder instillation. The patient is asked to ambulate and, after a period of time, the tampon is then removed and inspected for evidence of color-stained urine. Given this patient's symptoms and findings, a fistula is lower on the differential diagnosis and the narrow focus of this diagnostic study does not address this patient's hematuria and pain symptoms. In addition, the test is not feasible in the setting of vaginal agglutination and would not be the best next step.

A urine cytology examination can be an initial test when urothelial carcinoma or recurrent cancer involving the bladder is suspected. As with all cytology interpretation after radiation therapy, however, urine cytology as a screening test can be difficult to interpret due to radiation-induced changes. Moreover, this test addresses only one entity on the differential diagnosis and the acuity of this patient's presentation necessitates more immediate evaluation through cystoscopy where direct biopsy of visibly abnormal lesions can be undertaken. Therefore, urine cytology is not the best next step for this patient.

Urodynamic testing can assess bladder capacity, sphincter function, and detrusor instability. Such testing in a patient with chronic radiation cystitis may reveal reduced bladder capacity and compliance, increased bladder pressure, detrusor overactivity, incomplete bladder void, decreased urethral pressure profiles or urethral stricture. These are all relevant studies in a patient with chronic bladder symptoms but would not be useful in the evaluation of the patient's acute symptoms and is not the best next step.

Positron emission tomography–computed tomography (PET/CT) is very useful in the evaluation of suspected recurrent cervical cancer. In this scenario, CT has been undertaken for the evaluation of the acute symptoms, but it also has the ability to identify cancer recurrence, albeit with a slightly lower diagnostic sensitivity than PET/CT imaging. There were no additional abnormal findings outside the bladder. Moreover, recurrent cervical cancer is fairly low on the differential diagnosis at this point with this patient. Cervical cancer recurrence occurs within 5 years after completion of cancer therapy in most patients. The patient in this scenario is now 7 years from treatment completion, and her risk of cervical cancer recurrence is estimated to be less than 5%. For these reasons, the additional diagnostic sensitivity for detection of malignancy that is offered by PET/CT imaging is not the priority and is not the best next step.

Radiation-associated toxicities are common in patients treated for cervical cancer, and they can increase in severity over time. These late toxicities can have a significant effect on quality of life, functioning, and health care costs. Advances in techniques for radiation dosimetry and delivery are ongoing. All have the goal of allowing for more precise targeting of tumor while sparing nearby normal organs. Modifying patient risk factors, such as partnering for smoking cessation, also are important aspects of late radiation toxicity prevention.

Corbeau A, Heemsbergen WD, Kuipers SC, Godart J, Creutzberg CL, Nout RA, et al. Predictive factors for toxicity after primary chemoradiation for locally advanced cervical cancer: a systematic review. Int J Radiat Oncol Biol Phys 2024;119:127–42. doi: 10.1016/j.ijrobp.2023.11.010

Genitourinary. CT case studies. Accessed March 17, 2025. https://www.ctisus.com/teachingfiles/cases/genitourinary/383016

Ramaseshan AS, Felton J, Roque D, Rao G, Shipper AG, Sanses TV. Pelvic floor disorders in women with gynecologic malignancies: a systematic review. Int Urogynecol J 2018;29:459–76. doi: 10.1007/s00192-017-3467-4

Urinary incontinence in women. ACOG Practice Bulletin No. 155. American College of Obstetricians and Gynecologists. Obstet Gynecol 2015;126:e66–81. doi: 10.1097/AOG.0000000000001148

Vanneste BG, Van Limbergen EJ, Marcelissen TA, van Roermund JG, Lutgens LC, Arnoldussen CW, et al. Development of a management algorithm for acute and chronic radiation urethritis and cystitis. Urol Int 2022;106:63–74. doi: 10.1159/000515716

72 Receiver operator characteristic curve

The receiver operator characteristic (ROC) curve is one way to evaluate how well a test performs. A new cancer screening test is developed, and ROC curve is drawn to help select the optimal cut-point. The x and y axes represent

* (A) false-positive rate and true-positive rate
(B) prevalence and positive predictive value
(C) sensitivity and negative predictive value
(D) true negative rate and specificity

The original use of the ROC curve was to separate meaningful signals from unimportant noise in radar transmissions during wartime. The radar operator was tasked with deciding whether a blip indicated one of their own ships or planes or was an enemy. The method developed to accomplish this task consisted of comparing two probabilities (rates) termed operating characteristics. The probabilities were graphed in such a way as to compare the usefulness of applying particular criteria that permit selection of the best test and, once the test was selected, to determine the best cut-point that optimized the accuracy of deciding what produced the signal.

Each radar signal indicated an ally or an enemy and, for each signal, the radar operator's interpretation was either correct or incorrect. The frequencies of these four situations were sufficient statistics to determine the classic parameters of a test with a dichotomous outcome. These parameters are sensitivity (true-positive rate) and specificity (true-negative rate), positive and negative predictive values, and false-positive and negative rates.

Table 72-1 details the results of a hypothetical screening test and is an example of a straightforward presentation of the calculations needed to determine test parameters.

In medicine, it often is helpful to evaluate the usefulness of a screening (or other) test to accurately characterize individuals as having or not having a certain condition (eg, cancer, diabetes, fracture risk). Typically, the next step after a positive screening test is to offer a more precise diagnostic test to make a definitive determination of whether disease is present. Screening is similar to interpreting characteristics of radar signals to distinguish friend from foe. The best tests will be highly sensitive and highly specific.

The ROC curve is constructed by calculating false-positive and true-positive rates for each test subject and plotting them along the x and y axes, respectively. The x axis for the ROC curve is the false-positive rate (1 – specificity) and the y axis is the true-positive rate (sensitivity), and this is the correct answer to the question.

Once the curve is drawn, the test can be evaluated and compared with other candidate tests by calculating the area under the curve (AUC). The test with the highest AUC generally is the best option. A perfect test would detect all patients with the disease (sensitivity = 100%, for all values of [1 – specificity]) and all patients without disease would test negative ([1 – specificity] = 0%, for all values of sensitivity). Graphically, this would be shown as a line segment from the origin to (0,1) and a second line segment from (0,1) to (1,1). A useless test—one that is no better than flipping a coin—would demonstrate equal true-positive and false-positive rates throughout. The resulting ROC curve for a useless test will be the diagonal line segment from the origin to (1,1). The area under the ROC curve for the perfect test, therefore, is 1 and the area under a useless test (coin flip) is 0.5.

Figure 72-1 presents an example of how drawing an ROC curve has been applied in practice. The curve demonstrates the utility of the initial platelet count to separate neonates who have had a perinatal arterial ischemic stroke from those who have hypoxic-ischemic encephalopathy and who are undergoing

TABLE 72-1. Outcomes of a Screening Test

	DISEASE (+)	DISEASE (-)	TOTAL
Test (+)	a (true positives)	b (false positives)	(a+b) All who test positive
Test (–)	c (false negatives)	d (true negatives)	(c+d) All who test negative
Total	All with disease (a+c)	All without disease (b+d)	(a+b+c+d) All subjects

Positive predictive value = a/(a+b), the probability that a person who tests positive has disease.

Negative predictive value = d/(c+d), the probability that a person who tests negative does not have disease.

Sensitivity (true-positive rate) = a/(a+c), the probability that a person with disease will test positive.

Specificity (true-negative rate) = d/(b+d), the probability that a person without disease will test negative.

The false-negative rate = c/(a+c), the probability that a person with disease will test negative.

The false-positive rate (1 – specificity) = b/(b+d), the probability that a person without disease will test positive.

Disease prevalence = (a+c)/(a+b+c+d), the probability that person in the tested population will have disease.

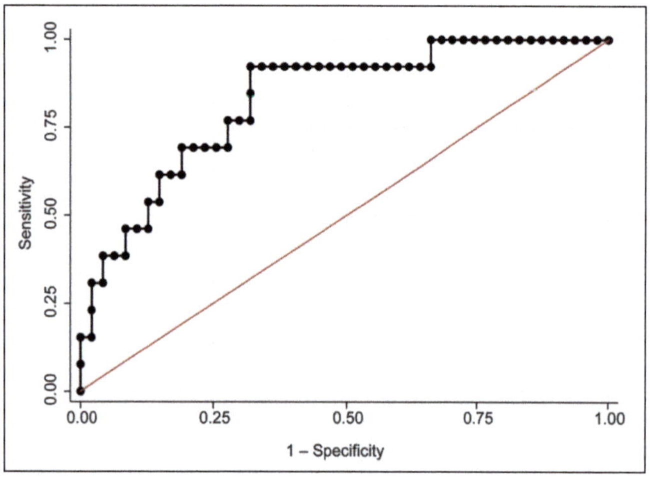

FIGURE 72-1. Receiver operating characteristic (ROC) curve for initial neonatal platelet count in distinguishing perinatal arterial ischemic stroke from hypoxic-ischemic encephalopathy treated with whole-body hypothermia with abnormal brain magnetic resonance imaging. Abbreviation: CI, confidence interval. (Reprinted from Adami RR, Grundy ME, Poretti A, Felling RJ, Lemmon M, Graham EM. Distinguishing Arterial Ischemic Stroke From Hypoxic-Ischemic Encephalopathy in the Neonate at Birth. Obstet Gynecol. 2016 Oct;128(4):704-712. doi: 10.1097/AOG.0000000000001631)

whole-body hypothermia. The diagonal, indicating the ROC curve for a useless test, is drawn in red.

Figure 72-1 shows the AUC of the platelet count test is 0.83. A test with an AUC of less than 0.83 will be inferior to using the platelet count to diagnose perinatal arterial ischemic, and a test with an AUC exceeding 0.83 will be superior.

Sensitivity and specificity are inherent properties of the test and independent of prevalence. Graphing sensitivity and prevalence, therefore, will not be informative because they are independent of each other. A graph between sensitivity and negative predictive value should correlate because a more sensitive test is more likely to identify individuals who do not have the disease, resulting in a higher negative predictive value. This would not be an ROC curve.

Positive and negative predictive values are conditional on disease prevalence because they account for persons who have disease and persons who do not have disease. Graphing the prevalence and positive predictive value will be informative as to the magnitude of the influence of prevalence on predictive value. This may be important when considering how to interpret screening tests in different populations and may affect choice of the cut point; however, this graph is not an ROC curve.

The true-negative rate and specificity are synonymous, so graphing them would be uninformative.

Baldessarini RJ, Finklestein S, Arana GW. The predictive power of diagnostic tests and the effect of prevalence of illness. Arch Gen Psychiatry 1983;40:569–73. doi: 10.1001/archpsyc.1983.01790050095011

Bharti B, Bharti S. Receiver-operating characteristic curve analysis in diagnostic, prognostic and predictive biomarker research: trade-off between sensitivity and specificity with change of test cut-offs. J Clin Pathol 2009;62:1051. doi: 10.1136/jcp.2009.069591

Brown CD, Davis HT. Receiver operating characteristics curves and related decision measures: a tutorial. Chemometrics Intellig Lab Syst 2006;80:24–38. doi: 10.1016/j.chemolab.2005.05.004

Jain S, Bharathi D. Receiver operating characteristic curve analysis and its application in dentistry. J Adv Med Dent Sci Res 2020;8:152–5.

Nahm FS. Receiver operating characteristic curve: overview and practical use for clinicians. Korean J Anesthesiol 2022;75:25–36. doi: 10.4097/kja.21209

73 Squamous dysplasia during pregnancy

A 34-year-old gravida 2, para 1, at 28 weeks of gestation undergoes colposcopy for high-grade squamous epithelial lesion (HSIL) cytology, human papillomavirus (HPV) type 16 positive. A colposcopic examination demonstrates dense acetowhite epithelium with coarse mosaicism at the 12:00 position of the cervix, and the lesion does not look concerning for invasion. The biopsy pathology shows cervical intraepithelial neoplasia 3 (CIN 3). The best next step in management is

(A) endocervical curettage
(B) excisional procedure
(C) HPV vaccine series
* (D) postpartum colposcopy

Cervical dysplasia is common in patients during their reproductive years, and these abnormalities may be detected during cervical cancer screening during pregnancy. Pregnancy physiology alters the size and appearance of the cervix, which may make colposcopic evaluation more challenging. For patients with high-grade lesions, colposcopic biopsy is safe during pregnancy and helps exclude invasive carcinoma. The rate of progression of CIN 3 to carcinoma appears to be similar in nonpregnant individuals and pregnant individuals; however, adequate follow-up during and after pregnancy is crucial to complete the appropriate evaluation.

This patient's colposcopic biopsy showed CIN 3, and clinical and pathologic examinations are not suggestive of invasive carcinoma. Based on these findings, the best next step for the patient in the scenario above is to repeat a colposcopic evaluation in 12–24 weeks, at which time this patient will be postpartum. The 2019 ASCCP Guidelines provide a range of surveillance options after colposcopy during pregnancy to account for a variety of gestational ages at the time of CIN diagnosis, the skill of the gynecologist, and the risks of losing the patient to follow up. If a repeat colposcopy result is concerning for invasive disease or progression of a lesion, repeat biopsy is recommended. Because this patient is at 28 weeks of gestation, repeating the colposcopy postpartum is most appropriate because she will be full term at the start of the recommended follow-up interval. The colposcopy should be performed at 6 weeks postpartum to allow for uterine involution and cervical stroma remodeling, but colposcopy can be performed as early as 4 weeks postpartum for patients at risk of losing their insurance or who may have other barriers to postpartum care.

Endocervical curettage is not recommended during pregnancy due to the risk of disruption of the pregnancy and is not the best next step. This procedure should be delayed until after delivery to avoid inadvertent instrumentation of the uterine cavity.

Although there are no known adverse effects of receiving the HPV vaccine series during pregnancy, there are a lack of safety data during pregnancy, and vaccination at this time is not recommended. Ideally completed before exposure occurs, HPV vaccination is estimated to prevent up to 90% of HPV-related cancer. This vaccination is recommended for all individuals aged 9–26 years, after shared decision making with their doctor. Patients aged 27–45 years may be considered if they were not adequately vaccinated earlier. Because the patient described above is pregnant, this is not the best next step for her; however, vaccination can be offered when she is no longer pregnant and after further evaluation and treatment of CIN 3 to potentially reduce the risk of re-infection with the same or other HPV types.

Excisional procedures, such as loop electrosurgical excision procedure or cold knife conization, are generally not recommended for CIN 3 during pregnancy. An excisional procedure is recommended during pregnancy if carcinoma is suspected on initial cytology, during the colposcopic examination, or on pathologic evaluation. The ideal timing of an excisional procedure is in the second trimester at which time the risk of hemorrhage, miscarriage, and preterm birth are lowest. Because this patient's clinical findings and pathology results are consistent with CIN 3 without concern for invasion, an excisional procedure is not the best next step and should not be performed at this time.

The decision to treat cervical dysplasia in pregnancy is indicated for individuals with cytologic, colposcopic, or histologic findings concerning for invasive disease. Lesions consistent with CIN 3 or lower can be managed with repeat colposcopy. Gynecologists should have systems in place to ensure adequate timely follow-up for these individuals, particularly for those needing postpartum evaluation.

American College of Obstetricians and Gynecologists. Adjuvant human papillomavirus vaccination for patients undergoing treatment for cervical intraepithelial neoplasia 2+. Practice Advisory. ACOG; 2023. Accessed March 13, 2025.

Gomez Y, Balaya V, Lepigeon K, Mathevet P, Jacot-Guillarmod M. Predictive factors involved in postpartum regressions of cytological/histological cervical high-grade dysplasia diagnosed during pregnancy. J Clin Med 2021;10:5319. doi: 10.3390/jcm10225319

Korenaga TK, Tewari KS. Gynecologic cancer in pregnancy. Gynecol Oncol 2020;157:799–809. doi: 10.1016/j.ygyno.2020.03.015

Stuebs FA, Mergel F, Koch MC, Dietl AK, Schulmeyer CE, Adler W, et al. Cervical intraepithelial neoplasia grade 3: development during pregnancy and postpartum. Arch Gynecol Obstet 2023;307:1567–72. doi: 10.1007/s00404-022-06815-7

74 Risk factors for patients on aromatase inhibitors

A 42-year-old surgically postmenopausal patient with recurrent low-grade serous ovarian cancer is initiating treatment with an aromatase inhibitor. She is taking no other medications, and her medical history is otherwise unremarkable. Before initiation of the aromatase inhibitor, the most appropriate baseline test for this patient is a (an)

* (A) bone mineral density scan
(B) echocardiogram
(C) estrogen level
(D) lipid panel
(E) liver function panel

Aromatase is an enzyme that mediates the conversion of androgens to estrogens. Aromatase inhibitors block the effects of aromatase, which decreases circulating and tissue estrogen levels in postmenopausal patients. In premenopausal women, compensatory physiological responses induce ovarian estrogen production, and the same effect is not seen. Low-grade serous ovarian cancer expresses estrogen receptors, and aromatase inhibitors often are used as a treatment in this disease.

However, because estrogen receptors are widely expressed in many other tissues, including bone, adverse bone effects can be observed with aromatase inhibitor use. Aromatase inhibitors potentiate a decrease in estrogen levels beyond that of menopause alone, leading to accelerated bone loss and an increased fracture risk. Studies have shown that the use of an aromatase inhibitor results in a twofold to fourfold increase in bone loss compared to untreated postmenopausal patients, resulting in a reported 10–20% increase in fracture risk.

Because of the high cost of fractures, including a high rate of disability, the National Comprehensive Cancer Network and other national cancer groups recommend that women initiating treatment with an aromatase inhibitor undergo baseline bone mineral density assessment. If bone mineral density is normal, repeat monitoring should be completed every 1–2 years while on aromatase inhibitor therapy. In addition, all patients beginning aromatase inhibitor therapy should be advised on strategies to increase bone mineral density including weight-bearing exercise and adequate dietary calcium and vitamin D intake with supplementation if necessary. Patients who meet diagnostic criteria for osteoporosis on bone mineral density testing should be treated with denosumab or bisphosphonate therapy. A proposed management algorithm in at-risk patients is presented in Figure 74-1.

This patient recently initiated therapy with an aromatase inhibitor and therefore should undergo baseline bone mineral density assessment, making this the correct answer. Aromatase inhibitors reliably decrease estrogen levels in postmenopausal patients and thus monitoring of estrogen levels is not indicated, so this is not the correct answer. Aromatase inhibitors can cause mild liver enzyme elevation; however, severe hepatotoxicity is rare. Liver function tests are not necessary when initiating aromatase inhibitor therapy; therefore, this is not the correct answer.

Postmenopausal status does increase the risks of cardiovascular disease, and adverse cardiovascular effects may be seen with the use of aromatase inhibitors. However, this is not mediated through a change in cholesterol levels and thus baseline lipid profile is not needed, so this is not the correct choice. In an asymptomatic patient initiating aromatase inhibitor therapy, a baseline echocardiogram is not indicated as this medication does not cause cardiotoxicity. However, if this patient were to receive a MEK inhibitor such as trametinib in a future line of therapy for her low-grade serous carcinoma, a baseline echocardiogram would be warranted as this class of medications does carry a risk of cardiotoxicity.

For this postmenopausal patient initiating aromatase inhibitor therapy, the best baseline test is bone mineral density due to the increased risk of bone mineral loss with this medication and the need for initiation of treatment in at-risk individuals. Monitoring of bone mineral density should be performed every 1–2 years while on therapy, as noted in Figure 74-1.

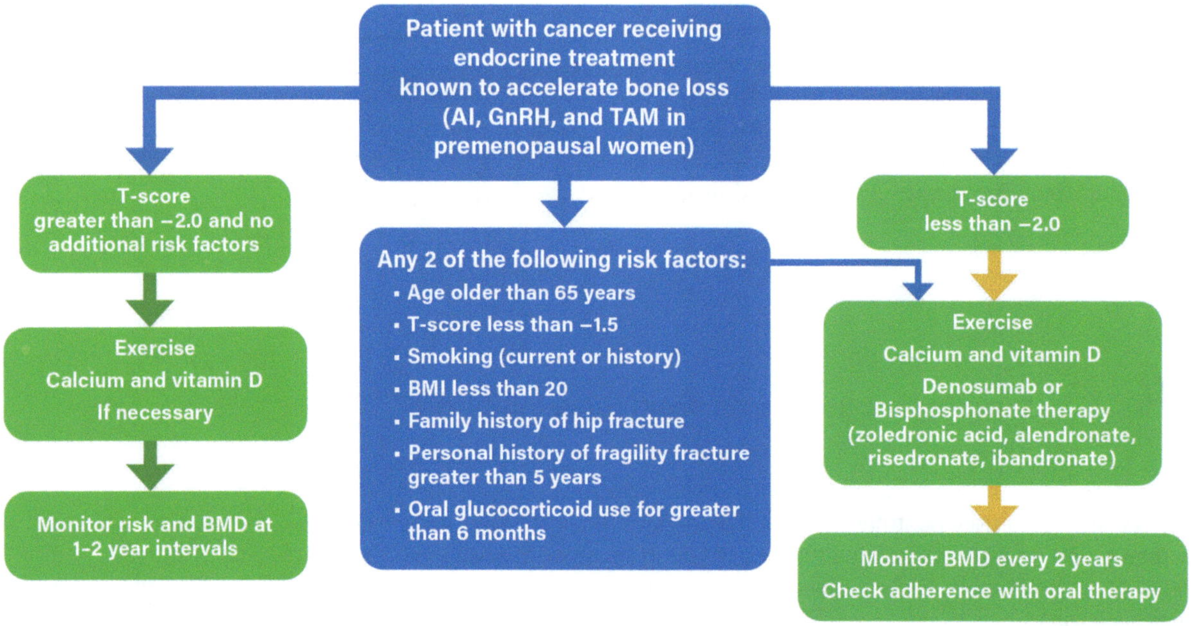

FIGURE 74-1. Recommended algorithm for managing bone health in patients receiving aromatase inhibitor therapy. Abbreviations: AI, aromatase inhibitor; BMD, bone mineral density; BMI, body mass index. If patients experience an annual decrease in bone mineral density (BMD) of 10% or more (using the same DXA absorptiometry machine), secondary causes of bone loss, such as vitamin D deficiency, should be evaluated and antiresorptive therapy initiated. Use the lowest T-score from three sites. (Reprinted from Hadji P, Aapro MS, Body J, Gnant M, Brandi ML, Reginster JY, et al. Management of aromatase inhibitor-associated bone loss [AIBL] in postmenopausal women with hormone sensitive breast cancer: joint position statement of the IOF, CABS, ECTS, IEG, ESCEO, IMS, and SIOG. J Bone Oncol 2017;7:1–12. doi: 10.1016/j.jbo.2017.03.001)

Gralow JR, Biermann JS, Farooki A, Fornier MN, Gagel RF, Kumar R, et al. NCCN task force report: bone health in cancer care. J Natl Compr Canc Netw 2013;11(suppl 3):S1–50; quiz S51. doi: 10.6004/jnccn.2013.0215

Hadji P, Aapro MS, Body J, Gnant M, Brandi ML, Reginster JY, et al. Management of aromatase inhibitor-associated bone loss (AIBL) in postmenopausal women with hormone sensitive breast cancer: joint position statement of the IOF, CABS, ECTS, IEG, ESCEO IMS, and SIOG. J Bone Oncol 2017;7:1–12. doi: 10.1016/j.jbo.2017.03.001

75 Types of clinical studies

A new drug is developed that targets a molecular abnormality occurring in many types of cancer. The most suitable study design to assess the activity of this drug in patients whose tumors have a mutation, irrespective of the primary tumor site, is

* (A) basket
  (B) noninferiority
  (C) phase IV
  (D) umbrella

Clinical research studies can be classified as either *observational* or *experimental*. In observational studies, the investigator does not assign the exposure. In experimental studies, the exposure is assigned by the research team. Clinical trials are experimental studies involving human subjects.

There are five phases of clinical trials that follow one after the other and commonly are used in the drug development process. In a phase 0 trial, a very small dose of a drug is given to a few patients for a short time period to evaluate pharmacokinetics and pharmacodynamics. Phase I trials determine the maximum tolerated dose, dose limiting toxicity, pattern of toxicity, and the most suitable dose to be carried forward to phase II studies. Phase II trials determine response rates and provide guidance on whether to proceed with a phase III study. Phase III trials are prospective and randomized and directly compare two treatments (experimental treatment versus standard of care treatment). Phase IV studies, also called *post-marketing surveillance trials*, are conducted after U.S. Food and Drug Administration approval and provide information on long-term effects. The goals of a phase IV trial are to learn about treatment-related adverse events that may not have been clear in earlier phase studies and to assess the real-world effectiveness of an approved agent.

Advances in molecular and genetic testing have resulted in a growing recognition that the long-standing practice of recommending systemic anticancer treatment based solely on primary site and cell type may not be the optimal approach. It is now common to consider oncologic treatments based more on specific drug targets or pathways than based on histologic appearance or organ of origin alone. The awareness that mechanisms of growth, metastasis, and other biologic processes are shared without respect to the traditional methods of classification has necessitated the development of novel clinical trial designs intended to facilitate the evaluation of targeted therapies. In response to this need, several types of clinical trials that can efficiently investigate more than one targeted treatment in a type of cancer or the activity of a single targeted agent in more than one disease have been developed.

A basket trial tests treatment for multiple cancer types with a common biomarker (Fig. 75-1). All potential participants are screened with testing for a specific molecular target; those whose tumors test positive may be eligible to enroll. Once enrolled, all patients receive the same treatment that is directed at the same, specific, molecular target. In their purest form, basket trials do not account for primary tumor site or histology. A well-known basket trial resulted in the approval of pembrolizumab for patients with metastatic or unresectable refractory cancer with mismatch repair deficient (MMRd)/microsatellite instability high (MSI-H) tumors, regardless of cell type or primary tumor site. A basket trial is the best study design for the scenario above because the novel agent is to be tested in patients whose tumors harbor the same target, regardless of cell type or primary tumor site.

Noninferiority studies are a good choice when comparing a treatment that is likely at least as effective as the standard treatment but may be preferred on the basis of tolerance, convenience, cost, or some other characteristic. Although a noninferiority design can be applied to phase II or IV studies, it is most often applied in phase III trials. There are several unique features, including statement of the hypothesis, that characterize noninferiority studies. The primary aim is to evaluate

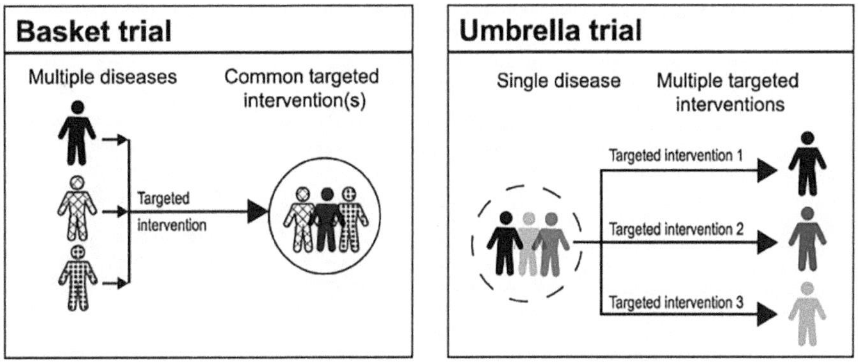

FIGURE 75-1. Comparison of basket trials versus umbrella trials. (Reprinted from Park JJ, Siden E, Zoratti MJ, Dron L, Harari O, Singer J, et al. Systematic review of basket trials, umbrella trials, and platform trials: a landscape analysis of master protocols. Trials 2019;20:572–1. doi: 10.1186/s13063-019-3664-1)

whether the outcome of interest (often survival or safety) with the new treatment is worse than the standard by less than an acceptable, prespecified, margin. This margin is termed the noninferiority margin. Therefore, for a noninferiority design, the null hypothesis is stated as follows: the primary outcome with the nonstandard (experimental) therapy is worse than the outcome with the standard by a margin that exceeds the noninferiority margin. Rejection of the null hypothesis permits concluding that the new treatment is not inferior to standard. A noninferiority trial is not the best type of study to assess the drug described above. Although it might be possible to design a noninferiority basket trial, there is no indication that such a design is required for this agent. The primary purpose of the study, to assess the activity of the novel agent, will likely be accomplished by evaluating response rate, clinical benefit rate, time to progression, or another standard phase II endpoint.

An umbrella trial investigates several targeted treatments in a single disease type (Table 75-1). In an umbrella design, patients are assigned to one of several study arms, each of which delivers a treatment directed at a different biomarker. An initial screening test is conducted and, if a target is identified, the patient is treated on the arm with the drug that targets their tumor biomarker. An umbrella type of study is not the best option for the scenario above that aims to test a single drug targeting one specific biomarker. Treatments are assigned according to biomarker testing and the study evaluates each agent according to appropriate phase II endpoints. Once evaluation of a particular drug is completed, the arm is closed and the agent may or may not move on to the next phase, depending on the results. As of 2019, 17 agents, or combinations of agents, have been evaluated, and seven have shown promising activity.

TABLE 75-1. Types of Master Protocols

TYPE OF TRIAL	OBJECTIVE
Umbrella	To study multiple targeted therapies in the context of a single disease
Basket	To study a single targeted therapy in the context of multiple diseases or disease subtypes
Platform	To study multiple targeted therapies in the context of a single disease in a perpetual manner, with therapies allowed to enter or leave the platform on the bases of a decision algorithm

Reprinted from Woodcock J, LaVange LM. Master protocols to study multiple therapies, multiple diseases, or both. N Engl J Med 2017;377:62–70. doi: 10.1056/NEJMra1510062

In the scenario above, the drug is not yet approved, or marketed, and a phase IV trial cannot be caried out because it cannot yet be used in the general population outside of the clinical trial setting.

Fountzilas E, Tsimberidou AM, Vo HH, Kurzrock R. Clinical trial design in the era of precision medicine. Genome Med 2022;14:101–1. doi: 10.1186/s13073-022-01102-1

Garralda E, Dienstmann R, Piris-Giménez A, Braña I, Rodon J, Tabernero J. New clinical trial designs in the era of precision medicine. Mol Oncol 2019;13:549–57. doi: 10.1002/1878-0261.12465

Mauri L, D'Agostino RB. Challenges in the design and interpretation of noninferiority trials. N Engl J Med 2017;377:1357–67. doi: 10.1056/NEJMra1510063

Woodcock J, LaVange LM. Master protocols to study multiple therapies, multiple diseases, or both. N Engl J Med 2017;377:62–70. doi: 10.1056/NEJMra1510062

76 Postmolar gestational trophoblastic neoplasia

A 21-year-old received a diagnosis of complete hydatidiform mole during a desired pregnancy and underwent a dilation and curettage. During the third month of post-procedure surveillance, the patient's quantitative serum human chorionic gonadotropin (hCG) values rose to 85,000, which represented an increase of greater than 10% in 2 weeks (measured over three tests). Her pelvic ultrasound is shown in Figure 76-1. Computed tomography (CT) of the patient's chest, abdomen, and pelvis is normal. The best next step in treatment is

* (A) chemotherapy
(B) dilation and curettage
(C) hysterectomy
(D) hysteroscopic resection
(E) pelvic radiotherapy

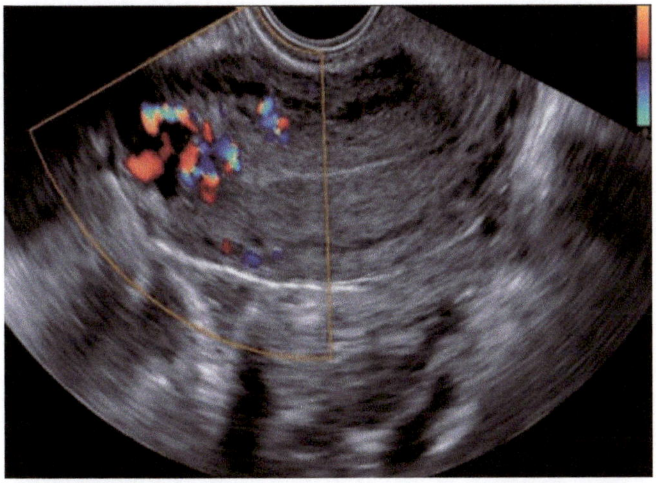

FIGURE 76-1. Three-centimeter mass extending to the uterine myometrium. (Reprinted from Lima LL, Parente RC, Maestá I, Amim Junior J, de Rezende Filho JF, Montenegro CA, Braga A. Clinical and radiological correlations in patients with gestational trophoblastic disease. Radiol Bras. 2016 Jul-Aug;49(4):241 250. doi: 10.1590/0100-3984.2015.0073)

The patient in the scenario above meets diagnostic criteria for postmolar gestational trophoblastic neoplasia (GTN). This diagnosis is based on weekly serum hCG evaluation. Established National Comprehensive Cancer Network (NCCN) criteria for evaluating serial serum-hCG trends allow gynecologic oncologists to accurately diagnose postmolar GTN early in the disease process (Appendix J). The diagnosis can be confirmed with pelvic ultrasound findings. Further confirmation of this diagnosis through direct biopsy is not recommended because it does not improve diagnostic accuracy and it increases the risk of bleeding.

Gestational trophoblastic neoplasia is described by stage of disease and through prognostic scoring systems. International Federation of Gynecology and Obstetrics (FIGO) staging of GTN is anatomic and based strictly on tumor location (Appendix H). Prognostic scoring systems, such as the World Health Organization (WHO) point-based scoring system (Appendix I) and the modified FIGO scoring system, incorporate additional clinical information. In the WHO system, a score of 6 or less is considered low-risk GTN and a score of 7 or higher is considered high-risk disease. For low-risk GTN, single-agent chemotherapy often is sufficient, whereas high-risk GTN requires multiagent chemotherapy to achieve the best outcomes. Stage IV disease also qualifies as high-risk disease and requires multiagent chemotherapy.

With rigorous adherence to post-evacuation serum hCG protocols, most cases of postmolar GTN are diagnosed early, with uterine confined disease and favorable prognostic scores. In the described patient, there is no evidence of metastatic disease on CT. Ultrasonography, however, depicts a heterogenous and highly vascular intracavitary mass with deep myometrial invasion.

Chemotherapy is the best next step in treatment for this patient with postmolar GTN who desires future fertility. In the scenario above, the patient's disease score is 3 and single-agent chemotherapy is her best option. A multitude of single-agent chemotherapy regimens and dosing schedules have been evaluated for treatment of low-risk GTN. Primary remission rates for each are high, with methotrexate ranging from 87% to 93% and dactinomycin ranging from 77% to 94% across studies. The efficacy of weekly methotrexate dosing is significantly lower, and is not currently recommended for treatment of GTN. Treatment efficacy is monitored by serial serum-hCG measurements. For disease that does not have a complete response to the first single-agent regimen, the crossover to the alternative regimen is recommended if the WHO prognostic re-scoring remains in the low-risk range.

For patients with high-risk disease, multiagent chemotherapy is recommended. Etoposide, methotrexate, actinomycin-D, cyclophosphamide, and vincristine (EMA-CO) chemotherapy is the standard treatment for high-risk GTN because it achieves remission in 80–90% of patients. Depending on the clinical presentation of high-risk GTN or in the case of persistent or recurrent disease, alternative regimens or localized interventions may be recommended and referral to, or consultation with, a center specializing in comprehensive GTN management should be considered.

The role of repeat dilation and curettage for low-risk non-metastatic GTN is controversial. Studies of secondary dilation and curettage in non-metastatic GTN report remission rates of approximately 40%, allowing for omission of chemotherapy in these patients. The patient described above has an invasive mole with deep myometrial invasion. The risks of uterine perforation and hemorrhage are anticipated to be higher in the setting of deep invasion, and the likelihood of complete resection with a second endometrial curettage is anticipated to be low. This is not the best next step in the scenario above.

The hysteroscopic resection of an invasive mole is contraindicated for many reasons, and this is not the best next step for the described patient. The primary benefit of hysteroscopic resection lies in its ability to selectively remove uterine masses under direct visualization while preserving as much myometrial tissue and endometrium as possible. Invasive moles are highly vascular and have an infiltrative growth pattern. Complete resection with myometrial preservation would be very difficult to achieve and would be associated with an unacceptably high risk of complications due to uterine perforation, organ injury, and hemorrhage. Hysteroscopic resection would introduce an additional risk of uterine synechiae and scar rupture that could compromise the implantation and safety of future pregnancies.

Hysterectomy is an effective surgical option for treatment of low-risk GTN, and it can be considered for uterine-confined disease if future fertility is not desired or in the setting of chemotherapy resistance. Hysterectomy, however, is not the best next step for this young patient who desires fertility.

Although radiotherapy has a potential role in the treatment of select metastasis in high-risk GTN, it is not employed for low-risk GTN that is confined to the uterus. In the patient above, the additional morbidity and fertility consequences from radiation exposure to the ovaries and endometrium outweigh the potential benefits, and radiotherapy is not the best next step.

Strict adherence to post-evacuation serum-hCG protocols allows early detection of postmolar GTN. More than 95% of patients with GTN will have low-risk disease at diagnosis, and survival rates are excellent if appropriate treatment is undertaken.

Kamijo K, Ishida K, Oide S, Anan K, Taito S, Kataoka Y, et al. Efficacy and safety of the surgery-first approach compared to the chemotherapy-first approach for treating low-risk gestational trophoblastic neoplasia: a systematic review and meta-analysis. Cureus 2023;15:e45726. doi: 10.7759/cureus.45726

National Comprehensive Cancer Network. Gestational trophoblastic neoplasia. Version 2.2025. NCCN Clinical Practice Guidelines in Oncology [after login]. NCCN; 2025. Accessed March 13, 2025. https://www.nccn.org/guidelines/guidelines-detail?category=1&id=1489

Osborne RJ, Filiaci VL, Schink JC, Mannel RS, Behbakht K, Hoffman JS, et al. Second curettage for low-risk nonmetastatic gestational trophoblastic neoplasia. Obstet Gynecol 2016;128:535–42. doi: 10.1097/AOG.0000000000001554

Soper JT. Gestational trophoblastic disease: current evaluation and management [published erratum appears in Obstet Gynecol 2022;139:149]. Obstet Gynecol 2021;137:355–70. doi: 10.1097/AOG.0000000000004240

77 Pulmonary evaluation

A 55-year-old underwent a hysterectomy and bilateral salpingectomy for symptomatic uterine fibroids 6 weeks ago. She now presents to the emergency department reporting 3 days of pleuritic chest pain, dyspnea, and cough. Her children are at home with upper respiratory infections. She takes no medications, reports an allergy to intravenous contrast, and has no other significant medical history. She felt fine, and was normally active, prior to the onset of symptoms. On physical examination, her temperature is 37.2 °C (99 °F), her heart rate is 90 beats per minute, her blood pressure is 130/80 mm Hg, and her oxygen saturation is 98% on room air. The remainder of her physical examination yields normal results. In addition to a respiratory panel, the best next step in evaluation is

(A) brain natriuretic peptide (BNP)
(B) chest radiograph
(C) computed tomography–pulmonary angiogram (CTPA)
* (D) serum D-dimer
(E) a ventilation perfusion (VQ) scan

Pulmonary embolism (PE) is a serious, potentially fatal, occurrence. Approximately 20% of patients die before or shortly after diagnosis. Evaluation frequently includes expensive imaging at an annual cost between $7 and $10 billion in the United States and often includes exposure to radiation and intravenous contrast.

The clinical diagnosis of PE is challenging. Presenting symptoms and physical findings are nonspecific and the differential diagnosis is broad, including pneumonia, bronchitis, pericarditis, angina, acute coronary syndrome, and heart failure. Because of the potential for life-threatening and fatal outcomes, there is a low threshold for evaluation of patients with suggestive symptoms. It has been estimated that the diagnosis of PE is confirmed in fewer than 10% of patients who undergo evaluation.

Although there are subtle differences in national and international guidelines, in general, a sensible and practical approach begins with application of one or more clinical decision tools, such as the modified Wells criteria (Box 77-1), the modified Geneva scores, the years rule, or the PE rule-out (PERC) criteria. A number of studies have shown that using a clinical decision rule early in the evaluation process avoids unnecessary and nondiagnostic studies and conserves resources (Table 77-1).

Calculating the PERC score is a reasonable initial step in estimating the probability of a pulmonary embolism based on clinical parameters. Depending on this score, additional testing can be avoided or recommended. The PERC score awards a point for each of the following: age older than 49 years, pulse more than 99 bpm, oxygen saturation greater than 95% on room air, hemoptysis, estrogen use, prior DVT or PE, unilateral leg swelling, or surgery/trauma with a hospital stay within 28 days. A PERC score of 0 excludes PE unless the clinical gestalt is that probability of an embolism exceeds 15%. Although the clinical suspicion of PE in this patient is relatively low, she has a PERC score of 1 based on her age. All other parameters are absent; however, a PERC score other than 0 indicates the need for further investigation. If her PERC score were 0, then no additional evaluation for PE would be recommended.

Because she has a PERC score of more than 0, an additional decision tool, such as the modified Wells or Geneva score, can be used. The modified Wells score includes a (subjective) clinical suspicion parameter, whereas the modified Geneva score does not have a clinical suspicion component. Regardless of whether Wells or Geneva is used, if the risk assessment is low or medium, the best next step is to obtain a serum D-dimer level.

If the D-dimer level is below the threshold, pulmonary embolus is essentially excluded and no additional evaluation is indicated. If it exceeds the threshold then further workup is required.

D-dimers are fragments of protein released from dissolving blood clots, are increased shortly after a pulmonary embolism, and are highly sensitive for diagnosis; however, increased D-dimer is a relatively nonspecific finding. Older age, recent operation, malignancy, and infection all are associated with increased levels. Unacceptably low specificity (approximating 10% in certain populations) has led to the recommendation that D-dimer be used in the evaluation for PE only along with a validated clinical decision tool, as described above. Some experts recommend using an age-adjusted threshold for D-dimer (for patients more than 50 years old, age × 10 ng/mL), and others recommend a higher threshold for those at the least risk based on clinical factors. Regardless, in this patient, obtaining a serum D-dimer is the best next step.

Chest imaging is indicated in two circumstances: 1) if the Wells or Geneva score suggests low or moderate risk and the D-dimer is above the threshold or 2) if the Wells or Geneva score suggests high risk (D-dimer is not helpful with a high-risk score).

BOX 77-1

Interpretation of Wells Criteria Scores

The interpretation can be applied in either three-tier (Wells Criteria) or two-tier models (modified Wells criteria).

Wells Criteria:

- High-risk patients: More than 6.0
  Recommended management: D-dimer not recommended
- Moderate-risk patients: 2.0–6.0
  Recommended management: Consider D-dimer or computed tomography–pulmonary angiography
- Low-risk patients: Less than 2.0
  Recommended management: Pulmonary embolism rule-out criteria (PERC) can be considered as well as D-dimer

Modified Wells Criteria:

- Unlikely: Clinical probability of pulmonary embolism score is 4.0 or less
  Recommended management: Consider D-dimer
- Likely: Clinical probability of pulmonary embolism if score is greater than 4.0
  Recommended management: Consider computed tomography–pulmonary angiography

Used with permission of Phil Wells, MD.

TABLE 77-1. Clinical Decision Rule According to the Modified Wells Criteria

CLINICAL FEATURES	SCORE
Clinical signs and symptoms of deep vein thrombosis	3.0
Pulmonary embolism likely or more likely than alternative diagnosis	3.0
Heart rate greater than 100 beats per minute	1.5
Immobilization for more than 3 days or surgery in the previous 4 weeks	1.5
Previously objectively diagnosed pulmonary embolism or deep vein thrombosis	1.5
Hemoptysis	1.0
Cancer	1.0

Used with permission of Phil Wells, MD.

If imaging were indicated, then a ventilation perfusion (VQ) scan could be considered; however, it is not the best next step in the above scenario. There are few, if any, contraindications to a VQ scan when indicated, and it is the modality of choice for patients who are unable to have CTPA. Ventilation perfusion scans are not widely available, cannot diagnose other conditions, and have a relatively low sensitivity. Many patients will have intermediate probability VQ scans, which do not rule in or rule out PE, necessitating additional testing or treatment based on clinical suspicion.

Brain natriuretic peptide is produced in the heart and involved in the regulation of blood pressure and fluid and sodium balance. Increased BNP levels frequently are present in patients with heart failure, and it has been used in diagnosis; however, increased BNP is nonspecific and may be associated with other conditions. Although BNP has been reported as prognostic for patients with pulmonary embolus, likely secondary to its association with right ventricular failure, it does not have a role in evaluation for PE.

Computed tomography–pulmonary angiography is used widely for diagnosis of pulmonary embolism. It has the advantages of high reliability and finding changes suggestive of alternative diagnoses. As discussed above, although chest imaging may be indicated depending on the D-dimer level, it is not the best next step. Computed tomography–pulmonary angiography requires intravenous contrast and would be relatively contraindicated in this patient due to her allergy; however, if the D-dimer were increased, desensitization before CTPA could be considered.

Chest radiograph may be obtained in the course of evaluating a patient with pulmonary symptom, and can diagnose pulmonary infarction or infection; however, it is neither sufficiently sensitive nor specific to be used as an early test in evaluation of patients with symptoms concerning for PE.

Di Nisio M, van Es N, Büller HR. Deep vein thrombosis and pulmonary embolism. Lancet 2016;388:3060–73. doi: 10.1016/S0140-6736(16)30514-1

Freund Y, Cohen-Aubart F, Bloom B. Acute pulmonary embolism: a review. JAMA 2022;328:1336–45. doi: 10.1001/jama.2022.16815

van der Hulle T, Cheung WY, Kooij S, Beenen LF, van Bemmel T, van Es J, et al. Simplified diagnostic management of suspected pulmonary embolism (the years study): a prospective, multicentre, cohort study [published erratum appears in Lancet 2017;390:230]. Lancet 2017;390:289–97. doi: 10.1016/S0140-6736(17)30885-1

78 HER2+ serous endometrial cancer

A 72-year-old patient presents for her postoperative follow-up after a robot-assisted total hysterectomy with bilateral salpingo-oophorectomy, partial omentectomy, and bilateral pelvic sentinel node mapping and biopsy. Her pathology shows a 4-cm serous adenocarcinoma of the endometrium with invasion into the myometrium and two positive lymph nodes. Today's testing reveals that her tumor is human epidermal growth factor 2 positive (HER2+). In addition to treatment with carboplatin and paclitaxel, the best next step is to administer

(A) doxorubicin
(B) external beam radiation therapy (EBRT)
(C) pembrolizumab
* (D) trastuzumab

Serous endometrial cancer comprises 10% of endometrial cancer and is an aggressive histologic subtype. It is estimated that 60% of cases of serous endometrial cancer are p53 mutated, and 30% are HER2 amplified. Serous endometrial cancer is frequently managed with surgical staging followed by systemic chemotherapy because of its high distant recurrence risk, even in early-stage disease.

Human epidermal growth factor 2 can be overexpressed in endometrial cancer. A tumor is considered HER2+ if the immunohistochemistry score is 3+ or if the score is 2+ and confirmed by fluorescence in situ hybridization. Human epidermal growth factor 2 amplification is mostly seen in serous endometrial cancer, yet HER2 can also be amplified in uterine carcinosarcomas and some high-grade endometrioid adenocarcinomas. In 2018, a randomized phase II trial demonstrated that the addition of anti-HER2 therapy (trastuzumab) to carboplatin and paclitaxel in the treatment of HER2+ serous endometrial cancer significantly improved progression-free and overall survival. The phase III trial GY026 is currently being conducted to confirm these results, and randomizes participants with HER2+ endometrial cancer to carboplatin and paclitaxel chemotherapy versus carboplatin, paclitaxel and trastuzumab versus carboplatin, paclitaxel and trastuzumab/pertuzumab. While awaiting these confirmatory results, the National Comprehensive Cancer Network guidelines include the addition of trastuzumab to carboplatin and paclitaxel chemotherapy for stage III–IV HER2+ serous carcinomas or carcinosarcomas. For the patient described above with HER2+ disease, the addition of trastuzumab is the most appropriate treatment addition. Trastuzumab is not used as a single-agent anti-neoplastic therapy for uterine cancer.

Radiation therapy may be offered as a complement to standard chemotherapy in advanced endometrial cancer. Data from PORTEC-3 showed combination radiation therapy and chemotherapy for advanced-stage disease improved progression-free survival, but data from the phase III GOG-258 trial showed no progression-free survival advantage with the addition of radiation therapy to chemotherapy. Radiation therapy can be added to chemotherapy in the form of external beam radiation therapy or, more commonly, vaginal brachytherapy, to help with local control in select cases. External beam radiation therapy alone is not sufficient for node-positive disease.

In the recurrent setting, after treatment with carboplatin, paclitaxel, and trastuzumab, multiple single-agent chemotherapy regimens can be offered. These agents, such as doxorubicin, have response rates of less than 20–30% and are not considered standard of care for first-line treatment.

The postoperative treatment of advanced endometrial cancer consists of systemic platinum-based chemotherapy; however, with a better understanding of the molecular differences of endometrial cancer histologic subtypes, therapy may include additional agents, such as immunotherapies or anti-HER2 therapies. Future trials will determine whether HER2 targeting therapies can be optimized for uterine serous and other subtypes of endometrial cancer.

Bogani G, Ray-Coquard I, Concin N, Ngoi NY, Morice P, Enomoto T, et al. Uterine serous carcinoma. Gynecol Oncol 2021;162:226–34. doi: 10.1016/j.ygyno.2021.04.029

Fader AN, Roque DM, Siegel E, Buza N, Hui P, Abdelghany O, et al. Randomized phase II trial of carboplatin-paclitaxel compared with carboplatin-paclitaxel-trastuzumab in advanced (stage III–IV) or recurrent uterine serous carcinomas that overexpress Her2/Neu (NCT01367002): updated overall survival analysis. Clin Cancer Res 2020;26:3928–35. doi: 10.1158/1078-0432.CCR-20-0953

National Comprehensive Cancer Network. Uterine neoplasms. Version 2.2025. NCCN Clinical Practice Guidelines in Oncology [after login]. NCCN; 2024. Accessed February 26, 2025. https://www.nccn.org/guidelines/guidelines-detail?category=1&id=1473

Oaknin A, Bosse TJ, Creutzberg CL, Giornelli G, Harter P, Joly F, et al. Endometrial cancer: ESMO clinical practice guideline for diagnosis, treatment and follow-up. ESMO Guidelines Committee. Ann Oncol 2022;33:860–77. doi: 10.1016/j.annonc.2022.05.009

Talhouk A, McConechy MK, Leung S, Li-Chang HH, Kwon JS, Melnyk N, et al. A clinically applicable molecular-based classification for endometrial cancer. Br J Cancer 2015;113:299–310. doi: 10.1038/bjc.2015.190

79 Postoperative complications

A 65-year-old woman, postoperative day 13 from an exploratory laparotomy, total abdominal hysterectomy, bilateral salpingo-oophorectomy, and tumor debulking, presents to the emergency department with a 2-day history of increasing intermittent abdominal pain, nausea, and vomiting. Her physical examination is notable for blood pressure of 90/52 mm Hg, heart rate of 123 beats per minute, abdominal distension, and decreased bowel sounds. Her abdominal radiograph is shown in Figure 79-1. The patient is transferred to the intensive care unit, a nasogastric tube is placed, and fluid resuscitation is initiated. Once the patient is stabilized, the best next step in evaluation is

* (A) computed tomography (CT)
(B) Gastrografin challenge
(C) MRI
(D) repeat radiograph
(E) ultrasonography

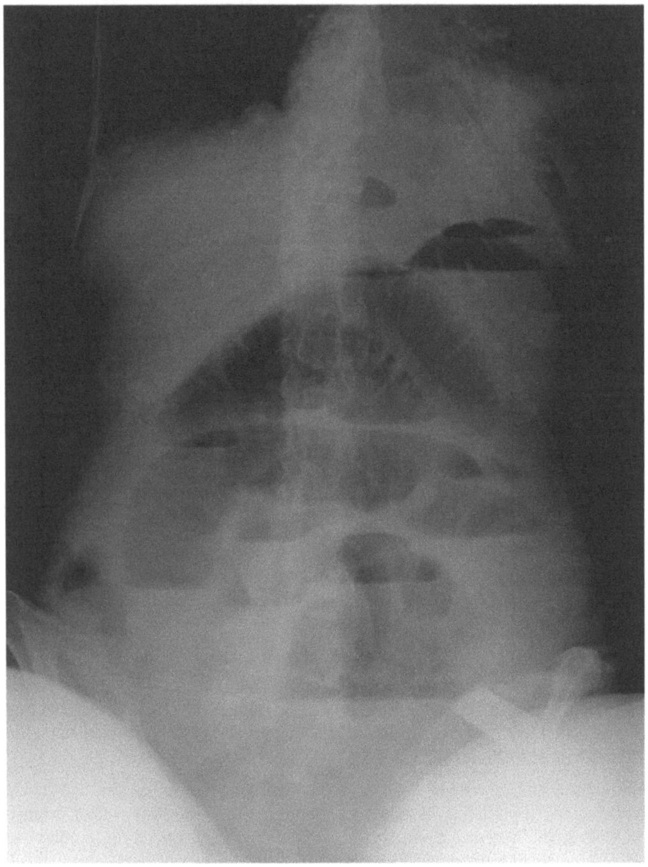

FIGURE 79-1. Abdominal radiograph.

Small bowel obstruction (SBO) is a potential complication after pelvic surgery and can lead to significant postoperative morbidity and mortality. Small bowel obstruction after hysterectomy is reported to be between 0.12% and 2%, depending on the route of surgery. Small bowel obstruction often is classified according to postoperative timing. Early SBO occurs within 30 days of surgery, and late SBO occurs after 30 days. Postoperative adhesions are the most common cause of SBO, and paralytic ileus should be considered as well, particularly with early SBO.

The classical clinical presentation of SBO includes colicky abdominal pain, nausea and vomiting, abdominal distention, and progressive constipation and obstipation. Abdominal pain may be described as crampy, constant, or intermittent and will become more constant if bowel ischemia or perforation develops (Box 79-1). Physical examination will reveal an acutely ill patient with possible signs of sepsis and shock due to dehydration including tachycardia, dry mucous membranes, poor skin turgor, and hypotension. Abdominal examination will show moderate to severe distention, high-pitched or hypoactive active bowel sounds, and tenderness to palpation. Differential diagnosis includes postoperative ileus, necrotic bowel, and acute colonic pseudo-obstruction (acute dilation of the colon in the absence of an anatomic lesion causing obstruction).

Laboratory evaluation for suspected SBO should include evaluation for dehydration and sepsis. Serum creatinine may be increased due to prerenal azotemia. Leukocytosis with leftward shift often is present. Lactate levels may be increased, particularly if intestinal ischemia is impending. Lactate also may be increased in the setting of dehydration accompanying SBO; however, if solely due to dehydration, lactate should improve to normal with fluid resuscitation. Abdominal radiographs, two views if possible, are the preferred initial imaging modality for diagnosis. As in this case, an abdominal X-ray reveals multiple loops of dilated small bowel, air-fluid levels, and trapped air in the "string of beads" sign.

Once SBO has been diagnosed, a nasogastric tube should be placed to decompress the dilated stomach and proximal small bowel loops. Intravenous fluid resuscitation should be initiated. If shock is present, patients may need admission to the intensive care unit for vasopressor therapy and closer monitoring. Serial abdominal examinations should be performed to evaluate for possible signs of bowel ischemia or perforation (Box 79-1). On stabilization, an abdominal CT with use of intravenous contrast and oral Gastrografin contrast should be obtained.

BOX 79-1

Signs of Bowel Ischemia and Perforation

- Fever
- Hypotension
- Increasing leukocytosis
- Increasing abdominal pain, at times out of proportion to examination
- Generalized guarding
- Rebound tenderness

Data from Rami Reddy SR, Cappell MS. A Systematic Review of the Clinical Presentation, Diagnosis, and Treatment of Small Bowel Obstruction. Curr Gastroenterol Rep. 2017 Jun;19(6):28. doi: 10.1007/s11894-017-0566-9

Computed tomography can provide information regarding the etiology of obstruction, the transition point, high- versus low-grade obstruction, and complete versus partial obstruction. In addition, CT is superior in demonstrating signs of bowel necrosis, ischemia, and perforation. Conservative management would not be prudent in individuals with such findings. The patient in this scenario has stabilized with initial measures and should undergo CT for further evaluation.

A Gastrografin challenge test is performed by administering Gastrografin through a nasogastric tube or orally followed by serial abdominal radiographs assessing for progression of contrast throughout the bowel. Gastrografin challenge tests are used as a therapeutic tool in patients with postoperative ileus, adhesive small bowel obstruction and refractory constipation. Although a Gastrografin challenge test may offer some benefit for this patient, it is not the optimal next step in evaluation, because it does not provide essential information on the underlying cause of the obstruction. This is a crucial factor to determine before initiating therapeutic interventions.

Magnetic resonance imaging is more time-consuming and costly than CT. Imaging quality can be more variable with MRI than CT. Computed tomography is preferred to MRI, particularly in the emergent setting, because it can detect perforation more accurately and quickly. Computed tomography can also identify pathology outside of the bowel, such as an ovarian mass in the pelvis, that may be causing symptoms. In contrast, although an abdominal MRI provides a detailed evaluation of the bowel, it may not capture potential pathology beyond the abdomen, such as in the pelvis. Although an MRI of the pelvis also could be obtained, this would be time and cost intensive without much added benefit over CT in evaluation of SBO.

Abdominal ultrasound is an option for patients who cannot undergo CT, such as children and pregnant patients, because it is noninvasive and devoid of radiation exposure. Ultrasonography has an 83% sensitivity and 100% specificity in diagnosing SBO. Ultrasonographic findings suggestive of the need for urgent surgical intervention include free fluid, mural thickness of greater than 4 mm and decreased or absent peristalsis. Ultrasonography has several limitations in evaluating SBO, including operator dependency, limited ability to determine the cause and level of obstruction, and difficulty in assessing complications at the obstruction site. Abdominal ultrasonography would not be the preferred imaging modality for this patient who is able to undergo CT.

A repeat abdominal radiograph can be useful in patients who are unable to undergo CT and when there is concern for worsening obstruction or possible sequelae. In this patient who has been stabilized, an abdominal X-ray would not provide additional clinically meaningful information and would not be the best next step for this scenario.

Small bowel obstruction is a known complication of gynecologic surgery and should remain on the top of the differential diagnosis when individuals present with symptoms and signs suggestive of SBO. Computed tomography is the preferred imaging modality for thoroughly evaluating SBO, because it provides detailed information on the etiology and potential complications, such as bowel ischemia and perforation.

Broek RP, Issa Y, van Santbrink EJ, Bouvy ND, Kruitwagen RF, Jeekel J, et al. Burden of adhesions in abdominal and pelvic surgery: systematic review and met-analysis. BMJ 2013;347:f5588. doi: 10.1136/bmj.f5588

Rami Reddy SR, Cappell MS. A systematic review of the clinical presentation, diagnosis, and treatment of small bowel obstruction. Curr Gastroenterol Rep 2017;19:28–9. doi: 10.1007/s11894-017-0566-9

Sheyn D, Bretschneider CE, Mahajan ST, Ridgeway B, Davenport A, Pollard R. Incidence and risk factors of early postoperative small bowel obstruction in patients undergoing hysterectomy for benign indications. Am J Obstet Gynecol 2019;220:251.e1–9. doi: 10.1016/j.ajog.2018.11.1095

80 Vaginal intraepithelial neoplasia

A 52-year-old patient presents for an annual well-woman examination. She reports having undergone a total hysterectomy at age 40 for management of cervical intraepithelial neoplasia 3. Vaginal cytology reveals high-grade squamous intraepithelial lesion (HSIL) with positive testing for high-risk human papillomavirus (HPV). The best next step is

(A) carbon dioxide laser ablation
(B) partial vaginectomy
(C) repeat cytology in 12 months
(D) topical 5% imiquimod therapy
* (E) vaginal colposcopy

Vaginal intraepithelial neoplasia (VaIN) is a rare entity with an incidence of 0.2–2 per 100,000 women per year. Vaginal intraepithelial neoplasia is a precursor to vaginal cancer with a rate of progression to invasive squamous carcinoma of about 2–7%. Most cases are related to HPV infection. Human papillomavirus 16, 33, and 45 are the genotypes found most commonly in high-grade (VaIN 2/3). Individuals with risk factors for persistent HPV infection, such as smoking, immunosuppression, and history of high-grade cervical dysplasia, are at an increased risk for vaginal precancerous lesions and cancer. Vaginal intraepithelial neoplasia 2/3 is most commonly found in association with previous or current cervical neoplasia. Risk factors for developing high-grade VaIN are listed in Box 80-1.

Most vaginal lesions will be diagnosed with cytology during cervical cancer screening or follow-up for cervical preinvasive or invasive disease in a patient who had a hysterectomy. Possible diagnoses with cytology are low-grade SIL and high-grade SIL. Vaginal atrophy may result in overreading of vaginal cytology. Therefore, histologic confirmation of vaginal neoplasia is necessary before any treatment planning. Colposcopy of the entire vagina is recommended and would be the appropriate next step for this individual. After application of 5% acetic acid, all vaginal walls, folds, and fornices should be completely visualized by rotating the speculum 360 degrees with blades open or dissembling the speculum and evaluating the anterior and posterior vagina independently. On colposcopy, VaIN usually is acetowhite with sharp borders and a granular surface appearance (Fig. 80-1). Occasional punctations are seen, but mosaicism and keratosis are rare. Biopsies should be taken of all lesions for histologic confirmation. The diagnostic criteria for both cytologic HSIL and histologic VaIN are listed in Box 80-2.

Carbon dioxide (CO_2) laser ablation, topical 5% imiquimod, and partial vaginectomy are treatment options for VaIN 2/3 once histologic diagnosis has been confirmed. It would not be appropriate to directly treat cytologic vaginal HSIL without histologic confirmation, given the diagnostic challenges

BOX 80-1

Risk Factors for Development of VaIN

- History of cervical cancer or cervical high-grade dysplasia
- History of hysterectomy for cervical high-grade dysplasia
- Prior radiation therapy for gynecologic malignancy
- Immunosuppression
- Postmenopausal status
- Exposure to diethylstilbestrol (DES)

Reprinted from Kesic V, Carcopino X, Preti M, Vieira-Baptista P, Bevilacqua F, Bornstein J, et al. The European Society of Gynaecological Oncology (ESGO), the International Society for the Study of Vulvovaginal Disease (ISSVD), the European College for the Study of Vulval Disease (ECSVD), and the European Federation for Colposcopy (EFC) consensus statement on the management of vaginal intraepithelial neoplasia. Int J Gynecol Cancer 2023;33:446–61. doi: 10.1136/ijgc-2022-004213

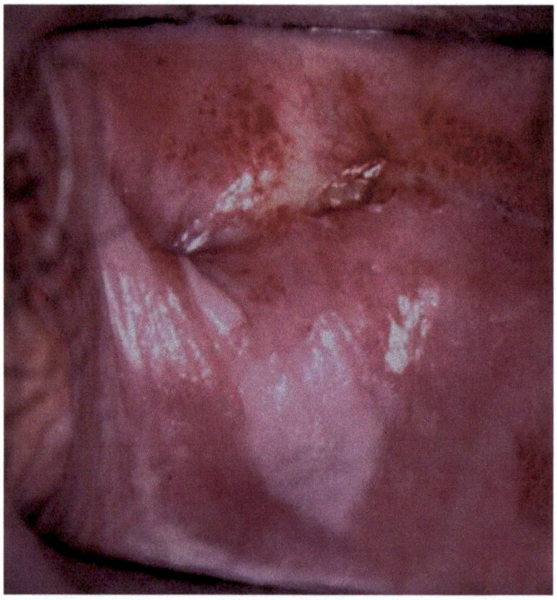

FIGURE 80-1. High-power image with crowded back-to-back glands with nuclear rounding, vesicular nuclei, small nucleoli, and squamous metaplasia. (Courtesy of Dr. Christine Bookhout, Department of Pathology, University of North Carolina.)

BOX 80-2

Diagnostic Criteria for High Grade Vaginal Dysplasia

Cytology

- Term: high-grade squamous intraepithelial lesion (HSIL)
- Diagnostic criteria
  - Nuclear changes: enlargement, irregular shape, hyperchromatic, irregular chromatin without nucleolus
  - High nuclear to cytoplasmic ratio
  - Individual cells or small flat clusters

Histology

- Term: vaginal intraepithelial neoplasia 2/3 or HSIL
- Diagnostic criteria
  - Nuclear changes: enlargement, irregular shape, hyperchromatic, irregular chromatin without nucleolus
  - Abnormal epithelium 2/3 or greater from the basement membrane

Data from World Health Organization. Female genital tumours. WHO classification of tumours. 5th ed. WHO; 2020. Accessed April 22, 2025. https://publications.iarc.fr/Book-And-Report-Series/Who-Classification-Of-Tumours/Female-Genital-Tumours-2020

with vaginal cytology, as mentioned above. In patients with histologically confirmed VaIN 2/3, treatment with partial vaginectomy, CO_2 laser ablation, or topical 5% imiquimod is recommended. Partial vaginectomy involves wide local excision of the involved vagina. Partial vaginectomy has the lowest risk of recurrence and should be considered in solitary lesions; however, applicability is limited as VaIN often is multifocal. Carbon dioxide laser ablation delivers a focused beam of infrared light that is highly absorbed by water within all cells, resulting in vaporization and destruction of cells. The CO_2 laser allows for extremely precise delivery to the target area of VaIN. Ablation to a depth of 1–1.5 mm is sufficient to treat VaIN. CO_2 laser often is used to treat multifocal lesions with limited morbidity. Topical 5% imiquimod is an immune response modifier that stimulates the release of proinflammatory cytokines that stimulate natural killer cells, promote Langerhans cells, and increase effectiveness of T-cell-mediated responses. Vaginal use of topical 5% imiquimod has been shown to be just as effective as CO_2 laser for VaIN 2/3 and often is used for multifocal lesions.

Repeat cytology in 12 months is not an appropriate next step for high-grade cytology. This patient should undergo vaginal colposcopy first with a directed biopsy, allowing for histologic confirmation of diagnosis before treatment planning. Depending on biopsy results and the extent of lesions, any of the treatment modalities discussed above may be considered in management.

Kesic V, Carcopino X, Preti M, Vieira-Baptista P, Bevilacqua F, Bornstein J, et al. The European Society of Gynaecological Oncology (ESGO), the International Society for the Study of Vulvovaginal Disease (ISSVD), the European College for the Study of Vulval Disease (ECSVD), and the European Federation for Colposcopy (EFC) consensus statement on the management of vaginal intraepithelial neoplasia. Int J Gynecol Cancer 2023;33:446–61. doi: 10.1136/ijgc-2022-004213

Perkins RB, Guido RS, Castle PE, Chelmow D, Einstein MH, Garcia F, et al. 2019 ASCCP risk-based management consensus guidelines for abnormal cervical cancer screening tests and cancer precursors. 2019 ASCCP Risk-Based Management Consensus Guidelines Committee [published erratum appears in J Low Genit Tract Dis 2020;24:427]. J Low Genit Tract Dis 2020;24:102–31. doi: 10.1097/LGT.0000000000000525

81 Nutritional intake after surgery

A 55-year-old woman is admitted to the hospital after undergoing optimal cytoreductive surgery for advanced ovarian cancer. Her body mass index is 27, and her past medical history is significant only for hypertension. On postoperative day 2, she develops nausea, an episode of emesis, decreased appetite, and bloating without passage of flatus or a bowel movement. Examination reveals abdominal distension and absent bowel sounds. Intravenous fluids are administered. The best management of her nutritional intake at this time is

(A) a clear liquid diet
* (B) nothing by mouth (NPO)
(C) placement of a feeding tube
(D) total parenteral nutrition (TPN)

This patient is showing signs and symptoms of postoperative ileus. Postoperative ileus is characterized by a delay in gastrointestinal motility after abdominal surgery causing obstipation and abdominal distension. Ileus is relatively common after cytoreductive surgery and is a frequent cause of poor tolerance of enteral diets in the immediate postoperative period. Postoperative ileus is managed expectantly with bowel rest and NPO. To prevent dehydration, intravenous fluids should be initiated. In most patients, postoperative ileus will resolve on its own within 1–3 days. Because of this short duration, an alternative source of nutrition is generally not indicated because patients will be able to return to normal oral intake within a few days. Historically, the use of nasogastric (NG) tubes—a tube inserted into the stomach through the nares—has been used for decompression of the stomach in postoperative ileus; however, contrary to their success in small bowel obstruction, NG tubes have delayed the return of bowel function in some studies. Furthermore, placement of an NG tube can cause discomfort and nasopharyngeal trauma. In patients with recurrent emesis, placement of an NG tube may be warranted to decrease persistent vomiting and resultant risk of aspiration. Placement of a nasogastric tube itself can precipitate an aspiration event, so the potential risks and benefits should be carefully weighed for each patient. For most patients, conservative management with intravenous hydration and NPO without other intervention is the most appropriate management. In making this determination, however, it is important to consider the patient's overall health and preoperative nutritional status.

Because nutritional status relates to wound healing and risks of perioperative complications, it is an important consideration in perioperative patients. Nutritional status is best assessed by history and physical examination with assessment of factors such as BMI, recent weight loss and food intake, gastrointestinal symptoms, and functional capacity. Preoperatively, nutritional status also can be assessed by validated nutritional assessment tools, such as the patient-generated subjective global assessment score (PG-SGA). These factors can identify patients with preoperative malnutrition or those who will be at high risk of malnutrition postoperatively and in whom earlier nutritional interventions might be considered.

Many laboratory values have been used as adjuncts for determination of nutritional status. Historically, serum proteins such as serum albumin and prealbumin have been used as proxy measures of nutritional status and in the diagnosis of malnutrition. However, more recently, the impact of inflammation on the accuracy of these values has refuted their use in the diagnosis of malnutrition. A decrease in albumin and prealbumin values is seen with acute inflammation such as with illness or after surgery. Thus, a decrease in these values does not necessarily reflect malnutrition but rather is the result of the underlying inflammatory response. As such, albumin laboratory values may be used as a component of the nutritional assessment of patients at risk for malnutrition but should not be used in isolation to determine the nutritional status of patients, to diagnose malnutrition, or to determine initiation of parenteral nutrition or follow patients' response to nutritional interventions.

Total parenteral nutrition is nutrition given intravenously. There is a lack of prospective studies comparing the routine use of parenteral nutrition in the immediate postoperative period to conservative management with intravenous fluids and nothing by mouth. Studies have shown the use of parenteral nutrition in selected patients at high risk of malnutrition to be a safe option in patients after cytoreductive surgery. Given the paucity of data to support a benefit, the use of TPN should be limited to patients who are severely malnourished, who have multiple organ failure, or who are not expected to tolerate oral intake for 7–10 days. Historically, TPN has been given exclusively through a central line due to high rates of thrombophlebitis with peripheral administration; however, newer techniques may allow short courses of parenteral nutrition to be given through peripheral venous access, often making peripheral administration of parenteral nutrition the preferred option when TPN is given in the postoperative period. Regardless of the route of administration, TPN is associated with risks such as catheter-related infections, hyperglycemia, cholestasis, and hypertriglyceridemia, among others. These potential risks associated with parenteral nutrition must be considered when deciding to pursue TPN in a postoperative patient with prolonged ileus. The described patient does not have a history that suggests preoperative malnutrition and has a postoperative ileus in the early postoperative period, which is likely to resolve by 7 days postoperatively. Thus, initiation of total parenteral nutrition is not the correct answer for this patient.

The other options provided, including a clear liquid diet and placement of a feeding tube, rely on enteral feeding (nutrition through the gastrointestinal tract). Postoperative ileus signifies decreased bowel motility, and avoiding enteral feeding is warranted. Conservative management with intravenous fluids and nothing by mouth is the most appropriate option for her immediate nutritional management.

Berlana D. Parenteral nutrition overview. Nutrients 2022;14:4480. doi: 10.3390/nu14214480

Evans DC, Corkins MR, Malone A, Miller S, Mogensen KM, Guenter P, et al. The use of visceral proteins as nutrition markers: an ASPEN position paper [published erratum appears in Nutr Clin Pract 2021;36:909]. Nutr Clin Pract 2021;36:22–8. doi: 10.1002/ncp.10588

Khan A, Beaumont A, Laing E, Guerra G, Jain A, Warrier S, et al. Parenteral nutrition after cytoreductive surgery for peritoneal malignancy: should it be administered routinely? Clin Nutr ESPEN 2023;57:487–93. doi: 10.1016/j.clnesp.2023.06.016

82 Back pain

A 54-year-old patient presents with acute onset of fecal incontinence and bilateral lower extremity weakness. She describes progressive lower back pain and a sharp shooting pain down both legs for the last 2 months. She has a history of endometrial cancer treated with chemotherapy 2 years ago and was last seen 6 months ago. Her physical examination is remarkable for point tenderness in the lumbar spine and a score of 3 out of 5 for strength in bilateral lower extremities. Laboratory studies are unremarkable. Magnetic resonance imaging of the lumbar spine is shown in Figure 82-1. You consult with a neurosurgeon and a radiation oncologist and determine that the best next step in treatment is to administer

(A) acetazolamide
* (B) dexamethasone
(C) gabapentin
(D) ketorolac
(E) morphine

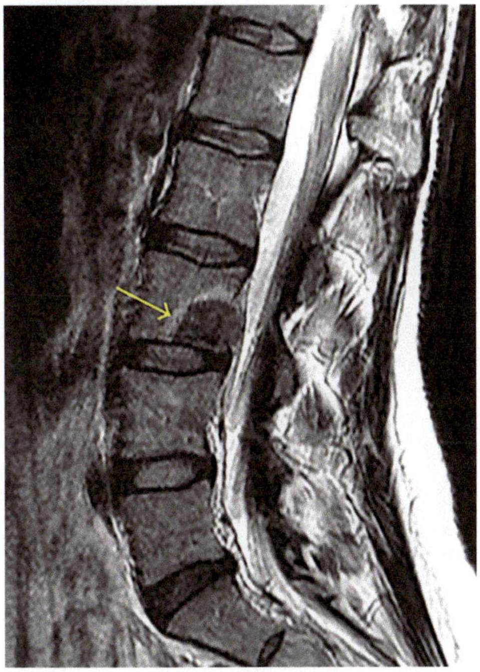

FIGURE 82-1. Magnetic resonance imaging of the lumbar spine. (Reprinted from Shah LM, Salzman KL. Imaging of spinal metastatic disease. Int J Surg Oncol 2011;2011:769753. doi: 10.1155/2011/769753)

Spinal cord compression due to metastatic disease is an uncommon occurrence in gynecologic cancer. Fewer than 2% of cases of gynecologic cancer present with a spinal cord metastasis. The most common presenting symptom is back pain. Motor loss, sensory deficits, and bowel and bladder dysfunction occur later. Spinal cord metastasis requires prompt diagnosis and treatment to prevent loss of neurologic function. The preferred method to diagnose spinal cord compression is imaging with MRI or computed tomography if MRI is contraindicated or not available.

There are several possible treatment options for spinal cord compression, including medical management, surgical resection, and radiotherapy. The initial therapy after diagnosis should focus on decreasing spinal cord edema and preserving neurologic function. Time is the most important factor in the preservation of neurologic function because prolonged nerve compression can cause irreversible neurologic damage. Corticosteroids reduce edema most effectively and quickly. Dexamethasone is the best corticosteroid choice for metastatic disease. Corticosteroids provide pain relief and can delay neurologic decline. In the scenario above, administering corticosteroids is the best next step to rapidly decrease edema and preserve neurologic function.

Opiates and opioids are beneficial for pain management in patients with spinal cord metastases but would not preserve neurologic function. Their use is secondary to corticosteroid administration, and morphine is not the best next option. For neuropathic pain, gabapentin and pregabalin may be useful and often are used for chemotherapy-induced neuropathy, but these drugs have not been studied for efficacy in the setting of spinal cord compression. Ketorolac is a nonsteroid anti-inflammatory drug that provides analgesic effects but also is secondary to corticosteroid administration. Acetazolamide is a diuretic used for reducing ocular edema that has been used to reduce visual symptoms in the setting of choroid metastatic disease. The described patient does not have visual symptoms, and the use of acetazolamide is not indicated.

Surgery for metastatic spinal lesions can play a pivotal role, particularly in the setting of spinal instability, spinal cord compression, or the presence of neurologic defects. Spinal stability is assessed with a scoring system that includes location, pain with movement, lytic versus blastic lesion, spinal alignment, vertebral body collapse, and involvement of vertebral pedicles or facets. Surgery significantly reduces pain and improves neurologic deficits and quality of life long-term; however, surgical intervention follows corticosteroid administration. Surgery takes time to arrange, and during this time, additional nerve function due to compression and edema can be lost without the protection of corticosteroids. Removal of the tumor can lead to spinal instability due to vertebral bone involvement, which may require additional surgical interventions, such as vertebroplasty or kyphoplasty.

Gynecologic cancer with spinal bone metastasis is generally thought to be very radiosensitive, and radiation is a mainstay of treatment for these lesions. Radiation may be administered with or without surgery. In some patients, spinal stability improves after radiation therapy due to bone re-ossification.

The long-term prognosis should be considered when deciding how to manage spinal metastases. Consideration of additional sites of metastatic disease, prior lines of therapy, anticipated response to the next line of therapy, and overall performance status is critical to determining the best management options for these patients.

For the patient described, who presents with symptomatic spinal cord metastasis, administration of corticosteroids is the best next step to minimize edema and preserve as much neurologic function as possible. Other supportive measures can be considered and administered after initiating corticosteroid therapy.

Foerster R, Habermehl D, Bruckner T, Bostel T, Schlampp I, Welzel T, et al. Spinal bone metastases in gynecologic malignancies: a retrospective analysis of stability, prognostic factors and survival. Radiat Oncol 2014;9:194. doi: 10.1186/1748-717X-9-194

Lawton AJ, Lee KA, Cheville AL, Ferrone ML, Rades D, Balboni TA, et al. Assessment and management of patients with metastatic spinal cord compression: a multidisciplinary review. J Clin Oncol 2019;37:61–71. doi: 10.1200/JCO.2018.78.1211

Liu S, Zhou X, Song A, Huo Z, Yao S, Wang Y, et al. Clinical characteristics and prognostic analysis of gynecologic cancer with spinal metastases: a single-center retrospective study. Cancer Manag Res 2020;12:7515–25. doi: 10.2147/CMAR.S268075

Sari R, Camci C, Kutlu R, Totan Y, Sevinc A, Buyukberber S. The efficacy of acetazolamide on visual functions in a patient with choroid metastasis of breast carcinoma. Int J Clin Pract 2001;55:488–90. doi: 10.1111/j.1742-1241.2001.tb11098.x

Tajima Y, Takahashi M, Kawai T, Higashi M, Sano H, Ichimura S, et al. Metastatic intradural extramedullary spinal cord tumor from ovarian cancer: a case report with a literature review. J Spinal Cord Med 2022;45:320–3. doi: 10.1080/10790268.2020.1739380

83 Regional anesthesia

A 54-year-old patient presents for an exploratory laparotomy for ascites, a large pelvic mass, and an increased CA 125 level. She has no allergies and has not had previous surgery. She is concerned about postoperative adverse effects and pain control. The best perioperative pain management strategy is

(A) erector spinae muscle block
* (B) incisional infiltration of bupivacaine
(C) intrathecal morphine injection
(D) thoracic epidural analgesia
(E) transversus abdominis plane (TAP) block

Enhanced Recovery After Surgery (ERAS) guidelines have been in place since 2016, and efforts are ongoing to improve postoperative recovery for gynecologic surgery patients. One of the main concerns for any surgical recovery is pain management. Opioid medications have long been used for pain control; however, concerns about adverse effects, such as nausea, slowed gut motility, sedation, and potential long-term addiction, have created a reluctance to rely on these medications.

Regional anesthesia has evolved during the last 10 years, and its use has alleviated some postoperative issues. Thoracic epidural analgesia has been shown to improve postoperative pain scores; however, it also is associated with postoperative nausea and vomiting, urinary retention, immobility, and, often, significant hypotension requiring fluid boluses or pressors. Intrathecal morphine has been shown to reduce the length of stay for patients post-laparotomy, but it did not result in lower pain scores compared to thoracic epidural analgesia. In addition, it may be associated with late-onset respiratory depression.

Erector spinae plane blocks also have been proposed as regional anesthesia. Although there is limited data in gynecologic surgery, small randomized controlled trials have shown improvement in pain scores over TAP blocks. Transversus abdominis plane blocks have been studied extensively and can help reduce opioid use, but the data on their exact usefulness for gynecologic surgery has been conflicting. Two studies in patients undergoing abdominal hysterectomy showed that in patients not receiving nonsteroidal anti-inflammatory drugs (NSAIDs), TAP was associated with decreased opiate use and shortened length of stay. In patients receiving scheduled NSAIDs, however, the same goals were met. Scheduled NSAID administration was more cost-effective and avoided the potential risks of TAP block placement. In addition, there have been several studies on the administration of TAP blocks, either by a surgeon or an anesthesia provider, as well as under ultrasound or laparoscopic guidance. None of these studies showed a significant improvement in pain scores or recovery over infiltration of the incision with bupivacaine. Transversus abdominis plane block and epidural block have not shown a significant improvement in postoperative recovery when compared with incisional infiltration. Incisional infiltration also has the advantage of being cost-effective and is easily administered with little to no adverse effects. Bupivacaine has been used for incisional infiltration to block the generation and conduction of nerve impulses for up to 8 hours of pain control. At the completion of surgery, 2–3 mL of bupivacaine can be injected in the subcutaneous tissue every 1–2 cm of the incision. Because incisional infiltration can be administered by the surgeon without additional equipment and because it does not cause major adverse effects as epidural does, the advantages of infiltration of the wound are easily seen.

For a patient concerned about postoperative nausea and pain control, such as the one in this scenario, incisional infiltration of bupivacaine is the best option. Thoracic epidural and intrathecal morphine may provide some pain control, but with the risk of major adverse effects, such as hypotension and respiratory depression, neither is the best choice for the described patient. Erector spinae blocks are not readily available, and there is limited data on TAP to support its use in patients undergoing midline laparotomy.

Ackroyd SA, Hernandez E, Roberts ME, Chu C, Rubin S, Mantia-Smaldone G, et al. Postoperative complications of epidural analgesia at hysterectomy for gynecologic malignancies: an analysis of the National Surgical Quality Improvement Program. Int J Gynecol Cancer 2020;30:1203–9. doi: 10.1136/ijgc-2020-001339

Bisch SP, Kooy J, Glaze S, Cameron A, Chu P, Ghatage P, et al. Impact of transversus abdominis plane blocks versus non-steroidal anti-inflammatory on post-operative opioid use in ERAS ovarian cancer surgery. Int J Gynecol Cancer 2019;29:1372–6. doi: 10.1136/ijgc-2019-000724

Black KA, Nelson G, Goucher N, Foley J, Pin S, Chong M, Ghosh S, Bisch SP. Effect of transversus abdominis plane block on postoperative outcomes in gynecologic oncology patients managed on an Enhanced Recovery After Surgery pathway. Gynecol Oncol. 2023 Nov;178:1-7. doi: 10.1016/j.ygyno.2023.09.003. Epub 2023 Sep 18. PMID: 37729808.

Nelson G, Fotopoulou C, Taylor J, Glaser G, Bakkum-Gamez J, Meyer LA, et al. Enhanced recovery after surgery (ERAS®) society guidelines for gynecologic oncology: addressing implementation challenges 2023 update. Gynecol Oncol 2023;173:58–67. doi: 10.1016/j.ygyno.2023.04.009

Perioperative pathways: enhanced recovery after surgery. ACOG Committee Opinion No. 750. American College of Obstetricians and Gynecologists [published errata appear in Obstet Gynecol 2019;133:1288; Obstet Gynecol 2019;134:1121]. Obstet Gynecol 2018;132:e120–30. doi: 10.1097/AOG.0000000000002818

Warner M, Yeap YL, Rigueiro G, Zhang P, Kasper K. Erector spinae plane block versus transversus abdominis plane block in laparoscopic hysterectomy. Pain Manag 2022;12:907–16. doi: 10.2217/pmt-2022-0037

84 Vulvar cancer lymph node evaluation

A 68-year-old with a history of lichen sclerosus presents to the clinic with worsening vulvar pruritus. On examination, there is a 1-cm lesion on the posterior left vulva crossing the midline (Fig. 84-1). A biopsy is performed and confirms invasive squamous cell carcinoma of the vulva with 1.5 mm of invasion. She is referred to a high-volume regional cancer center for disease management. Inguinal lymph nodes are normal to palpation bilaterally, and a radical vulvectomy is recommended. At the time of that procedure, the best recommendation regarding the inguinal-femoral lymph nodes is

(A) bilateral inguinal-femoral lymphadenectomy
* (B) bilateral sentinel lymph node biopsy
(C) ipsilateral inguinal-femoral lymphadenectomy
(D) ipsilateral sentinel lymph node biopsy
(E) no lymph node dissection

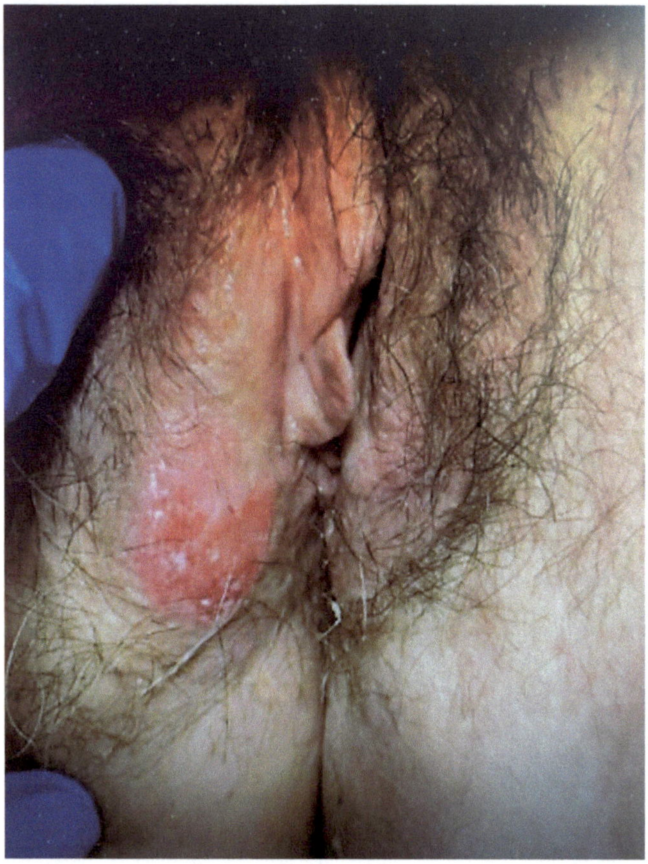

FIGURE 84-1. Vulvar lesion.

Vulvar cancer is relatively rare and accounts for fewer than 1% of cancer diagnoses in women in the United States (Fig. 84-1). The prognosis for vulvar cancer is generally favorable; however, lymph node involvement is a significant prognostic factor. It also is critical in planning appropriate therapy. Assessment of the local lymph nodes in at-risk patients is essential. When a vulvar cancer tumor is greater than 2 cm in diameter or has a depth of stromal invasion of greater than 1 mm, there is a reported 10% risk of lymph node involvement. Patients with tumors meeting these criteria require lymph node assessment to make appropriate treatment recommendations.

Lymphatic drainage of the vulva follows a predictable pattern from the vulva to the inguinal-femoral lymph nodes, making these the lymph nodes at the highest risk of metastasis. However, inguinal-femoral lymphadenectomy carries a high risk of morbidity, including postoperative infection and lymphedema. Studies of vulvar cancer have shown that sentinel lymph node mapping and biopsy are a reliable substitute for a full inguinal-femoral lymphadenectomy to determine whether cancer has spread to the lymph nodes when specific criteria are met. The sentinel lymph node is the first lymph node to which a tumor drains, making it the lymph node at the highest risk of containing metastatic disease. In a sentinel lymph node biopsy, the sentinel lymph node is identified and removed so that it can be examined to determine whether the cancer has spread to the lymph nodes.

The procedure for sentinel lymph node biopsy of vulvar cancer involves the intradermal injection of a radioactive tracer, such as technetium-99, at the tumor border nearest the groin. If tumors cross the midline, both sides of the tumor are injected. Commonly, imaging to identify accumulation of the tracer within the lymphatic system is then performed. Just before the sentinel lymph node biopsy, blue dye is injected in the same fashion at the border of the tumor and adjacent skin. During the sentinel lymph node biopsy, a gamma probe, which can detect technetium-99, is used to help identify the sentinel lymph node within the inguinal-femoral lymph node basin. The blue dye allows for visual identification of the sentinel lymph node within the groin, and the combination of a radiotracer and dye has been shown to have the highest detection rates. For this reason, the combination is the preferred method for sentinel lymph node biopsy. In any patient in whom a sentinel lymph node is not identified, a full inguinal-femoral lymphadenectomy should be performed on the tumor's side. Because there is a learning curve for performing sentinel lymph node mapping and biopsy, this technique should be performed by a high-volume surgeon experienced in this procedure.

The Gynecologic Oncology Group (GOG) 173 study evaluated sentinel lymph node biopsy in patients who had vulvar tumors measuring 2–6 cm in diameter with invasion of at least 1 mm and clinically negative nodes. Patients underwent sentinel lymph node biopsy using the process described above. After the sentinel lymph node was removed, a full inguinal-femoral lymphadenectomy was performed. In those patients with a tumor measuring 2 cm to less than 4 cm, the sensitivity of the sentinel lymph node to detect lymphatic metastasis was 92%. The false-negative rate was 2%. Tumors measuring 4 cm or greater had a substantially higher false-negative rate of 7.4%; therefore, sentinel lymph node biopsy is not recommended for tumors 4 cm or larger.

Building upon this information, the Groningen International Study on Sentinel Nodes in Vulvar Cancer (GROINSS-V) I examined outcomes after sentinel lymph node biopsy in patients who had vulvar tumors measuring less than 4.0 cm. When the sentinel lymph node(s) were negative for metastatic disease, full inguinal-femoral lymphadenectomy was omitted. This study design allowed the comparison of morbidity between patients who only underwent sentinel lymph node biopsy and those who had a full inguinal-femoral lymphadenectomy. Short-term morbidity, such as wound breakdown (11.7% versus 34.0%) and cellulitis (4.5% versus 21.3%), was significantly lower in the group who underwent sentinel lymph node biopsy compared with those who underwent full lymphadenectomy. Long-term lymphedema risk was also significantly decreased (1.9% versus 25.2%) with sentinel lymph node biopsy.

Based on these data, sentinel lymph node biopsy is the preferred method of lymph node assessment in patients who have a unifocal tumor (depicted in Fig. 84-1) that is less than 4 cm in diameter with clinically negative lymph nodes. For *lateralized vulvar tumors* (defined variably in the literature as greater than 1–2 cm from the midline), unilateral lymph node dissection is appropriate because the risk of contralateral lymph node metastasis is low. For tumors involving the midline, bilateral lymph node assessment should be performed. Tumors within 1–2 cm of midline, termed *lateral ambiguous* or *near midline*, historically have been treated as midline lesions; however, data regarding the management of these tumors are limited. An ancillary analysis of the aforementioned GOG 173 study revealed that in lesions less than 2 cm from the midline but not involving the midline, there were no contralateral positive lymph nodes if preoperative lymphoscintigraphy showed only unilateral drainage. More recently, the GROINSS-V II study allowed unilateral sentinel lymph node biopsy for tumors less than 1 cm from midline but not involving the midline if lymphoscintigraphy showed only unilateral drainage; thus, in lateral ambiguous tumors, ipsilateral lymph node evaluation alone can be considered if preoperative lymphoscintigraphy demonstrates only ipsilateral drainage.

In the scenario above, the patient's vulvar cancer has a depth of invasion of more than 1 mm, and lymph node evaluation should be performed. Foregoing lymph node dissection is not correct. Removal of only the primary tumor is reserved for tumors with a depth of invasion 1 mm or less that also are 2 cm or less in size. Because the tumor crosses the midline, lymphatic drainage from the tumor could go to either groin, and bilateral nodal assessment is indicated, making both of the choices with only ipsilateral nodal evaluation incorrect due to the risk of missing metastatic disease in the contralateral lymph nodes.

This patient is being treated at a high-volume center, with surgeons experienced in performing sentinel lymph node biopsy will be available. For the patient described above, bilateral sentinel lymph node biopsy is the best procedure because it has the potential to spare her the morbidity of a full inguinal-femoral lymphadenectomy. This is the preferred approach for lymph node evaluation at the time of her vulvar procedure.

Coleman RL, Ali S, Levenback CF, Gold MA, Fowler JM, Judson PL, et al. Is bilateral lymphadenectomy for midline squamous carcinoma of the vulva always necessary? An analysis from Gynecologic Oncology Group (GOG) 173. Gynecol Oncol 2013;128:155–9. doi: 10.1016/j.ygyno.2012.11.034

Levenback CF, Ali S, Coleman RL, Gold MA, Fowler JM, Judson PL, et al. Lymphatic mapping and sentinel lymph node biopsy in women with squamous cell carcinoma of the vulva: a gynecologic oncology group study. J Clin Oncol 2012;30:3786–91. doi: 10.1200/JCO.2011.41.2528

National Comprehensive Cancer Network. Vulvar cancer. Version 4.2024. NCCN Clinical Practice Guidelines in Oncology [after login]. NCCN; 2024. Accessed January 22, 2025. https://www.nccn.org/guidelines/guidelines-detail?category=1&id=1476

Van der Zee AG, Oonk MH, De Hullu JA, Ansink AC, Vergote I, Verheijen RH, et al. Sentinel node dissection is safe in the treatment of early-stage vulvar cancer. J Clin Oncol 2008;26:884–9. doi: 10.1200/JCO.2007.14.0566

85 Hypoxia

A 72-year-old woman with platinum-resistant ovarian cancer presents with shortness of breath. Her physical examination reveals decreased breath sounds in the right lung. Her oxygen saturation is 94% at rest. Her chest X-ray is shown in Figure 85-1. The best next step to manage this condition is to

(A) administer antibiotics
(B) administer diuretics
(C) perform pleurodesis
* (D) perform thoracentesis
(E) provide oxygen supplementation

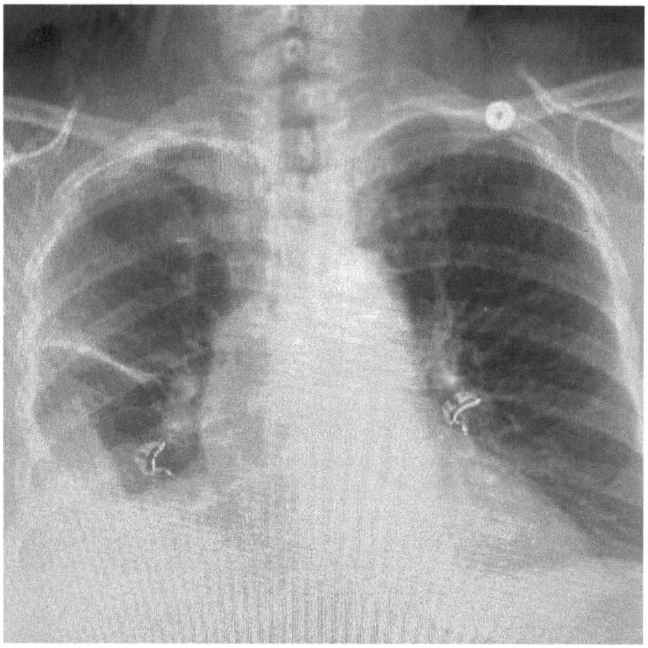

FIGURE 85-1. Patient's chest X-ray with blunting of the costophrenic angle with dependent opacity.

Malignant pleural effusion is a buildup of fluid in the pleural space due to malignancy. Malignant pleural effusions occur in up to 15% of patients with cancer. Most malignant pleural effusions are exudative and unilateral, although bilateral effusions can be seen. Malignant effusions develop from an imbalance in the production and absorption of pleural fluid. Increased permeability of the pleural and tumor vessels due to malignancy causes increased fluid production while impaired lymphatic flow and pleural-based cancer impede outflow. The most common symptoms of pleural effusion are shortness of breath and cough. A physical examination revealing decreased breath sounds at the lung base and dullness to percussion, in addition to imaging, can help identify a malignant effusion. A chest radiograph can detect an effusion of 200 mL or greater and is usually adequate for diagnosis. Computed tomography may provide further information about the pleural cavity and disease burden.

The treatment goals are palliation of symptoms and improvement in patient quality of life. In a patient presenting with dyspnea and a new pleural effusion, the standard first-line treatment is aspiration with thoracentesis to relieve symptoms and facilitate cytologic evaluation; therefore, thoracentesis is the best next step for the patient in the scenario above. Ultrasound guidance can be used for the procedure but is not required for large effusions when lung percussion can be performed. The patient is seated with a tabletop or pillow used to help them bend forward to expand the intercostal spaces. The location of needle insertion is identified with ultrasonography or percussion. After administration of local anesthesia, a needle is gently inserted into the pleural space while aspirating a syringe in the mid-scapular line until fluid is withdrawn. After pleural entry, fluid aspiration can be performed. Active aspiration and gravity drainage have been shown to be similar in procedural risk with lower procedural time with active aspiration. There is a higher risk of recollection of fluid after aspiration of more than 1.5 L.

Antibiotics are appropriate in the treatment of pneumonia and are not the best next step for this patient with a pleural effusion without evidence of infection. Pneumonia typically presents with fever, cough, muscle pain, and weakness. Classic chest X-ray findings for pneumonia include patchy airway infiltrates. Although parapneumonic effusion could present with a unilateral effusion, signs of infection were not present in the described patient, and malignant pleural effusion is more likely. Gram stain and culture of thoracentesis fluid, as well as obtaining a fluid glucose level and cytology, can distinguish a malignant effusion from a parapneumonic effusion.

Diuretics are appropriate for the treatment of fluid overload. Fluid overload has classic X-ray findings of increased vascular markings, peribronchial cuffing, thickening of the interlobular septa, and interstitial edema. It likely includes bilateral effusions as opposed to the unilateral effusion seen in the described patient. Additional clinical signs of fluid overload include lower extremity swelling and weight gain, which are not described in this patient. Diuretics are not the best next step in the treatment of this patient's shortness of breath.

Supplemental oxygen is used in patients with oxygen saturation less than 90%. This patient's oxygen saturation is greater than 90%, and providing supplemental oxygen is not the best next step. Rather, drainage of the effusion will provide symptomatic relief and improve oxygenation.

Fluid reaccumulation after thoracentesis is common until disease control has been obtained. In patients with recurrent malignant pleural effusions, chemical pleurodesis or an indwelling pleural catheter can be considered. *Pleurodesis* is obliteration of the pleural space through the apposition of the parietal and visceral pleura with a sclerosing agent. Multiple sclerosing agents are available, but currently talc is the most used and most cost effective. Antibiotics, bacterial agents, and silver nitrate also have been studied as sclerosing agents. Success rates for this procedure in preventing reaccumulation range from 70% to 90%. Another option for recurrent effusion is placement of indwelling pleural catheters, which can be placed percutaneously and allow for intermittent drainage while also causing some pleural space obliteration. There is no evidence to indicate the superiority of pleurodesis or indwelling catheters, and each patient should be evaluated on a case-by-case basis. The patient described above is not experiencing recurrent pleural effusions at this time, and pleurodesis would not be the best next step in treatment.

Ferreiro L, Suárez-Antelo J, Álvarez-Dobaño JM, Toubes ME, Riveiro V, Valdés L. Malignant pleural effusion: diagnosis and management. Can Respir J 2020;2020:2950751. doi: 10.1155/2020/2950751

Gayen S. Malignant pleural effusion: presentation, diagnosis, and management. Am J Med 2022;135:1188–92. doi: 10.1016/j.amjmed.2022.04.017

Lentz RJ, Shojaee S, Grosu HB, Rickman OB, Roller L, Pannu JK, et al. The impact of gravity vs suction-driven therapeutic thoracentesis on pressure-related complications: the GRAVITAS multicenter randomized controlled trial. Interventional Pulmonary Outcomes Group. Chest 2020;157:702–11. doi: 10.1016/j.chest.2019.10.025

86 Ovarian cancer

A 71-year-old woman presents for evaluation of abdominal distention, bloating, and early satiety. Abdomen and pelvic computed tomography reveal a left ovarian mass invading the rectosigmoid, large-volume ascites, and a tumor replacing the omentum and involving the splenic hilum and the small bowel mesentery. Her serum CA 125 concentration is 6,500 IU/mL. A biopsy of the omental mass confirms high-grade serous cancer consistent with a gynecologic primary. You recommend neoadjuvant platinum-based chemotherapy. The disease factor that best predicts the inability of complete primary tumor resection is

(A) ascites
(B) CA 125 concentration
* (C) mesenteric involvement
(D) rectosigmoid involvement
(E) splenic hilum involvement

Epithelial ovarian cancer is the most common cause of death for women with a gynecologic malignancy and ranks fifth as the leading cause of cancer-related death in women in the United States. Effective primary screening for successful detection of early-stage tumors still is lacking, and, as a result, an estimated 75–80% of patients present with advanced-stage (ie, International Federation of Gynecology and Obstetrics [FIGO] stage III and stage IV) disease (Appendix H). The mainstay of primary treatment for patients with advanced stage disease is a combination of surgical primary resection and platinum-based adjuvant therapy or neoadjuvant chemotherapy with interval cytoreduction.

The amount of residual disease left after primary debulking surgery is inversely correlated to survival. Although the definition of optimal surgical cytoreduction has changed over time, complete resection to no gross residual disease, rather than 1 cm or less, is preferred. Primary surgical debulking is recommended for women who are deemed medically fit and in whom complete cytoreduction (ie, no residual visible disease present) or optimal cytoreduction (ie, 1 cm or less residual disease) can be achieved. In a 2011 review of 11 retrospective studies, optimal debulking (ie, less than 1 cm) resulted in significant improvements in overall survival (hazard ratio [HR] 1.36; 95% CI, 1.10–1.68) when compared with suboptimal cytoreduction (1 cm or more). A greater improvement in overall survival was seen in patients undergoing complete tumor resection to no gross residual disease compared with those who had an optimal cytoreductive procedure (HR 2.20; 95% CI, 1.90–2.54).

Neoadjuvant chemotherapy is an appropriate alternative for women who are not good candidates for primary surgery or when tumor extension is likely to result in suboptimal primary debulking. Studies have aimed at defining patient-related or tumor-related features that may identify patients best suited for neoadjuvant chemotherapy. In an exploratory analysis released by the European Organization and Research for the Treatment of Cancer, biomarkers, including the Eastern Cooperative Oncology Group performance status, tumor grade, histology, pretreatment serum CA 125 concentration, ascites, and the presence of omental disease were not predictive of 5-year overall survival by modality of treatment. Similarly, tumor involvement of the splenic hilum or rectosigmoid do not predict tumor resectability. Although the described patient's biomarkers indicate extensive disease, they do not necessarily indicate lower tumor resectability. In addition to patient history and tumor-related factors, the feasibility of complete cytoreduction also depends on the surgeon's expertise and available institutional infrastructure.

Several studies have evaluated the role of diagnostic laparoscopy in assessing the likely success of optimal primary surgical resection. In a study of 113 women with a preoperative clinical or radiologic diagnosis (or both) of advanced stage ovarian cancer (International Federation of Gynecology and Obstetrics [FIGO] stage III and stage IV), diagnostic laparoscopy detected features such as omental cake, extensive carcinomatosis, mesenteric involvement, stomach or bowel infiltration, and splenic or hepatic superficial metastasis. Given this capability, the diagnostic laparoscopy is an accurate predictor of optimal resectability. Most experts agree that the following tumor factors are predictive of lack of resectability at the time of primary surgery:

- small bowel mesentery
- duodenum or pancreas
- the hepatoduodenal ligament, celiac trunk, or behind the porta hepatis
- liver parenchyma

Of the described patient's clinical findings, the small bowel mesentery found on computed tomography indicates the highest prediction of primary tumor resectability.

A European Organization for the Research and Treatment of Cancer trial included 670 women with FIGO stage IIIC or stage IV epithelial ovarian cancer. The women were randomized to either primary debulking surgery after six cycles of platinum-based chemotherapy or to neoadjuvant chemotherapy with carboplatin and paclitaxel for three cycles followed by interval surgical cytoreduction and adjuvant chemotherapy. Neoadjuvant chemotherapy was associated with a lower rate of complications, including fewer postoperative deaths, infections, hemorrhage, and thrombotic events. A higher rate of optimal cytoreduction (ie, less than 1 cm) also was seen in the neoadjuvant chemotherapy group (81%), compared with the primary debulking one (42%). Overall and progression-free survival rates were similar in the two groups (12 months in each arm; HR 1.01; 95% CI, 0.86–1.17; and 29 versus 30 months, HR 0.98; 95% CI, 0.82–1.18, respectively). Other studies have demonstrated similar findings. Despite lower complication rates reported with neoadjuvant chemotherapy, evidence showing that neoadjuvant chemotherapy improves overall survival compared with primary debulking surgery is lacking. Therefore, neoadjuvant chemotherapy is preferred in high-risk patients who cannot undergo debulking surgery or in whom optimal disease resection is unlikely.

Elattar A, Bryant A, Winter-Roach BA, Hatem M, Naik R. Optimal primary surgical treatment for advanced epithelial ovarian cancer. Cochrane Database of Systematic Reviews 2011, Issue 8. Art. No.: CD007565. doi: 10.1002/14651858.CD007565.pub2

Fagotti A, Ferrandina G, Fanfani F, Garganese G, Vizzielli G, Carone V, et al. Prospective validation of a laparoscopic predictive model for optimal cytoreduction in advanced ovarian carcinoma. Am J Obstet Gynecol 2008;199:642.e1–6. doi: 10.1016/j.ajog.2008.06.052

Kehoe S, Hook J, Nankivell M, Jayson GC, Kitchener H, Lopes T, et al. Primary chemotherapy versus primary surgery for newly diagnosed advanced ovarian cancer (CHORUS): an open-label, randomised, controlled, non-inferiority trial. Lancet 2015;386:249–57. doi: 10.1016/S0140-6736(14)62223-6

van Meurs HS, Tajik P, Hof MH, Vergote I, Kenter GG, Mol BW, et al. Which patients benefit most from primary surgery or neoadjuvant chemotherapy in stage IIIC or IV ovarian cancer? An exploratory analysis of the European Organisation for Research and Treatment of Cancer 55971 randomised trial. Eur J Cancer 2013;49:3191–201. doi: 10.1016/j.ejca.2013.06.013

Vergote I, Trope CG, Amant F, Kristensen GB, Ehlen T, Johnson N, et al. Neoadjuvant chemotherapy or primary surgery in stage IIIC or IV ovarian cancer. European Organization for Research and Treatment of Cancer-Gynaecological Cancer Group, NCIC Clinical Trials Group. N Engl J Med 2010;363:943–53. doi: 10.1056/NEJMoa0908806

87 Malignant ascites

A 58-year-old woman with a history of ovarian cancer presents for a surveillance visit with concerns of abdominal swelling, nausea, and bloating. Her last chemotherapy cycle with platinum and taxane was completed 4 months ago. Her examination is notable for a distended abdomen with a fluid wave. Computed tomography of her abdomen and pelvis is consistent with recurrence, revealing large-volume ascites and peritoneal carcinomatosis. In addition to taxol and carboplatin, the most effective therapeutic agent to improve her symptoms is

(A) acetazolamide
(B) albumin
* (C) bevacizumab
(D) furosemide
(E) spironolactone

The development of malignant ascites is common in ovarian cancer in the primary and recurrent settings. Ascites can cause a significant decrease in quality of life for the patient. Ascites can cause symptoms such as shortness of breath, abdominal discomfort, nausea, and vomiting, which may impair some patients' ability to perform activities of daily living.

Malignant ascites is thought to accumulate because of an increase in the production of peritoneal fluid and obstruction of outflow. Peritoneal fluid is normally produced by capillary membranes and reabsorbed through the lymphatic channels. Tumor obstructs this normal pathway, preventing reabsorption. There also is increased vascular permeability due to inflammation and vasodilation mediators and tumor production of vascular endothelial growth factor (VEGF). Management of symptomatic ascites should include preventing and removing excess fluid accumulation.

Debulking surgery, particularly to no residual disease, will significantly reduce ascites, but systemic therapy is generally needed to prevent reaccumulation. In patients who receive neoadjuvant chemotherapy, a reduction in ascites is typically seen within the first few weeks. For recurrent disease or those in whom surgery is not feasible, systemic therapy is the best option. The patient may also need paracentesis for mechanical drainage of the ascites while waiting for the effect of medical therapy or as best supportive care when systemic therapy is no longer being administered. Paracentesis is most commonly performed under ultrasound guidance with a one-time abdominal puncture. Most studies suggest that removal of up to 5 L of ascites in a single paracentesis can be done with minimal risk of hypotension. This may need to be repeated serially, especially in the recurrent setting when the tumor may be more resistant to therapy.

In patients with a need for serial paracenteses, peritoneal catheter placement may be an option. This is an implanted tunneled catheter that can be used for repeated drainage outside of the hospital or clinic and may be a significant method of palliation for patients enrolled in hospice care. Peritoneovenous shunts also have been evaluated and can be successful in removing the ascites but have higher rates of complications such as pulmonary edema and embolization compared to tunneled catheters.

Although mechanical options are used to drain the ascites, prevention or treatment of the cause is achieved with medical therapy. Some patients will also develop loculated ascites, which makes drainage a challenge or not possible. Diuretics have been used in nongynecologic malignancies with some success. Spironolactone is a mineralocorticoid receptor antagonist and functions as a diuretic to promote excretion of water and sodium. Furosemide is a loop diuretic that promotes water excretion by inhibiting reabsorption in the proximal and distal tubules of the nephrons. Both of these drugs can be used to reduce edema but have little efficacy in the setting of malignant ascites. Acetazolamide is a carbonic anhydrase inhibitor diuretic used for reducing ocular edema and has been used to reduce visual symptoms in the setting of choroid metastatic disease.

Albumin may be given to patients with liver cirrhosis who undergo paracentesis. Albumin increases the colloid pressure of the blood, which can help prevent reaccumulation of ascites by decreasing fluid leakage out of the blood vessels. A systematic review and meta-analysis in patients with cirrhosis undergoing paracentesis found that there was a significant reduction in the risk of circulatory dysfunction when patients were given albumin. In the setting of spontaneous bacterial peritonitis, albumin administration significantly reduced mortality. This does not hold true for patients with ovarian cancer. Giving albumin after paracentesis may increase colloid pressure, but it does not significantly decrease reaccumulation or improve gastrointestinal symptoms in the malignant setting.

Systemic therapy is the primary therapeutic method to prevent reaccumulation of ascites. Bevacizumab is a monoclonal antibody that inhibits the binding of normal VEGF ligand to its receptor and consequently inhibits angiogenesis and tumor proliferation, which play a role in the development of malignant ascites. In the primary setting, bevacizumab was added to combination platinum and taxane chemotherapy in two large, randomized control trials (ICON7 and GOG 218).

Although these trials showed improvements in progression-free survival, no survival benefit was seen in oxygen saturation for optimally debulked stage III patients. In a subset of patients at higher risk of progression, including those who were stage IV or inoperable stage III, or those who were suboptimally debulked, oxygen saturation was improved with the addition of bevacizumab in ICON 7. The GOG 218 study was not able to validate this finding, but there was a trend toward improved survival in patients who had stage IV disease. Bevacizumab in the recurrent setting also has been studied in GOG 213 in combination with a surgical arm to evaluate secondary debulking, the OCEANS trial for patients with platinum-sensitive disease, and in the AURELIA trial for patients with platinum-resistant disease. The AURELIA trial evaluated quality of life and found that patients who received bevacizumab had improved abdominal and gastrointestinal (GI) symptoms versus those who did not. Although there was no survival advantage, the number of paracenteses needed decreased and GI symptoms improved. In total, these studies indicate that bevacizumab may play a role in the reduction of ascites and improvement in quality of life.

The patient in this scenario has platinum-resistant disease, given that her last chemotherapy was 4 months ago (less than 6 months ago). Acetazolamide, spironolactone, and furosemide have limited effects on ascites for ovarian cancer, and none of these is the best next option for this patient. Albumin will not improve her GI symptoms.

Bevacizumab is the best therapy because it is a VEGF inhibitor and has been shown to improve quality of life in patients with GI symptoms stemming from malignant ascites and recurrent ovarian cancer.

Malayev Y, Levene R, Gonzalez F. Palliative chemotherapy for malignant ascites secondary to ovarian cancer. Am J Hosp Palliat Care 2012;29:515–21. doi: 10.1177/1049909111434044

Meyer L, Suidan R, Sun C, Westin S, Coleman RL, Mills GB. The management of malignant ascites and impact on quality of life outcomes in women with ovarian cancer. Expert Rev Qual Life Cancer Care 2016;1:231–8. doi: 10.1080/23809000.2016.1185369

National Comprehensive Cancer Network. Ovarian cancer/fallopian tube cancer/primary peritoneal cancer. Version 3.2024. NCCN Clinical Practice Guidelines in Oncology [after login]. NCCN; 2024. Accessed January 22, 2025. https://www.nccn.org/guidelines/guidelines-detail?category=1&id=1453

Quan Q, Zhou S, Liu Y, Yin W, Liao Q, Ren S, et al. Relationship between ascites volume and clinical outcomes in epithelial ovarian cancer. J Obstet Gynaecol Res 2021;47:1527–35. doi: 10.1111/jog.14682

Rickard BP, Conrad C, Sorrin AJ, Ruhi MK, Reader JC, Huang SA, et al. Malignant ascites in ovarian cancer: cellular, acellular, and biophysical determinants of molecular characteristics and therapy response. Cancer (Basel) 2021;13:4318. doi: 10.3390/cancer13174318. doi: 10.3390/cancer13174318

88 Postoperative fever

A 49-year-old woman presents to the emergency department 5 days after an uncomplicated total laparoscopic hysterectomy and bilateral salpingo-oophorectomy. She reports 2 days of fever, diffuse abdominal pain, and generalized malaise. Her medical history includes obesity, hypertension, and type 2 diabetes mellitus. On examination, her vital signs include a temperature of 38.8 °C (101.9 °F), a blood pressure of 91/47 mm Hg, a heart rate of 123 beats per minute, a respiratory rate of 18 breaths per minute, and oxygen saturation 95% on room air. She appears uncomfortable and has diffuse abdominal tenderness. A genitourinary examination demonstrates purulent drainage from the vaginal cuff and a fluctuant mass palpable superior to the vaginal cuff. Laboratory values are shown in Table 88-1. In addition to starting antibiotics, the best next step is

(A) computed tomography
* (B) fluid resuscitation
(C) subcutaneous insulin
(D) surgical exploration
(E) vasopressors

TABLE 88-1. The Described Patient's Laboratory Study Results

TEST	RESULT
White blood cell count	18,000 micrograms/L
Hemoglobin	12.3 g/dL
Platelets	216,000/microliter
Glucose	237 mg/dL
Creatinine	1.1 mg/dL
Lactate	1.7 mmol/L

This patient presents with sepsis likely due to a vaginal cuff abscess after hysterectomy. Sepsis results from an infectious process causing a dysregulated host response, resulting in end organ dysfunction. Prompt recognition and intervention are crucial to limiting morbidity and mortality. Sepsis can be life threatening and is a leading cause of mortality worldwide. Guidelines recommend a standardized sepsis bundle to aid in early diagnosis and intervention (Box 88-1).

Multiple screening tools for sepsis exist and vary in their sensitivity and specificity. None of these tools has demonstrated

BOX 88-1

Surviving Sepsis Campaign

Hour-1 Bundle: Initial Resuscitation for Sepsis and Septic Shock

1. Measure lactate level.*
2. Obtain blood cultures before administering antibiotics.
3. Administer broad-spectrum antibiotics.
4. Begin rapid administration of 30 mL/kg crystalloid for hypotension or lactate 4 or more mmol/L.
5. Apply vasopressors if hypotensive during or after fluid resuscitation to maintain a mean arterial pressure 65 or more mm Hg.

*Remeasure lactate if initial lactate increased (more than 2 mmol/L).

Reprinted from Surviving Sepsis Campaign. Hour-1 bundle: initial resuscitation for sepsis and septic shock. Society of Critical Care Medicine; 2019. Accessed August 14, 2025. https://sccm.org/SCCM/media/SCCM/PDFs/Surviving-Sepsis-Campaign-Hour-1-Bundle.pdf.

superiority. Signs or symptoms of sepsis in patients with suspected or confirmed infection that should prompt further evaluation and initiation of the sepsis protocol include temperature higher than 38 °C (100 °F) or lower than 35 °C (95 °F), increased respiratory rate, hypotension, tachycardia, hypoxia, and altered mental status. Initial intervention bundles typically include, in addition to early recognition of sepsis, immediate bloodwork, including lactate and blood cultures; initiation of antibiotics; and initiation of fluid resuscitation. Incorporation of sepsis bundles into standard practice in the hospital setting is associated with decreased mortality.

Prompt initiation of antibiotics is crucial to aid in treating the underlying disease process. In addition, those with hypotension or evidence of hypoperfusion, such as this patient, should receive fluid resuscitation with crystalloid at a minimum of 30 mL/kg of ideal body weight. There is no clear benefit of using colloid solution for initial resuscitation compared with crystalloid solution, the latter of which is readily available and inexpensive. Therefore, crystalloid solution is recommended. This early resuscitation is associated with decreased in-hospital mortality and decreased length of intensive care stay. Patients with sepsis may require additional fluid resuscitation beyond this initial bolus and care should be individualized, with the option of either continued crystalloid resuscitation or vasopressor infusion.

Abdominal and pelvic computed tomography are important to investigate the etiology of sepsis; however, given evidence of hypotension, fluid resuscitation should occur first, and imaging is not the best next step. Imaging should be obtained soon after the initial resuscitation and stabilization to confirm the source of the underlying infection, which will assist in tailoring antibiotic and additional treatment.

Subcutaneous insulin is not the best next step for this patient. This patient will benefit from insulin administration once her initial treatment and stabilization have occurred. In patients with sepsis, insulin therapy should be initiated if the blood glucose level exceeds 180 mg/dL with a goal level of 144–180 mg/dL after fluid resuscitation and repeat blood sugar.

Surgical exploration is not the most appropriate next step in this patient. Imaging and other clinical findings may lead to procedural intervention; however, resuscitation should occur first.

Vasopressor initiation is not the most appropriate next step for this patient. Initial resuscitation should occur with crystalloid fluids. Patients who have persistent hypotension or hypoperfusion despite crystalloid resuscitation warrant initiation of vasopressors. Norepinephrine is the first-line choice, with a target mean arterial pressure of 65 mm Hg. Patients requiring vasopressors may benefit from invasive hemodynamic monitoring for close monitoring of response to therapy.

Sepsis is a common cause of in-hospital mortality worldwide and should be recognized and treated early. Initial interventions focus on stabilization and include supportive care, such as fluid resuscitation and broad-spectrum antibiotics. Once the patient's condition has stabilized, focus can shift to identification and treatment of the underlying source.

Adams R, Henry KE, Sridharan A, Soleimani H, Zhan A, Rawat N, et al. Prospective, multi-site study of patient outcomes after implementation of the TREWS machine learning-based early warning system for sepsis. Nat Med 2022;28:1455–60. doi: 10.1038/s41591-022-01894-0

Evans L, Rhodes A, Alhazzani W, Antonelli M, Coopersmith CM, French C, et al. Surviving sepsis campaign: international guidelines for management of sepsis and septic shock 2021. Intensive Care Med 2021;47:1181–247. doi: 10.1007/s00134-021-06506-y

Preparing for clinical emergencies in obstetrics and gynecology. Committee Opinion No. 590. American College of Obstetricians and Gynecologists. Obstet Gynecol 2014;123:722–5. doi: 10.1097/01.AOG.0000444442.04111.c6

Yu SC, Shivakumar N, Betthauser K, Gupta A, Lai AM, Kollef MH, et al. Comparison of early warning scores for sepsis early identification and prediction in the general ward setting. JAMIA Open 2021;4:ooab062. doi: 10.1093/jamiaopen/ooab062

89 Vulvar dermatoses

A 65-year-old patient presents with concerns of persistent, generalized vulvar itching during the last 6 months. Her physical examination findings are noted in Figure 89-1, and the vulvar biopsy result is shown in Figure 89-2. The best next step in treatment is topical

(A) antifungal
* (B) corticosteroid
(C) estrogen
(D) petroleum jelly
(E) tacrolimus

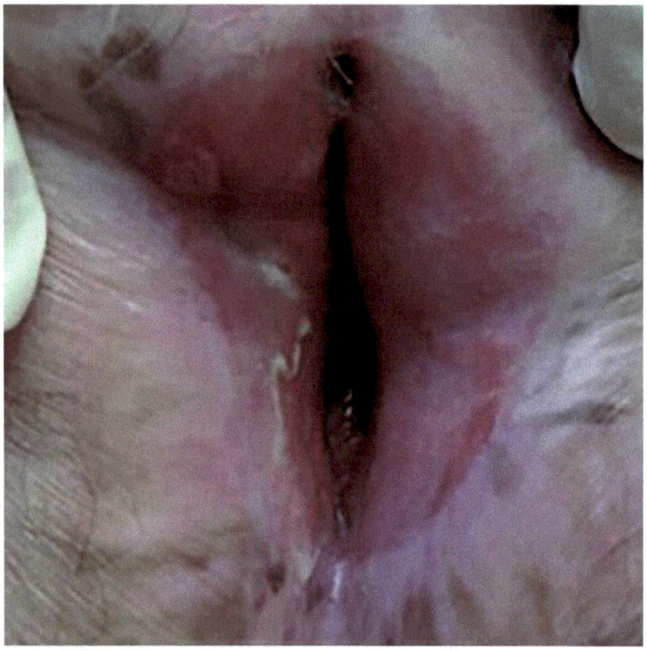

FIGURE 89-1. Physical examination findings. (Reprinted from Howard M, Hall A. Vulval lichen planus–lichen sclerosus overlap. Int J STD AIDS 2018;29:1017–23. doi: 10.1177/0956462418758777)

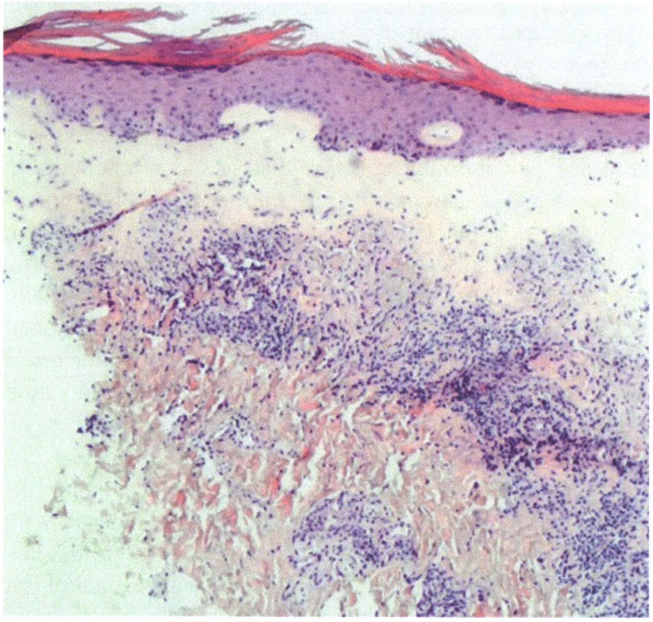

FIGURE 89-2. Patient's vulvar biopsy. (Reprinted from Huvila J, Gilks CB. Lichen sclerosus. PathologyOutlines.com. Accessed July 11, 2025. https://www.pathologyoutlines.com/topic/vulvalichensclerosus.html)

Lichen sclerosus is a chronic, scarring dermatological disorder that most commonly affects postmenopausal women and prepubertal girls. Although lichen sclerosus can develop on any skin surface, the anogenital region is the most common site of clinical presentation. Despite being one of the most common conditions treated in vulvar clinics, the true prevalence is unknown, with estimates ranging from 1 out of 30 among older adult women to 1 out of 60 in general gynecologic clinics. In pediatric vulvar clinics, the estimate is 1 out of 900 patients. Adults with vulvar lichen sclerosus are at a slightly higher risk of vulvar squamous cell carcinoma. The risk estimate for associated squamous cell carcinoma is less than 5%.

The etiology of lichen sclerosus is unknown but is likely multifactorial. Familial factors, immunologic abnormalities including autoimmune diseases, and hormonal factors have been observed in patients with lichen sclerosus. Vulvar pruritus is the most common presenting symptom, as presented in this scenario. Patients may also experience perianal involvement and develop dyschezia or form anal fissures. Dyspareunia and dysuria may also be presenting symptoms. A physical examination is important because some findings of lichen sclerosus may only be detected among asymptomatic individuals.

Classic vulvar lichen sclerosus presents as white or pale papules that may coalesce into plaques. Ecchymoses or purpura may also be present. The labia minora and majora are the most common sites of disease, with the skin in these areas appearing thinned, whitened, and crinkled, often like tissue paper. The disease can spread to involve the clitoris and the perineum in a keyhole or "figure-of-eight" fashion. Over time, plaques may become thickened because of repeated scratching and excoriations. Fusion of tissues can occur, and phimosis of the clitoral hood may be observed. Even though lichen sclerosus can be suspected on physical examination, biopsy should be considered because high-grade squamous intraepitheliel neoplasia (HSIL) and malignant conditions can mimic lichen sclerosus. A biopsy will reveal epidermal atrophy, hyperkeratosis, hyalinization of the upper dermis, and a lymphocytic infiltrate in the dermal layer, as illustrated in this scenario.

Treatment of vulvar lichen sclerosus involves controlling symptoms and preventing disease progression. Patient education is an important component of managing this chronic disease, including discussion regarding disease chronicity, the expectation that existing scarring or vulvar architectural changes will persist, and that pharmacotherapy can improve symptoms. A medium- or high-potency topical corticosteroid, such as clobetasol propionate (0.05%) or mometasone furoate (0.1%), is recommended for initial treatment. Although the optimal dosing, potency, and duration of clobetasol propionate (0.05%) ointment use are not known, experts recommend once daily at night for 4 weeks, then alternate nights for 4 weeks, and then twice weekly for an additional 4 weeks. Alternatively, patients can apply the topical therapy nightly for 12 weeks. Tapering regimens have demonstrated success in treating lichen sclerosus. During follow-up, biopsies should be performed of any new lesions to evaluate for high-grade squamous intraepithelial lesion because they are precursors to vulvar cancer.

Low-potency topical treatments are not recommended as first-line treatment in a patient with vulvar lichen sclerosus. Low-potency topical corticosteroids can be used first-line in patients with mild vulvar symptoms, such as in contact dermatitis, or as maintenance therapy for patients in whom lichen sclerosus has been controlled and is currently very mild. Examples of corticosteroid classifications are noted in Box 89-1.

Antifungal medications are used for patients with evidence of vulvar and vaginal candidiasis. They can be prescribed as both topical or oral regimens. Patients typically present with itching, erythema, and white thick discharge; however, the described patient has lichen sclerosus confirmed by biopsy, and topical antifungal treatment is not the best next step for the described patient.

Lichen sclerosus usually occurs in patients with low estrogen concentrations, and adding vaginal estrogen can improve symptoms of genitourinary syndrome. Vaginal estrogen may be used as an adjunct therapy in lichen sclerosus, but it is not an effective treatment option for the patient in the scenario above.

Application of petroleum jelly to the affected area often is recommended to help decrease symptoms but is not a treatment for lichen sclerosis. Other options, such as using oral antihistamines and avoiding soaps and scented or dyed toilet tissue may be recommended, but. none of these measures effectively treat lichen sclerosis.

Tacrolimus (0.1%) is a topical calcineurin inhibitor and is a treatment option when topical corticosteroid therapy is ineffective or poorly tolerated. An advantage to its use is the absence of risk of drug-induced cutaneous atrophy, which is associated with topical corticosteroid use. Because the patient in this scenario has not had prior therapy, this would not be the best next step in treatment.

BOX 89-1

Common Topical Corticosteroid Ointments for Vulvar Skin Disorders*

High Potency
- betamethasone dipropionate 0.05%
- clobetasol propionate 0.05%
- halobetasol propionate 0.05%
- fluocinonide 0.05%
- triamcinolone acetonide 0.5%

Medium Potency
- desoximetasone 0.05%
- hydrocortisone butyrate 0.1%
- hydrocortisone valerate 0.2%
- mometasone furoate 0.1%
- triamcinolone acetonide 0.025%, 0.1%

Low Potency
- desonide 0.05%
- hydrocortisone 1%, 2.5%

*A topical corticosteroid ointment is preferable to other formulations (cream, gel, lotion), which often contain alcohol or preservatives that can cause or exacerbate irritation.

Data from Stockdale CK, Boardman L. Diagnosis and treatment of vulvar dermatoses. Obstet Gynecol 2018;131:371–86; Thorstensen KA, Birenbaum DL. Recognition and management of vulvar dermatologic conditions: lichen sclerosus, lichen planus, and lichen simplex chronicus. J Midwifery Womens Health 2012;57:260–75; *and* Ference JD, Last AR. Choosing topical corticosteroids. Am Fam Physician 2009;79:135–40.

Reprinted from Diagnosis and management of vulvar skin disorders. ACOG Practice Bulletin No. 224. American College of Obstetricians and Gynecologists. Obstet Gynecol 2020;136:e1–14. doi: 10.1097/AOG.0000000000003944

After initial treatment for lichen sclerosus with high-potency corticosteroids, patients should be monitored in 3 months to assess response. In patients with well-controlled disease, follow-up may occur again at 3–6 months. Patients should be counseled that maintaining use of topical therapy may be required after initial treatment. Because adult-onset lichen sclerosus is associated with an increased risk of differentiated vulvar intraepithelial neoplasia and development of squamous cell carcinoma, additional follow-up visits should occur every 6–12 months, and patients should be encouraged to perform self-examinations and return for evaluation sooner if they note recurrence or return of symptoms.

Diagnosis and management of vulvar skin disorders. ACOG Practice Bulletin No. 224. American College of Obstetricians and Gynecologists. Obstet Gynecol 2020;136:e1–14. doi: 10.1097/AOG.0000000000003944

Lee A, Bradford J, Fischer G. Long-term management of adult vulvar lichen sclerosus: a prospective cohort study of 507 women. JAMA Dermatol 2015;151:1061–7. doi: 10.1001/jamadermatol.2015.0643

Lewis FM, Tatnall FM, Velangi SS, Bunker CB, Kumar A, Brackenbury F, et al. British Association of Dermatologists guidelines for the management of lichen sclerosus, 2018. Br J Dermatol 2018;178:839–53. doi: 10.1111/bjd.16241

Vieira-Baptista P, Pérez-López FR, López-Baena MT, Stockdale CK, Preti M, Bornstein J. Risk of development of vulvar cancer in women with lichen sclerosus or lichen planus: a systematic review. J Low Genit Tract Dis 2022;26:250–7. doi: 10.1097/LGT.0000000000000673

90 Positive and negative predictive values

A direct-to-consumer marketed blood test is advertised as a screening test for ovarian cancer for women aged 50 and older in the United States and reportedly has 90% sensitivity and 80% specificity. If this test is adopted for screening, and the test result is positive, what are the chances that the patient actually has ovarian cancer? The information you need to answer this question is

(A) false-negative rate
(B) false-positive rate
(C) incidence
(D) population size
* (E) prevalence

The clinical utility of a screening test is determined by its sensitivity, specificity, positive predictive value (PPV), and negative predictive value (NPV). An understanding of these terms is essential when deciding whether to adopt a screening test into clinical practice.

Sensitivity is the proportion of people with a condition who are correctly identified by the test as having that condition. The sensitivity of the test is 90%, meaning the test correctly identifies 90% of people with ovarian cancer. *Specificity* is the proportion of people without the condition who are correctly identified by the test as not having the condition. The test in the scenario above has an 80% specificity and correctly identifies 80% of healthy individuals as not having ovarian cancer. *Positive predictive value* is the probability that someone with a positive test actually has the disease, and negative predictive value is the probability that someone with a negative test actually is disease free. Unlike sensitivity and specificity, PPV and NPV vary depending on the prevalence of disease in the population.

Although related to PPV and NPV, sensitivity and specificity examine the test from different perspectives, which is a common source of confusion. When determining the sensitivity and specificity of a test, one takes the perspective of knowing who actually has the disease and then assessing the ability of the test to correctly identify people with the disease (sensitivity) and correctly identify people without the disease (specificity). Sensitivity and specificity relate to a test's fundamental relationship to the condition it is evaluating and do not change depending on the prevalence of disease in the population. When determining PPV and NPV, one takes the perspective of *not* knowing who actually has the disease in a population and assessing the *probability* that a person with a positive test actually has the disease (PPV) and the *probability* that a person with a negative test does not have the disease (NPV). Because this situation reflects what is usually the case in actual clinical practice, PPV and NPV are more useful indicators of the clinical value of the test. Appendix B, Table B-1 shows the relationship between sensitivity, specificity, PPV, and NPV for a screening test for ovarian cancer.

To illustrate how PPV and NPV change depending on the prevalence of disease for the test described, Appendix B, Table B-2 shows what the PPV and NPV would be if the test were used in a population of 1,000 patients in which the prevalence of ovarian cancer is 40%. In this scenario, the likelihood that someone with a positive test actually has ovarian cancer (PPV) would be 75%, whereas the likelihood that someone with a negative test does not have cancer (NPV) would be 92%.

Table 90-1 shows what would happen if the same test were used in a population in which the prevalence of ovarian cancer is 2%. Although the sensitivity and specificity of the test remain the same, the PPV decreases to 8.4%, meaning the likelihood that an individual with a positive test has cancer is only 8.4%. In this case, the NPV increases to 99.7%, which may sound impressive but the a priori likelihood that someone in the population is cancer-free, independent of the test, is 98% because only 2% of patients have ovarian cancer.

In the United States, the actual prevalence of ovarian cancer is approximately 1 out of 2,500. This extremely low prevalence makes it challenging to identify a test aimed at identifying ovarian cancer with a high enough PPV to be clinically useful.

To know the predictive value of a screening test, gynecologic oncologists must know the prevalence of disease, because PPV is calculated from sensitivity, specificity, and disease

TABLE 90-1. Calculation of Positive Predictive Value and Negative Predictive Value for an Ovarian Cancer Screening Test With 90% Sensitivity and 80% Specificity in a Population With 2% Ovarian Cancer Prevalence

	OVARIAN CANCER PRESENT (20)	OVARIAN CANCER ABSENT (980)	FORMULA
Test positive	True positive (A=18)	False positive (B=196)	PPV=A/A+B=18/18+196=8.4%
Test negative	False negative (C=2)	True negative (D=784)	NPV=D/D+C=784/784+2=99.7%
Formula	Sensitivity= A/A+C=18/20=90%	Specificity=D/B+D=784/980=80%	

prevalence. The size of the population is not needed to determine the PPV because sensitivity, specificity, and prevalence do not depend on population size.

The incidence of ovarian cancer is the rate of new ovarian cancer diagnoses over time. Although incidence rates together with mortality rates will ultimately determine disease prevalence, PPV is based on the prevalence of disease at a given point in time and cannot be determined from disease incidence.

The false-negative rate of a test is another way of describing the sensitivity of the test. A highly sensitive test will have a low false-negative rate because it will correctly identify persons with the disease as having the disease. The sensitivity of the test is already known.

The false-positive rate of a test is another way of describing the specificity of the test. A highly specific test will have a low false-positive rate. The specificity of the test is already known.

Elias KM, Guo J, Bast RC Jr. Early detection of ovarian cancer. Hematol Oncol Clin North Am 2018;32:903–14. doi: 10.1016/j.hoc.2018.07.003

Mallett S, Halligan S, Thompson M, Collins GS, Altman DG. Interpreting diagnostic accuracy studies for patient care. BMJ 2012;345:e3999. doi: 10.1136/bmj.e3999

Trevethan R. Sensitivity, specificity, and predictive values: foundations, pliabilities, and pitfalls in research and practice. Front Public Health 2017;5:307. doi: 10.3389/fpubh.2017.00307

91 Cancer diagnosis

A 37-year-old patient presents with several months of worsening abdominal distension and discomfort. Computed tomography is shown in Figure 91-1. Her CA 125 level is 108 U/mL, her carcinoembryonic antigen (CEA) level is 20.7 ng/mL, and CA 19-9 level is 195 U/mL. Based on these findings, the most likely primary site of disease is the

* * (A) appendix
* (B) breast
* (C) ovary
* (D) pancreas
* (E) uterus

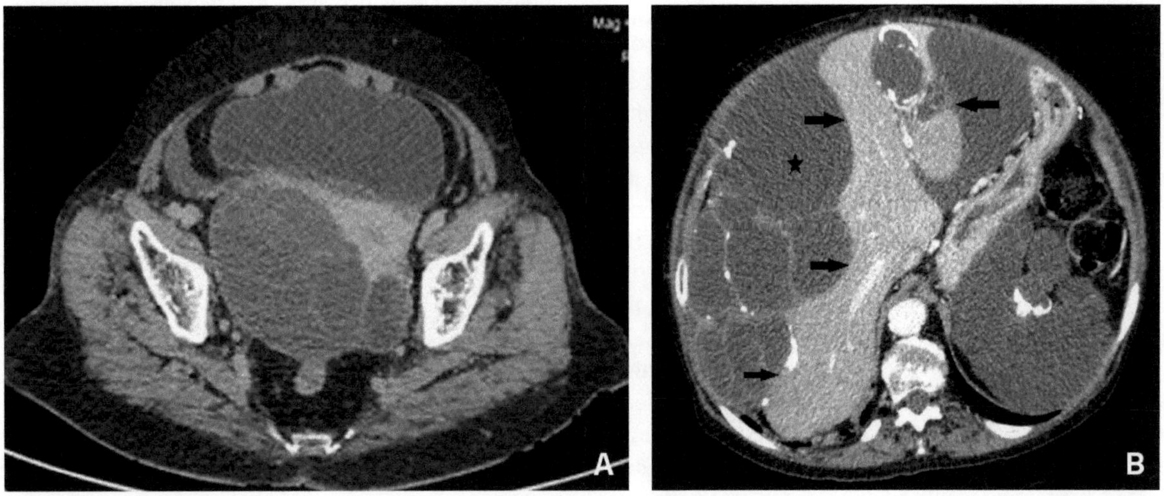

FIGURE 91-1. A. Computed tomography of the pelvis (Reprinted from Joseph R, Sathiamoorthy R, Gnanasekaran R, Gunasekaran L, Ilangovan G. A case report of pseudomyxoma peritonei arising from primary mucinous ovarian neoplasms. Cureus 2022;14:e29309. doi: 10.7759/cureus.29309). B. Upper abdomen showing liver scalloping characteristic of pseudomyxoma peritonei. (Reprinted from Allart K, Sabbagh C, Regimbeau J. Liver scalloping: pseudomyxoma peritonei liver compression. J Visc Surg 2019;156:75–6. doi: 10.1016/j.jviscsurg.2018.09.001)

Pseudomyxoma peritonei is a disease characterized by mucinous implants involving the peritoneum along with mucinous ascites originating from a perforated mucinous neoplasm, most commonly a low-grade neoplasm in the appendix. Previously, when mucinous ascites was encountered with a mucinous borderline ovarian tumor, the ovary was thought to be the originating site of disease. With greater use of immunohistochemistry and molecular genetic analyses, it is now clear that the ovary is secondarily involved with the primary site of disease in the gastrointestinal tract in almost all instances; therefore, inspection of the appendix in patients with right-sided or bilateral ovarian mucinous borderline tumors is advisable.

The location of tumor implants in the abdomen is influenced primarily by routes of peritoneal circulation and gravity rather than cell adhesion in what is termed the *redistribution phenomenon*. Implants accumulate primarily in the omentum, diaphragmatic surface, paracolic gutters, or pouch of Douglas (rectovaginal pouch), with relative sparing of the bowel. The tumor often is low grade, and progression of disease is relatively slow. Many patients are asymptomatic early in the course of disease. The most common presentations among women are detection of an abnormal ovarian mass (39%), acute appendicitis (27%), or abdominal distension (23%). The diagnosis may be made incidentally on imaging or at abdominal surgery for what would seem to be an unrelated concern, such as ventral hernia repair.

In the above scenario, the patient has computed tomography (CT) findings of a cystic right-sided ovarian mass (Fig. 91-1A) and scalloping ascites around the liver (Fig. 91-1B). Scalloping ascites is considered a pathognomonic finding of pseudomyxoma because only mucinous ascites causes indentation of the liver surface. The appendix is the most common primary site of disease in pseudomyxoma peritonei and, therefore, it is the most likely primary site of her disease.

The patient described has a mildly increased CA 125 level of 108 U/mL. Although CA 125 is most commonly high in cases of ovarian cancer, mild increases in the 100–200 U/mL range are nonspecific and can be seen in many benign conditions as well as in any condition in which the peritoneum is inflamed or irritated. Carcinoembryonic antigen is a tumor marker most commonly increased in gastrointestinal cancer, whereas CA 19-9 is most commonly increased in biliary cancer. High CEA and CA 19-9 are frequently seen in pseudomyxoma, and higher CEA and CA 19-9 levels are associated with poorer prognosis. Because the normal range for CEA is 0–5 ng/mL and the normal range for CEA is 0–37 U/mL, these markers are more significantly increased compared with the CA 125 level in the patient described above.

Although this patient also has a right-sided ovarian mass, the combination of mucinous ascites and the high levels of CEA and CA 19-9 indicates a high likelihood of malignancy that is metastatic to the ovary rather than primary ovarian cancer. Therefore, ovary is incorrect. Although breast and uterine cancer can metastasize to the ovary, neither would be associated with mucinous ascites and would be unlikely to cause increases in CEA and CA 19-9 levels. Breast and uterus are not the most likely primary sites for the described patient's disease. Metastatic pancreatic cancer would be potentially associated with high CA 19-9 levels, but it is not typically associated with mucinous ascites.

The nomenclature used to describe pseudomyxoma peritonei has evolved over time. In 2016, the Peritoneal Surface Oncology Group proposed the term *low-grade appendiceal mucinous neoplasm* to replace *appendiceal adenoma*, which differentiates it from high-grade appendiceal mucinous neoplasms. Peritoneal disease is classified according to clinical aggressiveness, in four categories:

- acellular mucin
- low-grade mucinous carcinoma peritonei (previously referred to as *adenomucinosis*)
- high-grade mucinous carcinoma peritonei
- high-grade mucinous carcinoma peritonei with signet ring cells

Optimal treatment is complete cytoreductive surgery, ideally to no visible disease, which typically involves peritonectomy, diaphragmatic stripping, omentectomy. If not previously done, right colectomy and hysterectomy with bilateral salpingo-oophorectomy (in women) will be undertaken. Splenectomy and cholecystectomy also may be necessary. Often a chest tube is placed prophylactically in anticipation of potential pneumothorax from diaphragmatic stripping.

In addition to cytoreduction, hyperthermic intraperitoneal chemotherapy (HIPEC) may be administered with the goal of eradicating residual microscopic disease. Hyperthermic intraperitoneal chemotherapy uses multiple chemotherapeutic agents that are heated, typically to 42–43 °C and instilled into the abdominal cavity for 60–120 minutes after surgery has been completed. The described patient has a classic presentation of pseudomyxoma peritonei originating in an appendiceal tumor with secondary involvement of the right ovary. In addition to cytoreductive surgery, the best treatment is HIPEC.

Several HIPEC regimens and techniques have been reported and a standard has not been established. The two most common chemotherapeutic agents used intraperitoneally are mitomycin C and oxaliplatin, which are sometimes given in conjunction with intravenous 5-fluorouracil. Retrospective studies have not found a significant difference in outcomes in patients receiving oxaliplatin versus mitomycin C, and prospective studies comparing the regimens are needed. Some centers administer HIPEC with the abdomen open (*colosseum technique*), and others administer it with a catheter after closing the abdomen (*closed technique*).

These extensive cytoreductions—with or without HIPEC—are complex and require multidisciplinary coordination among surgeons, anesthesiologists, intensivists, and other members of the care team to prevent complications and minimize morbidity.

Allart K, Sabbagh C, Regimbeau J. Liver scalloping: pseudomyxoma peritonei liver compression. J Visc Surg 2019;156:75–6. doi: 10.1016/j.jviscsurg.2018.09.001

Carr NJ, Finch J, Ilesley IC, Chandrakumaran K, Mohamed F, Mirnezami A, et al. Pathology and prognosis in pseudomyxoma peritonei: a review of 274 cases. J Clin Pathol 2012;65:919–23. doi: 10.1136/jclinpath-2012-200843

Hübner M, van Der Speeten K, Govaerts K, de Hingh I, Villeneuve L, Kusamura S, et al. 2022 Peritoneal Surface Oncology Group international consensus on HIPEC regimens for peritoneal malignancies: colorectal cancer. Ann Surg Oncol 2024;31:567–76. doi: 10.1245/s10434-023-14368-5

Taflampas P, Dayal S, Chandrakumaran K, Mohamed F, Cecil TD, Moran BJ. Pre-operative tumour marker status predicts recurrence and survival after complete cytoreduction and hyperthermic intraperitoneal chemotherapy for appendiceal pseudomyxoma peritonei: analysis of 519 patients. Eur J Surg Oncol 2014;40:515–20. doi: 10.1016/j.ejso.2013.12.021

Van der Speeten K, Lemoine L, Sugarbaker P. Overview of the optimal perioperative intraperitoneal chemotherapy regimens used in current clinical practice. Pleura Peritoneum 2017;2:63–72. doi: 10.1515/pp-2017-0003

92 Ovarian cancer screening

A 57-year-old patient presents for her annual examination. She is asymptomatic and has a past medical history remarkable for hypertension. She reports a family history of colon cancer in a paternal aunt. She requests ovarian cancer screening because she is anxious after her older sister received a diagnosis of ovarian cancer. Compared with no screening, available screening strategies for ovarian cancer are associated with

* (A) increased likelihood of unnecessary surgery
(B) lower ovarian cancer mortality
(C) reduced patient anxiety
(D) similar stage at diagnosis

Ovarian cancer has the highest mortality rate of gynecologic cancer. It is estimated that 19,680 patients received diagnoses of ovarian cancer in 2024, and 12,740 patients with ovarian cancer died. Given these statistics, anxiety regarding ovarian cancer, as reported by the patient in this scenario, is common. No effective screening strategy has been identified. Three randomized controlled trials of ovarian cancer screening—the UK Collaborative Trial of Ovarian Cancer Screening (UKCTOCS), the Prostate, Lung, Colorectal, Ovarian cancer screening trial (PLCO), and the Shizuoka Cohort Study of Ovarian Cancer Screening (SCSOCS)—concluded that screening using transvaginal ultrasound and CA 125 tumor marker testing does not reduce the likelihood of death from ovarian cancer.

The largest and most recent screening trial is the UKCTOCS trial which, from 2001 to 2005, enrolled 202,638 postmenopausal women aged 50–74 years and randomized them into three groups: no screening (control), multimodal screening (using longitudinal CA 125 algorithm with repeat CA 125 testing and transvaginal scan), or ultrasound screening using transvaginal scan alone (with repeat scan to confirm abnormality). With a median follow-up of 16.4 years, outcomes data published in 2020 demonstrated no difference in mortality from ovarian or fallopian tube cancer in either the multimodal or ultrasound group compared with the no screening group.

The UKCTOCS trial did find that multimodal screening was associated with a 39% increase in diagnoses at stages I and II, and a 10% decrease in diagnoses at stages III and IV, whereas ultrasound screening alone was not associated with a difference in stage at diagnosis compared with the no-screening group; therefore, current screening strategies have not been associated with similar stage at diagnosis, and the modest stage migrations from screening have not been sufficient to reduce mortality. The reasons are complex but are in part explained by the fact that high-grade serous cancer, which is responsible for approximately 75% of ovarian cancer deaths, tends to metastasize early and is associated with an approximately 25% rate of relapse even when diagnosed at an early stage. Ovarian cancer screening is not associated with lower ovarian cancer mortality.

A consistent finding across screening trials is that screening is associated with an increased risk of surgery for benign findings. A meta-analysis of the three screening trials concluded that screening using ultrasonography and CA 125 tumor marker testing resulted in 13 surgeries for every cancer detected. The rate of major complications from these surgeries for benign findings ranged from 3.5% to 15%, with hemorrhage, infection, and injury to hollow viscus being the most common complications. Screening is associated with an increased likelihood of unnecessary surgery.

Psychological morbidity was assessed in the UKCTOCS and PLCO trials. Although being screened was itself not a cause of distress, patients in the screening groups who required follow-up for an abnormal screening result demonstrated higher levels of anxiety-related psychological morbidity for up to 2 years after screening. Screening is not associated with lower anxiety.

The patient in this scenario does not report a significant family history of breast or ovarian cancer, although this does not rule out the possibility that she carries a *BRCA* or other deleterious mutation resulting in high cancer risk. Even among patients with high hereditary risk of ovarian cancer, studies have found that screening for CA 125 tumor marker and ultrasonography is equally ineffective at reducing ovarian cancer mortality.

Screening strategies to date have failed to demonstrate an improvement in mortality from ovarian cancer but have increased the likelihood of surgery and anxiety. Because the patient described above has no obvious risk factors for ovarian or fallopian tube cancer, routine follow-up is warranted.

Menon U, Gentry-Maharaj A, Burnell M, Singh N, Ryan A, Karpinskyj C, et al. Ovarian cancer population screening and mortality after long-term follow-up in the UK Collaborative Trial of Ovarian Cancer Screening (UKCTOCS): a randomised controlled trial. Lancet 2021;397:2182–93. doi: 10.1016/S0140-6736(21)00731-5

Reade CJ, Riva JJ, Busse JW, Goldsmith CH, Elit L. Risks and benefits of screening asymptomatic women for ovarian cancer: a systematic review and meta-analysis. Gynecol Oncol 2013;130:674–81. doi: 10.1016/j.ygyno.2013.06.029

The role of the obstetrician-gynecologist in the early detection of epithelial ovarian cancer in women at average risk. Committee Opinion No. 716. American College of Obstetricians and Gynecologists. Obstet Gynecol 2017;130:e146–9. doi: 10.1097/AOG.0000000000002299

93 Clinical findings and associated hereditary cancer syndromes

A 38-year-old patient presents for her annual examination. The physical examination is remarkable for macrocephaly. Mucosal findings (Fig. 93-1) and skin findings (Fig. 93-2) also are appreciated with an otherwise unremarkable examination. After confirmatory genetic testing, the patient undergoes screening for cancer genetically linked with her condition. The screening test most likely to detect an associated cancer is a(n)

(A) colonoscopy
(B) endometrial biopsy
* (C) mammogram
(D) renal ultrasonography
(E) thyroid ultrasonography

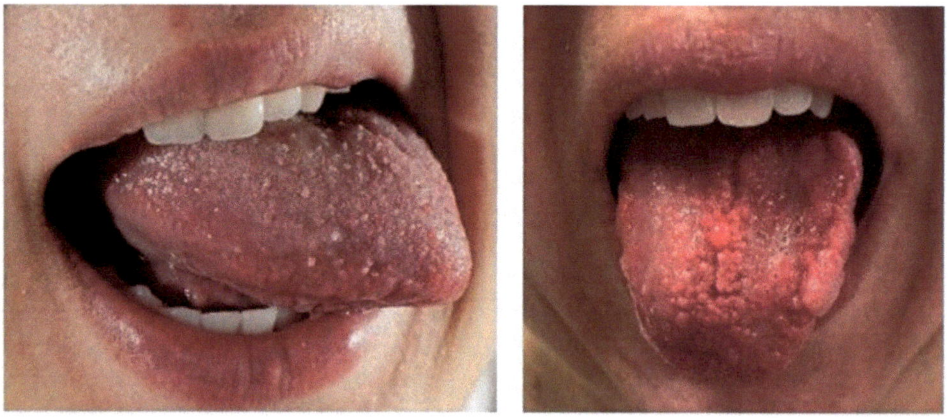

FIGURE 93-1. Extensive oral papillomas resulting in cobblestone appearance of tongue. (Reprinted from National Cancer Institute. Oral papilloma. In: NCI dictionary of genetics terms. Accessed June 3, 2025. https://www.cancer.gov/publications/dictionaries/genetics-dictionary/def/oral-papilloma)

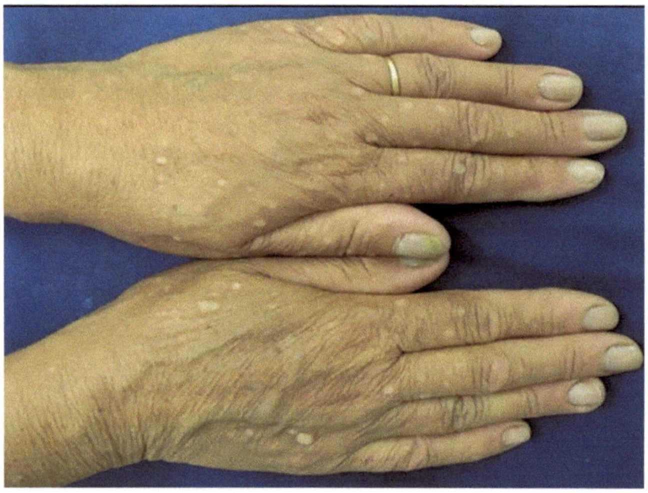

FIGURE 93-2. Warty appearing acral keratosis on the hands. (Reprinted from Flores IL, Romo SA, Tejeda Nava FJ, Roger dos Santos Silva A, Vargas PA, Paes de Almeida O, et al. Oral Surg Oral Med Oral Pathol Oral Radiol 2014;117:E301-10. doi: 10.1016/j.oooo.2014.01.015)

The phosphate and tensin homolog tumor suppressor gene (*PTEN*) is located on chromosome 10q23.3 and controls apoptosis of the cell cycle through the phosphatidylinositol 3-kinase (PI3K)/AKT/mammalian target of rapamycin (mTOR) pathways. Germline mutations in *PTEN* have been associated with a group of syndromes termed *PTEN hamartoma tumor syndrome*. Although originally referred to as *Cowden syndrome*, it is now recognized as a variety of syndromes associated with mutations in *PTEN*.

The clinical manifestations of *PTEN* hamartoma tumor syndrome typically present in young adulthood and may include a constellation of cutaneous, mucocutaneous, and malignant conditions. Cutaneous manifestations include papules near the eyelids, forehead, nose, mouth, or hands and feet, flesh-colored hamartomas near the hairline, angiomas, dermal fibromas, lipomas, and neurofibromas. Mucocutaneous lesions include trichilemmomas, oral papillomas, and acral keratoses.

The diagnosis of *PTEN* hamartoma tumor syndrome is based on specific major and minor criteria (Table 93-1) and requires either three or more major criteria, with one including macrocephaly, Lhermitte-Duclos disease, or gastrointestinal hamartomas; or two major and three minor criteria. If one individual in a family meets *PTEN* hamartoma tumor syndrome clinical diagnostic criteria or has a *PTEN* pathogenic or likely pathogenic mutation, diagnosis can be made with any two major criteria with or without minor criteria, one major and two minor criteria, or three minor criteria.

These patients are at a high lifetime risk of several types of cancer, including breast, thyroid, endometrial, and renal cancer. Patients also have a higher-than-population-level risk of colorectal cancer and melanoma. Recommended screening studies in these patients are summarized in Table 93-2. Breast cancer is the most common cancer seen in *PTEN* hamartoma tumor syndrome, with up to an 85% lifetime risk. The most appropriate screening test for breast cancer is mammography starting at ages 30–35 years, and patients with *PTEN* hamartoma tumor syndrome should undergo screening every 6 months with alternating mammography and breast magnetic resonance imaging; therefore, this is the best next step for the described patient.

Thyroid cancer is the second most common cancer in this patient population. Follicular and papillary histology are associated with *PTEN* hamartoma tumor syndrome, but medullary thyroid cancer is not. Cumulative lifetime risk of thyroid cancer is up to 38%. Annual thyroid ultrasonography is recommended beginning at age 7 years.

Renal cancer incidence is increased by up to 34% during a life span in this population. National Comprehensive Cancer Network guidelines recommend baseline renal ultrasonography at age 40 years followed by repeat renal ultrasonography every 1–2 years.

TABLE 93-1. Major and Minor Criteria for Diagnosis of *PTEN* Hamartoma Tumor Syndrome

MAJOR CRITERIA	MINOR CRITERIA
Breast cancer	Autism spectrum disorder
Endometrial cancer	Colon cancer
Follicular thyroid cancer	Esophageal glycogenic acanthoses
Multiple gastrointestinal hamartomas	Lipomas
Lhermitte-Duclos disease	Intellectual disability (IQ less than 75)
Macrocephaly	Papillary or follicular variant of thyroid cancer
Macular pigmentation of glans penis	Thyroid structural lesions (adenoma, modules, goiter)
Mucocutaneous lesions:	Renal cell carcinoma
Biopsy proven trichilemmoma	Single gastrointestinal hamartoma or ganglioneuroma
Multiple palmoplantar keratoses	Testicular lipomatosis
Extensive oral mucosal papillomas	Vascular anomalies
Multiple cutaneous facial papules	

Data from National Comprehensive Cancer Network. Genetic/familial high-risk assessment: breast, ovarian, pancreatic, and prostate. Version 2.2025. NCCN Clinical Practice Guidelines in Oncology [after login]. NCCN; 2024. Accessed January 28, 2025.

TABLE 93-2. Cancer Screening in *PTEN* Hamartoma Tumor Syndrome

ASSOCIATED CANCER	APPROXIMATE LIFETIME RISK	SURVEILLANCE METHOD	INTERVAL	STARTING AGE, IN YEARS
Breast	67–85%	Mammogram	Yearly	30–35
		Magnetic resonance imaging	Yearly	30–35
		Risk-reducing surgery	—	—
Thyroid	25–38%	Ultrasonography	Yearly	7
Renal	9–34%	Ultrasonography	Every 1–2 years	40
Colorectal	9–20%	Colonoscopy	Every 5 years	35*
Melanoma	2–6%	Skin examination	Yearly	30
Endometrial	21–28%	Can consider transvaginal ultrasonography in postmenopausal patients	—	—

*Screening should be initiated 5–10 years before the earliest year a known family member received a cancer diagnosis.

Modified from Dragoo DD, Taher A, Wong VK, Elsaiey A, Consul N, Mahmoud HS, et al. PTEN hamartoma tumor syndrome/Cowden syndrome: genomics, oncogenesis, and imaging review for associated lesions and malignancy. Cancer (Basel) 2021;13:3120. doi: 10.3390/cancers13133120

Patients with *PTEN* hamartoma tumor syndrome may have an up to 28% risk of developing endometrial cancer. Screening for endometrial cancer in patients with this syndrome is somewhat controversial. The National Comprehensive Cancer Network recommends screening with endometrial biopsy beginning at age 35 years; however, routine screening without signs of abnormal uterine bleeding is of unproven benefit given that endometrial biopsy has low sensitivity and specificity for the diagnosis of endometrial cancer in the absence of abnormal uterine bleeding. Although annual transvaginal ultrasonography after menopause can be considered, this has not shown sufficient sensitivity for detecting endometrial cancer in the absence of abnormal uterine bleeding.

Hysterectomy has not been shown to reduce morbidity from uterine cancer, but it can reduce its incidence and may be considered in asymptomatic patients with the *PTEN* mutation.

An increased risk of colorectal cancer is possible in patients with *PTEN* hamartoma tumor syndrome. Reported rates of colon cancer in patients with this syndrome range from 9% to 20% compared with 4% in the general population. Due to the moderate increase in risk, colonoscopy is recommended every 5 years beginning at age 35 years. Screening guidelines also recommend consideration of colonoscopy initiation 5–10 years before the youngest age at which a relative was diagnosed with colon cancer.

Melanoma risk also is reported to be slightly increased from baseline population risk in this syndrome. Patients have a 2–6% lifetime risk of melanoma compared to 0.5–1.5% in the general population. As such, an annual skin cancer screening by a dermatologist is recommended.

Patients with cutaneous and mucocutaneous signs of *PTEN* hamartoma tumor syndrome, or relatives of individuals with known *PTEN* hamartoma tumor syndrome, may benefit from genetic counseling and testing. Identification of this genetic cancer syndrome and adherence to screening guidelines can help reduce the risk of cancer and improve early detection in patients with genetic syndromes.

Dragoo DD, Taher A, Wong VK, Elsaiey A, Consul N, Mahmoud HS, et al. PTEN hamartoma tumor syndrome/Cowden syndrome: genomics, oncogenesis, and imaging review for associated lesions and malignancy. Cancer (Basel) 2021;13:3120. doi: 10.3390/cancer13133120

Hendricks LA, Hoogerbrugge N, Mensenkamp AR, Brunet J, Lleuger-Pujol R, Høberg-Vetti H, et al. Cancer risks by sex and variant type in PTEN hamartoma tumor syndrome. PTEN Study Group. J Natl Cancer Inst 2023;115:93–103. doi: 10.1093/jnci/djac188

Mester J, Eng C. Cowden syndrome: recognizing and managing a not-so-rare hereditary cancer syndrome. J Surg Oncol 2015;111:125–30. doi: 10.1002/jso.23735

National Comprehensive Cancer Network. Genetic/familial high-risk assessment: breast, ovarian, pancreatic, and prostate. Version 2.2025. NCCN Clinical Practice Guidelines in Oncology [after login]. NCCN; 2024. Accessed January 28, 2025. https://www.nccn.org/guidelines/guidelines-detail?category=2&id=1545

94 Pulmonary complications after surgery

A 64-year-old with no significant cardiac or pulmonary history undergoes an abdominal hysterectomy for symptomatic benign leiomyoma. In the recovery room, she had several episodes of vomiting immediately after surgery. On postoperative day 2, she develops a fever of 38.6 °C (101.4 °F) and worsening shortness of breath. On examination, her heart rate is 100 beats per minute, her blood pressure is 110/60 mm Hg, crackles are present at both lung bases, and her respiratory rate is 32 breaths per minute. Her oxygen saturation is 88% on 6 L of high-flow oxygen by nasal cannula. An electrocardiogram shows sinus tachycardia but no other abnormalities, and a chest X-ray (Fig. 94-1) is performed. You initiate broad-spectrum antibiotics. The best next step is

(A) high-dose corticosteroids
(B) incentive spirometry
* (C) mechanical ventilation
(D) nebulizer treatment
(E) thrombolytic therapy

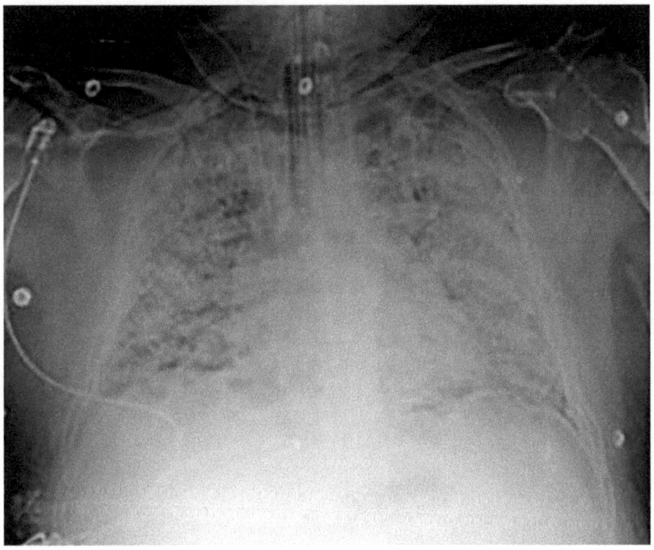

FIGURE 94-1. Chest X-ray.

Respiratory failure is defined as the inability to maintain adequate gas exchange with spontaneous respirations. *Type 1* respiratory failure refers to the inability to maintain adequate oxygenation (hypoxemia) indicated by an arterial partial pressure of oxygen (PaO_2) of less than 60 mm Hg, whereas *type 2* respiratory failure, also known as *ventilatory failure*, is the inability to adequately expel carbon dioxide (*hypercapnia*) indicated by an arterial partial pressure of CO_2 ($PaCO_2$) of greater than 45 mm Hg with a pH less than 7.35 due to inadequate respiratory effort. The decision to place a patient on mechanical ventilation is based on evidence of respiratory failure, an assessment of the overall clinical picture, and the expected course of the underlying cause of the respiratory distress. The goals of mechanical ventilation are to correct hypoxemia and respiratory acidosis while treating the underlying cause of respiratory failure and allowing the respiratory muscles to rest.

The described patient is experiencing respiratory failure with low oxygenation despite receiving supplemental oxygen. An oxygen saturation level of 90% on pulse oximetry correlates with a PaO_2 of 60 mm Hg. The fact that the patient is unable to maintain PaO_2 of 60 mm Hg despite supplemental oxygen is an indication of respiratory failure. A respiratory rate of greater than 30 breaths per minute is an additional sign of respiratory failure. It indicates that there is increased work of respiration required to maintain PaO_2 leading to an increased risk of respiratory muscle fatigue.

Although there are several potential underlying causes of respiratory failure in the postoperative setting, the described patient's chest X-ray demonstrates bilateral pulmonary opacities, which in addition to the other described parameters, is consistent with acute respiratory distress syndrome (ARDS). Acute respiratory distress syndrome is a condition that typically starts with an initial insult or injury to the lung that triggers an inflammatory response causing endothelial damage, increased pulmonary capillary permeability, and flooding of alveolar air spaces. The inciting event can be a direct (as with trauma, toxins, or aspiration) or indirect injury to the lung from systemic inflammatory response (as with sepsis, hemorrhagic shock, or multiple transfusions), and the course of progression can vary from as few as 6 hours to 2–3 days. A study of patients with ARDS found that among those who did not have ARDS on admission, the median time from admission to development of ARDS was 30 hours. In the above scenario, the patient may have had an aspiration event, which is a leading cause of ARDS. Because of the rapid deterioration of lung function often observed in patients with ARDS, and its tendency to be associated with multi-organ system failure, mechanical ventilation is generally required.

In the patient described, given the evidence of respiratory failure of low oxygen saturation despite supplemental oxygen, a respiratory rate greater than 30, risk factors for and evidence of ARDS on chest X-ray, intubation and mechanical ventilation are the best next step.

It can be challenging to distinguish ARDS from other causes of respiratory failure, particularly acute cardiogenic pulmonary edema. Previously, the diagnosis of ARDS depended on demonstrating a pulmonary capillary wedge pressure of less than 18 mm Hg; however, meta-analyses have found that pulmonary artery catheterization, which is invasive and potentially morbid, was not associated with improved outcomes. Currently, ARDS is most commonly defined by the Berlin criteria published in 2012, which eliminated pulmonary capillary wedge pressure and relies on clinical assessment to exclude cardiac failure or fluid overload as the cause of respiratory failure. A systematic review of methods used to distinguish between cardiogenic pulmonary edema and ARDS concluded that there are no biomarkers or tools with high-quality evidence for differentiating ARDS from cardiogenic pulmonary edema, although several biomarkers show promise. The distinction, therefore, relies on a critical review of clinical information and the patient's response to therapy (including diuretics).

Incentive spirometry is commonly used in the postoperative setting to encourage patients to take deep breaths to prevent and treat atelectasis, or partial collapse of the lung, which typically occurs as a result of anesthesia and shallow breathing. It is not an effective treatment for patients with evidence of respiratory failure; therefore, incentive spirometry is not the best next step for the described patient.

Thrombolysis is the administration of thrombolytic agents to dissolve blood clots and is used in clinically serious cases of pulmonary embolism. Although fever, tachycardia, hypotension, tachypnea, and hypoxia can occur in cases of pulmonary embolism, a chest X-ray is usually clear without opacities. The constellation of signs and symptoms in the patient described, together with a history of aspiration, is more consistent with ARDS, and thrombolysis is not the best next step.

Nebulizer treatment with albuterol is used to treat acute bronchoconstriction in patients with asthma exacerbation. The described patient does not have a history of asthma or other reactive airway disease and does not exhibit wheezing on examination, and asthma exacerbation is extremely unlikely. Although tachycardia, tachypnea, and hypoxia can be seen in cases of asthma exacerbation, fever and hypotension are not typically present and a chest X-ray is usually clear; therefore, nebulizer treatment is not the best next step.

High-dose corticosteroids also are used in cases of severe acute bronchoconstriction. A meta-analysis of 61 trials concluded that corticosteroids reduced 28-day mortality from sepsis but did not improve long-term mortality, and current guidelines recommend considering corticosteroids in patients with septic shock who require ongoing support with vasopressors. For ARDS specifically, clinical trials have yielded conflicting results with some showing benefit in early ARDS and others showing harm. Although debate continues, if corticosteroids were to be used, they would not be used before initiation of mechanical ventilation, and high-dose corticosteroids are not the best next step for the patient described above.

Fan E, Brodie D, Slutsky AS. Acute respiratory distress syndrome: advances in diagnosis and treatment. JAMA 2018;319:698–710. doi: 10.1001/jama.2017.21907

Ferguson ND, Fan E, Camporota L, Antonelli M, Anzueto A, Beale R, et al. The Berlin definition of ARDS: an expanded rationale, justification, and supplementary material [published erratum appears in Intensive Care Med. 2012;38:1731-2]. Intensive Care Med 2012;38:1573–82. doi: 10.1007/s00134-012-2682-1

Komiya K, Akaba T, Kozaki Y, Kadota J, Rubin BK. A systematic review of diagnostic methods to differentiate acute lung injury/acute respiratory distress syndrome from cardiogenic pulmonary edema. Crit Care 2017;21:228–8. doi: 10.1186/s13054-017-1809-8

Kuperminc E, Heming N, Carlos M, Annane D. Corticosteroids in ARDS. J Clin Med 2023;12:3340. doi: 10.3390/jcm12093340

95 Hemodynamic monitoring

A patient with a diagnosis of advanced-stage ovarian cancer is admitted to the intensive care unit in septic shock. A pulmonary artery catheter is placed and initial values of systemic vascular resistance (SVR), pulmonary vascular resistance (PVR), cardiac index (CI), and pulmonary capillary wedge pressure (PCWP) are obtained. The combination of hemodynamic parameters that is most consistent with septic shock is

(A) increased SVR, normal PVR, decreased CI, increased PCWP
* (B) decreased SVR, normal PVR, increased CI, normal PCWP
(C) increased SVR, normal PVR, decreased CI, decreased PCWP
(D) normal SVR, increased PVR, decreased CI, normal PCWP

Hemodynamic monitoring permits evaluation and tracking of volume status and heart function and frequently is essential to the treatment of critically ill patients, including those in shock. Monitoring may be accomplished with either noninvasive or invasive techniques; however, certain parameters are commonly measured, including CI, SVR and PVR, mixed venous oxygen saturation, arterial and venous pressures, and PCWPs. One of the most frequent indications for hemodynamic monitoring is circulatory shock.

Circulatory shock occurs when oxygen demand exceeds oxygen delivery and, if not addressed promptly and adequately, may result in catastrophic end-organ damage and death. The clinical presentation of a patient with shock can vary but may include altered mental status, increased serum lactic acid level, and skin changes. Shock is classified into one of four types: cardiogenic, distributive, hypovolemic, or obstructive. Distinguishing one type of shock from the others is important because management may vary considerably depending on the underlying cause.

Distributive shock is the most common form of shock. It is the result of fluid shifts (redistribution) from the intravascular space into the extracellular, interstitial space. The characteristic hemodynamic profile of distributive shock includes normal-to-increased cardiac index and mixed venous oxygen saturation, normal PVR, normal-to-decreased right atrial and venous pressures and PCWPs, and decreased SVR. The three types of distributive shock are anaphylactic, neurogenic, and septic. Anaphylactic shock typically is due to a hypersensitivity reaction with histamine release.

Neurogenic shock is caused by disruption of the normal sympathetic and parasympathetic vascular tone, resulting in vasodilation and resultant hypoperfusion.

The combination of hemodynamic parameters that is typical of a patient in *septic shock* is decreased SVR, normal PVR, increased CI, and normal PCWP. This profile is the result of overwhelming infection, release of proinflammatory mediators resulting in decreased vascular tone, and capillary leakage as seen in the patient described above.

Cardiogenic shock results from diminution of the heart's ability to pump blood, leading to a lower ejection fraction, lower ventricular filling, or hypotension. The causes of cardiogenic shock include myocardial infarction, valvular disease, cardiomyopathy, arrythmias, cardiotoxins, and trauma. Cardiogenic shock is characterized by decreased CI and mixed venous oxygen saturation, increased SVR, right atrial and venous pressures and pulmonary artery wedge pressures, and normal peripheral vascular resistance. Management is directed at re-establishing end-organ perfusion by medical management with catecholamines, vasodilators, antiarrhythmic medications, or other drugs, and mechanical means (such as intra-aortic balloon pumps or extracorporeal membrane oxygenation [ECMO]). Treatment of the underlying cause also is needed and may include cardiac revascularization, ablation, or pacemaker placement.

The combination of increased SVR, normal PVR, decreased CI, and increased PCWP is not the best choice for the patient described above. This combination of hemodynamic parameters is most consistent with a patient in cardiogenic shock. The patient described above is not in cardiogenic shock, and this is not the best combination for her.

Hypovolemic shock results from inadequate intravascular volume, frequently from hemorrhage, but may also be caused by reduced plasma volume in the absence of bleeding (eg, fluid loss from vomiting or diarrhea), or from soft tissue trauma leading to cytokine release and loss of fluid (eg, large burns). Hypovolemic shock is characterized by decreased CI, mixed venous oxygen saturation, and right atrial and venous pressures, in addition to pulmonary artery wedge pressures, increased SVR, and normal PVR. Acute management is focused on volume resuscitation, as well as treatment of the underlying cause of intravascular volume depletion. The combination of increased SVR, normal PVR, decreased CI, and decreased PCWP is most consistent with a patient presenting with hypovolemic shock, and this is not the best choice for the patient described above.

Obstructive shock results from blockage of major blood vessels or of the cardiac chambers leading to decreased preload or increased afterload. Etiologies include pneumothorax, pericardial tamponade, compression of the vena cava, pulmonary embolism, or intracardiac masses. Obstructive shock is characterized by decreased CI, normal to increased mixed venous oxygen saturation and normal to decreased pulmonary artery wedge pressure, normal SVR, increased PVR and right atrial and venous pressures. Management is directed at relieving the obstruction with interventions such as pulmonary endarterectomy, thrombolytics, or chest tube placement. The combination of normal SVR, increased PVR, decreased CI, and normal PCWP is most consistent with a patient presenting in obstructive shock.

Adler A, Sharma R, Higgins T, McGee WT. Hemodynamic assessment and monitoring in the intensive care unit: an overview. Enliven J Anesth Crit Care Med 2014;1:1–13. doi: 10.18650/2374-4448.14010

Kashani K, Omer T, Shaw AD. The intensivist's perspective of shock, volume management, and hemodynamic monitoring. Clin J Am Soc Nephrol 2022;17:706–16. doi: 10.2215/CJN.14191021

Standl T, Annecke T, Cascorbi I, Heller AR, Sabashnikov A, Teske W. The nomenclature, definition and distinction of types of shock. Dtsch Arztebl Int 2018;115:757–68. doi: 10.3238/arztebl.2018.0757

96 Surgery for leiomyosarcoma

A 40-year-old is scheduled for a total laparoscopic hysterectomy for a uterine mass. Pelvic ultrasonography confirms that the mass has increased in size from 8 to 12 cm during the last 6 months. The growing mass is increasing the patient's symptoms of pelvic pressure and abdominal discomfort. Due to the rapid increase in size, there is concern about the possibility of leiomyosarcoma. During the hysterectomy, it is noted that the uterus is enlarged with no disease outside of the uterus. Leiomyosarcoma is confirmed intraoperatively. The best next step in surgical management is

* (A) bilateral salpingectomy
(B) bilateral salpingo-oophorectomy
(C) omentectomy
(D) pelvic lymphadenectomy
(E) peritoneal biopsies

Leiomyosarcoma (LMS) accounts for approximately 1–2% of uterine malignancy. The average age at diagnosis is 51 years, and, for reasons that are not fully understood, Black patients are diagnosed twice as frequently as white patients. Despite advances in systemic and radiation therapy, the mortality rate for patients with uterine LMS has changed little over time, with an overall 5-year survival rate of only 60% for patients with localized disease and 12% for patients with distant disease.

Leiomyosarcoma is a malignancy that originates from uterine myometrial cells and often is difficult to differentiate from benign leiomyoma preoperatively. Preoperative symptoms overlap with those caused by benign leiomyomas. Even among patients with apparent rapidly enlarging fibroids, the reported incidence of LMS is less than 1%. Although older age is associated with a higher incidence of LMS, no preoperative factors or tests have proved reliable in differentiating LMS from leiomyoma. Several retrospective cohort studies have suggested various radiologic scoring systems for differentiating leiomyomas from LMS, but these studies are generally small and lack prospective validation. A negative endometrial biopsy does not rule out LMS, but it can reveal LMS in a subset of patients in whom the tumor impinges on the endometrium.

Surgical removal of the intact tumor with complete hysterectomy is the recommended primary therapy; however, more than 50% of cases of LMS are diagnosed postoperatively, necessitating additional surgery in patients who have undergone subtotal hysterectomy or myomectomy. Because approximately 33% of patients with LMS have metastatic disease at diagnosis, evaluation with either positron emission tomography (PET) combined with computed tomography (CT) or CT evaluation of the chest, abdomen, and pelvis is recommended. Because there are many variants of sarcomas, it can be challenging to differentiate them pathologically, and expert gynecologic pathology confirmation of the diagnosis is recommended.

Recognizing that the prognostic factors for uterine sarcoma differ from those of endometrial carcinoma, the International Federation of Gynecology and Obstetrics (FIGO) introduced a separate staging system for uterine sarcomas in 2009 (Box 96-1). The FIGO system reflects the importance of tumor size in addition to extension of disease beyond the uterus.

Although the staging system includes lymph node status, in the absence of gross involvement, routine staging with pelvic or para-aortic lymphadenectomy and peritoneal biopsies and omentectomy has not been associated with improvements in survival and is not recommended. Thus, these are not best next steps for the patient in the above scenario.

Although postmenopausal patients may undergo bilateral salpingo-oophorectomy at the time of hysterectomy for presumed leiomyoma, ovarian conservation among premenopausal patients does not appear to compromise survival, and bilateral salpingo-oophorectomy is no longer considered a mandatory component of surgical management. In the scenario described above, if a leiomyosarcoma is diagnosed intraoperatively, complete hysterectomy would be adequate surgical management, and no additional surgery, such as opportunistic salpingectomy, would be required.

BOX 96-1

International Federation of Gynecology and Obstetrics (FIGO) Leiomyosarcoma Staging

I Tumor limited to uterus
- **IA** 5 cm or less
- **IB** More than 5 cm

II Tumor extends beyond the uterus, within the pelvis
- **IIA** Adnexal involvement
- **IIB** Involvement of other pelvic tissues

II Tumor invades abdominal tissues (not just protruding into the abdomen)
- **IIIA** One site
- **IIIB** More than one site
- **IIIC** Metastasis to pelvic and/or para-aortic lymph nodes

IV
- **IVA** Tumor invades bladder and/or rectum
- **IVB** Distant metastasis

For patients with disease confined to the uterus, observation is recommended because adjuvant treatment with either radiation or chemotherapy has not been shown to improve survival. In patients with advanced or recurrent disease not amenable to surgery, treatment is palliative. Anthracycline-based chemotherapy has traditionally been used but has low response rates in the 10–15% range and short duration of response. A recent trial (LMS-04) reported a response rate of 36% for doxorubicin and trabectedin, a novel alkylating agent, compared with 13% for doxorubicin alone. The improvement in progression-free survival from 6.2 months to 12.2 months make this regimen an attractive first-line treatment for patients with metastatic disease. Response rates to immune checkpoint inhibitors have been disappointing, although trials evaluating response to combinations of checkpoint inhibitors and other anti-neoplastic agents are underway.

Kapp DS, Shin JY, Chan JK. Prognostic factors and survival in 1396 patients with uterine leiomyosarcomas: emphasis on impact of lymphadenectomy and oophorectomy. Cancer 2008;112:820–30. doi: 10.1002/cncr.23245

Lacuna K, Bose S, Ingham M, Schwartz G. Therapeutic advances in leiomyosarcoma. Front Oncol 2023;13:1149106. doi: 10.3389/fonc.2023.1149106

Parker WH, Fu YS, Berek JS. Uterine sarcoma in patients operated on for presumed leiomyoma and rapidly growing leiomyoma. Obstet Gynecol 1994;83:414–8.

Pautier P, Italiano A, Piperno-Neumann S, Chevreau C, Penel N, Firmin N, et al. Doxorubicin alone versus doxorubicin with trabectedin followed by trabectedin alone as first-line therapy for metastatic or unresectable leiomyosarcoma (LMS-04): a randomised, multicentre, open-label phase 3 trial. Lancet Oncol 2022;23:1044–54. doi: 10.1016/S1470-2045(22)00380-1

Roberts ME, Aynardi JT, Chu CS. Uterine leiomyosarcoma: a review of the literature and update on management options. Gynecol Oncol 2018;151:56272. doi: 10.1016/j.ygyno.2018.09.010

97 Obstipation

A 68-year-old woman with recurrent high-grade serous ovarian cancer presents to the emergency room with severe abdominal pain, nausea, vomiting, and obstipation. She received cycle 2 of carboplatin and paclitaxel 7 days ago. She has otherwise tolerated her treatment and has an Eastern Cooperative Oncology Group performance status of 1. Her vital signs are listed in Table 97-1. A physical examination is notable for moderate abdominal distention, hyperactive bowel sounds, tympany to percussion, and tenderness to palpation in the bilateral lower quadrants. Computed tomography (CT) is shown in Figure 97-1. The best next step in management is a (an)

(A) cecostomy tube
(B) endoscopic stent
(C) enema
(D) nasogastric tube
* (E) surgical diversion

TABLE 97-1. The Described Patient's Vital Signs

Temperature	37.3 °C (99.3 °F)
Heart rate	110 beats per minute
Blood pressure	110/70 mm Hg
Respiratory rate	16 breaths per minute
Oxygen saturation on room air	97%

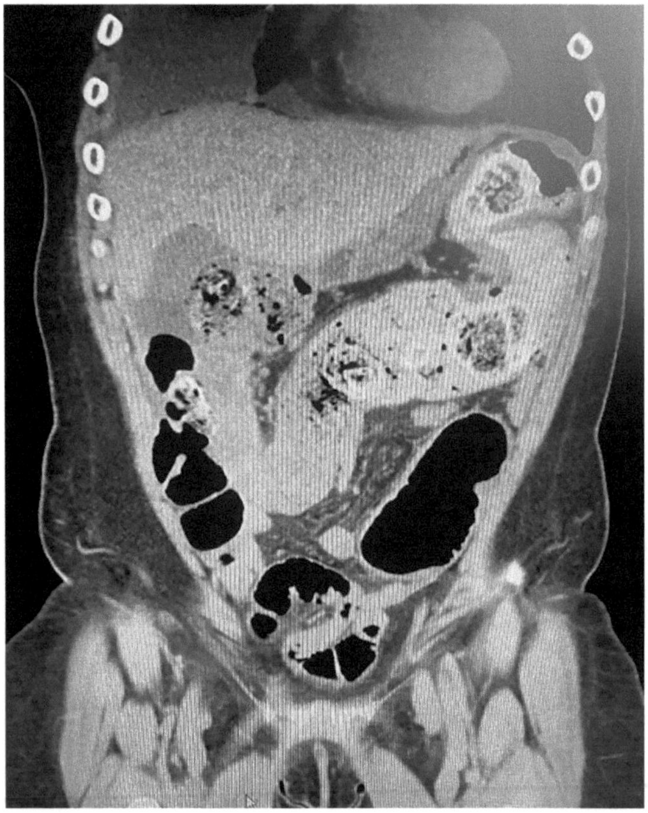

FIGURE 97-1. Patient's computed tomography.

Malignant bowel obstruction occurs in up to 50% of patients with advanced and recurrent ovarian cancer. Large-bowel obstruction constitutes approximately 25% of all intestinal obstructions, most occurring in the distal or transverse colon where the colonic lumen is smaller. Obstruction can be caused by peritoneal carcinomatosis or an intra-abdominal tumor mass. Typical management of malignant bowel obstruction is based on clinical and prognostic factors.

The patient in this scenario has a malignant large-bowel obstruction diagnosed by CT, demonstrating a collapsed rectum with a tumor surrounding the sigmoid colon. The classic patient presentation includes abdominal pain, distention, and failure to pass stool or gas. Major diagnostic findings for bowel obstruction on CT imaging include proximal dilation with distal decompression. Intestinal dilation is noted with a colon diameter greater than 6 cm and a cecal diameter greater than 9 cm.

In patients expected to live months to years, surgery, including resection, bypass, or diverting ostomy, can improve quality of life. Patients should be considered potential surgical candidates unless they are critically ill, have poor performance status or extremely limited life expectancy, or decline surgery. Because this patient has an obstruction at the rectosigmoid colon, surgical intervention and diverting ostomy would allow control of symptoms and allow her to continue chemotherapy; therefore, this is the best choice in this scenario. If the patient is able to continue chemotherapy, she could experience additional tumor response and be a candidate for reversal of the ostomy at a later date.

A venting percutaneous cecostomy tube allows for nonsurgical decompression of the gastrointestinal tract at the level of the cecum. It is an option for patients who are poor surgical candidates or have limited life expectancy. The main goal of cecostomy tube placement is to prevent bowel perforation by allowing for decompression of the colon. Placement of a cecostomy tube would allow resumption of oral intake for the patient and allow a longer-term solution for symptom management while also relieving bloating and discomfort associated with obstruction. If a patient declines surgical intervention to bypass the obstruction or is a poor surgical candidate, a venting cecostomy tube would be a long-term solution for controlling symptoms.

Colonic stents allow for short-term management of obstruction and may be used with patients who are not surgical candidates due to medical comorbidities, do not have a long-term survival estimate, or have declined surgical intervention. Colonic stents are placed endoscopically through the rectum. Long-term success of stents is limited, and up to a third of patients may require repeat intervention. Additionally, a meta-analysis comparing palliative surgery to stent placement among patients with malignant bowel obstruction found stents to be less effective at relieving obstruction. Because the patient in this scenario is early in her treatment course after recurrence of ovarian cancer and has no contraindications to surgery, the most definitive way to relieve her current symptoms while continuing chemotherapy would be through surgical colon diversion; therefore, endoscopic stent placement is not the correct answer.

Enemas often are used to treat chronic constipation or fecal impaction and should be used with caution among patients receiving chemotherapy who may be neutropenic. Liquid from an enema softens stool, can draw water to rectal tissues to help stool soften further, and by increasing pressure in the rectum, can trigger a bowel movement. The patient in this scenario has extrinsic compression of the colon, and an enema will not relieve her symptoms and may increase pain. An enema is not the recommended management.

Nasogastric (NG) tube placement is the recommended initial management for patients with a small-bowel obstruction, but it is less effective for the management of a large-bowel obstruction due to the presence of the ileocecal valve, which prevents the retrograde flow of colonic contents. Nasogastric tubes often are used for symptom control through the evacuation of gastrointestinal secretions and the reduction of nausea, vomiting, and pain. However, NG tubes may become occluded and require flushing or replacement, which may be uncomfortable for patients. When placed for long periods, the NG tube can interfere with cough reflexes, cause nasal cartilage erosion or otitis media, and place patients at risk for aspiration, esophagitis, and bleeding. Given these associated risks and lack of efficacy for the resolution of a large-bowel obstruction, NG tubes should be considered a temporizing measure in the initial evaluation and treatment of malignant large-bowel obstructions and be removed as soon as feasible. As this patient has a large-bowel obstruction, an NG tube is unlikely to cause significant improvement and provide long-term management; therefore, it is not the correct answer in this scenario.

The management of malignant large-bowel obstruction requires an individualized approach and is dependent on a patient's performance status, current disease status and prognosis, and goals of care. If a patient is willing to undergo surgery, is a reasonable surgical candidate, and is expected to live months to years, surgical diversion with ostomy formation is the best recommendation.

Cousins SE, Tempest E, Feuer DJ. Surgery for the resolution of symptoms in malignant bowel obstruction in advanced gynaecological and gastrointestinal cancer. Cochrane Database of Systematic Reviews 2016, Issue 1. Art. No.: CD002764. Doi: 10.1002/14651858.CD002764.pub2.

Jansen J, Oldenburger E, Jansen J, Wolthuis A, Van Nieuwenhuysen E, Neven P, et al. Bowel obstruction in advanced tubo-ovarian cancer: a retrospective cohort study. Ann Med Surg (Lond) 2023;85:1539–45. doi: 10.1097/MS9.0000000000000660

National Comprehensive Cancer Network. Palliative care. Version 1.2025 NCCN Clinical Practice Guidelines in Oncology [after login]. NCCN; 2024. Accessed March 13, 2025. https://www.nccn.org/professionals/physician_gls/pdf/palliative.pdf

Nelson G, Fotopoulou C, Taylor J, Glaser G, Bakkum-Gamez J, Meyer LA, et al. Enhanced recovery after surgery (ERAS®) society guidelines for gynecologic oncology: addressing implementation challenges 2023 update. Gynecol Oncol 2023;173:58–67. doi: 10.1016/j.ygyno.2023.04.009

Zhao X, Cai B, Cao R, Shi R. Palliative treatment for incurable malignant colorectal obstructions: a meta-analysis. World J Gastroenterol 2013;19:5565–74. doi: 10.3748/wjg.v19.i33.5565

98 Ovarian vein thrombosis

A 63-year-old with advanced ovarian cancer underwent complete cytoreductive surgery followed by six cycles of chemotherapy with carboplatin and paclitaxel. She presents to your office after completing chemotherapy for post-therapy computed tomography (CT). She has no bothersome symptoms, and her physical examination is unremarkable. The CT is notable for a left ovarian vein thrombosis that does not extend into the renal vein. There are no other findings and no evidence of residual malignancy. The best next step in management is

(A) antibiotics
(B) low-dose aspirin
* (C) routine ovarian cancer surveillance
(D) therapeutic anticoagulation
(E) thrombectomy

Ovarian vein thrombosis is a rare thrombotic event generally associated with the postpartum period. However, ovarian vein thrombosis also has been associated with other conditions such as pelvic inflammatory disease, inflammatory bowel disease, abdominopelvic surgery, and malignancy. Ovarian vein thrombosis outside of the puerperium is a distinct clinical entity that is managed differently than thromboses in postpartum patients.

Ovarian vein thrombosis has been associated with debulking or cytoreductive surgery for ovarian cancer. A retrospective review of patients who had undergone ovarian cancer cytoreductive surgery showed approximately 25% developed an ovarian vein thrombus postoperatively. Cytoreductive surgery for the treatment of ovarian cancer includes removal of the ovaries, and ligation of the ovarian vessels results in absent blood flow through the vessels and a high rate of thrombosis. Other contributing factors include manipulation of the vessels during surgery and the hypercoagulable state associated with malignancy and the postoperative period. Ovarian vein thrombosis in this setting is most often diagnosed incidentally on imaging for other indications because many patients are asymptomatic, as was the case with the patient in this scenario.

In most patients, thrombosis is limited to the ovarian vein without propagation into the deep veins of the abdomen, such as the inferior vena cava or left renal vein. Isolated ovarian vein thrombosis has not been shown to be associated with concurrent existence of thromboses at other sites. Furthermore, these patients are not at an increased risk for subsequent development of venous thromboembolism. Therefore, the finding of an isolated ovarian vein thrombus does not warrant treatment with anticoagulation.

If the ovarian vein thrombus extends into the renal vein or inferior vena cava at the time of diagnosis, treatment with therapeutic anticoagulation is indicated in accordance with usual practice for the treatment of deep vein thrombosis. Because the patient in this scenario has an isolated ovarian vein thrombosis without extension into the inferior vena cava or left renal vein, she does not need therapeutic anticoagulation. Low-dose aspirin often is used to prevent arterial clots that can lead to stroke and other morbidity. It also has been studied for its potential to prevent recurrent deep vein thrombosis in patients who have completed treatment for deep vein thrombosis. These scenarios do not apply to the described patient; therefore, low-dose aspirin is not the best next step for a patient with an asymptomatic ovarian vein thrombosis.

Thrombectomy is a procedure to remove or break up a clot to restore blood flow within a deep vein and is done when an occlusive deep vein thrombosis is causing severe symptoms or leading to tissue damage or patient compromise. The patient in this scenario is asymptomatic and does not have a thrombus within the larger deep veins; thus, a thrombectomy is not the best next step.

Antibiotic therapy is used in the treatment of some patients with postpartum ovarian vein thrombosis; however, the pathophysiology of peripartum ovarian vein thrombosis is distinct from that of a postoperative thrombus. Antibiotic therapy is not indicated in the treatment of postoperative ovarian vein thrombosis in patients with ovarian cancer.

Because the described patient has an asymptomatic postoperative ovarian vein thrombus that does not extend into the deep veins of the abdomen, routine ovarian cancer surveillance in accordance with usual practice is the best next step..

Cunningham FG, Leveno KJ, Dashe JS, Hoffman BL, Spong CY, Casey BM. Puerperal infection. In: Williams obstetrics, 26th ed. McGraw Hill; 2022. Accessed March 13, 2025.

Lenz CJ, Wysokinski WE, Henkin S, Cohoon KP, Casanegra A, Simmons BS, et al. Ovarian vein thrombosis: incidence of recurrent venous thromboembolism and survival. Obstet Gynecol 2017;130:1127–35. doi: 10.1097/AOG.0000000000002319

Mantha S, Sarasohn D, Ma W, Devlin SM, Chi DS, Roche KL, et al. Ovarian vein thrombosis after debulking surgery for ovarian cancer: epidemiology and clinical significance. Am J Obstet Gynecol 2015;213:208.e1–4. doi: 10.1016/j.ajog.2015.02.028

99 Uterine bleeding in patients receiving cancer treatment

A 15-year-old adolescent with Hodgkin lymphoma who is undergoing chemotherapy presents to the emergency department with acute-onset heavy vaginal bleeding. She has a history of a deep venous thrombosis while using the birth control patch last year and is not on anticoagulation currently. On examination, her blood pressure is 100/60 mm Hg, and her pulse is 102 beats per minute. She is pale but otherwise in no acute distress. A pelvic examination is notable for active bleeding from the cervical os. Her hemoglobin is 6.8 g/dL, and a urine pregnancy test is negative. In addition to intravenous (IV) fluid resuscitation and blood transfusion, the best next step in treatment is

(A) depot leuprolide acetate
(B) dilation and curettage
(C) intravenous estrogen
(D) levonorgestrel-releasing intrauterine device (LNG-IUD)
* (E) oral progestin

Approximately 4% of all new cancer diagnoses are among female and male adolescents and young adults, including individuals aged 15–39 years. This timeframe represents a major component of reproductive life, and it is likely that female patients will menstruate during treatment. Patients undergoing cancer treatment, particularly those with hematologic malignancies, are at risk of abnormal bleeding due to adverse effects from treatment of the underlying disease. Female adolescents and young women with cancer may benefit from menstrual suppression, which can reduce the risk of clinically significant bleeding, but they may also need treatment for acute vaginal bleeding during their disease course. Various treatment options exist for management of acute bleeding and must be tailored to the specific clinical scenario (Fig. 99-1).

The patient in the above scenario presented with acute vaginal bleeding in the context of treatment for a hematologic malignancy. First-line treatment includes resuscitation and medical treatment. Either IV estrogen or oral progestin can be administered for rapid cessation of bleeding. Given this patient's history of venous thromboembolism while using combined hormonal contraception, estrogen should be avoided, and oral progestin therapy is the best next step. This approach can be used as a bridge to longer-term menstrual suppression. One option for treatment is medroxyprogesterone acetate 60–80 mg twice daily until cessation of bleeding, then 10 mg every 4–6 hours as tolerated based on bleeding symptoms. Adding estrogen can further increase the risk of venous thromboembolism; however, if the patient's bleeding does not respond to oral progestin therapy, reassessment of the risks and benefits of short-term intravenous estrogen therapy should be considered for management of acute bleeding. Importantly, oral progestins used for the management of acute bleeding do not function as contraception.

Depot leuprolide acetate is effective in suppressing menstruation in individuals undergoing treatment for malignancies, particularly in those in whom thrombocytopenia is anticipated around the time of menstruation. This treatment is effective in creating amenorrhea and does not increase the risk of venous thromboembolism. However, initiation of this method of menstrual suppression can lead to a "flare" response in which patients may have increased bleeding initially. This intervention is more effective for menstrual suppression rather than treatment of acute bleeding, and is not the best next step. Additionally, depot leuprolide acetate is not effective for contraception. Data regarding the utility of depot leuprolide acetate for ovarian protection during chemotherapy are mixed, and its use is controversial for this purpose.

Dilation and curettage is an effective method to treat acute heavy bleeding that does not respond to medical therapies, as is in patients who are not clinically stable. This patient is clinically stable and is a candidate for medical therapy; therefore, dilation and curettage is not the recommended first-line treatment. Given her age and concurrent medical conditions, it is unlikely that her bleeding is due to a structural cause; however, dilation and curettage can control acute heavy bleeding that does not respond to initial medical therapy or progresses to life-threatening bleeding. Preoperative ultrasonography can be considered if the bleeding does not respond to initial medical therapy. Curettage can be performed with suction evacuation or with sharp curettage. If heavy bleeding persists, an intrauterine Foley balloon can be placed to provide tamponade as a temporary bridge to other forms of menstrual suppression and further resuscitation. Surgical management should be paired with discussion of options for menstrual suppression to avoid the need for repeated procedures.

Levonorgestrel-releasing intrauterine device placement is not recommended for management of acute bleeding. Although these devices can lead to menstrual suppression and amenorrhea, this effect is typically delayed for weeks to months after placement. If a patient requires dilation and curettage for management of acute bleeding, concurrent placement of an LNG-IUD for menstrual suppression can occur at the time of

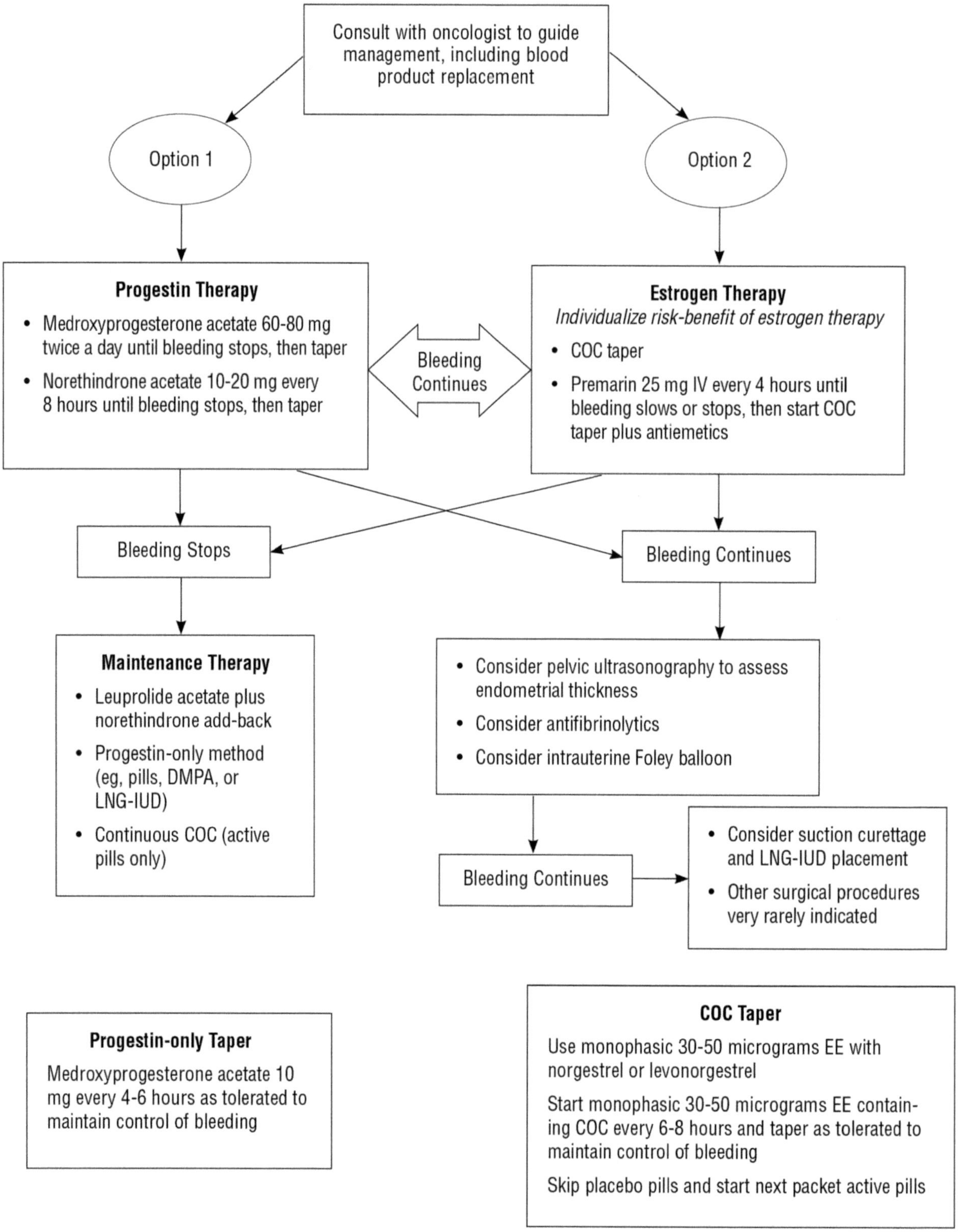

FIGURE 99-1. Emergent treatment for acute heavy uterine bleeding in adolescents with cancer. Abbreviations: COC, combined oral contraceptive; DMPA, depot medroxyprogesterone acetate; EE, ethinyl estradiol; IV, intravenous; LNG-IUD, levonorgestrel-releasing intrauterine device. (Reprinted from Options for prevention and management of menstrual bleeding in adolescent patients undergoing cancer treatment. ACOG Committee Opinion No. 817. American College of Obstetricians & Gynecologists [published erratum appears in Obstet Gynecol 2022;140:344]. Obstet Gynecol 2021;137:e7–15. doi: 10.1097/AOG.0000000000004209)

surgery. Preoperative counseling should include discussion of the increased risk of IUD expulsion when the device is placed during an acute bleeding episode.

Adolescents and young adults with cancer may present with acute vaginal bleeding during the course of their care. Medical therapy is typically considered first line, and the best initial approach depends on the patient's characteristics and presentation. Due to the increased risk of comorbid conditions related to cancer or cancer treatment, such as thrombosis risk, the patient's individual risks should be considered when choosing a medical therapy. Surgical intervention is occasionally needed as a bridge to longer-term menstrual suppression to attempt to avoid recurrence of acute bleeding. In addition to menstrual suppression, an assessment of contraceptive use is appropriate in the context of the treatment provided.

Cancer and Contraception. Society of Family Planning Guideline 20121. Society of Family Planning. Contraception 2012;86(3): 191-198. doi: 10.1016/j.contraception.2012.05.008

Fertility preservation in patients undergoing gonadotoxic therapy or gonadectomy: a committee opinion. Practice Committee of the American Society for Reproductive Medicine. Fertil Steril 2019;112:1022–33. doi: 10.1016/j.fertnstert.2019.09.013

Gynecologic issues in children and adolescent cancer patients and survivors. ACOG Committee Opinion No. 747. American College of Obstetricians and Gynecologists. Obstet Gynecol 2018;132:e67–77. doi: 10.1097/AOG.0000000000002763

Nguyen AT, Curtis KM, Tepper NK, Kortsmit K, Brittain AW, Snyder EM, et al. US medical eligibility criteria for contraceptive use, 2024. MMWR Recomm Rep 2024;73(RR-4):1–126. doi: 10.15585/mmwr.rr7304a1

Options for prevention and management of menstrual bleeding in adolescent patients undergoing cancer treatment. ACOG Committee Opinion No. 817. American College of Obstetricians and Gynecologists [published erratum appears in Obstet Gynecol 2022;140:344]. Obstet Gynecol 2021;137:e7–15. doi: 10.1097/AOG.0000000000004209

Patel A, Schwarz EB. Cancer and contraception. SFP Guideline #20121. Society of Family Planning. Contraception 2012;86:191–8. doi: 10.1016/j.contraception.2012.05.008

Screening and management of bleeding disorders in adolescents with heavy menstrual bleeding. ACOG Committee Opinion No. 785. American College of Obstetricians and Gynecologists. Obstet Gynecol 2019;134:e71–83. doi: 10.1097/AOG.0000000000003411

100 Vaginal dysplasia

A 46-year-old gravida 4, para 4, underwent a total laparoscopic hysterectomy for abnormal uterine bleeding. Pathology was notable for benign uterine fibroids. Her cervical cancer screening was up to date at the time of surgery, and she does not have a history of cervical dysplasia. Two years after the hysterectomy, her primary care doctor performs cervical cytology with human papillomavirus (HPV) testing. The results indicate low-grade squamous intraepithelial lesion (LSIL) and return positive for high-risk HPV type. Her pelvic examination reveals a normal-appearing, well-healed vaginal cuff. The best next step in management is

(A) HPV vaccination
(B) laser ablation of vaginal cuff
* (C) repeat vaginal cytology and HPV co-testing in 1 year
(D) vaginal colposcopy

Hysterectomy for benign indications is one of the most common procedures performed on reproductive-aged women in the United States. After a total hysterectomy, if a patient has had appropriate cervical cancer screening with no history of moderate-severe cervical dysplasia (cervical intraepithelial neoplasia 2+ [CIN 2+]) in the last 25 years and no additional risk factors, they can defer any further cervical cancer screening.

The patient in this scenario has had routine cervical cancer screening with no history of CIN 2+ and underwent a benign total hysterectomy; therefore, she does not qualify for continued cervical cytology testing or HPV testing. For patients who have not been appropriately screened and have abnormalities on their vaginal cytology or HPV testing, guidance on how to proceed is available. According to the American College of Obstetricians & Gynecologists (ACOG), women who have had a hysterectomy without a history of cervical cancer or cervical changes do not need cancer screening of the vaginal cuff. However, women who have had a hysterectomy to treat cervical cancer or moderate to severe cervical changes should continue screening for 20 years after the surgery. The described patient was inappropriately screened after hysterectomy, and abnormalities are detected on the screening tests; therefore, reassurance only with routine care is not an appropriate option at this point. In this situation, LSIL on vaginal cytology with high-risk HPV positivity warrants repeat cytology in 1 year (repeated again in 1 year) or repeat co-testing in 1 year. If abnormalities persist or cytology indicates disease more severe than LSIL, a vaginal colposcopy is recommended (Table 100-1).

Human papillomavirus vaccination would not be considered for a patient who is 46 years old (outside the approved age range of 9–45 years). The recommended age range for vaccination is 9–26 years; however, some women aged 27–45 years

TABLE 100-1. U.S. Preventive Services Task Force Recommendations for Routine Cervical Cancer Screening

POPULATION*	RECOMMENDATION	USPSTF RECOMMENDATION GRADE
Aged less than 21 years	No screening	D
Aged 21–29 years	Cytology alone every 3 years	A
Aged 30–65 years	Any one of the following: Cytology alone every 3 years FDA-approved primary hrHPV testing alone every 5 years Cotesting (hrHPV testing and cytology) every 5 years	A
Aged greater than 65 years	No screening after adequate negative prior screening results	D
Hysterectomy with removal of the cervix	No screening in individuals who do not have a history of high-grade cervical precancerous lesions or cervical cancer	D

Abbreviations: FDA, U.S. Food and Drug Administration; hrHPV, high-risk human papillomavirus testing.

*These recommendations apply to individuals with a cervix who do not have signs or symptoms of cervical cancer, regardless of their sexual history or HPV vaccination status. These recommendations do not apply to individuals who are at high risk of the disease, such as those who have previously received a diagnosis of a high-grade precancerous cervical lesion. These recommendations also do not apply to individuals with in utero exposure to diethylstilbestrol or those who have a compromised immune system (eg, individuals with human immunodeficiency virus).

Reprinted from American College of Obstetricians and Gynecologists. Updated cervical cancer screening guidelines. Practice Advisory. ACOG; 2021. Accessed February 24, 2025.

who are previously unvaccinated may use shared clinical decision making with their gynecologist to decide whether to have the vaccination.

Laser ablation of the vaginal cuff is not indicated in the absence of vaginal intraepithelial neoplasia (VaIN). The patient in this scenario has a normal-appearing vaginal cuff, but if an abnormality is found, it should be biopsied. Treatments for vaginal dysplasia include laser ablation, excision, or topical therapies (including 5-fluorouracil, imiquimod, or trichloroacetic acid). Vaginal estrogen can be considered in cases of atrophy that cause persistent low-grade cytology changes that are not associated with HPV-related pathology.

This patient should not undergo immediate vaginal colposcopy because no abnormality is visible on speculum examination. If a gross abnormality is found, it should be biopsied regardless of cytologic and HPV test results. If abnormalities on cytology or HPV testing persist (any cytologic abnormality or persistent HPV positivity) on repeat testing, a vaginal colposcopy should be performed. If the initial cytology reveals high-grade abnormalities or atypical glandular cells, an immediate vaginal colposcopy is indicated.

The incidence of vaginal cancer is significantly lower than cervical cancer, and it is important not to overscreen patients who are not at high risk. Established management algorithms (Fig. 100-1) should be followed for patients who are inappropriately screened after total hysterectomy, and vaginal colposcopy should be performed if indicated.

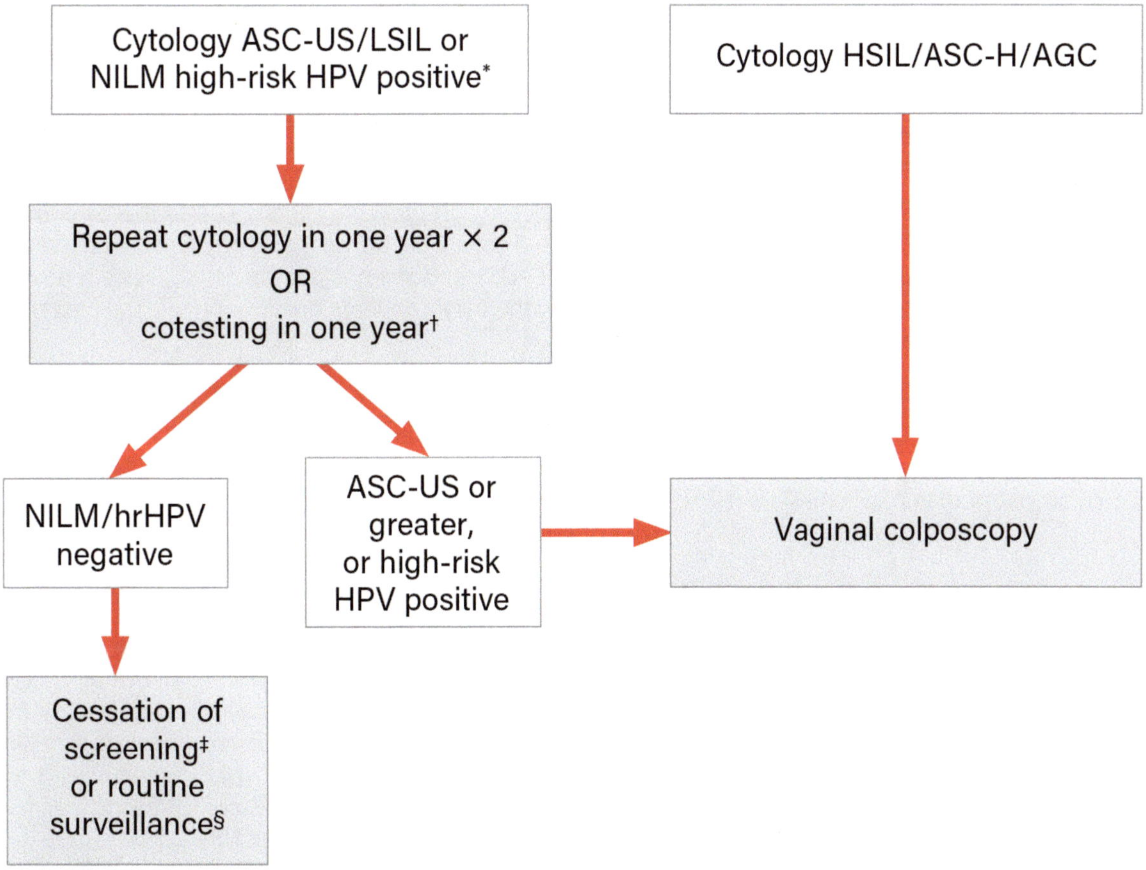

FIGURE 100-1. Proposed management for abnormal vaginal cancer screening tests in women with a history of hysterectomy. Abbreviations: ASC-US, atypical squamous cells of undetermined significance; LSIL, low-grade squamous intraepithelial lesion; HSIL, high-grade squamous intraepithelial lesion; ASC-H, atypical squamous cells cannot rule out high-grade; AGC, atypical glandular cells; NILM, negative for intraepithelial lesion or malignancy. (Reprinted from Khan MJ, Massad LS, Kinney W, Gold MA, Mayeaux EJ Jr, Darragh TM, et al. A common clinical dilemma: management of abnormal vaginal cytology and human papillomavirus test results. Gynecol Oncol 2016;141:364–70. doi: 10.1016/j.ygyno.2015.11.023)

American College of Obstetricians and Gynecologists. Updated cervical cancer screening guidelines. Practice Advisory. ACOG; 2021. Accessed February 24, 2025.

Human papillomavirus vaccination. ACOG Committee Opinion No. 809. American College of Obstetricians and Gynecologists. Obstet Gynecol 2020;136:e15–21. doi: 10.1097/AOG.0000000000004000

Khan MJ, Massad LS, Kinney W, Gold MA, Mayeaux EJ Jr, Darragh TM, et al. A common clinical dilemma: management of abnormal vaginal cytology and human papillomavirus test results. Gynecol Oncol 2016;141:364–70. doi: 10.1016/j.ygyno.2015.11.023

Perkins RB, Guido RS, Castle PE, Chelmow D, Einstein MH, Garcia F, et al. 2019 ASCCP risk-based management consensus guidelines for abnormal cervical cancer screening tests and cancer precursors. 2019 ASCCP Risk-Based Management Consensus Guidelines Committee [published erratum appears in J Low Genit Tract Dis 2020;24:427]. J Low Genit Tract Dis 2020;24:102–31. doi: 10.1097/LGT.0000000000000525

101 Cervical cancer screening

A 40-year-old patient has a history of a loop electrosurgical excision procedure (LEEP) performed 8 years ago for the treatment of cervical intraepithelial neoplasia 2–3 (CIN 2-3). Cervical cytology 5 years ago showed atypical squamous cells of undetermined significance (ASC-US), and she has had no testing since then. Her physical examination is notable for vaginal candidiasis, but the cervix appears grossly normal. The best next step for cervical cancer screening is

(A) colposcopy
(B) cytology
(C) endocervical curettage (ECC)
* (D) high-risk human papillomavirus (HPV)-based testing

The recognition that HPV is the causative agent for 98–99% of cervical carcinomas has led to the incorporation of HPV testing into cervical cancer screening, first as a triage test for minor cytologic abnormalities, and later in conjunction with cytology and as stand-alone screening. Evolving national cervical cancer screening guidelines are increasingly recommending primary HPV testing. Because the lead time from HPV infection to development of cancer is estimated to be at least 10 years, a negative HPV test confers reassurance for a longer period of time, allowing screening intervals using HPV to be extended compared to cytology. Primary HPV testing is noninferior to co-testing (simultaneous cytology and HPV testing) and less costly. Although cytology every 3 years is considered acceptable for patients aged 30–65, multiple clinical trials have demonstrated that HPV testing provides 60–70% greater protection against cervical cancer. The retention of cytology as an option is in recognition that some practice settings may not be resourced to provide HPV testing.

The described patient is 5 years from her last screening by cytology and is overdue for follow-up screening. Although cervical cytology alone or as part of co-testing is a screening option, the presence of vaginal candida increases the likelihood of a false-positive cytologic result, most commonly ASC-US. Screening methods using cervical cytology are not optimal for this patient; therefore, primary HPV testing is the best screening method in this scenario and is the best next step for her.

Whereas HPV-based screening methods are more sensitive than cytology for detection of CIN 3, they are not necessarily more specific, and most patients who test positive for high-risk HPV will not have CIN 3. Referral of all patients testing positive for HPV to colposcopy would result in excessive harms in the form of patient anxiety, discomfort, and potential overtreatment of less severe lesions that would otherwise regress, including cervical excisions that are associated with an increased likelihood of obstetric complications. A means of effective triage to colposcopy is needed to mitigate potential harms of HPV-based screening. Colposcopy is recommended for individuals whose estimated risk of CIN 3 is 4% or greater.

Currently, there are three HPV assays that are U.S. Food and Drug Administration-approved for use in primary screening, all of which identify HPV types 16 and 18 separately from the other 12 high-risk types. Patients testing positive for HPV 16 and 18 should undergo colposcopy because the risk of CIN 3 associated with these types is sufficiently high, whereas additional triage to colposcopy is needed for patients testing positive for the 12 other high-risk HPV types.

In addition to the identification of HPV types 16 and 18 (limited genotyping), there are three tools available to assist with triage of patients testing positive for one or more of the 12 other high-risk HPV types: cytology, dual stain, and extended genotyping. If using cytology, patients with ASC-US or worse are usually directed to colposcopy. An alternative to cytology is dual stain, an immunohistochemical stain for p16 and Ki-67 proteins. Dual stain has been shown in several studies to be more sensitive and specific than cytology in identifying patients with CIN 3. The tumor suppressor protein p16 is upregulated in cells in which normal mechanisms of cell cycle regulation have been disrupted, whereas Ki-67 is expressed in dividing cells. Cells expressing both p16 and Ki-67 expression (dual-stain-positive cells) have been transformed by HPV and are dividing. If using dual stain, patients testing positive are directed to colposcopy. Extended genotyping refers to HPV tests that identify types other than 16, 18, and 45, either individually or in groups. Currently, extended genotyping has the potential to change management if the test identifies HPV types 56, 59, 66, either alone or in combination, and no other high-risk types, because 56, 59, and 66 are associated with very low risk. In this situation, patients can return in 1 year for repeat HPV testing without additional triage testing provided concurrent cytology. Management guidelines will continue to evolve as triage testing strategies provide more precise risk estimates.

The patient described requires screening and potentially additional triage testing to determine whether colposcopy is warranted; therefore, colposcopy at this time is not the best next step for this patient.

Endocervical curettage is not used for routine screening. It is used to evaluate the cervical canal at the time of colposcopy or for surveillance to detect glandular dysplasia in patients with a history of endocervical dysplasia, such as adenocarcinoma in situ. Neither of these situations applies to this patient at this time.

Curry SJ, Krist AH, Owens DK, Barry MJ, Caughey AB, Davidson KW, et al. Screening for cervical cancer: US Preventive Services Task Force recommendation statement. US Preventive Services Task Force. JAMA 2018;320:674–86. doi: 10.1001/jama.2018.10897

Fontham ET, Wolf AM, Church TR, Etzioni R, Flowers CR, Herzig A, et al. Cervical cancer screening for individuals at average risk: 2020 guideline update from the American Cancer Society. CA Cancer J Clin 2020;70:321–46. doi: 10.3322/caac.21628

Gage JC, Schiffman M, Katki HA, Castle PE, Fetterman B, Wentzensen N, et al. Reassurance against future risk of precancer and cancer conferred by a negative human papillomavirus test. J Natl Cancer Inst 2014;106:dju153. doi: 10.1093/jnci/dju153

Perkins RB, Guido RS, Castle PE, Chelmow D, Einstein MH, Garcia F, et al. 2019 ASCCP risk-based management consensus guidelines: updates through 2023. J Low Genit Tract Dis 2024;28:3–6. doi: 10.1097/LGT.0000000000000788

102 Low-grade serous ovarian cancer

A 23-year-old underwent a diagnostic laparoscopy with unilateral salpingo-oophorectomy, omentectomy, and drainage of ascites. Her final pathology was notable for stage IIIC low-grade serous ovarian cancer. Next-generation sequencing is notable for a *BRAF* v600e mutation. Postoperatively, she received chemotherapy with carboplatin and paclitaxel. Before cycle 4 of chemotherapy, she presented with worsening abdominal distension and decreased breath sounds bilaterally. Computed tomography of the chest, abdomen, and pelvis demonstrated bilateral pleural effusions, ascites, and multiple peritoneal implants. The best next step in her treatment is to

(A) add bevacizumab to chemotherapy
(B) begin an aromatase inhibitor
(C) continue paclitaxel and carboplatin
* (D) initiate molecular targeted therapy
(E) perform secondary cytoreduction

For epithelial ovarian cancer, histology can be used to predict the response to treatment and outcomes. Of the various epithelial subtypes, ovarian carcinosarcoma, clear cell, mucinous, or low-grade serous endometrioid can be particularly difficult to treat. Less than 10% of ovarian cancer is low grade. Low-grade serous ovarian cancer typically occurs in younger patients and has longer survival rates because of its frequent presentation at an early stage and the more indolent nature of the cancer. These tumors are very unlikely to be related to germline *BRCA* mutations. Unlike high-grade serous cancer, which commonly has mutations in p53, low-grade serous cancer is more likely to have *KRAS* or *BRAF* mutations. These differences support consideration for different treatment approaches to these distinct cancer subtypes.

Until recently, the same primary treatment was used for high-grade and low-grade serous ovarian cancer. The response to carboplatin and paclitaxel in the low-grade serous subtypes has been described to be far less than the 80% response rate in high-grade serous tumors. Thus, alternatives to traditional platinum-doublet therapy are needed. In the setting of recurrent cancer, the anti-angiogenic agent bevacizumab has been explored retrospectively and has demonstrated some activity; however, this effect needs to be confirmed in patients with a new diagnosis who are treatment naive.

Low-grade serous tumors have strong estrogen receptor positivity. For this reason, endocrine therapy, such as the aromatase inhibitor letrozole, often is used as maintenance therapy after completion of cytotoxic chemotherapy. This therapy is based on retrospective analyses that have shown improvements in progression-free survival and overall survival with maintenance endocrine therapy. A phase III noninferiority trial of frontline and maintenance letrozole compared with carboplatin and paclitaxel chemotherapy followed by letrozole maintenance therapy for stage II–IV low-grade serous carcinoma postsurgical cytoreduction is currently ongoing. At this time, the use of aromatase inhibitors is not the best choice of treatment for this patient.

Secondary cytoreduction can be considered in patients with low-grade serous ovarian cancer. In fact, frequently, a surgical debulking attempt is the best next step for these patients because of the lack of effective systemic therapies. Although cytoreductive surgery can be considered for disease that is resectable, multifocal disease, including disease in the chest and peritoneal carcinomatosis, is unlikely to benefit from a surgical approach without systemic therapy. Multifocal disease recurrence and pleural effusions eliminate cytoreductive surgery as the best next step, especially in a patient with biomarker status (such as a *BRAF* mutation) that would allow for treatment with targeted therapies.

Targeted molecular therapies, which are geared toward specific proliferation pathways in these tumors, are promising treatment options for this type of ovarian cancer. This is especially true if the disease is refractory to traditional chemotherapy. Targeted molecular therapies that have been described include MEK inhibitors, BRAF inhibitors, mTOR inhibitors, and CDK 4/6 inhibitors. In treatment-refractory patients, these targeted therapies currently play an important role. In patients with low-grade serous ovarian cancer, up to 20% carry a BRAF v600e mutation. Both BRAF and MEK are involved in the mitogen-activated protein kinase (MAPK) pathway, and BRAF and MEK inhibitors are now used to treat low-grade serous ovarian cancer in patients with these biomarkers. A phase II/III trial by the Gynecologic Oncology Group found a 52% reduction in the risk of progression or death with the use of a MEK inhibitor compared with physician-choice chemotherapy in recurrent or progressed disease after platinum-based chemotherapy. In addition, BRAF inhibitors also have demonstrated efficacy in this patient population. Further research will indicate whether MEK and BRAF inhibitors should be used together to treat recurrent disease. Currently, the U.S. Food and Drug Administration has approved BRAF inhibitors for use in patients with low-grade serous ovarian cancer who harbor a BRAF v600e mutation. Targeted molecular therapy, such as a BRAF inhibitor, is the best next step for this patient with platinum-refractory low-grade disease.

Low-grade serous ovarian cancer is a rare subtype. It is clear that the biology of these tumors differs greatly from the traditional high-grade types. Alternatives to the standard platinum-taxane approach have been explored and appear promising either in combination or as maintenance.

Cobb L, Gershenson D. Novel therapeutics in low-grade serous ovarian cancer. Int J Gynecol Cancer 2023;33:377–84. doi: 10.1136/ijgc-2022-003677

Grisham RN, Slomovitz BM, Andrews N, Banerjee S, Brown J, Carey MS, et al. Low-grade serous ovarian cancer: expert consensus report on the state of the science. Int J Gynecol Cancer 2023;33:1331–44. doi: 10.1136/ijgc-2023-004610

Slomovitz B, Gourley C, Carey MS, Malpica A, Shih I, Huntsman D, et al. Low-grade serous ovarian cancer: state of the science. Gynecol Oncol 2020;156:715–25. doi: 10.1016/j.ygyno.2019.12.033

Westin SN, Wong KK, Gershenson DM. Low-grade serous ovarian cancer: expert consensus report on the state of the science. Int J Gynecol Cancer. 2023 Sep 4;33(9):1331–1344. doi: 10.1136/ijgc-2023-004610.

103 Maintenance therapy in ovarian cancer

A 55-year-old patient underwent a genomic evaluation that revealed a somatic *BRCA2*. After primary optimal debulking surgery for stage IIIC high-grade serous ovarian cancer, she completed six cycles of carboplatin and paclitaxel chemotherapy. Computed tomography after cycle 6 revealed no evidence of disease. The best agent for maintenance therapy is

(A) bevacizumab
(B) mirvetuximab
* (C) olaparib
(D) pazopanib
(E) pembrolizumab

At diagnosis, approximately 50% of patients with epithelial ovarian cancer exhibit a deficiency in repairing double-strand DNA breaks due to alterations in homologous recombination repair pathway genes. The most prominent deficiencies are *BRCA* mutations. In epithelial ovarian cancer, germline *BRCA* mutations (present in every cell of the body and passed from generation to generation) are identified in up to 15% of cases and somatic mutations (limited to the tumor and not heritable) are present in up to 10% of patients. Poly(ADP-ribose) polymerase (PARP) inhibitors trap enzymes PARP1 and PARP2 on DNA, leading to PARP–DNA complexes. Formation of these complexes inhibits DNA single-strand break repairs, which results in cell death. Poly(ADP-ribose) polymerase inhibitors work particularly well in cells with *BRCA* mutations or other homologous repair deficiencies because as unrepaired single-strand breaks accumulate the DNA replication fork collapses causing double-strand breaks. Inability of these cells to repair double-strand breaks enhances cell death; this strategy is called *synthetic lethality*. Once ovarian pathology is confirmed at diagnosis, patients should be referred for genetic risk evaluation and counseling regarding genetic testing as these results can inform maintenance therapy after primary therapy to delay the progression or relapse of disease. Approximately 80% of patients with ovarian cancer will have a complete disease response to frontline therapy; however, many patients will relapse within 5 years of primary therapy. The goal of maintenance therapy is to delay or prevent recurrence.

Poly(ADP-ribose) polymerase inhibitors inhibitor maintenance therapy should be considered for patients with stage III–IV epithelial ovarian cancer who have a partial or complete disease response to frontline platinum-based chemotherapy. Olaparib was the first PARP inhibitor to be approved as frontline maintenance monotherapy in the United States for patients with *BRCA* mutations or *BRCA*-mutated tumors based on the results of the phase III SOLO1 trial. Among patients with germline or somatic *BRCA* mutations, a statistically significant improvement in progression-free survival was observed with olaparib maintenance compared with placebo (median not reached versus 13.8 months). At 3 years of follow-up, 60% of patients in the olaparib group versus 27% in the placebo group remained disease free.

Use of PARP inhibitors for first-line maintenance therapy is now considered a standard of care among patients with *BRCA*-mutated ovarian cancer. Olaparib also is U.S. Food and Drug Administration (FDA) approved in combination with bevacizumab for frontline maintenance therapy for homologous repair-deficient tumors demonstrating response to first-line chemotherapy with bevacizumab; this patient did not receive bevacizumab therapy, so single-agent olaparib maintenance is the correct choice. Niraparib is another PARP inhibitor that is FDA approved for first-line maintenance therapy irrespective of *BRCA* or homologous repair deficiency status, although the PRIMA trial showed the greatest progression-free survival benefit for *BRCA*-mutated tumors followed by homologous repair-deficient tumors, and the least benefit for non-*BRCA*, non-homologous repair-deficient tumors. Of the choices listed, olaparib is the only medication that is a PARP inhibitor, and this is the best next step in treatment.

Bevacizumab is a vascular endothelial growth factor inhibitor and was approved in 2018 by the FDA for use in combination with carboplatin and paclitaxel followed by bevacizumab maintenance therapy. The Gynecologic Oncology Group (GOG) study 218 noted a 3-month improvement in progression-free survival in patients who received bevacizumab plus chemotherapy followed by maintenance bevacizumab compared to chemotherapy alone. This patient did not receive bevacizumab with primary therapy, and the addition of bevacizumab as maintenance therapy alone has not been studied in a randomized controlled trial. Furthermore, with the development of PARP inhibitors, bevacizumab monotherapy is no longer favored for patients with homologous recombination-deficient tumors but can be used for primary maintenance therapy in combination with olaparib in this setting.

Mirvetuximab soravtansine is an antibody–drug conjugate targeting folate receptor α. It has been FDA approved for use in patients with recurrent platinum-resistant ovarian cancer that is folate receptor α positive. For this patient, who has just completed primary platinum-based chemotherapy and has no evidence of disease, mirvetuximab is not the best next therapy.

Pazopanib is a tyrosine kinase inhibitor. A randomized phase III trial showed improved progression-free survival with pazopanib compared with placebo as first-line maintenance therapy; however, there was no increase in overall survival and the safety profile was concerning. Patients noted poorer quality of life, often due to persistent diarrhea. It was previously recommended as an option for patients with stage II–IV disease after complete disease response to first-line chemotherapy but is no longer recommended given the availability of better drug options and it is not the best next step.

Pembrolizumab targets and blocks programmed death-ligand 1 (PD-L1) on the surface of T cells. Among patients with recurrent ovarian cancer, pembrolizumab monotherapy has been associated with only modest antitumor activity, and studies are ongoing to improve ovarian cancer response to checkpoint inhibition. Pembrolizumab has shown tumor response and favorable progression-free survival benefit in combination with other chemotherapeutic agents in the recurrent setting, but is not currently used for primary maintenance therapy; clinical trials of anti-PD-L1 therapy in combination with chemotherapy followed by anti-PD-L1 maintenance therapy in the first-line setting are ongoing; therefore, pembrolizumab is not the best next treatment option for this patient.

Matulonis UA, Shapira R, Santin A, Lisyanskaya AS, Pignata S, Vergote I, et al. Final results from the KEYNOTE-100 trial of pembrolizumab in patients with advanced recurrent ovarian cancer. JCO 2020;38(suppl):6005. doi: 10.1200/JCO.2020.38.15_suppl.6005

Nag S, Aggarwal S, Rauthan A, Warrier N. Maintenance therapy for newly diagnosed epithelial ovarian cancer- a review. J Ovarian Res 2022;15:88–1. doi: 10.1186/s13048-022-01020-1

National Comprehensive Cancer Network. Ovarian cancer including fallopian tube cancer and primary peritoneal cancer. Version 1.2025 NCCN Clinical Practice Guidelines in Oncology. NCCN; 2025. Accessed March 25, 2025. https://www.nccn.org/professionals/physician_gls/pdf/ovarian.pdf

Nishio S, Matsumoto K, Takehara K, Kawamura N, Hasegawa K, Takeshima N, et al. Pembrolizumab monotherapy in Japanese patients with advanced ovarian cancer: subgroup analysis from the KEYNOTE-100. Cancer Sci 2020;111:1324–32. doi: 10.1111/cas.14340

Tew WP, Lacchetti C, Kohn EC. Poly (ADP-Ribose) polymerase inhibitors in the management of ovarian cancer: ASCO guideline rapid recommendation update. PARP Inhibitors in the Management of Ovarian Cancer Guideline Expert Panel. J Clin Oncol 2022;40:3878–81. doi: 10.1200/JCO.22.01934

104 Microinvasive cervical cancer

A 28-year-old nulligravida receives a diagnosis of cervical adenocarcinoma on biopsy during colposcopy. There is no visible lesion on her physical examination. Cervical cold knife conization is performed, and the result is notable for a 4-mm grade 1 cervical adenocarcinoma with 4-mm depth of invasion, negative lymphovascular space invasion (LVSI), 2-mm negative surgical margins, and benign endocervical curettage. Computed tomography and surgical lymph node assessment are negative for metastatic disease. The patient was undergoing a fertility evaluation before her colposcopy, and she wants to retain her ability to have children. The best next step in management is

* (A) cervical cancer surveillance
(B) radical trachelectomy
(C) repeat cold knife conization
(D) total hysterectomy

Cancer of the cervix is the third most common gynecologic malignancy in the United States and is a significant cause of morbidity and mortality worldwide, with more than 85% of cases occurring in developing countries. The prognosis is favorable when patients are diagnosed with stage I disease, with 5-year survival rates more than 90%. This patient has an International Federation of Gynecology and Obstetrics (FIGO) 2018 stage IA2 low-grade cervical adenocarcinoma (Appendix G), which has been completely excised with negative surgical margins.

Fertility preservation can be an option for patients with tumors sized 2 cm or less who meet additional criteria. Lymph node assessment is recommended in all patients with greater than stage IA1 disease. The patient in the scenario above underwent lymph node assessment, which yielded no metastatic disease. She fulfills standards for fertility-sparing treatment: low-grade squamous cell or adenocarcinoma, lack of LVSI, negative conization margins, tumor size of 2 cm or less, and negative imaging for deep invasion or metastatic disease. Recent studies have suggested that less radical procedures (conization or extrafascial hysterectomy with lymph node assessment) can be performed with reduced morbidity and fewer detrimental effects on future pregnancies. Because of these factors and in accordance with the National Comprehensive Cancer Network Guidelines, the best next step in management is cervical cancer surveillance. The Society of Gynecologic Oncology surveillance guidelines for cervical cancer include office visits every 3–6 months for review of symptoms, a pelvic examination, and cytologic screening if indicated.

Repeat cold knife conization or trachelectomy is indicated when a patient does not desire future fertility, but the surgical margins were positive in the initial procedure (stage IA1–IA2), including some stage IB1 if LVSI is negative. Negative margins are considered at least 1 mm in a nonfragmented specimen with no invasive cancer or high-grade dysplasia. Endocervical curettage should be performed with conization procedures and used as additional information about margin status, except during pregnancy. In the Prospective Trial of Conservative Surgery for Low-risk Early-stage Cervical Cancer (ConCerv), follow-up after cervical conization was performed every 3 months for 2 years after treatment with pelvic examination and cytology, then followed per standard cervical cancer guidelines. Radical trachelectomy is an option in early-stage squamous cell or adenocarcinoma with LVSI (stage IA1 or IA2) or those with smaller visible tumors limited to the cervix (stage IB1). This patient did not have LVSI, but if she did, a cervical conization would still be an option if able to achieve negative margins per the ConCerv trial. A radical trachelectomy involves removal of the cervix, upper vagina, and parametria. The morbidity associated with radical trachelectomy, such as urinary tract injury, fistula formation, hemorrhage, and pelvic autonomic dysfunction, is similar to radical hysterectomy.

This patient desires to retain her options for future pregnancies, and performing a simple extrafascial hysterectomy is not the best next step. If she did not desire fertility preservation, this would be the best next step along with the lymph node assessment.

Surgical treatment with radical hysterectomy is reserved for patients in whom fertility preservation is either not desired or not an option, starting with patients that have stage IB1 cancer that do not meet conservative surgical criteria for extrafascial hysterectomy, as outlined in the National Comprehensive Cancer Network guidelines. Radical hysterectomy involves removal of parametria, uterosacral ligaments, and the upper vagina to ensure negative margins and evaluate for microscopic disease spread. Alternatively, these patients can be treated with pelvic external beam radiation therapy and brachytherapy with curative intent and equivalent survival outcomes, balancing toxicity profiles of surgery versus radiation.

Abu-Rustum NR, Yashar CM, Arend R, Barber E, Bradley K, Brooks R, et al. NCCN Guidelines Insights: cervical cancer, version 1.2024. J Natl Compr Canc Netw 2023;21:1224–33. doi: 10.6004/jnccn.2023.0062

Bhatla N, Berek JS, Cuello Fredes M, Denny LA, Grenman S, Karunaratne K, et al. Revised FIGO staging for carcinoma of the cervix uteri [published erratum appears in Int J Gynaecol Obstet 2019;147:279-80]. Int J Gynaecol Obstet 2019;145:129–35. doi: 10.1002/ijgo.12749

National Comprehensive Cancer Network. Cervical cancer. Version 3.2025. NCCN Clinical Practice Guidelines in Oncology [after login]. NCCN; 2025. Accessed February 26, 2025. https://www.nccn.org/guidelines/guidelines-detail?category=1&id=1426

Schmeler KM, Pareja R, Lopez Blanco A, Humberto Fregnani J, Lopes A, Perrotta M, et al. ConCerv: a prospective trial of conservative surgery for low-risk early-stage cervical cancer. Int J Gynecol Cancer 2021;31:1317–25. doi: 10.1136/ijgc-2021-002921

105 Ovarian cancer risk reduction

A 47-year-old patient presents to the office for a preoperative visit before planned total laparoscopic hysterectomy for abnormal uterine bleeding secondary to fibroids. Her history is notable for well-controlled hypertension and a cesarean delivery. She shares that her friend's mother recently received a diagnosis of ovarian cancer and asks if there is anything that can reduce her own risk. The best next step is to recommend a (an)

(A) aromatase inhibitor
* (B) bilateral salpingectomy
(C) bilateral salpingo-oophorectomy
(D) combined oral contraceptive pill
(E) selective estrogen receptor modulator (SERM)

Ovarian cancer is the second most common gynecologic malignancy, and 75% of patients with ovarian cancer present with advanced-stage disease. Epithelial ovarian cancer is the most common type of ovarian cancer. Nine out of 10 tumors of the ovary (90%) are epithelial. The 5-year overall survival rate for epithelial ovarian cancer is less than 50%. Ovarian cancer symptoms often are vague or nonspecific, and there are no effective screening tests for detection of early-stage disease. Attempts at developing screening tests for ovarian cancer have been limited by high false-positive rates leading to unnecessary surgeries and increased health care expenditures (Box 105-1) Additionally, the ovarian cancer tumor marker CA 125 level is high in only 50% of cases of early-stage ovarian cancer, and the time between discovery of radiographically detectable localized disease and the onset of metastatic disease is short, leaving little time for an effective intervention once cancer is present. Strategies for prevention are crucial to reduce risk.

Data from molecular studies support the theory that most epithelial ovarian cancer originates from the fallopian tube and secondarily involves the ovary. Additionally, fallopian tubes from patients with increased risk of hereditary ovarian cancer often contain occult serous carcinomas that appear to be ovarian carcinomas or serous tubal intraepithelial carcinoma lesions. These lesions are precursors to ovarian carcinoma. The presence of occult carcinoma and serous tubal intraepithelial carcinoma lesions in tubal specimens support the theory that epithelial ovarian carcinogenesis originates from the fallopian tube; therefore, opportunistic salpingectomy is an option for ovarian cancer risk reduction. The Society for Gynecologic Oncology and the American College of Obstetricians & Gynecologists recommend opportunistic salpingectomy for patients with an average risk of ovarian cancer who are undergoing pelvic surgery for benign disease, including hysterectomy. These societies also recommend salpingectomy rather than tubal ligation for sterilization of women.

For this average-risk patient undergoing planned hysterectomy for benign disease, the addition of bilateral salpingectomy will reduce her risk of ovarian cancer, and this is the best option. Salpingectomy at the time of hysterectomy or for sterilization in an average-risk patient does not increase the risk of complications or alter ovarian function but does increase operative time (16 minutes with hysterectomy; 10 minutes with sterilization). A study performed in Sweden found a decreased risk of ovarian cancer among patients who had bilateral salpingectomy compared with those who had tubal ligation (65% versus 28% ovarian cancer risk reduction, respectively). Similarly, salpingectomy at the time of hysterectomy is associated with decreased risk of ovarian cancer compared with those who did not have salpingectomy. Population-based studies in Canada also support these findings. Despite increased operative time, opportunistic salpingectomy reduces the risk of ovarian cancer and is cost effective compared with usual care. Gynecologists should counsel their patients on the risks and benefits of opportunistic salpingectomy as part of the informed consent process for patients undergoing pelvic surgery. Because this procedure does not eliminate the risk of

BOX 105-1

Criteria for Further Genetic Evaluation for Hereditary Breast and Ovarian Cancer

Women affected with one or more of the following have an increased likelihood of having an inherited predisposition to breast* and ovarian, tubal, or peritoneal cancer and should receive genetic counseling and be offered genetic testing:

- Epithelial ovarian, tubal, or peritoneal cancer
- Breast cancer at age 45 years or less
- Breast cancer and have a close relative† with breast cancer at age 50 years or less or close relative† with epithelial ovarian, tubal, or peritoneal cancer at any age
- Breast cancer at age 50 years or less with a limited or unknown family history‡
- Breast cancer and have two or more close relatives† with breast cancer at any age
- Breast cancer and have two or more close relatives† with pancreatic cancer or aggressive prostate cancer (Gleason score 7 or greater)
- Two breast cancer primaries, with the first diagnosed before age 50 years
- Triple-negative breast cancer at age 60 years or less
- Breast cancer and Ashkenazi Jewish ancestry at any age
- Pancreatic cancer and have two or more close relatives† with breast cancer; ovarian, tubal, or peritoneal cancer; pancreatic cancer; or aggressive prostate cancer (Gleason score 7 or greater)

Women unaffected with cancer, but with one or more of the following have an increased likelihood of having an inherited predisposition to breast and ovarian, tubal, or peritoneal cancer and should receive genetic counseling and be offered genetic testing:

- A first-degree or several close relatives† that meet one or more of the aforementioned criteria
- A close relative† carrying a known *BRCA1* or *BRCA2* mutation§
- A close relative† with male breast cancer

*Invasive ductal carcinoma in situ breast cancer.

†*Close relative* is defined as first degree (parent, sibling, offspring), second degree (grandparent, grandchild, aunt, uncle, and nephew, niece, half-sibling), or third degree (first cousin, great-grandparent or great-grandchild).

‡Limited family history includes fewer than two first-degree or second-degree female relatives surviving beyond age 45 years.

§Or carrying another known actionable deleterious mutation associated with hereditary breast and ovarian cancer syndrome.

Reprinted from Hereditary breast and ovarian cancer syndrome. Practice Bulletin No. 182. American College of Obstetricians and Gynecologists. Obstet Gynecol 2017;130:e110–26. doi: 10.1097/AOG.0000000000002296

BOX 105-2

Evaluation for Ovarian Cancer

New onset (less than 12 months) of the following signs and symptoms occurring 12 days per month or more should prompt evaluation

- bloating
- increased abdominal girth
- abdominopelvic pain
- early satiety
- decreased appetite

ovarian cancer, individuals with signs and symptoms of ovarian cancer should undergo the appropriate evaluation for this disease (Box 105-2).

Chemoprevention with aromatase inhibitors and SERMs is associated with decreased risk of breast cancer among patients at increased risk. Specifically, tamoxifen, a SERM, decreases breast cancer risk by 62% in patients with *BRCA2* mutations. It is not effective in patients with *BRCA1* mutations. Selective estrogen receptor modulators can also decrease breast cancer risk among other high-risk individuals. Aromatase inhibitors also decrease the risk of breast cancer in those at increased risk, and their use is appropriate in the postmenopausal period. The patient in this scenario is at average risk of breast cancer; therefore, they are not the best next step. Additionally, these medications have not been studied for chemoprevention for ovarian cancer, which is her primary concern.

Oophorectomy leads to surgical menopause, which increases risks of cardiovascular disease, other cancer, osteoporosis, and all-cause mortality. Oophorectomy is recommended for certain patients, including those with hereditary breast and ovarian cancer syndromes, those with hormonally responsive malignancies, and those with ovarian pathology. It can be considered for patients aged 50 and older. This patient's family history is not suggestive of a hereditary breast and ovarian cancer syndrome, and in the absence of another indication, performing a bilateral salpingo-oophorectomy at the time of her hysterectomy, with the goal of reducing ovarian cancer risk, is not the best next step.

Combined oral contraception is associated with a reduced risk of ovarian cancer (odds ratio 0.73 compared to nonuse). Those who use combined oral contraception for more than 10 years have about a 50% decreased incidence of ovarian cancer. Decreased rates of ovarian cancer also are seen among patients with *BRCA* mutations who use combined oral contraception. Despite this benefit, the Centers for Disease Control and Prevention recommends that combined hormonal contraception should generally be avoided in patients with hypertension because the risks (acute myocardial infarction and stroke) outweigh theoretical or proven benefit. Although the risks of using a method of contraception are typically weighed against the risk of pregnancy, this patient will not be at risk of pregnancy after hysterectomy, and her risk of acute myocardial infarction or stroke must be weighed against the risk of ovarian cancer. Because her risk of ovarian cancer is average, her risk of complications from combined hormonal contraception outweighs the benefit of decreased ovarian cancer risk. Combined hormonal contraceptive pills are not an appropriate choice in this scenario.

Havrilesky LJ, Moorman PG, Lowery WJ, Gierisch JM, Coeytaux RR, Urrutia RP, et al. Oral contraceptive pills as primary prevention for ovarian cancer: a systematic review and meta-analysis. Obstet Gynecol 2013;122:139–47. doi: 10.1097/AOG.0b013e318291c235

Hereditary breast and ovarian cancer syndrome. Practice Bulletin No. 182. American College of Obstetricians and Gynecologists. Obstet Gynecol 2017;130:e110–26. doi: 10.1097/AOG.0000000000002296

Opportunistic Salpingectomy as a Strategy for Epithelial Ovarian Cancer Prevention. Committee Opinion 774. American College of Obstetricians and Gynecologists. Obstet Gynecol 2019;133(4):e279-284. doi:10.1097/AOG.0000000000003164

Rush SK, Ma X, Newton MA, Rose SL. A revised Markov model evaluating oophorectomy at the time of hysterectomy for benign indication: age 65 years revisited. Obstet Gynecol 2022;139:735–44. doi: 10.1097/AOG.0000000000004732

The role of the obstetrician-gynecologist in the early detection of epithelial ovarian cancer in women at average risk. Committee Opinion No. 716. American College of Obstetricians and Gynecologists. Obstet Gynecol 2017;130:e146–9. doi: 10.1097/AOG.0000000000002299

106 Posttreatment surveillance of cervical cancer

A 56-year-old woman who recently completed primary chemoradiotherapy treatment for stage IIIC1 squamous cell carcinoma of the cervix presents for post-therapy follow-up care. You discuss the signs and symptoms of cervical cancer recurrence and the potential benefits of surveillance strategies. The most effective modality for local cancer recurrence detection is

(A) cervical biopsy
(B) cervical cytology
(C) colposcopy
(D) high-risk human papillomavirus (HPV) testing
* (E) pelvic examination

One of the primary goals of surveillance protocols after completing primary treatment for cancer is to detect recurrence early enough to implement therapies that could improve clinical outcomes. The protocols developed for cancer surveillance are informed by our understanding of recurrence risks and the patterns of recurrence that are associated with the specific type of cancer. In turn, protocols also are influenced by the potential clinical effects that available cancer therapies may have for recurrent disease.

Resources in cancer surveillance are most concentrated toward the detection of recurrences in which curative or highly effective palliative therapies are available. The types of recurrent cervical cancer can be broadly categorized according to location. Recurrences may be central pelvic, lateral pelvic, or extra-pelvic. Central pelvic recurrences may involve the vaginal vault or native cervix and uterus, the parametria, the bladder, or the rectum. Central pelvic recurrences have potential curative options, but other types of recurrence are not typically considered curable. For local cervical cancer recurrences after hysterectomy in a patient who has had no prior radiation, chemoradiation is an option. If prior radiation was given, the patient may be a candidate for pelvic exenteration. Outlining the best methods to detect local recurrence is essential to improving outcomes in patients treated for cervical cancer.

A pelvic examination includes visual inspection of the lower genital tract, bimanual examination, and rectovaginal examination, and it is the most effective primary surveillance tool for detecting local cancer recurrence. It is diagnostically sensitive for detecting local recurrence of cervical cancer and is cost-effective. Surveillance examinations are recommended at greater frequency in the first 2 years after treatment, given higher rates of recurrence in this period. National Comprehensive Cancer Network (NCCN) and Society of Gynecologic Oncology (SGO) guidelines recommend examinations every 3–6 months for 2 years and every 6 months for years 3–5 after treatment. Abnormalities identified by pelvic examination require further evaluation with biopsy.

Routine surveillance imaging is not recommended after treatment for cervical cancer because it is costly and does not measurably improve the diagnostic sensitivity of pelvic examination for detecting central recurrence; however, it can be obtained at the discretion of the treating gynecologic oncologist to further characterize abnormal physical examination findings or to explore new patient symptoms.

Annual cytology of the cervix and vagina is recommended by the SGO and NCCN in patients who have been treated for cervical cancer; however, the likelihood of detecting recurrence of cervix cancer in an otherwise asymptomatic patient with normal pelvic examination findings is quite low. Studies have shown that cytology does not improve diagnostic sensitivity compared with pelvic examination alone, and this is not the best surveillance method for the patient in the above scenario. Nonetheless, patients with a history of HPV-associated cancer will be at risk of a second primary cancer due to HPV, and annual screening in these patients is a reasonable recommendation. However, radiation causes inflammatory changes as well as cytoplasmic and nuclear alterations, such as bizarre and pleomorphic cell shapes, nuclear enlargement, increased nucleoli, and loss of polarity, and these radiation-induced features on cytology can result in costly high false-positive rates. For this reason, some clinicians elect to forgo cervical cytology in patients who have had prior chemoradiation. For patients undergoing cytology surveillance after treatment for cervical cancer, the SGO recommends colposcopic evaluation only for the finding of high-grade cytology (eg, high-grade squamous intraepithelial lesion, atypical squamous cells—cannot exclude HSIL, or abnormal glandular cells).

Abnormal findings that are identified on pelvic examination should be further characterized through biopsy; however, the diagnostic yield of random routine cervix biopsy in the absence of abnormal pelvic examination findings is exceedingly low. There is real danger in loss of follow-up if patients can expect painful biopsies at each surveillance visit. Routine cervix biopsy is not recommended for cancer surveillance. Likewise, abnormal findings identified on cytology can be further characterized through colposcopy; however, routine colposcopy also is not recommended.

The identification of high-risk subtypes of HPV also is an inefficient surveillance tool in patients previously treated for cervical cancer. Because HPV is noted in most patients with cervical cancer, this test lacks sufficient specificity in this population for effective triage of patients to further testing. Human papillomavirus testing is not recommended.

Serial pelvic examinations conducted at specified intervals after treatment for cervical cancer are a sensitive and low-cost method for detecting central recurrence. Patients should be educated about symptoms of potential recurrence, which allows self-monitoring for cancer recurrence. Optimal posttreatment care requires cooperation and communication among caregivers focused on reducing health risks going forward. Practices such as smoking cessation are central to achieving positive long-term outcomes.

National Comprehensive Cancer Network. Cervical cancer. Version 3.2025. NCCN Clinical Practice Guidelines in Oncology [after login]. NCCN; 2025. Accessed February 26, 2025. https://www.nccn.org/guidelines/guidelines-detail?category=1&id=1426

Rimel BJ, Ferda A, Erwin J, Dewdney SB, Seamon L, Gao F, et al. Cervicovaginal cytology in the detection of recurrence after cervical cancer treatment. Obstet Gynecol 2011;118:548–53. doi: 10.1097/AOG.0b013e3182271fdd

Salani R, Khanna N, Frimer M, Bristow RE, Chen L. An update on post-treatment surveillance and diagnosis of recurrence in women with gynecologic malignancies: Society of Gynecologic Oncology (SGO) recommendations. Gynecol Oncol 2017;146:3–10. doi: 10.1016/j.ygyno.2017.03.022

107 Respiratory distress

A 78-year-old patient with a medical history of hypertension underwent her first cycle of neoadjuvant chemotherapy for stage IV ovarian cancer. Two days later, she presented to the emergency department with shortness of breath, cough, and heart palpitations. Relevant vital signs and laboratory findings are listed in Table 107-1. An electrocardiogram demonstrates right bundle branch block and sinus tachycardia. Chest computed tomography (CT) is depicted in Figure 107-1. In addition to supplemental oxygen, the best next step is

(A) antibiotics
* (B) anticoagulation
(C) diuretics
(D) granulocyte colony-stimulating factor (G-CSF)
(E) thoracentesis

TABLE 107-1. The Described Patient's Vital Signs and Laboratory Study Results

Temperature	37.8 °C (100.04 °F)
Blood pressure	92/60 mm Hg
Heart rate	130 bpm
Oxygen saturation	88%
Hemoglobin	8.2 mg/dL
Absolute neutrophil count	2.0 (x 10^9/L)

New-onset dyspnea is exceedingly common in patients with advanced cancer. The differential diagnosis is wide ranging and can include pulmonary, cardiac, and infectious causes. This patient's chest CT, however, demonstrates a pulmonary embolism.

Thromboembolic events frequently occur in malignancy and are the second leading cause of death in patients with cancer. Ovarian cancer has one of the highest venous thromboembolism (VTE) rates among all types of cancer. Up to 20% of patients with advanced ovarian cancer present with VTE at diagnosis, and the incidence increases by 10% during neoadjuvant chemotherapy treatment. Sudden-onset dyspnea is the most common presenting symptom for pulmonary embolism. When complicated by pulmonary infarction, pleuritic chest pain can occur.

Clinical prediction tools, such as the Wells criteria or the Geneva score, are commonly employed in the emergency department setting to determine the necessity for further diagnostic testing in patients when VTE is on the differential diagnosis (Box 107-1). D-dimer, a plasmin-derived degradation product, has a high sensitivity and negative predictive value in diagnosis of VTE and often is used in conjunction with these scoring systems to further improve risk stratification. In this patient, the pretest probability of VTE is sufficiently high to justify imaging without additional triage. D-dimer is associated with higher false-positive rates in patients with malignancy, limiting its discriminatory value in this context.

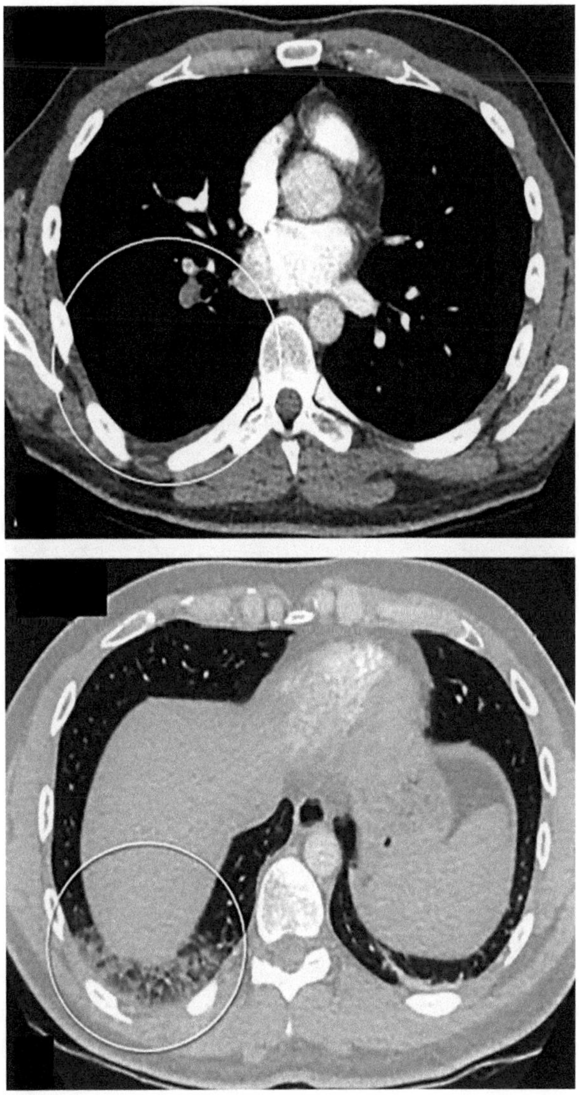

FIGURE 107-1. Chest CT depicting both soft tissue and lung windows. The circles represent the area of interest.

BOX 107-1

Differential diagnosis of new-onset shortness of breath in patients with cancer

Pulmonary
- Pulmonary embolism
- Pneumonia
- Pleural effusion and ascites that reduces lung capacity
- Pulmonary metastases
- Pulmonary fibrosis
- Airway obstruction

Cardiac
- Pericardial effusion, cardiac tamponade
- Superior vena cava syndrome
- New coronary event
- Chemotherapy-associated cardiac toxicity

Other
- Anemia
- Sepsis
- Anxiety, panic attacks

Imaging plays a central role in further evaluating the most likely and highest-risk entities on the differential diagnosis. Computed tomography pulmonary angiography (CTPA) is the imaging modality of choice for the workup of patients with suspected acute pulmonary embolism. Its reported diagnostic sensitivity and specificity are 83% and 96%, respectively. Additionally, it can simultaneously evaluate the other entities in the differential diagnosis, including pulmonary infection, pleural effusion, and pulmonary edema.

The diagnostic sensitivity of CTPA is highest when there is optimal opacification of the pulmonary arterial vasculature, allowing for clear differentiation between the intravascular thrombus and intraluminal contrast material. An iodine-containing contrast agent is injected at a high rate and images are rapidly acquired during the time of maximum concentration of contrast within the pulmonary arteries. Images are displayed on different grayscales for interpretation, and soft tissue and lung windows are utilized. Soft tissue windows provide good contrast resolution to optimize visualization of the vascular anatomy. The lung windows, on the other hand, are specialized settings that enhance contrast between air-filled structures and surrounding tissues and allow for improved evaluation of the pulmonary parenchyma and the airways. As noted above, the patient's CTPA findings depicted in Figure 107-1 reveal a pulmonary embolism.

In the soft tissue windows, a non-opacified pulmonary vessel is noted in the left lung, whereas contrast material is evident within all surrounding pulmonary vessels. In the lung windows, a wedge-shaped opacity is noted peripheral to the pulmonary embolism. This suggests an associated pulmonary infarct—a notable consequence of acute pulmonary embolism. There are pertinent negative findings on this patient's imaging, including the absence of pleural effusion. Although a pulmonary infarct suggests a heightened cardiovascular risk associated with pulmonary embolism, there does not appear to be cardiac enlargement or pulmonary edema to suggest overt myocardial strain or cardiac failure.

In this patient with radiographic confirmation of a pulmonary embolism, anticoagulation therapy is the best next step. It prevents further clot formation and reduces the risk of clot propagation.

In patients with a larger and more centrally located pulmonary embolism, or in whom multiple emboli and a higher clotting risk are identified, the risk of circulatory collapse attributable to right heart failure is increased. In that setting, thrombolytic therapy may be considered. Data on thrombolytic therapy show improvements in patient symptoms without associated improvements in mortality. Right ventricular strain is best evaluated with echocardiography; however, the patient in this scenario is hemodynamically stable and there is no evidence for right ventricular dilation on CT. The additional risk of hemorrhage with thrombolytic therapy is not justified at this time in this hemodynamically stable patient and is not the best next step.

This patient has recently received chemotherapy, and infectious complications also are on the differential diagnosis; however, the data do not support a diagnosis of infection or neutropenia, and neither antibiotics nor G-CSF is warranted. There is a focal lung opacification shown on imaging, but it is attributed to infarction secondary to pulmonary embolism, rather than pulmonary infection. Although this patient's absolute neutrophil count is somewhat low at 2,000/mm^3, she is not considered neutropenic (defined as an absolute neutrophil count less than 1,500/mm^3), and she does not require G-CSF treatment.

Because there is no evidence for pulmonary edema on the described patient's imaging, diuretic therapy is not indicated. Pleural effusions are very common in advanced ovarian cancer but are not identified on this patient's CT and thoracentesis is not warranted.

Acute pulmonary embolism is common in patients with ovarian cancer and can be a fatal complication of the cancer and its therapy. Timely diagnosis and implementation of effective anticoagulation therapy in patients with pulmonary embolism are essential. Computed tomography pulmonary angiography for patients presenting with a high likelihood of pulmonary embolism is the diagnostic modality of choice, having the notable advantages of being fast, readily available and possessing a high diagnostic accuracy; moreover, CTPA allows for the simultaneous evaluation of other cardiac and pulmonary entities on the differential diagnosis of patients with shortness of breath and can facilitate timelier implementation of therapeutics.

Black KA, Bowden S, Chu P, McClurg C, Pin S, Metcalfe A. Incidence of venous thromboembolism in patients with ovarian cancer receiving neoadjuvant chemotherapy: systematic review and meta-analysis. Int J Gynecol Cancer 2024;34:855–62. doi: 10.1136/ijgc-2023-005166

Harvey JJ, Huang S, Uberoi R. Catheter-directed therapies for the treatment of high risk (massive) and intermediate risk (submassive) acute pulmonary embolism. Cochrane Database of Systematic Reviews 2022, Issue 8. Art. No.: CD013083. doi: 10.1002/14651858.CD013083.pub2

Moore AJ, Wachsmann J, Chamarthy MR, Panjikaran L, Tanabe Y, Rajiah P. Imaging of acute pulmonary embolism: an update. Cardiovasc Diagn Ther 2018;8:225–43. doi: 10.21037/cdt.2017.12.01

108 Timing of delivery in pregnancies affected by cervical cancer

A 38-year-old gravida 1 at 28 weeks of gestation presents with new vaginal spotting. Her physical examination reveals a 1-cm irregular mass on the cervix with smooth parametria and a normal rectovaginal septum. Biopsy of the mass reveals invasive squamous cell carcinoma. She elects to delay cancer treatment for pregnancy continuation. Her pelvic MRI is notable for the known cervical tumor and otherwise negative. The most appropriate delivery plan is

(A) preterm cesarean
(B) preterm vaginal
* (C) term cesarean
(D) term vaginal

Cervical cancer is the most commonly diagnosed gynecologic malignancy in pregnancy with an incidence rate of 1.5–12 per 100,000 live births. Approximately 1–3% of all cervical cancer is diagnosed during pregnancy or the postpartum period. Survival outcomes of pregnant individuals diagnosed with cervical cancer match those of nonpregnant individuals stage for stage. Treatment planning will depend on gestational age, extent of disease, and the patient's desire for pregnancy preservation. A multidisciplinary team including obstetricians, pediatricians, and oncologists should be utilized when managing cervical cancer due to the inherent complexities in treatment.

Evaluation and staging are the same for pregnant and nonpregnant individuals diagnosed with cervical cancer. Evaluation of lymph node status is a key factor in the prognosis and treatment of cervical cancer. Pelvic MRI without gadolinium contrast and ultrasonography are options for the evaluation of lymph node status and urinary system in pregnant individuals. If more advanced disease is suspected, a chest X-ray to evaluate for pulmonary metastasis can be performed. The patient in this scenario has International Federation of Gynecology and Obstetrics (FIGO) stage IB1 disease (tumor limited to the cervix with a visible lesion less than 2 cm). Once the stage is determined, management options are the same as those for nonpregnant individuals and will depend on the patient's desire for pregnancy preservation and gestational age. Patients diagnosed in early pregnancy should be offered pregnancy termination along with a discussion of treatment options.

The management of early-stage cervical cancer (FIGO stage IA1–IB1), is largely determined by gestational age in individuals desiring pregnancy preservation. For individuals with early-stage cervical cancer and negative lymph nodes diagnosed at 22–25 weeks of gestation or later, treatment can be safely delayed until after delivery without adverse oncologic outcomes. The patient in this scenario has FIGO stage IB1 squamous cell carcinoma of the cervix with a negative workup for metastatic disease. Given a gestational age of 28 weeks, it is appropriate to delay treatment until after delivery. Delivery should not be scheduled before fetal lung maturity solely for oncologic indications. When feasible, delivery should be planned after 37 weeks of gestation with a goal of avoiding active labor. Delivery before 37 weeks of gestation should be considered for obstetric indications; therefore, in the scenario given, this patient should have a term delivery.

The mode of delivery in pregnant individuals with cervical cancer is determined by the FIGO stage. Patients with FIGO stage IA1 disease without lymphovascular space invasion may undergo vaginal delivery. Cesarean delivery is the delivery mode of choice for individuals with stage IA2–IIA disease due to the possibilities of infection, hemorrhage, and possible dissemination of tumor cells. Several studies have shown increased risk of disease recurrence and decreased overall survival with vaginal delivery compared to cesarean delivery. Because this patient has stage IB1 cancer, vaginal delivery options are not appropriate. Professional societies and clinical experts recommend that cancer-specific treatment be initiated immediately after delivery, and a term cesarean delivery with concomitant hysterectomy would be recommended for this patient.

The management of early-stage cervical cancer diagnosed during pregnancy is dependent on the stage of disease and gestational age at the time of diagnosis. Treatment planning with a multidisciplinary team is paramount to optimize oncologic, obstetric, and neonatal outcomes.

Cibula D, Raspollini MR, Planchamp F, Centeno C, Chargari C, Felix A, et al. ESGO/ESTRO/ESP guidelines for the management of patients with cervical cancer—update 2023. Int J Gynecol Cancer 2023;33:649–66. doi: 10.1136/ijgc-2023-004429

Cordeiro CN, Gemignani ML. Gynecologic malignancies in pregnancy: balancing fetal risks with oncologic safety. Obstet Gynecol Surv 2017;72:184–93. doi: 10.1097/OGX.0000000000000407

Gungorduk K, Sahbaz A, Ozdemir A, Gokcu M, Sancı M, Köse MF. Management of cervical cancer during pregnancy. J Obstet Gynaecol 2016;36:366–71. doi: 10.3109/01443615.2015.1065235

Korenaga TK, Tewari KS. Gynecologic cancer in pregnancy. Gynecol Oncol 2020;157:799–809. doi: 10.1016/j.ygyno.2020.03.015

109 Database research

The Surveillance, Epidemiology, and End Results (SEER) Program provides cancer statistics in an effort to reduce the cancer burden in the U.S. population. The linked SEER Medicare Cancer database includes data pertaining to the clinical setting, incidence, and survival information from cancer registries that cover a substantial proportion of the U.S. population and links the data to Medicare claims data. A study that analyzed information in this data file reported that women with ovarian cancer who were prescribed metformin do not have improved survival compared with women with ovarian cancer who were not prescribed metformin. The inherent design limitation of this study is that it is

(A) inaccurate
(B) incomplete
* (C) not generalizable
(D) subject to information bias

All database research is retrospective and does not provide the same level of evidence as prospective clinical trials. Although well-conducted retrospective analyses can describe associations, they cannot determine cause and effect. Analyses of high-quality databases can be conducted economically and expeditiously, may provide useful insights, and often generate hypotheses for future prospective research. Dataset analyses facilitate characterizing geographic, demographic, or other variations in care and outcome and lend themselves to development of risk-adjusted models.

Databases typically are classified as either clinical or administrative. These types of datasets are derived from different sources, serve different purposes, and can be most effectively utilized to address different types of inquiries.

Clinical cancer databases are developed from patient level care data submitted from local, regional, or national tumor registries, or from information shared by practitioners or health care system or national organizations. Advantages of clinical databases are inclusion of information regarding incidence, survival, stage, grade, and treatment. Limitations of clinical databases include lack of generalizable conclusions from studies conducted in regional, or otherwise limited, registries. The study in this scenario is of limited utility because the data are not generalizable, and this is the limitation in the study's design.

Administrative databases are derived either from claims placed by practitioners to third-party payers or from the payers themselves. Advantages of administrative databases include the ability to address questions addressing charges and costs of care and provide data according to International Classification of Diseases, Ninth Revision, Clinical Modification (ICD-9-CM) and Current Procedural Terminology (CPT) codes. Limitations of administrative databases include reliance on input from professional coders, rather than clinicians, and the database may lack clinically meaningful patient-specific information, such as cancer stage, grade, and performance status. In addition, long-term follow-up data, including complications and survival, may be missing.

The SEER Program dataset offers the advantage of combining clinical and administrative datasets to facilitate investigations that require both types of information. It is ideally suited to address research questions focused on cost, use, quality, and delivery of health care. The results of this study are not generalizable to the ovarian cancer population as a whole because the linked data are almost exclusively derived from patients aged 65 or older, and the findings may not apply to younger patients.

Hospital medical records, abstracted by specially trained cancer registrars, serve as the primary source for information recorded in SEER. Research has demonstrated a high degree of accuracy for services provided in a hospital; however, data regarding cancer care given outside the hospital setting may be less accurate. Still, Medicare claims data are relatively reliable to identify payment for medications among beneficiaries (reportedly close to 90%). Mortality data for all causes of death in the United States are collected by the National Center for Health Statistics and are, in general, accurate. Inaccuracy of data is not a limitation of the study described above.

In the United States, cancer is a reportable disease, and all cases must be reported to a state or regional cancer registry. Typically, SEER Program registries demonstrate case ascertainment rates in excess of 95%. With such a high ascertainment rate, the study described above is not limited because of incomplete data.

Research bias is defined as a systematic error that may adversely affect a study's findings by altering assessments, thereby reducing the validity of findings. There are two broad categories of bias, and several specific types of bias within each category. The broad categories are termed *selection bias* and *information bias*. Selection bias occurs when the procedures for inclusion in a study result in a group that is not representative of the population from which it is drawn. Information bias occurs when the manner in which data obtained from, or regarding, study subjects is not uniform. It seems unlikely that information regarding survival was collected differently from patients depending on whether or not they were prescribed metformin. Differences in collecting information can result in misclassifying patients regarding exposures or disease status, introducing inaccuracies in findings and conclusions. Although there is evidence that bias exists in some of the SEER Program data, overall the chance of bias is relatively small. In this scenario described above, the probability of bias is minimized by the research question itself and linkage of the SEER Program to the Medicare claims data.

Abdel-Kader AK, Eisenkraft JB, Katz DJ. Overview and limitations of database research in anesthesiology: a narrative review. Anesth Analg 2021;132:1012–22. doi: 10.1213/ANE.0000000000005346

Cook JA, Collins GS. The rise of big clinical databases. Br J Surg 2015;102:e93–101. doi: 10.1002/bjs.9723

Murphy M, Alavi K, Maykel J. Working with existing databases. Clin Colon Rectal Surg 2013;26:5–11. doi: 10.1055/s-0033-1333627

110 Vulvar cancer

An 82-year-old patient with hypertension presents to the office with vaginal bleeding and vulvar pain. She reports that she has never had surgery and walks 2 miles every day. She has had vulvar pain for 6 months, and she noticed an ulcer 3 months ago. Her physical examination is notable for a 1.5-cm ulcerative lesion on the left labium majus approximately 1 cm from the clitoris. There are no palpable inguinal lymph nodes. Biopsy results indicate squamous cell carcinoma of the vulva with 4 mm of invasion. The best next step in cancer treatment is

(A) complete radical vulvectomy with bilateral inguinal lymphadenectomy
(B) neoadjuvant chemotherapy with cisplatin and paclitaxel
(C) radiation therapy with concurrent cisplatin
* (D) radical local excision with bilateral sentinel inguinal lymph node biopsies
(E) radical vulvectomy with postoperative radiation therapy

Vulvar cancer (Fig. 110-1) is a rare disease that primarily affects women aged 65 years and older. Its risk factors include older age, history of tobacco use, and the presence of human papillomavirus (HPV) infection or lichen. In disease that is clinically confined to the vulva, a staging surgery is indicated; however, certain features, such as patient frailty, comorbidities, and involvement of or proximity to the anus or urethra, may make a surgical approach difficult. In those situations, radiation with sensitizing chemotherapy is the more appropriate initial management.

Delays in the diagnosis of vulvar cancer are common. Any suspicious lesion should be promptly biopsied to facilitate timely surgical management. Preferably, the lesion should not be completely excised to allow for a sentinel node biopsy technique at the time of vulvectomy. It is acceptable to use the scar of the previous biopsy or excision during the sentinel lymph node biopsy procedure. If there are multifocal lesions, each lesion should be biopsied because multifocal tumors are not eligible for a sentinel node mapping procedure. Treatment of vulvar cancer is dependent on the initial clinical, pathologic, and radiographic staging. If the disease is truly confined to the vulva, without obvious extension into the regional lymph nodes, vagina, urethra, or anus, primary surgical intervention is the recommended management.

Surgical intervention should be completed with a radical local excision. The objective is to achieve a tumor-free margin of more than 2–3 mm, and some surgeons advocate for an 8-mm margin. This margin may be difficult to achieve if the primary tumor approximates the clitoris and urethra or anus.

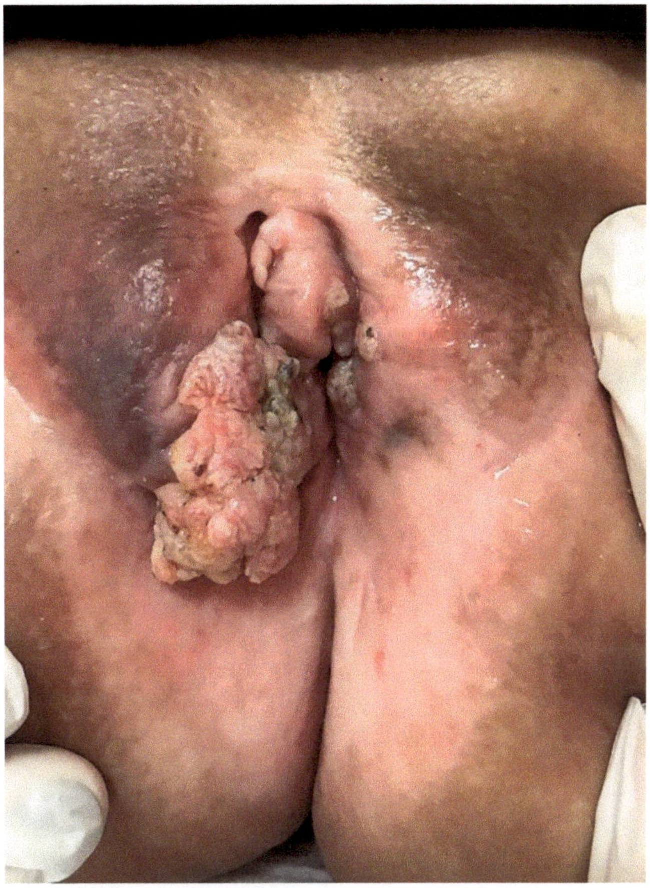

FIGURE 110-1. Vulvar cancer.

If the preoperative biopsy demonstrates a depth of invasion of 1 mm or less (International Federation of Gynecology and Obstetrics [FIGO] stage IA), the inguinal lymph nodes do not need to be assessed, but for tumors that have a depth of invasion of greater than 1 mm, inguinal lymph node assessment is recommended.

A sentinel lymph node procedure involves injecting a radiologic substance or blue dye in the primary tumor (or scar) to identify the most proximal lymph node, which is the lymph node most likely to have metastatic disease. Sentinel lymph nodes are identified during surgery by using a gamma tracer or visualizing the dye in the lymph node or lymphatic channel, or a combination of both. Lymphoscintigraphy may be used before surgery to help localize the sentinel lymph node. This approach should only be considered if the following criteria are met: 1) No suspicious or enlarged lymph nodes are identified preoperatively, and 2) the tumor is less than 4 cm in diameter and unifocal (Box 110-1). Bilateral sentinel lymph nodes should be identified and removed if the tumor lies within 2 cm of the midline. Because this patient has a relatively small midline tumor (1.5 cm), a radical local excision with sentinel node biopsy is the appropriate surgical approach.

Complete radical vulvectomy with en bloc full inguinal node dissection is no longer considered standard of care due to morbidity. Inguinofemoral lymphadenectomy should be performed if a sentinel lymph node is not identified.

Neoadjuvant (or preoperative) systemic chemotherapy has been studied but not in a randomized trial, and it is not currently the standard of care. This therapy may be considered in unique situations when neither surgery nor radiation is feasible due to tumor size. Because the patient in this scenario has a small tumor that is amenable to resection, neoadjuvant systemic chemotherapy is not the best next step.

In the setting of advanced-stage disease, such as disease that extends into nearby or distant structures, combined chemotherapy and radiation therapy is the most appropriate approach to minimize morbidity. Primary chemoradiation therapy has been shown to result in a complete clinical response in 80% of patients and a complete pathologic response in 50% of patients. If there is residual disease after primary chemoradiation therapy, surgical resection of residual disease can be considered. Because the described patient has a small tumor with no involvement of surrounding structures, this is not the best next step in her treatment.

The management of vulvar cancer involves preoperative clinical and pathologic assessment and thoughtful surgical planning. In the preoperative assessment, the patient's functional status and tumor location should be considered.

BOX 110-1

Sentinel lymph node criteria for vulvar cancer

- Unifocal cancer
- Tumor size less than 4 cm
- Negative results from groin examination, imaging of the groin, or both
- No prior vulvar surgery that would disrupt vulvar lymphatic channels
- High-volume sentinel lymph node surgeon available

Lukovic J, Han K. Postoperative management of vulvar cancer. Int J Gynecol Cancer 2022;32:338–43. doi: 10.1136/ijgc-2021-002463

National Comprehensive Cancer Network. Vulvar cancer. Version 4.2024. NCCN Clinical Practice Guidelines in Oncology [after login]. NCCN; 2024. Accessed January 22, 2025. https://www.nccn.org/guidelines/guidelines-detail?category=1&id=1476

Oonk MH, Planchamp F, Baldwin P, Mahner S, Mirza MR, Fischerová D, et al. European Society of Gynaecological Oncology guidelines for the management of patients with vulvar cancer update 2023. Int J Gynecol Cancer 2023;33:1023–43. doi: 10.1136/ijgc-2023-004486

Oonk MH, Slomovitz B, Baldwin PJ, van Doorn HC, van der Velden J, de Hullu JA, et al. Radiotherapy versus inguinofemoral lymphadenectomy as treatment for vulvar cancer patients with micrometastases in the sentinel node: results of GROINSS-V II. J Clin Oncol 2021;39:3623–32. doi: 10.1200/JCO.21.00006

111 Endometriosis-associated ovarian cancer

A 47-year-old patient with a history of biopsy-proven endometriosis was noted 1 year ago to have a 4-cm left adnexal mass. Ultrasound imaging of the mass at that time is shown in Figure 111-1A, and her current ultrasound is shown in Figure 111-1B. She now reports pelvic pain, and her CA 125 level, which was previously in the normal range, is 362 U/mL. Other than endometrioid adenocarcinoma, the most likely cancer histology of this mass is

(A) carcinosarcoma
* (B) clear cell
(C) high-grade serous
(D) low-grade serous
(E) mucinous

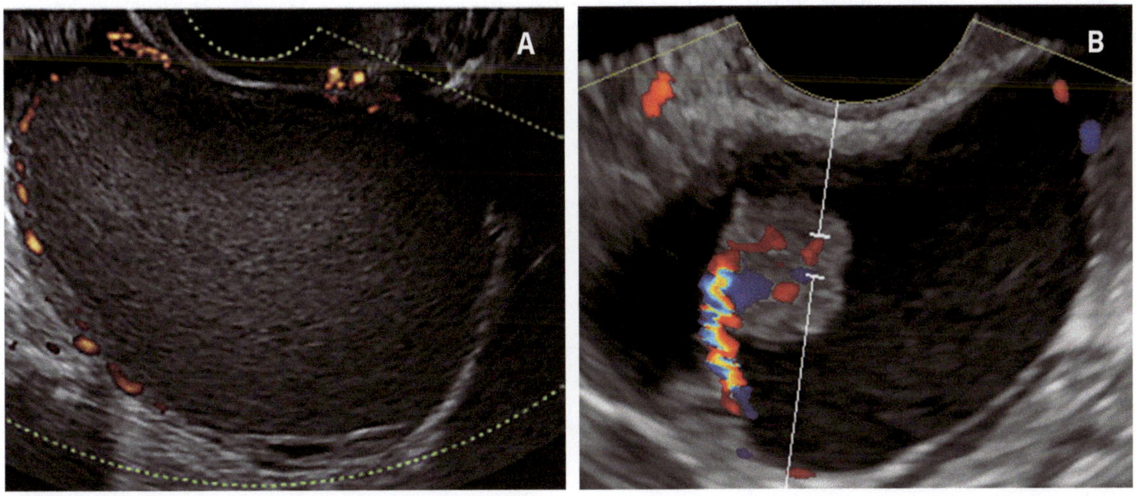

FIGURE 111-1. A and B. Past and current ultrasound images of left adnexal mass. (Figure 111-1A reprinted from Exacoustos C, Manganaro L, Zupi E. Imaging for the evaluation of endometriosis and adenomyosis. Best Pract Res Clin Obstet Gynaecol. 2014 Jul;28(5):655-81. doi: 10.1016/j.bpobgyn.2014.04.010.)

Endometriosis is a surgically diagnosed, chronic inflammatory gynecologic condition of widely varying severity in which endometrial tissue is found outside the uterus. The ovaries are commonly involved, and the tissue may develop endometriomas. Although itself benign, endometriosis is associated with an increased risk of developing gynecologic malignancy. *Endometriosis-associated malignancy* refers to malignancy that is found adjacent to endometriosis. When cancer is contiguous with endometriosis, clonal analysis has demonstrated common mutations in the *ARID1A* tumor suppressor gene, supporting endometriosis as the putative precursor lesion.

Among the histologic types of ovarian cancer, the two types most commonly diagnosed in association with endometriosis are endometrioid and clear cell carcinoma. A recent large population-based case–control study in the Netherlands found that patients with histologically confirmed endometriosis had an age-adjusted incidence risk ratio (IRR) of 29.06 (95% CI, 20.66–40.87) for endometrioid ovarian carcinoma, followed by an IRR of 21.34 (95% CI, 14.01–32.51) for clear cell carcinoma.

In the scenario above, the patient has a presumptive diagnosis of an endometrioma. The typical ultrasound appearance of an endometrioma, as shown in Figure 111-1A, is a cystic mass with homogeneous ground glass echoes. Although endometriomas are common benign neoplasms and clear cell carcinoma is rare, the development or growth of a solid vascular nodule in a presumed endometrioma, as shown in Figure 111-1B, should raise concern about the possibility of clear cell carcinoma. Clear cell carcinomas have been reported to be diagnosed in association with endometriomas in up to 50% of patients. In the above scenario, apart from endometrioid adenocarcinoma, the patient's history and current ultrasonography are most consistent with clear cell carcinoma.

Whereas the average age of diagnosis of ovarian cancer is 63 years, patients with clear cell and endometrioid carcinomas diagnosed in association with endometriosis are approximately 10 years younger at diagnosis and more likely to be diagnosed with early-stage disease compared with patients with cancer that is not associated with endometriosis.

Currently, the role of adjuvant chemotherapy for patients with stage I clear cell carcinoma is controversial, with either adjuvant chemotherapy or observation considered acceptable options for patients with stage IA, 1B, and 1C1 clear cell carcinoma with complete surgical staging. For patients with stages IA or IB grade 1 endometrioid ovarian carcinoma, observation is recommended and is an option for patients with stage IC disease. For patients with apparent early-stage clear cell or endometrioid ovarian cancer, complete staging is essential because negative staging may indicate that chemotherapy can be avoided. Advanced-stage clear cell carcinomas are treated with a similar strategy as high-grade serous cancer, but prognosis tends to be worse due to lower response rates to chemotherapy. Randomized trials comparing irinotecan plus cisplatin versus paclitaxel and cisplatin have not demonstrated a significant difference in survival; however, cytoreduction to no residual disease has been associated with survival benefit.

High-grade serous carcinoma, which is responsible for approximately 75% of ovarian cancer deaths, is the most common histologic type of ovarian cancer and the type most strongly associated with *BRCA* mutations or hereditary high-risk syndromes. Mucinous carcinoma and carcinosarcomas are rare histologic types, each accounting for approximately 1–3% of ovarian cancer. Low-grade serous carcinoma comprises 5–10% of ovarian cancer, is relatively indolent, and is generally resistant to chemotherapy. As a result, they are treated primarily with surgery. The incidence of these other histologic types has been reported in association with endometriosis to a much lower degree compared with endometrioid and clear cell carcinomas. In the Netherlands study, an increase in the incidence of other types of ovarian cancer among patients with endometriosis was observed only among patients who received a synchronous diagnosis of endometriosis and cancer.

Anglesio MS, Bashashati A, Wang YK, Senz J, Ha G, Yang W, et al. Multifocal endometriotic lesions associated with cancer are clonal and carry a high mutation burden. J Pathol 2015;236:201–9. doi: 10.1002/path.4516

Hermens M, van Altena AM, Nieboer TE, et al. Incidence of endometrioid and clear-cell ovarian cancer in histological proven endometriosis: the ENOCA population-based cohort study. Am J Obstet Gynecol 2020;223:107.e1–107.e11

Kim HS, Kim TH, Chung HH, Song YS. Risk and prognosis of ovarian cancer in women with endometriosis: a meta-analysis. Br J Cancer 2014;110:1878–90. doi: 10.1038/bjc.2014.29

Pearce CL, Templeman C, Rossing MA, Lee A, Near AM, Webb PM, et al. Association between endometriosis and risk of histological subtypes of ovarian cancer: a pooled analysis of case-control studies. Lancet Oncol 2012;13:385–94. doi: 10.1016/S1470-2045(11)70404-1

Pozzati F, Moro F, Pasciuto T, Gallo C, Ciccarone F, Franchi D, et al. Imaging in gynecological disease (14): clinical and ultrasound characteristics of ovarian clear cell carcinoma. Ultrasound Obstet Gynecol 2018;52:792–800. doi: 10.1002/uog.19171

112 Tumor markers

A 59-year-old presents with a 2- to 3-month history of persistent lower abdominal pain, hematochezia, and nausea. She is afebrile with normal vital signs, and her abdominal examination is notable for mild tenderness to deep palpation across the lower abdomen. Laboratory test results are listed in Table 112-1. Imaging of the abdomen and pelvis with computed tomography (CT) is obtained (Fig. 112-1A and -1B). To determine a diagnosis, the best additional tumor marker to evaluate is

(A) α-fetoprotein (AFP)
(B) CA 15-3
* (C) carcinoembryonic antigen (CEA)
(D) human chorionic gonadotropin (hCG)
(E) human epididymis protein 4 (HE4)

TABLE 112-1. The Described Patient's Laboratory Study Results

White blood cell count	7,200/microliter
Hematocrit	28.6%
Blood urea nitrogen	10 mg/dL
Creatinine	0.9 mg/dL
CA 125	142 U/mL
CA 19-9	34 U/mL

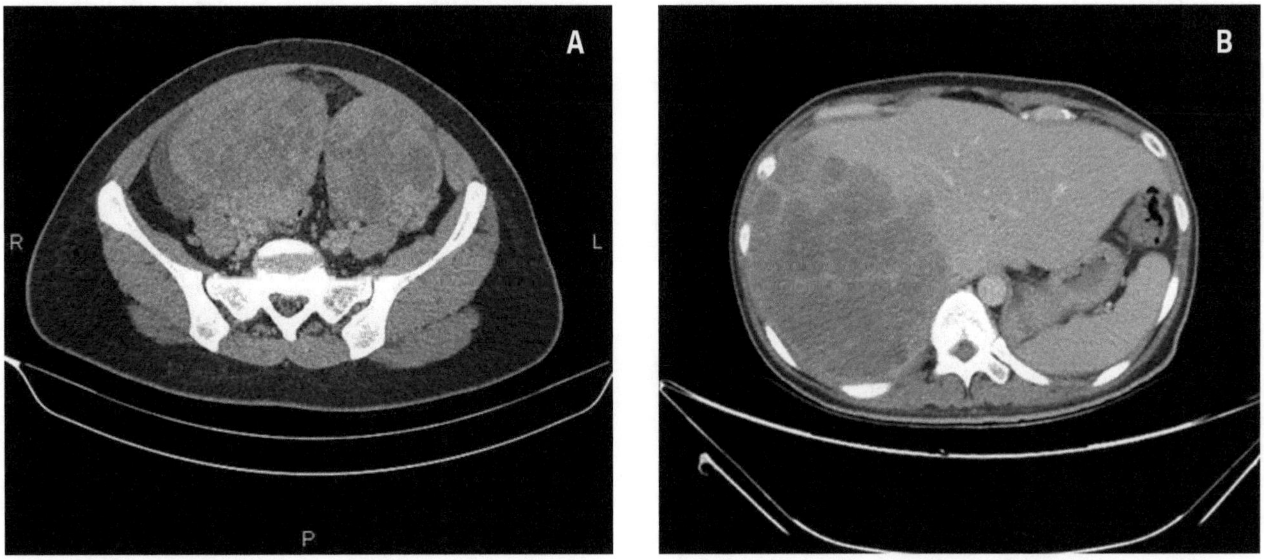

FIGURE 112-1. A and B. Described patient's computed tomography results. (A. Reprinted from Molinari A. Krukenberg tumor. Radiopaedia. Accessed June 3, 2025. https://radiopaedia.org/articles/krukenberg-tumor-2. B. Reprinted from Wang W, Lin CC, Liang WY, Chang SC, Jiang JK. Adenocarcinoma of sigmoid colon with metastasis to an ovarian mature teratoma: A case report. World J Clin Cases. 2024 Feb 6;12(4):853–858. doi: 10.12998/wjcc.v12.i4.853)

Tumor markers are secreted or membrane-associated glycoproteins produced by cancer cells. The degree to which they are clinically useful depends on the sensitivity and specificity of a high tumor marker level for a particular disease and how it will be used, whether for screening, as a follow-up test to aid in triage for patients who already have evidence of disease, or disease monitoring after diagnosis.

The patient in this scenario has multiple findings suggestive of a primary gastrointestinal malignancy, including hematochezia, bilateral solid adnexal masses, and liver lesions on

CT suggestive of liver metastases. Bilateral solid adnexal masses are a classic finding with associated with Krukenberg tumor or metastasis from a primary gastrointestinal neoplasm. Intraparenchymal liver metastases are commonly associated with a gastrointestinal or biliary primary but not with primary ovarian cancer. Given these findings, in addition to CA 125 and CA 19-9, CEA is the best tumor marker to further evaluate the described patient's ovarian masses for malignancy. Carcinoembryonic antigen is a tumor marker with levels that often are increased in gastrointestinal cancer; however, increased levels also can be associated with lung, thyroid, biliary, breast, bladder, and ovarian tumors.

CA 125 is expressed on ovarian epithelium but also in small amounts in many other tissues, including the peritoneum, lung, colon, gallbladder, kidney, breast, and stomach. Although it is not useful as a screening test, a CA 125 level is commonly used in patients diagnosed with ovarian cancer to assess response to therapy or recurrence. It can also be useful as a triage tool in patients for whom there is suspicion for cancer based on other factors, such as indeterminate or suspicious adnexal masses or other evidence of malignancy, to assist in directing the patient toward the best management. In the scenario above, the patient is postmenopausal and has bilateral solid adnexal masses and evidence of a metastatic process; therefore, evaluation of CA 125 is appropriate.

CA 19-9, like CA 125, is expressed in a wide range of tissues and can be a nonspecific marker of inflammation. A false-positive increase of CA 19-9 is reported in a diverse set of benign conditions, including pancreatitis, hepatitis, poorly controlled diabetes mellitus, diffuse lung disease, collagen vascular disease, and endometriosis. Although not recommended as a screening test, it is most often used to assist in diagnosis of patients suspected of having pancreatic or other biliary cancer. Because hepatic metastases are frequently seen in biliary cancer, it is reasonable to evaluate it in the patient described, although in the absence of evidence of a pancreatic mass or other hepatobiliary primary on imaging, a gastrointestinal primary tumor is more likely.

Alpha-fetoprotein is produced by liver tissue with increased levels seen in cirrhosis and viral hepatitis as well as liver cancer. It is used for monitoring response to therapy in patients with hepatocellular carcinoma. In patients with an adnexal mass, AFP is useful if a germ cell tumor is suspected, because AFP is frequently increased in germ cell tumors, particularly yolk-sac tumors, which most commonly occur in reproductive-aged women. Germ cell tumors are extremely rare after age 40 years, with peak incidence occurring between the ages of 15 and 19 years. Although levels are normally increased in pregnancy, extremely high levels (eg, 10,000 ng/mL) in a pregnant patient should raise concern regarding a possible germ cell tumor. Alpha-fetoprotein testing is not appropriate in this scenario because the patient is 59 years old and is unlikely to have a germ cell tumor.

CA 15-3 can be used to assess treatment response and to monitor patients with breast cancer for recurrence. Although CA 15-3 also can be overexpressed in other malignancies, including ovarian cancer, it is less sensitive and specific for ovarian cancer than CA 125 and rarely provides useful additional information.

Human chorionic gonadotropin is a heterodimeric protein that includes α and β subunits. It is expressed in placental tissue and used to diagnose pregnancy. The β subunit of hCG is frequently increased in malignant germ cell tumors, particularly choriocarcinoma. Again, given the patient's age, it is extremely unlikely that her adnexal masses represent a germ cell tumor.

Human epididymis protein 4 is a biomarker of ovarian cancer that also is expressed in normal tissues in the reproductive and respiratory tract. It has a reported sensitivity of 75% and specificity of 92.3% in postmenopausal patients and a sensitivity of 75% and specificity of 76.5% in premenopausal patients. It is not recommended as a screening test for ovarian cancer but is U.S. Food and Drug Administration approved for assisting with diagnostic evaluation and monitoring for relapse of disease. In the described patient, who is postmenopausal, it is unlikely that HE4 would significantly affect the CA 125 assessment of the likelihood that the patient has ovarian cancer versus another primary cancer.

Evaluation and management of adnexal masses. Practice Bulletin No. 174. American College of Obstetricians and Gynecologists. Obstet Gynecol 2016;128:e210–26. doi: 10.1097/AOG.0000000000001768

Henderson JT, Webber EM, Sawaya GF. Screening for ovarian cancer: updated evidence report and systematic review for the US Preventive Services Task Force. JAMA 2018;319:595–606. doi: 10.1001/jama.2017.21421

Kodama M, Grubbs BH, Blake EA, Cahoon SS, Murakami R, Kimura T, et al. Feto-maternal outcomes of pregnancy complicated by ovarian malignant germ cell tumor: a systematic review of literature. Eur J Obstet Gynecol Reprod Biol 2014;181:145–56. doi: 10.1016/j.ejogrb.2014.07.047

Matsas A, Stefanoudakis D, Troupis T, Kontzoglou K, Eleftheriades M, Christopoulos P, et al. Tumor markers and their diagnostic significance in ovarian cancer. Life (Basel) 2023;13:1689. doi: 10.3390/life13081689

Xie H, Erickson BJ, Sheedy SP, Yin J, Hubbard JM. The diagnosis and outcome of Krukenberg tumors. J Gastrointest Oncol 2021;12:226–36. doi: 10.21037/jgo-20-364.

113 Hospice

A 68-year-old woman with recurrent ovarian cancer is undergoing fourth-line chemotherapy. At the time of her scheduled follow-up, she reports mild fatigue and intermittent nausea that has been well managed with palliative care. She states that she is able to garden daily, enjoys walks with her spouse, and likes to cook family dinners. The most recent imaging studies reveal progression of the disease. She explains that she would like to continue to feel well and does not want to continue cytotoxic treatment. For this patient, the best type of institution for hospice referral is

(A) assisted-living facility
* (B) patient's home
(C) inpatient facility
(D) long-term nursing facility

Obstetrician–gynecologists care for women throughout their entire life span. This relationship places the obstetrician–gynecologist in the ideal position to have ongoing conversations with patients regarding their values and wishes for future end-of-life care. End-of-life care fluctuates considerably depending on the setting, degree of disease invasiveness, and intensity of care. Good end-of-life care requires an intra- and interdisciplinary approach with the patient at the center.

Opting for less invasive and intensive medical treatment at the end of life improves quality of life and reduces the patients' health care costs. Patients with high symptom burden who utilize hospice services have improved symptom management. Acceptance of hospice care is increasing within the United States, including among patients with ovarian cancer; however, early referral rates remain low, with 56% of hospice enrollees referred within 1 month of death. Referrals are most commonly made from the inpatient hospital setting rather than the outpatient clinic. These referral timings and trends have not changed much over a 10-year period. Patients referred to hospice from an inpatient setting have greater than six times the odds of referral within the last 3 days of life as compared to more than 90 days before death in the outpatient setting. Early referral to hospice is key in improving hospice enrollment while allowing the patient maximum benefit to quality of life.

In this scenario, the patient does not desire further invasive or intensive cancer treatment; therefore, early referral to hospice from the outpatient setting should be made. She is ready to transition from palliative care management of symptoms while undergoing treatment to hospice management of symptoms at the end of life. Furthermore, she is able to perform both activities of daily living and instrumental activities of daily living and wishes to continue with her hobbies. Outpatient home hospice would be the most appropriate referral to make. If she were unable to care for herself, or her family were unable to care for her, referral to hospice in an assisted living facility or nursing home may occur depending on her level of function. Inpatient hospice care is generally reserved for patients who require intravenous medications or other intensive palliative care, and thus inpatient hospice referral would not be appropriate for this patient at this time.

Early referral to hospice improves quality of life for patients, reduces invasive and intensive care that may be of no benefit, and reduces health care costs. It is important to begin conversations regarding values and goals for end-of-life care early in the disease process; this will allow for appropriately timed referrals to hospice.

End-of-life decision making. Committee Opinion No. 617. American College of Obstetricians and Gynecologists. Obstet Gynecol 2015;125:261 7. doi: 10.1097/01.AOG.0000459869.98866.91

Mullins MA, Ruterbusch J, Cote ML, Uppal S, Wallner LP. Trends in hospice referral timing and location among individuals dying of ovarian cancer: persistence of missed opportunities. Int J Gynecol Cancer 2023;33:1099–105. doi: 10.1136/ijgc-2023-004405

Taylor JS, Zhang N, Rajan SS, Chavez-MacGregor M, Zhao H, Niu J, et al. How we use hospice: hospice enrollment patterns and costs in elderly ovarian cancer patients. Gynecol Oncol 2019;152:452–8. doi: 10.1016/j.ygyno.2018.10.041

114–117 Checkpoint inhibitor toxicity

Choose the most appropriate intervention (A–D) in the setting of toxicity caused by checkpoint inhibitor therapy for the described patient (114–117).

(A) Administer intravenous (IV) corticosteroids
(B) Permanently discontinue checkpoint inhibitor therapy
(C) Administer oral corticosteroids
(D) Proceed with next cycle

114. A. A 55-year-old presents for cycle 2 of maintenance therapy with a checkpoint inhibitor. She reports 10 non-bloody stools a day for the past week.

115. C. A 62-year-old presents for cycle 4 of platinum, taxane, and a checkpoint inhibitor. She reports that since cycle 3 she has experienced joint pain that limits her ability to dress herself.

116. B. A 45-year-old presents for cycle 6 of maintenance therapy with a checkpoint inhibitor. She was recently treated and discharged from the hospital for a diagnosis of grade 4 checkpoint inhibitor hepatitis.

117. D. A 70-year-old presents for cycle 4 of maintenance checkpoint inhibitor therapy. Her pretreatment thyroid-stimulating hormone (TSH) concentration is 5.6 micro-international units/mL but her T_4 level is within normal range.

Checkpoint inhibitors, such as pembrolizumab or dostarlimab, are a type of immunotherapy being assessed or recommended for multiple clinical scenarios in gynecologic cancer, including endometrial, vulvar, ovarian, and cervical cancer. This therapy targets checkpoint proteins, which typically facilitate cancer cells to evade the immune system. Blocking these proteins leads to recognition of the tumor by the immune system and an immune response that leads to cell death. In addition, these medications can increase autoimmune-like reactions in healthy tissue. Checkpoint inhibitor therapy (specifically related to single-agent PD-(L)1 inhibition overall is well-tolerated with more than 80% of toxicities being low grade. Ten to 20% percent of patients will experience grade 3 or 4 toxicities and may require intervention, including oral or IV corticosteroids, hospitalizations, permanent discontinuation of therapy, or a mix of these options. Common toxicities include thyroiditis, colitis, or dermatitis. Less common toxicities include hepatitis, nephritis, pneumonitis, or encephalitis. For some patients, checkpoint inhibitor therapy leads to long-lasting remission and provides a survival benefit; therefore, management of these immune mediated toxicities is important. Early recognition and prompt management is critical because these effects can be fatal when unrecognized.

Colitis is an inflammation of the colon, whereas *diarrhea* is defined as watery or loose stools. Any grade diarrhea (and colitis) will occur in roughly 10% of patients on checkpoint inhibitors. Of these, less than 1% are grade 3 or 4. Immune-mediated diarrhea can progress to colitis and include nausea and abdominal pain, or both. A diagnosis of colitis requires colonoscopy; however, findings on computed tomography can also suggest colitis. *Grade 1 diarrhea* is defined as fewer than four episodes per day over baseline, whereas *grade 2* is four to six episodes per day, and *grade 3* is seven or more episodes per day. *Grade 4 diarrhea* includes life-threatening consequences requiring urgent intervention. For grade 3 or 4 diarrhea, colitis, or both, patients should be admitted to the hospital to receive IV systemic corticosteroids, IV fluids, and electrolyte replacement. If a patient has grade 3 diarrhea or colitis, or both, consideration can be given to retreatment with checkpoint inhibitor if the colitis resolves to grade 1 or less. For the patient in Scenario 114, the appropriate management for grade 3 diarrhea is to hold checkpoint therapy and treat with IV corticosteroids.

The frequency of immune checkpoint inhibitor arthralgia or arthritis, or both, can range from 1% to approximately 40%. Most commonly, joint pain occurs after 2 to 3 months of checkpoint inhibitor therapy, and some patients exhibit symptoms after the therapy has been discontinued. Patients with grade 1 arthralgia present with mild pain. When pain affects instrumental activities of daily living, arthralgia is grade 2. Grade 3 limits self-care activities of daily living. Although grade 1 arthralgia can be treated with nonsteroidal anti-inflammatory drugs, for grade 2 or higher, checkpoint inhibitor therapy should be withheld and oral corticosteroids are indicated. Referral to a rheumatologist could be useful to determine efficacy of treatment and resumption of therapy. For the patient in Scenario 115, the appropriate intervention is to administer oral corticosteroids for grade 2 arthritis.

Immune checkpoint inhibitor therapy also can increase liver enzymes and hepatitis. This adverse event has been reported in up to 10% of patients in clinical trials. Most patients present with increased liver enzymes. Mild increases (grade 1, less than three times upper limit normal) in liver enzymes do not require interruptions in therapy. Despite some limited data suggesting the feasibility of re-challenge with immune checkpoint inhibitor therapy after grade 3 or 4 hepatitis, guidelines continue to recommend permanent discontinuation after symptomatic grade 3 or any grade 4 hepatotoxicity. For the patient in Scenario 116, the appropriate intervention is to permanently discontinue therapy for hepatotoxicity.

Thyroid dysfunction related to immune checkpoint inhibitors is a common adverse event. Hypothyroidism is typical, but hyperthyroidism also can occur. Guidelines recommend thyroid function tests monthly. Most cases of thyroiditis occur within 1–2 months of starting treatment and are grade 1 or 2. *Thyrotoxicosis* is defined as a suppressed level of TSH and high free thyroxine or triiodothyronine, whereas with hypothyroidism, TSH is increased and free thyroxine is decreased. American Society of Clinical Oncology (ASCO) guidelines define hypothyroidism only in terms of TSH: Grade 2 includes TSH levels greater than 10, and grades 3–4 indicate severe symptoms. Common terminology criteria for adverse events is entirely based on symptoms. Per ASCO, one can consider holding immune checkpoint inhibitors for grade 2 and definitely hold for grades 3–4. If this criterion is not met, immune checkpoint inhibitor therapy does not need to be held. In Scenario 117, the patient's TSH level is classified as grade 1, and she can continue therapy.

Despite the toxicities associated with immune checkpoint inhibitor therapy, patients can tolerate long treatment intervals and multiple cycles of therapy. In the appropriate patient, these therapies have led to improved outcomes in several clinical settings in gynecologic cancer. With close surveillance and careful management strategies, toxicities can be managed, and patients can be continued on treatment. Management strategies can include holding therapy, treating with corticosteroids or other agents, consulting specialty services to co-manage toxicities, or using a combination of these.

Chan KK, Bass AR. Monitoring and management of the patient with immune checkpoint inhibitor-induced inflammatory arthritis: current perspectives. J Inflamm Res 2022;15:3105–18. doi: 10.2147/JIR.S282600

Miah A, Tinoco G, Zhao S, Wei L, Johns A, Patel S, et al. Immune checkpoint inhibitor-induced hepatitis injury: risk factors, outcomes, and impact on survival. J Cancer Res Clin Oncol 2023;149:2235–42. doi: 10.1007/s00432-022-04340-3

Nielsen DL, Juhl CB, Chen IM, Kellermann L, Nielsen OH. Immune checkpoint inhibitor-induced diarrhea and colitis: incidence and management. A systematic review and meta-analysis. Cancer Treat Rev 2022;109:102440. doi: 10.1016/j.ctrv.2022.102440

Schneider BJ, Naidoo J, Santomasso BD, Lacchetti C, Adkins S, Anadkat M, et al. Management of immune-related adverse events in patients treated with immune checkpoint inhibitor therapy: ASCO guideline update [published erratum appears in J Clin Oncol 2022;40:315]. J Clin Oncol 2021;39:4073–126. doi: 10.1200/JCO.21.01440

Terrin M, Migliorisi G, Dal Buono A, Gabbiadini R, Mastrorocco E, Quadarella A, et al. Checkpoint inhibitor-induced colitis: from pathogenesis to management. Int J Mol Sci 2023;24:11504. doi: 10.3390/ijms241411504

118–121 Granulosa cell ovarian tumor

Match the correct management (A–F) of the granulosa cell tumor with each patient scenario (118–121).

(A) Aromatase inhibitor
(B) Bleomycin, etoposide, and cisplatin
(C) Endometrial sampling and surgical staging
(D) Hysterectomy with oophorectomy and surgical staging
(E) Paclitaxel and carboplatin
(F) Surveillance examinations and serum inhibin B

118. F. A 56-year-old patient underwent a robot-assisted laparoscopic hysterectomy with bilateral salpingo-oophorectomy and surgical staging for a 4-cm solid mass of the ovary. The ovary was intact, cytology was negative for malignant cells, and there was no other evidence of disease.

119. D. A 42-year-old gravida 3, para 3, with a past surgical history of bilateral tubal ligation underwent an oophorectomy with bilateral salpingectomy for ovarian torsion. The 12-cm ovarian mass was removed intact.

120. C. A 28-year-old nulligravida undergoes surgery for a 6-cm cystic and solid adnexal mass found during infertility evaluation. No other visible disease is present. She undergoes a unilateral oophorectomy with a frozen section, which confirms a sex cord-stromal tumor.

121. E. A 61-year-old with stage IIIC disease undergoes a hysterectomy and bilateral salpingo-oophorectomy with suboptimal tumor debulking.

Granulosa cell tumors are a rare type of ovarian cancer classified as sex cord-stromal tumors. Sex cord-stromal tumors can be benign, malignant, or of uncertain malignant potential. Benign tumors include fibromas, thecomas, and well-differentiated Sertoli–Leydig tumors. Malignant tumors are granulosa cell tumors, moderate and poorly differentiated Sertoli–Leydig tumors, malignant steroid cell tumors, and fibrosarcomas. Several of the sex cord-stromal tumors, both benign and malignant, can be hormonally active, producing androgens, estrogen, or inhibins. Patients may present with signs of excess hormonal activity, including precocious puberty, virilization, hirsutism, abnormal uterine bleeding, or postmenopausal bleeding. Due to the production of excessive estrogen, a number of patients will also have abnormal endometrial pathology at the time of presentation. Endometrial hyperplasia has been found in 25–50% of patients, and endometrial cancer has been found in up to 10% of patients with granulosa cell tumors.

Malignant sex cord-stromal tumors are typically indolent tumors with a potential for late recurrence for as long as 30 years after the initial diagnosis. There are two histologic hallmarks for granulosa cell tumors: Call–Exner bodies and "coffee bean" nuclei. Call–Exner bodies are rosettes of cells around a fluid-filled space. The nuclei of granulosa cells appear as an elongated central depression creating the appearance of a coffee bean. Approximately 95% of adult-type granulosa cell tumors have a genetic mutation in the *FOXL2* gene, which may be used to confirm the diagnosis.

Surgical staging is typically recommended, and the types of procedures performed are based on the patient's desires for fertility. Staging for sex cord-stromal tumors is similar to that for epithelial ovarian cancer, but lymphadenectomy may be omitted when the disease appears to be confined to the ovary because the rates of lymph node metastasis are exceedingly low. Hysterectomy with bilateral salpingo-oophorectomy is recommended for those not desiring fertility. Granulosa tumors are not commonly bilateral, and if the contralateral ovary is normal appearing, they may be safely left in situ in a younger patient. Endometrial sampling should be included for fertility-sparing surgeries, given the potential for endometrial pathology due to excess estrogen secretion.

Most granulosa cells are diagnosed as stage I, and survival for these is high, with greater than 90% survival rates at 5 years. Adjuvant chemotherapy may be considered for high-risk stage I disease (ie, tumor rupture, stage IC, poorly differentiated tumors, size greater than 10–15 cm). Survival for patients with advanced disease (stages II–IV) is lower, and adjuvant therapy is typically recommended, although the benefit is uncertain. A SEER database analysis with 907 patients with stage I–IV disease did not show a survival benefit to chemotherapy in the adjuvant setting. These results are supported by a matched cohort analysis from the National Cancer Database, which also did not show a survival benefit with the addition of chemotherapy.

Chemotherapy is typically reserved for patients with advanced-stage disease, recurrence, or unresectable disease. Granulosa cell tumors generally have low rates of response to chemotherapy, but current literature and National Comprehensive Cancer Network guidelines support the use of platinum-based chemotherapy with either bleomycin, etoposide, cisplatin, or paclitaxel and carboplatin. Trials that directly compare the two chemotherapy regimens have been slow to accrue, but both regimens have shown activity in this setting. The side effect profile for paclitaxel and carboplatin is generally preferred when compared to bleomycin, etoposide, and cisplatin. Because these tumors typically express hormone receptors, the use of endocrine therapy (eg, tamoxifen, anastrozole) also should inhibit proliferation of tumors. A review of 19 trials with 31 patients treated with endocrine therapy for granulosa cell tumors showed an overall response rate of 71% (complete response, 25.8%; partial response, 42.5%). The PARAGON (ANZGOG-0903) trial evaluated 38 patients with recurrent estrogen receptor, progesterone-positive granulosa cell tumors. This was a phase 2 trial of anastrozole, and after 12 weeks, 76.3% of patients had stable disease. At 6 months on anastrozole, 59% of patients were progression free. Single-agent bevacizumab also has been shown to induce response and may be an option in the recurrent setting but would not be indicated for primary treatment. A phase 2 trial of single-agent bevacizumab showed stable disease in 77.8% of patients after a median of nine cycles of treatment. The challenge in studying the efficacy of systemic therapy in an indolent tumor is that it is unclear how much benefit is due to the therapy versus the slow-growing nature of the tumor itself.

In the primary and recurrent settings, survival benefits have been seen in the patients who receive complete surgical resection, and surgical resection of all visible disease continues to be the mainstay of granulosa cell treatment. For the patient in Scenario 118, who has a stage IA tumor with no high-risk features with adequate surgical staging, surveillance without adjuvant treatment is recommended, and this is the best option for her. For the first 2 years, surveillance with physical examination is recommended every 6–12 months for patients at low risk of recurrence and every 4–6 months for patients at higher risk of recurrence. Serum tumor markers can also be followed with a similar schedule. Monitoring serum levels of inhibin A and B can also be considered. Inhibin B is more sensitive and may be preferred, particularly if concentrations were high before surgery. Routine imaging is generally not recommended and should occur only if clinically indicated. Given the late risk of recurrence, surveillance should continue annually long term.

The patient in Scenario 119 underwent an oophorectomy and does not desire fertility, and hysterectomy with surgical staging including omentectomy and peritoneal biopsies is the best option for her. The patient in the third scenario was diagnosed with a granulosa cell tumor during an infertility workup. The best option for her includes endometrial sampling based on higher rates of abnormal endometrial pathology and complete surgical staging. The patient in Scenario 121 has metastatic disease that was not completely resected at the time of surgery, and chemotherapy is indicated. Carboplatin and paclitaxel is the best option because this therapy entails fewer adverse effects and is easier to administer compared with bleomycin, etoposide, and cisplatin.

Al Harbi R, McNeish IA, El-Bahrawy M. Ovarian sex cord-stromal tumors: an update on clinical features, molecular changes, and management. Int J Gynecol Cancer 2021;31:161–8. doi: 10.1136/ijgc-2020-002018

Banerjee SN, Tang M, O'Connell RL, Sjoquist K, Clamp AR, Millan D, et al. A phase 2 study of anastrozole in patients with oestrogen receptor and/progesterone receptor positive recurrent/metastatic granulosa cell tumours/sex-cord stromal tumours of the ovary: the PARAGON/ANZGOG 0903 trial. PARAGON investigators. Gynecol Oncol 2021;163:72–8. doi: 10.1016/j.ygyno.2021.07.024

Zhuang Y, Zhang S, Liu Y, Yang H. Can adjuvant chemotherapy improve the prognosis of adult ovarian granulosa cell tumors? A narrative review. Medicine (Baltimore) 2022;101:e29062. doi: 10.1097/MD.0000000000029062

122–127 Genitourinary injury

Match the appropriate surgical intervention (A–F) to each ureteral injury (122–127) and the corresponding site indicated in Figure 122–127-1.

(A) Cystoscopy with ureteral stent placement
(B) Percutaneous nephrostomy tube placement with delayed ureteroneocystostomy
(C) Ureteroneocystostomy
(D) Ureteroneocystostomy with psoas hitch
(E) Ureteroneocystostomy with Boari flap
(F) Uretero-ureteral anastomosis

122. F. Ureter transected with scissors during mobilization of the peritoneum in attempt to remove para-aortic lymph nodes (location 1)

123. E. Extensive thermal injury during dissection for endometriosis (location 2)

124. D. Ureter transected using electrosurgery taking down the posterior peritoneum during surgery for leiomyoma (location 3)

125. A. Ureter clamped in attempt to control bleeding at uterine vessels, recognized, and released before suture, with no devascularization noted (location 4)

126. C. Ureter incorporated into suture for hemostasis after sacrificing the uterine vessels with devascularization noted (location 4)

127. B. Worsening flank pain 3 weeks after laparoscopic hysterectomy with a computed tomography urogram showing left hydroureteronephrosis and a contrast defect (near location 3).

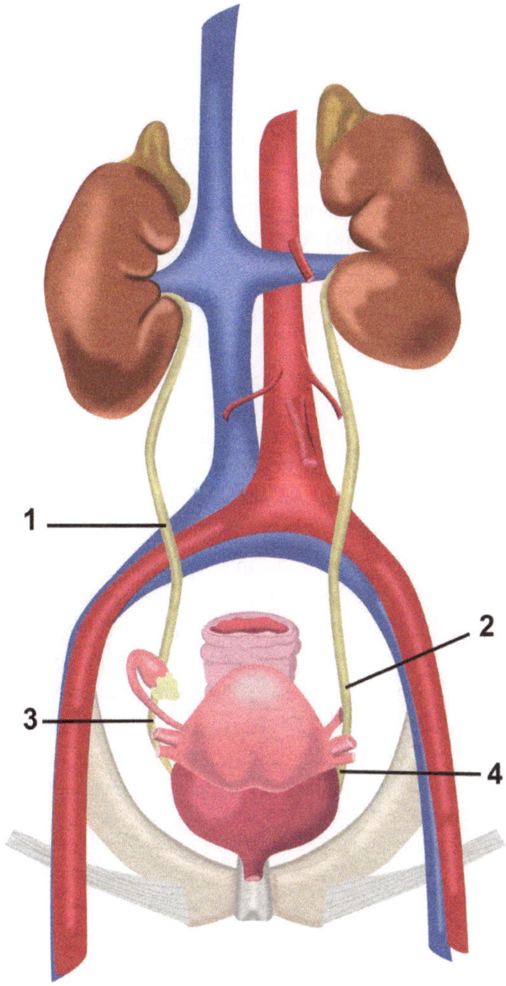

FIGURE 122-127-1. Female pelvic organs. Used with permission from Keytha Collins.

Gynecologic and obstetric surgeries are the most common cause of iatrogenic genitourinary injury apart from urologic surgery. Rates of injury vary by procedure type and surgical approach. After a hysterectomy, the incidence of bladder injury ranges from 0.2% to 1.8%, whereas the incidence of ureteral injury varies between 0.03% and 4.4%. Genitourinary injury increases postoperative morbidity and health care costs.

Treatment of genitourinary injury is largely determined by the timing of injury recognition and the type of injury.

Ureteral injury can be diagnosed intraoperatively (40% of injuries) or, more commonly, postoperatively (60% of injuries). Intraoperative recognition of ureteral injury allows for immediate repair and treatment, decreasing morbidity and risk of potential long-term complications. Intraoperative management of ureteral injury is determined by the mechanism of injury and location of injury. Injury types include laceration, transection, crush, kinking, ligation, and thermal injury. The most common procedures associated with ureteral injury during a hysterectomy are ligation of the ovarian vessels at the pelvic brim, ligation of the uterine vessels, mobilization of the bladder, and closure of the vaginal cuff. Recognition of ureteral injury can be through direct observation or at the time of cystoscopy.

Laceration and transection injuries require ureteral repair, and the type of repair is determined by the location of the injury. When transection of the ureter occurs in its upper and middle thirds, uretero-ureteral anastomosis over a ureteral stent is the recommended repair. To be successful, the repair should be tension-free with minimal use of suture. A drain to closed suction also should be placed. If more mobility of the ureter is needed, the kidney or distal ureter can be mobilized. If a tension-free repair is not feasible, a ureteroneocystostomy is the standard management. Ureteroneocystostomy is performed by employing a segment of distal ileum to bridge the gap from the proximal ureter to the bladder. In Scenario 122, a complete transection of the ureter is immediately recognized in the middle one-third, and this would be repaired with uretero-ureteral anastomosis with stent placement as a tension-free repair is highly likely.

Within the lower third of the ureter, transection and thermal injuries each raise concern for vascular compromise in its distal portion; therefore, a direct ureteroneocystostomy is the standard repair in such cases. Similarly, the ureteral reimplantation should be tension-free and over a stent. When injury occurs within close proximity to the bladder, such as those at location 4 (Fig. 122–127-1), the ureter can be directly anastomosed to the bladder over a ureteral stent without difficulty. The bladder can be mobilized, and a psoas hitch can be performed to allow for tension-free ureteroneocystostomy, when necessary, depending on the injury's location, as in Scenario 124. A psoas hitch involves complete mobilization of the bladder by freeing it from the areolar attachment anteriorly in the retropubic space; once freed, the bladder is entered at the dome, ureterostomy is done at 90 degrees to the direction desired to elongate the bladder, and the bladder is then stitched to the psoas tendon with permanent suture. For ureteral defects more than 6–8 cm from the bladder that cannot be bridged by the psoas hitch, as in Scenario 123, a Boari flap is a viable option. The Boari flap is performed by making a rhombic-shaped flap in the anterior bladder, rotating and fixating the bladder to the psoas tendon, and then re-implanting the ureter into the bladder flap allowing for a tension-free ureteral implantation.

Individuals with ureteral transection or laceration with delayed recognition can present with abdominopelvic or flank pain, peritonitis, ileus, fever, and hematuria. A high degree of suspicion for genitourinary injury should be maintained in the postoperative period, and imaging should be completed to evaluate for such injury. The patient in Scenario 127 has a delayed recognition of ureteral injury, most likely a transection or laceration with leakage of urine into the pelvis. Once confirmed, some form of immediate intervention must be undertaken. A percutaneous nephrostomy tube should be placed for urinary diversion. Although the optimal timing for repair can be debated, most experts recommend waiting several weeks to allow postoperative inflammatory changes to subside, facilitating a smoother repair.

Crushing, kinking, and ligation of the ureter can ultimately result in obstruction. If recognized intraoperatively, the offending suture or instrument should be removed and a ureteral stent placed to prevent the development of obstruction. Ureteral crush injury recognized intraoperatively, as in Scenario 125, can be managed conservatively if there is no evidence of devascularization. A ureteral stent should be placed via cystoscopy and remain in place for 7–10 days. If devascularization is noted, as in Scenario 126, the damaged portion of ureter should be resected and reimplantation with ureteroneocystostomy should be performed. Postoperatively, patients with these types of ureteral injury will present with obstruction and flank pain. Preferred management remains ureteral stent placement, either antegrade with cystoscopy or retrograde with percutaneous nephrostomy, if feasible. If ureteral stenting is impossible, urinary diversion with percutaneous nephrostomy and delayed ureteral reimplantation often is used.

Ureteral injuries are a well-known complication of gynecologic surgery. Although prevention with strong knowledge of anatomy and meticulous surgical technique is paramount, gynecologic surgeons must be able to recognize and manage these complications intraoperatively and postoperatively.

Burks FN, Santucci RA. Management of iatrogenic ureteral injury. Ther Adv Urol 2014;6:115–24. doi: 10.1177/1756287214526767

De Cicco C, Ret Dávalos ML, Van Cleynenbreugel B, Verguts J, Koninckx PR. Iatrogenic ureteral lesions and repair: a review for gynecologists. J Minim Invasive Gynecol 2007;14:428–35. doi: 10.1016/j.jmig.2007.01.003

Sharp HT, Adelman MR. Prevention, recognition, and management of urologic injuries during gynecologic surgery. Obstet Gynecol 2016;127:1085–96. doi: 10.1097/AOG.0000000000001425

Stein R, Rubenwolf P, Ziesel C, Kamal MM, Thüroff JW. Psoas hitch and Boari flap ureteroneocystostomy. BJU Int 2013;112:137–55. doi: 10.1111/bju.12103

128–132 Cervical cancer screening in patients with human immunodeficiency virus/immunocompromised status

Choose the best testing (A–E) option for each clinical scenario (128–132).

(A) Cervical cytology with human papillomavirus (HPV) testing now
(B) Cervical cytology with HPV testing in 12 months
(C) Cervical cytology with HPV testing in 3 years
(D) Cervical cytology with HPV testing in 5 years
(E) Colposcopy now with endocervical curettage

128. A. A 35-year-old woman presents for a well-woman examination after a new diagnosis of HIV. Her last cervical cytology was 2 years ago and was negative for intraepithelial lesion or malignancy (NILM).

129. C. A 45-year-old woman with HIV presents to follow up on cervical cytology results. She has had two prior screenings that returned normal cytology with negative HPV testing. Her most recent result is NILM cytology, HPV negative.

130. B. A 32-year-old women diagnosed with HIV 1 year ago, with normal cervical cytology and HPV testing at that time, has a repeat screening that indicates NILM cytology, HPV negative.

131. E. A 55-year-old woman living with HIV presents to discuss the results of her recent cervical cancer screening, which indicated atypical squamous cells of undetermined significance (ASC-US) cytology and non-HPV 16/18 positive status. One year ago, her screening results were NILM cytology and HPV negative status.

132. C. An 18-year-old woman with newly diagnosed HIV presents for a routine gynecology appointment and has no prior cervical cancer screening. She is not currently sexually active.

Individuals who are immunocompromised are at risk of HPV persistence and development of cervical cancer. In the United States, women living with HIV have a significantly higher prevalence of cervical cancer when compared to women in the general population. Human immunodeficiency virus infection and low CD4 cell count have been associated with HPV infection persistence and pre-cancer. Given this, screening occurs at more frequent intervals.

Multiple groups have devised consensus guidelines for cervical cancer screening in patients with HIV (Table 128–132-1). Historically, screening was initiated early (before age 21 years), but development of cervical cancer before age 21 is rare. Some societies recommend that screening start at the time of HIV diagnosis but no sooner than age 21 years. A 2019 study published by the HIV/AIDS Cancer Match Study included 160,000 women living with HIV, and 552 developed cervical cancer, but none of these individuals developed cancer before age 21 years. In 2021, the Centers for Disease Control and Prevention (CDC), National Institutes of Health (NIH), and HIV Medicine Association of the Infectious Diseases Society of America (HIVMA) recommended screening women with HIV at the time of diagnosis only starting at age 21, regardless of sexual activity.

After initial cervical cancer screening with normal results, screening with cytology alone in individuals under the age of 30 years should be performed annually for 3 years followed by screening every 3 years until age 30. In patients over age 30, screening may continue with cytology alone or with co-testing every 3 years; primary HPV testing guidelines for immunocompromised populations have not yet been developed (Fig. 128–132-1). In general, colposcopy is recommended for all HPV-positive results, persistent ASC-US cytology over 6–12 months, and any low-grade squamous intraepithelial lesion or higher-grade cytology.

The patient in Scenario 128 is presenting after a new diagnosis of HIV. Despite having completed screening within the last 3 years, because she now has a new diagnosis of HIV, cervical cytology and HPV testing are recommended. This recommendation is in accordance with the CDC, NIH, and HIVMA.

The patient in Scenario 129 has a known HIV diagnosis. Including her most current result, she has now completed three annual routine screenings. Because she has had three normal results over three consecutive years since initial normal screening, she may now space screening to every 3 years.

The patient in Scenario 130 was diagnosed with HIV 1 year ago and now has completed two screening examinations,

TABLE 128-132-1. Overview of Cervical Cancer Screening Guidelines Among People With HIV/Immunocompromised by Society Recommendations

OVERVIEW OF CERVICAL CANCER SCREENING GUIDELINES					
	LESS THAN 21 YEARS	**21-24 YEARS**	**25-29 YEARS**	**30 YEARS OR OLDER**	**COMMENTS**
NIH OAR Adult and Adolescent OI Guidelines (specific to people with HIV)	No screening recommended	**Cytology Only** • Cytology yearly — If normal cytology on 3 consecutive annual tests, adjust to every 3 years	**Cytology Only** • Cytology yearly — If normal cytology on 3 consecutive annual tests, adjust to every 3 years	**Co-testing*** • Co-testing yearly — If normal cytology and hr-HPV negative on 3 consecutive years, adjust to every 3 years **Cytology Only** • Cytology yearly • If normal cytology on 3 consecutive years, adjust to every 3 years	
USPSTF (no HIV-specific guidance)	No screening recommended	• Cytology every 3 years	• Cytology every 3 years	**Cytology Only** • Every 3 years **hr-HPV Testing Only** Every 5 years co-testing* Every 5 years	Not specific to people with HIV
ASCCP					Same as USPSTF
ACOG					Same as USPSTF
ACS (no HIV-specific guidance)	No screening recommended	No screening recommended	**Preferred** • Primary HPV test† every 5 years **Acceptable** • Co-testing every 5 years • Cytology alone every 3 years	**Preferred** • Primary HPV test† every 5 years **Acceptable** • Co-testing every 5 years • Cytology alone every 3 years	Updated July 2020 Not specific to people with HIV
WHO (HIV-specific guidance)	No screening recommended	No screening recommended	**Preferred** • Primary HPV test† (provider-obtained or self-collection every 3–5 years)	**Preferred** • Primary HPV test† (provider-obtained or self-collection every 3–5 years)	Updated July 2021

Abbreviations: ACOG, American College of Obstetricians and Gynecologists; ACS, American Cancer Society; ASCCP, American Society for Colposcopy and Cervical Pathology; HPV, human papillomavirus; hr-HPV, high-risk HPV; NIH OAR, National Institutes of Health Office of AIDS Research; OI, opportunistic infection; USPSTF, United States Preventive Services Task Force; WHO, World Health Organization.

*Co-testing refers to combined cytology and high-risk HPV (hr-HPV) testing.

†Primary HPV testing is hr-HPV testing alone.

Reprinted from Office of AIDS Research. Overview of cervical cancer screening guidelines. In: Guidelines for the prevention and treatment of opportunistic infections in adults and adolescents with HIV. National Institutes of Health; 2024. Accessed March 13, 2025. https://clinicalinfo.hiv.gov/en/guidelines/hiv-clinical-guidelines-adult-and-adolescent-opportunistic-infections/human

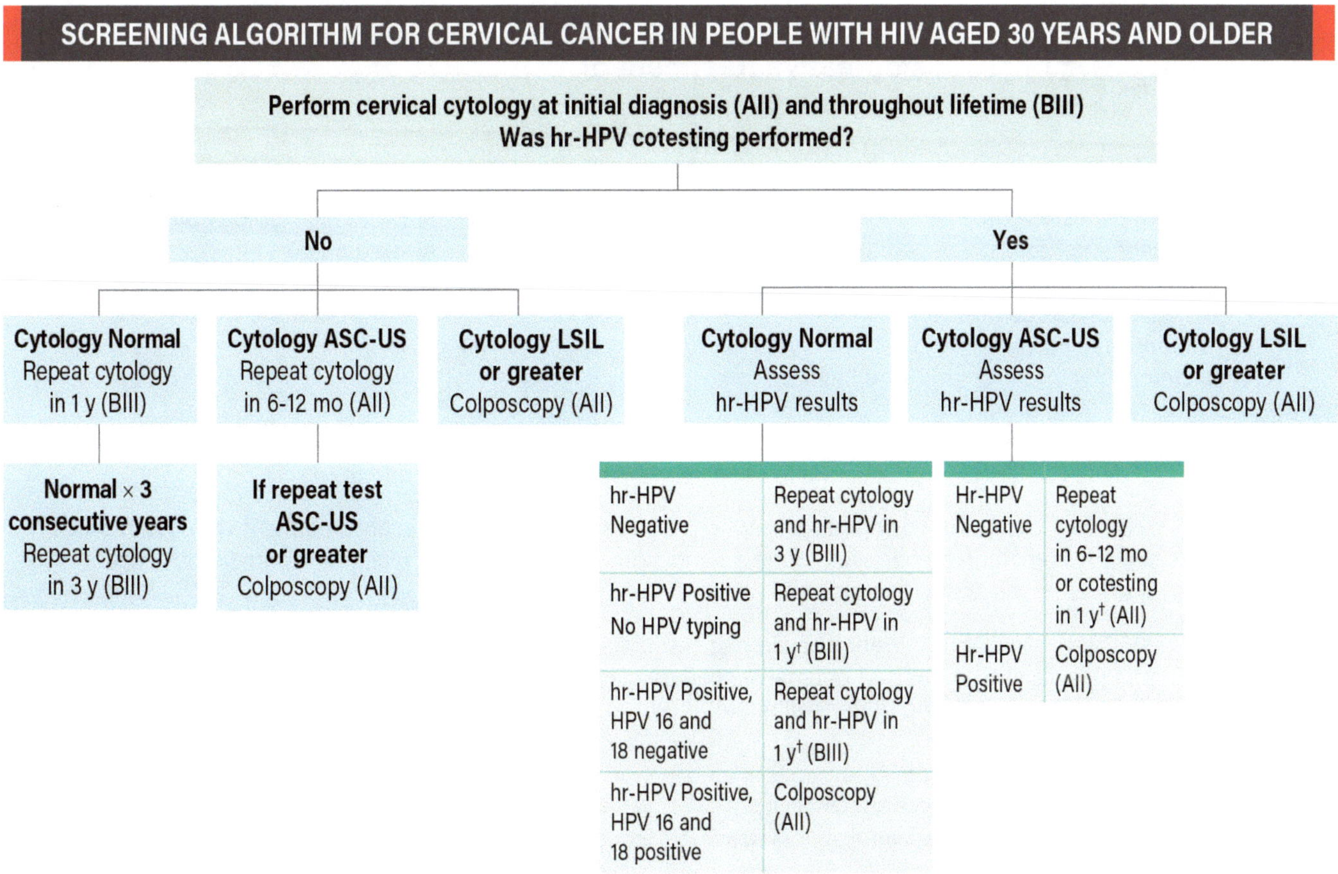

FIGURE 128-132-1. Screening algorithm for cervical cancer in people with HIV aged 30 years and older. (Reprinted from Budak JZ. Basic HIV primary care: primary care management. In: Spach DH, Wood BR, Budak JZ, Kalapila AG, editors. National HIV curriculum. 3rd ed. University of Washington Infectious Diseases Education & Assessment (IDEA) Program; 2025. Accessed September 8, 2025.)

that returned negative. She requires additional follow-up in 12 months with cervical cytology and HPV testing.

The patient in Scenario 131 has an ASC-US, non-HPV 16/18 cervical cytology result. Given HPV positivity, colposcopy is recommended. Positive HPV screening test results are more common in women living with HIV, and up to 35% of women with HIV will have an abnormal cytology (ASC-US positive) at each clinical visit.

The patient in Scenario 132 is presenting at age 18 years with a new diagnosis of HIV. Screening may begin in 3 years at age 21 given her age and the rarity of cervical cancer cases in women with HIV less than age 21. This is in accordance with recommendations by the CDC, NIH, and HIVMA.

Women with HIV should not space out screening to 5-year increments, given their increased risk for progression to cervical intraepithelial neoplasia and cervical cancer. Additionally, women older than 65 years who have a diagnosis of HIV should continue screening, given their higher risk for cervical cancer. Patients with HIV do not qualify for primary HPV testing. Clinicians should discuss prevention strategies for cervical cancer with patients including HPV vaccination, smoking cessation, and condom use.

Cervical cancer screening guidelines for adolescents. Contemp Ob Gyn 2022;67(8):24–8.

Office of AIDS Research. Guidelines for the prevention and treatment of opportunistic infections in adults and adolescents with HIV. National Institutes of Health; 2024. Accessed March 13, 2025.

Timoney MT, Atrio JM, McGowan JP, Fine SM, Vail R, Merrick ST, et al. Screening for cervical dysplasia and cancer in adults with HIV. Johns Hopkins University; 2022.

133–135 Postoperative treatment of ovarian cancer

Choose the most appropriate treatment (A–C) for each of the patients (133–135) with high-grade epithelial ovarian cancer and Eastern Cooperative Oncology Group (ECOG) performance status of 0.

(A) Paclitaxel and carboplatin
(B) Liposomal doxorubicin
(C) Gemcitabine, carboplatin, and bevacizumab

133. A. A 60-year-old-presents with stage III disease. She is chemotherapy naive and has undergone optimal primary cytoreduction. She has hypertension and nephrotic syndrome.

134. B. A 62-year old with recurrent disease who progressed on her most recent treatment with platinum-based chemotherapy has undergone an end sigmoid colostomy for malignant sigmoid obstruction. She has no medical comorbidities.

135. C. A 63-year old with recurrent disease had complete response to her last course of carboplatin and paclitaxel. She has had optimal secondary cytoreduction. Today she presents with grade III chemotherapy-induced peripheral neuropathy.

Patients presenting with newly diagnosed advanced high-grade ovarian cancer are best treated with a combination of surgical cytoreduction and combined platinum-based systemic chemotherapy.

For decades, the first step in treatment of a patient with suspected ovarian cancer had been an exploratory operation intended to simultaneously confirm the diagnosis and remove as much cancer as feasible, ideally leaving no gross residual disease. The amount of disease remaining at the completion of surgery is recognized as the most important prognostic factor for survival. The tumor's responsiveness to platinum also is critical for achieving long-term remission and cure.

The 2010 Gynecologic Cancer Intergroup study randomized more than 600 patients with advanced ovarian cancer to either primary cytoreductive surgery followed by at least six courses of platinum-based chemotherapy or to three courses of neoadjuvant platinum-based chemotherapy followed by interval debulking surgery and at least three postoperative courses of platinum-based chemotherapy. The study concluded that neoadjuvant chemotherapy followed by surgery and additional chemotherapy was not inferior to the traditional approach of upfront surgery followed by chemotherapy. This publication altered the approach to patients with advanced ovarian cancer. Currently, although primary surgery remains a mainstay of treatment, patients who are medically unfit to tolerate a major cytoreductive procedure and those whose disease is unlikely to be optimally cytoreduced are treated with neoadjuvant chemotherapy followed by planned interval surgery and additional chemotherapy.

Even though response to platinum-based chemotherapy is high and patients often have no detectable disease at the completion of primary treatment, recurrence is common among patients with advanced ovarian cancer. Treatment of recurrence nearly always includes systemic therapy and is highly individualized. The approach to a patient with recurrence is influenced by a number of factors including site and number of metastases, medical comorbidities, performance status, preexisting toxicities, genetic and molecular profile, and predicted sensitivity to retreatment with platinum (which correlates with responsiveness to many other drugs as well). Characteristics of recurrent disease that are correlated with a higher probability of response to chemotherapy include longer disease-free interval, prior complete response, and homologous repair deficiency. Recurrent disease is typically classified as platinum sensitive (platinum free interval of 6 months or more), platinum resistant (platinum free interval of less than 6 months), or platinum refractory (progression of tumor during the most recent course of platinum-based chemotherapy). Prognosis is best for patients with platinum-sensitive disease because their disease is far more likely to respond to second line treatment than resistant or refractory disease.

The role of surgery in treatment of patients with recurrent ovarian cancer is controversial. The literature includes reports of a few prospective, randomized clinical trials with conflicting results. Although recommendations of surgery for recurrent disease are individualized, factors that favor surgery include an intent to palliate a patient with a malignant large bowel obstruction and resection of an isolated metastasis in a patient with excellent performance status and a long platinum-free interval who is an excellent candidate for postoperative systemic treatment.

The cornerstone of primary systemic treatment for ovarian cancer is platinum. Carboplatin is preferred over cisplatin because of a more favorable adverse effect profile, including lower incidences of nausea and vomiting, nephrotoxicity, and neuropathy. It is standard to combine carboplatin with a taxane (paclitaxel or docetaxel) for initial systemic treatment. Depending on the clinical circumstance, bevacizumab, an anti-vascular endothelial growth factor (VEGF) antibody, concurrently and as maintenance may be used as a third component of first line therapy. Certain patients may be considered for post chemotherapy maintenance. A number of agents may be considered for maintenance, depending on individual tumor characteristics. A poly(ADP-ribose) polymerase inhibitor is recommended for maintenance in patients with homologous repair deficient tumors, including those with mutations in *BRCA1* or *BRCA2*.

Systemic treatment of recurrent disease also is highly individualized. In general, patients with platinum-sensitive disease recurrence are treated with a combination of carboplatin and another agent. Liposomal doxorubicin, paclitaxel, and gemcitabine are commonly recommended. Bevacizumab may be added to any of the platinum combinations. In addition to platinum combinations, there are a number of other options for single agent treatment for recurrence.

Treatment of patients with platinum-resistant disease is challenging. Response rates are in the range of 20%. Options include a variety of single-agent cytotoxic and biologic agents, including mirvetuximab for patients whose tumor expresses folate receptor α. Checkpoint inhibitor immunotherapy (pembrolizumab or dostarlimab) may be considered for the few patients with mismatch repair deficient (MMRd) or microsatellite instability high (MSI-H) tumors or with tumor mutation burden high (TMB-H) disease.

The patient in Scenario 133 is best treated with paclitaxel and carboplatin. Although bevacizumab could be considered, its side effects include hypertension and proteinuria, which could exacerbate her medical comorbidities. Because this patient had an optimal cytoreduction, it would be reasonable to avoid exposing her to the risks of adding bevacizumab.

In Scenario 134, the patient has recurrent chemo-refractory disease and has undergone a diverting colostomy for malignant bowel obstruction. Although a discussion of best supportive care is appropriate, treatment also is an option. A non-platinum single agent, such as liposomal doxorubicin, is a suitable choice. Because she has a tumor on the colon wall, bevacizumab should be avoided given that it is associated with an increased risk of intestinal perforation, particularly in areas of tumor involvement.

The patient in Scenario 135 has platinum-sensitive recurrence and significant preexisting neuropathy that might be exacerbated by administration of paclitaxel. Although docetaxel could be considered, substituting gemcitabine for paclitaxel, as described in the OCEANS study, will provide a similar response rate. In OCEANS, the addition of bevacizumab concurrently with chemotherapy and as subsequent maintenance therapy significantly improved progression-free survival compared with chemotherapy alone.

Aghajanian, Carol, et al. Final overall survival and safety analysis of OCEANS, a phase 3 trial of chemotherapy with or without bevacizumab in patients with platinum-sensitive recurrent ovarian cancer. Gynecologic oncology 139.1 (2015): 10-1

National Comprehensive Cancer Network. Ovarian cancer: including fallopian tube cancer and primary peritoneal cancer. Version 1.2025. NCCN Clinical Practice Guidelines in Oncology [after login]. NCCN; 2025. Accessed April 22, 2025. https://www.nccn.org/guidelines/guidelines-detail?category=1&id=1453

Vergote I, Tropé CG, Amant F, Kristensen GB, Ehlen T, Johnson N, et al. Neoadjuvant chemotherapy or primary surgery in stage IIIC or IV ovarian cancer. N Engl J Med 2010;363:943–53. doi: 10.1056/NEJMoa0908806

136–139 Cancer syndromes

Choose the most likely germline mutation (A–F) for each clinical scenario (136–139).

(A) *BRCA1*
(B) *DICER1*
(C) *MSH6*
(D) *PTEN*
(E) *STK11*
(F) *TP53*

136. E. A 21-year-old nulligravida receives a diagnosis of cervical adenocarcinoma on biopsy. She has areas of increased pigmentation on their fingers, toes, and inside the mouth.

137. A. A 35-year-old gravida 2, para 2, undergoes a bilateral salpingectomy for sterilization. Final pathology reveals serous tubal intraepithelial carcinoma (STIC). The patient reports that her mother has a history of triple-negative breast cancer at age 42 years.

138. F. A 28-year-old gravida 1, para 1, has a history of childhood soft tissue sarcoma and receives a diagnosis of breast cancer on biopsy.

139. B. A 15-year-old nulligravida presents with clitoromegaly, voice deepening, male-pattern baldness, and amenorrhea. Her pelvic ultrasonography demonstrates a complex mass on the right ovary.

The patient in Scenario 136, with cervical adenocarcinoma and skin hyperpigmentation, most likely has Peutz–Jeghers syndrome, which is caused by an autosomal dominant germline mutation in the tumor suppressor gene *STK11*. Hyperpigmentation of mucosa is present in more than 95% of patients with Peutz–Jeghers syndrome, and they usually dissipate with age. These patients have an increased risk of cancer of the gastrointestinal tract as well as many types of gynecologic cancer, including cervical adenoma malignum (a specific type of adenocarcinoma), ovarian sex-cord stromal tumors, endometrial cancer, and breast cancer (Appendix K, Table K-1).

The patient in Scenario 137 has a diagnosis of STIC and first-degree family history of premenopausal triple-negative breast cancer, which is suggestive of hereditary breast and ovarian cancer syndrome, such as a *BRCA1* mutation. Hereditary breast and ovarian cancer syndrome can be caused by several germline pathogenic variants, most notably *BRCA1* and *BRCA2*, but also *ATM, BRIP1, PALB1, RAD51C,* and *RAD51D,* among others. Patients with autosomal dominant germline mutations in tumor suppressor *BRCA1* mutation have a 64–75% lifetime risk of breast cancer and 39–46% lifetime risk of ovarian cancer. The American College of Obstetricians & Gynecologists recommends affected patients to undergo risk-reducing bilateral salpingo-oophorectomy between ages 35–40 years or when childbearing is completed (Appendix K, Table K-2). In contrast, *BRCA2*-related ovarian cancer occurs later than *BRCA1*, and risk-reducing surgery can be delayed until she is aged 40–45 years. This patient also should undergo enhanced breast cancer screening with mammography and MRI of the breasts annually, with consideration for risk-reducing mastectomy.

The patient in Scenario 138 has a history of childhood soft tissue sarcoma, and a new diagnosis of breast cancer is suggestive of Li–Fraumeni syndrome, an autosomal dominant hereditary cancer caused by germline mutation in tumor suppressor *TP53*. This can increase the risk of malignancy up to 50 times that of the general population and is more common in women. A variety of malignancies can occur and most commonly include sarcomas, brain tumors, premenopausal breast cancer, and gastrointestinal cancer. Early-onset cancer is more common, and more than 50% of patients are diagnosed before they are 30 years old. The risk of malignancy is greater than 90% by age 70 years.

The patient in Scenario 139 has evidence of hyperandrogenism in addition to a complex adnexal mass. Frequently, Sertoli–Leydig ovarian tumors can lead to virilization, caused by an autosomal dominant mutation in *DICER1*. This rare condition is associated with an increased risk of pleuropulmonary blastoma, Wilms tumor, thyroid cancer, cervical embryonal rhabdomyosarcoma, gynandroblastomas, Sertoli–Leydig ovarian tumors, and others. Most Sertoli–Leydig cancer attributable to *DICER1* mutation are stage I at diagnosis, occur in adolescence, and present with virilization or amenorrhea.

None of the clinical scenarios are suggestive of either an *MSH6* or *PTEN* mutation.

An *MSH6* mutation is associated with Lynch syndrome and an increased risk of endometrial, colon, and ovarian cancer. Approximately 3–5% of all endometrial cancer is hereditary, and most types are due to Lynch syndrome, which is caused by mutations in DNA mismatch repair genes *MLH1, MSH2, MSH6, PMS2,* and *EPCAM*. The lifetime risks of endometrial (30–71%) and ovarian cancer (4–24%) vary, with risk of colorectal cancer as high as 85%, depending on the specific mutation.

Mutations in the tumor suppressor *PTEN* are present in *PTEN* hamartoma tumor syndrome (formerly referred to as *Cowden syndrome*), and cause characteristic hamartomas and mucocutaneous lesions. Breast cancer risk approaches 85%, whereas the risk of endometrial cancer is 13–28%, usually premenopausal onset, and is inherited in an autosomal dominant fashion.

Hampel H, Bennett RL, Buchanan A, Pearlman R, Wiesner GL. A practice guideline from the American College of Medical Genetics and Genomics and the National Society of Genetic Counselors: referral indications for cancer predisposition assessment. Genet Med 2015;17:70–87. doi: 10.1038/gim.2014.147

Hereditary cancer syndromes and risk assessment. ACOG Committee Opinion No. 793. American College of Obstetricians and Gynecologists. Obstet Gynecol 2019;134:e143–9. doi: 10.1097/AOG.0000000000003562

Kostov S, Watrowski R, Kornovski Y, Dzhenkov D, Slavchev S, Ivanova Y, et al. Hereditary gynecologic cancer syndromes a narrative review. Onco Targets Ther 2022;15:381–405. doi: 10.2147/OTT.S353054

140–143 High-risk gestational trophoblastic neoplasia

Choose the most appropriate treatment (A–D) for each of the patients with gestational trophoblastic neoplasia (GTN) (140–143).

(A) Hysterectomy
(B) Reduced-dose induction multiagent chemotherapy
(C) Immunotherapy
(D) Single-agent chemotherapy

140. B. A 39-year-old woman had evacuation of a hydatidiform mole 4 months ago. Her human chorionic gonadotropin (hCG) concentration is 1,100,000 mIU/mL. She has nine metastases to the liver, spleen, and peritoneum, the largest of which is 10 cm. She has had no prior chemotherapy.

141. C. A 25-year-old woman had evacuation of a hydatiform mole 20 months ago. Her hCG is 200,000 mIU/mL. She has seven lung metastases, the largest of which is 2 cm. She declines cytotoxic chemotherapy.

142. A. A 50-year-old woman had evacuation of a hydatidiform mole 14 months ago and subsequent treatment with single-agent methotrexate followed by single-agent actinomycin-D. The hCG plateaued at 900 (units). Repeat computed tomography shows a mass in the uterus and no evidence of metastatic disease.

143. D. A 37-year-old woman with low-risk (stage I) GTN is undergoing treatment with actinomycin D. Her β-hCG nadir was 60 mIU/mL and subsequent values plateaued over 3 weeks. She is asymptomatic. Imaging reveals disease confined to the uterus. During counseling, she reports completed childbearing, and she chooses to undergo a hysterectomy and bilateral salpingectomy.

Gestational trophoblastic disease comprises several tumors of placental origin that result from disorders of fertilization. The benign forms include complete and partial hydatidiform moles and placental nodules. Malignant gestational trophoblastic disease, also known as *gestational trophoblastic neoplasia*, most frequently follows a molar pregnancy but may occur after any type of gestation, including term or preterm births, abortions, or ectopic pregnancies. Types of GTN include postmolar disease, invasive mole, choriocarcinoma, placental site trophoblastic tumor, and epithelioid trophoblastic tumor.

With the exception of placental site trophoblastic tumor and epithelioid trophoblastic tumor, both of which are quite uncommon, GTN are classified according to International Federation of Gynecology and Obstetrics (FIGO) stage (Appendix H) and WHO score (Appendix I). Patients with FIGO stage I GTN and those with FIGO stages II or III and a WHO score of 6 or less have low-risk disease. These patients are treated with single-agent chemotherapy, typically methotrexate or actinomycin D, and have an excellent prognosis. For most patients with low-risk GTN, these treatments are curative, but some will require second-line treatment or more. For those with WHO scores of 5 or 6, the single-agent treatments are at a particularly high risk of failure. Up to 70% of tumors do not respond to single-agent treatment.

Patients with FIGO stage IV disease and those with any stage disease with a WHO score of 7 or more have high-risk GTN. High-risk disease requires more aggressive treatment, typically with combination chemotherapy. The most commonly utilized regimen for patients with high-risk GTN is EMA-CO, which consists of etoposide, methotrexate, and actinomycin-D on day 1, and cyclophosphamide and vincristine on day 8, repeated every 14 days.

Patients with a WHO score of 13 or greater are considered ultra-high risk. These individuals are at exceptionally high risk of life-threatening complications. Initial treatment with induction chemotherapy has resulted in better outcomes due to a reduction in the risk of hemorrhage or other life-threatening consequences of therapy.

Surgery and radiation each have a role in selected patients with GTN. Recommendations are individualized according to site(s) of metastases, reproductive goals, and other considerations.

The best treatment choice for the patient in Scenario 140 is reduced-dose induction multiagent chemotherapy. She has a WHO score of 14: her hCG is 100,000 mUI/mL (4 points), she has a 10-cm tumor (2 points), she has liver metastases (4 points), and she has nine metastatic lesions (4 points). She is considered ultra-high risk, and literature suggests that risk of hemorrhage and other life-threatening adverse events may be mitigated by a course of low-dose induction chemotherapy. This approach, giving reduced doses of etoposide and cisplatin for 1 to 2 weeks before initiating full-dose EMA-CO, has been used at the Charing Cross Gestational Trophoblastic Center in London for a number of years and has been associated with a dramatic reduction in early death. This patient's liver disease poses a particularly high risk of bleeding, and radiation therapy, embolization, or even resection may be considered as well.

Immunotherapy is the best treatment choice for the patient in Scenario 141. She has a WHO score of 11: she is 20 months from the antecedent pregnancy to diagnosis (4 points), her hCG is 200,000 mIU/mL (4 points), and she has seven metastatic lesions (3 points.) She would have a relatively high chance of cure, approximately 80%, if she were to accept conventional multiagent chemotherapy. Her declining response to standard treatment compels consideration of alternative systemic therapies. There are published reports of successful treatment of patients with chemo-refractory GTN who have responded to immunotherapy (checkpoint inhibition). Pembrolizumab (anti-PD-1) and avelumab (anti-PD-L1) each have been described as active in patients with GTN. Although additional research is needed before these drugs can be considered standard treatment, success in small series of selected patients is encouraging and merits consideration for this patient who declines traditional chemotherapy.

In Scenario 142, the patient should undergo a hysterectomy. Presuming she is a suitable candidate for surgery, hysterectomy is the best option because it avoids exposure to the adverse effects of combination chemotherapy. She has a WHO score of 9: she is 50 years old (1 point), molar pregnancy was the antecedent pregnancy (0 point), more than 12 months have passed from the antecedent pregnancy to her diagnosis (4 points), and two previous chemotherapy regimens failed (4 points). Because she has no obvious metastases on computed tomography, it is likely that the uterus is the site of a residual tumor. Her hCG levels should be monitored after surgery to ensure complete normalization. If she were of childbearing age and desirous of preserving fertility, combination chemotherapy without hysterectomy would be recommended. Hysterectomy also is an option for selected patients with low-risk disease confined to the uterus.

The patient in Scenario 143 has low-risk GTN and is undergoing single-agent treatment with actinomycin D. She had an initial response to treatment but her β-hCG has plateaued, and she has disease confined to the uterus on imaging. Given these features and her completed childbearing, she opted for hysterectomy. An alternative option for patients who prefer to maintain fertility is to change therapy to single-agent methotrexate. The National Comprehensive Cancer Network guidelines recommend that patients who undergo hysterectomy in this scenario also should receive the single-agent chemotherapy not used in initial treatment. Presumably, hysterectomy would decrease the number of chemotherapy cycles needed for treatment; however, there is insufficient evidence to confirm this theory. This patient should receive methotrexate and β-hCG monitoring for response with continuation of chemotherapy until β-hCG is undetectable for two to three cycles after normalization, then monthly for 1 year.

Horowitz NS, Eskander RN, Adelman MR, Burke W. Epidemiology, diagnosis, and treatment of gestational trophoblastic disease: a Society of Gynecologic Oncology evidenced-based review and recommendation. Gynecol Oncol 2021;163:605–13. doi: 10.1016/j.ygyno.2021.10.003

Ngan HY, Seckl MJ, Berkowitz RS, Xiang Y, Golfier F, Sekharan PK, et al. Diagnosis and management of gestational trophoblastic disease: 2021 update. Int J Gynaecol Obstet 2021;155(suppl 1):86–93. doi: 10.1002/ijgo.13877

Soper JT. Gestational trophoblastic disease: current evaluation and management [published erratum appears in Obstet Gynecol 2022;139:149]. Obstet Gynecol 2021;137:355–70. doi: 10.1097/AOG.0000000000004240

144–147 Optimal modality of breast imaging

Choose the correct breast imaging modality (A–D) for each clinical scenario (144–147).

(A) Mammography
(B) Mammography and ultrasonography
(C) Ultrasonography
(D) Magnetic resonance imaging with contrast

144. C. A 25-year-old woman presents with a new breast lump that has been present for 4 months. Her maternal grandmother had breast cancer at age 67 years.

145. A. A 51-year-old asymptomatic patient presents for her annual examination. She is adopted and does not know her family history.

146. A. A 47-year-old woman has a new breast lump that is palpable on clinical breast examination. She has no family history of breast or ovarian cancer.

147. D. A 27-year-old asymptomatic woman presents for her annual examination. She is a *BRCA1* mutation carrier.

Breast symptoms should be elicited at annual gynecologic examinations and when patients present reporting specific breast concerns. A breast symptom history should include any symptoms or changes the patient has had, including pain, changes in the appearance or feel of breast tissue, duration of these changes, the area of concern, the presence of nipple discharge, and any changes over time. The initial evaluation also should include an assessment of the individual's risk of breast cancer based on the personal and family history as well as a clinical breast examination to evaluate for abnormalities. A clinical breast examination is used for initial evaluation of a patient's symptoms and can be offered to asymptomatic patients of average risk. The optimal breast imaging modality to evaluate a given patient differs based on the indication for testing as well as her personal risk for breast cancer.

Breast imaging is an important screening tool that is used to identify breast cancer in asymptomatic patients. The goal of breast screening imaging modalities is to detect early-stage disease to improve outcomes and survival. Screening tests for asymptomatic patients may lead to false-positive results that may have negative psychosocial effects on an individual patient, including increased anxiety related to abnormal results, increased cost, and potential overtreatment, and screening recommendations must balance the risks and benefits for individual patients. The American College of Obstetricians & Gynecologists recommends a shared decision-making approach to counseling regarding a patient's options for breast screening. Generally, screening mammography should be offered or recommended to average-risk individuals at age 40 years. Mammography results are categorized based on findings, and the recommended management strategies vary based on the likelihood of a malignancy (Table 144–147-1).

Screening mammography in individuals found to have *dense breasts*, defined as Breast Imaging-Reporting and Data System (BI-RADs) category C or D (Table 144–147-2), is less sensitive at detecting breast cancer. These individuals are at increased risk of breast cancer, but available data have not found that additional screening with other modalities offers additional benefit. Nevertheless, some states have laws that require gynecologists to discuss these increased risks and offer screening with breast ultrasonography for patients with dense breasts.

Patients with hereditary breast and ovarian cancer syndromes are at increased risk of breast cancer. By age 70 years, 45–85% of patients who are carriers of *BRCA1* or *BRCA2* will be diagnosed with breast cancer. The screening approach for these patients differs compared with those of average risk. Patients aged 25–29 with *BRCA* mutations should undergo a clinical breast examination every 6–12 months and breast MRI with contrast annually. Those aged 30 years and older should undergo annual screening mammography and breast MRI, alternating every 6 months, along with annual clinical breast examinations.

Diagnostic imaging options for patients with breast symptoms differ based on the patient's age and presenting symptoms. Patients younger than 30 years with a breast mass should be managed based on clinical suspicion of disease. Those with low suspicion of malignancy can be observed for 1–3 menstrual cycles and if the mass persists, diagnostic ultrasonography is indicated. Those with high clinical suspicion for malignancy should proceed to directly diagnostic ultrasonography. Further management depends on the ultrasound findings and may include routine observation, interval surveillance imaging, diagnostic mammography, or tissue sampling. Individuals

TABLE 144-147-1. Breast Imaging-Reporting and Data System (BI-RADS) Categories for Mammography Assessment

ASSESSMENT	MANAGEMENT	LIKELIHOOD OF CANCER
Category 0: Incomplete—need additional imaging evaluation and/or prior mammograms for comparison	Recall for additional imaging and/or comparison with prior examination(s)	N/A
Category 1: Negative	Routine mammography screening	Essentially 0% likelihood of malignancy
Category 2: Benign	Routine mammography screening	Essentially 0% likelihood of malignancy
Category 3: Probably benign	Short-interval (6-month) follow-up or continued surveillance mammography	Greater than 0% but 2% or lower likelihood of malignancy
Category 4: Suspicious	Tissue diagnosis	Greater than 2% but less than 90% likelihood of malignancy
Category 4A: *Low suspicion* for malignancy		Greater than 2% to 10% or lower likelihood of malignancy
Category 4B: *Moderate suspicion* for malignancy		Greater than 10% to 50% or lower likelihood of malignancy
Category 4C: *High suspicion* for malignancy		Greater than 50% to less than 95% likelihood of malignancy
Category 5: Highly suggestive of malignancy	Tissue diagnosis	95% or higher likelihood of malignancy
Category 6: Known biopsy-proven malignancy	Surgical excision when clinically appropriate	N/A

Reprinted from American College of Radiology. ACR BI-RADS mammography. In: ACR BI-RADS atlas: breast imaging reporting and data system. 5th ed. ACR; 2013. p. 1–175.

TABLE 144-147-2. Breast Imaging-Reporting and Data System (BI-RADS) Categories for Breast Composition

BREAST COMPOSITION CATEGORIES
a. The breasts are almost entirely fatty.
b. There are scattered areas of fibroglandular density.
c. The breasts are heterogeneously dense, which may obscure small masses.
d. The breasts are extremely dense, which lowers the sensitivity of mammography.

Reprinted from American College of Radiology. ACR BI-RADS mammography. In: ACR BI-RADS atlas: breast imaging reporting and data system. 5th ed. ACR; 2013. p. 1–175.

aged 30 years and older with a breast mass should undergo diagnostic mammography first, followed by either diagnostic ultrasound or tissue biopsy depending on the findings from the initial mammography.

The patient in Scenario 144 should undergo diagnostic breast ultrasonography due to the presence of a palpable mass that has persisted for 4 months. Next steps in the evaluation will depend on the result of this testing. The patient in Scenario 145 is asymptomatic and has an average risk of breast cancer; therefore, she should undergo screening breast mammography. In the Scenario 146, the patient has a new palpable mass on examination and, based on her age, should undergo diagnostic mammography. The best next step will depend on the result of this testing. The patient in Scenario 147 has hereditary breast and ovarian cancer syndrome. Based on her age, she should undergo screening breast MRI with contrast.

Breast cancer risk assessment and screening in average-risk women. Practice Bulletin No. 179. American College of Obstetricians and Gynecologists. Obstet Gynecol 2017;130:e1–16. doi: 10.1097/AOG.0000000000002158

Diagnosis and management of benign breast disorders. Practice Bulletin No. 164. American College of Obstetricians and Gynecologists [published erratum appears in Obstet Gynecol 2021;137:382]. Obstet Gynecol 2016;127:e141–56. doi: 10.1097/AOG.0000000000001482

Hereditary breast and ovarian cancer syndrome. Practice Bulletin No. 182. American College of Obstetricians and Gynecologists. Obstet Gynecol 2017;130:e110–26. doi: 10.1097/AOG.0000000000002296

Management of women with dense breasts diagnosed by mammography. Committee Opinion No. 625. American College of Obstetricians and Gynecologists [published erratum appears in Obstet Gynecol 2016;127:166]. Obstet Gynecol 2015;125:750–1. doi: 10.1097/01.AOG.0000461763.77781.79

148–151 Adnexal masses

For each clinical scenario and image (148–151), choose the best next step (A–D):

(A) Gynecologic oncology referral
(B) Interval pelvic ultrasound (US)
(C) Image-guided (RI) biopsy of mass
(D) Magnetic resonance imaging (MRI)

148. A. A 66-year-old woman presents with 3 months of bloating and lower abdominal pain. Her pelvic examination is significant for a right adnexal mass that is solid and fixed. Her CA 125 concentration is 120 U/mL. Pelvic ultrasonography is performed, and the result is shown in Figure 148–151-1.

149. D. A 38-year-old woman presents with heavy menstrual bleeding and a firm palpable mass on bimanual examination. She has future fertility desires. Ultrasound imaging is shown in Figure 148–151-2. A urine human chorionic gonadotropin test is negative.

150. B. A 50-year-old patient presents with recent imaging demonstrating an 8-cm adnexal mass. Her CA 125 concentration is 28 U/mL. Ultrasound imaging is shown in Figure 148–151-3.

151. A. A 45-year-old patient undergoes pelvic ultrasonography because of heavy menses and right-sided pelvic pain for the past 6 months. Her urine pregnancy test is negative and her CA 125 concentration is 200 U/mL. Imaging of the ovary is shown in Figure 148–151-4.

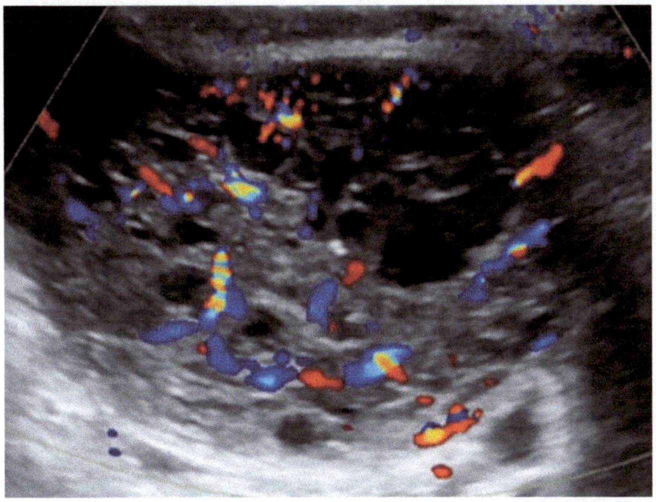

FIGURE 148-151-1. Ultrasonography showing an adnexal mass. (Reprinted from Strachowski LM, Jha P, Phillips CH, Blanchette Porter MM, Froyman W, Glanc P, et al. O-RADS US v2022: an update from the American College of Radiology's Ovarian-Adnexal Reporting and Data System US Committee. Radiology 2023;308:e230685. doi: 10.1148/radiol.230685)

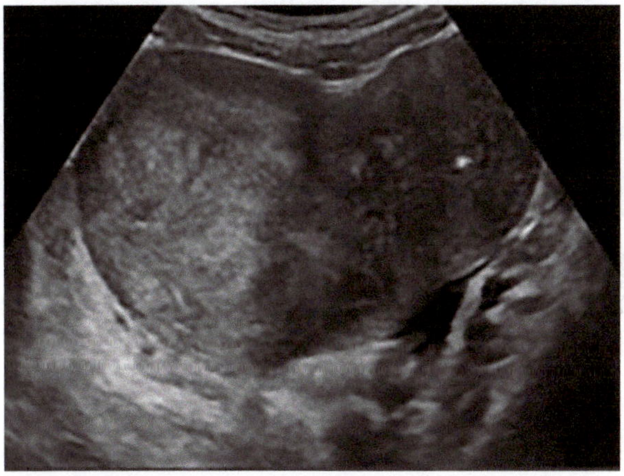

FIGURE 148-151-2. Pelvic ultrasound image for the patient in Scenario 149. (Reprinted from Geertsma T. Uterine fibroids leiomyomas. Ultrasound Cases. Accessed March 17, 2025. https://www.ultrasoundcases.info/uterine-fibroids---leiomyomas-6697/)

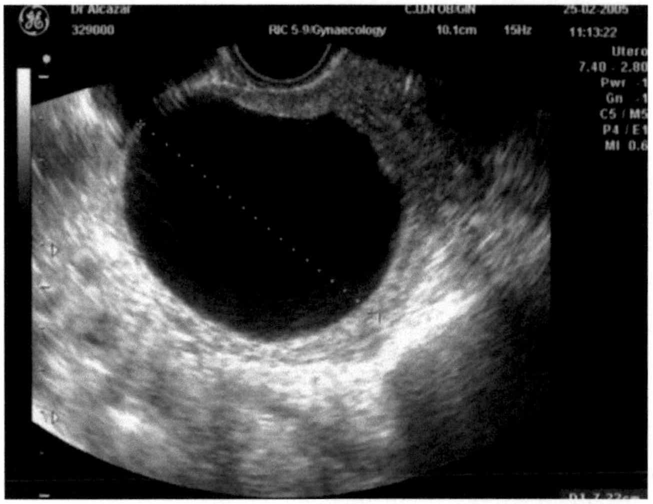

FIGURE 148-151-3. Ultrasound image for the patient in Scenario 150 showing an 8-cm ovarian cyst. (Reprinted from Alcazar JL, Martinez N, Juez L, Caparros M, Salas A, Errasti T. Ovarian simple cysts in asymptomatic postmenopausal women detected at transvaginal ultrasound: A review of literature. World J Obstet Gynecol 2015; 4(4): 108-112. doi: 10.5317/wjog.v4.i4.108)

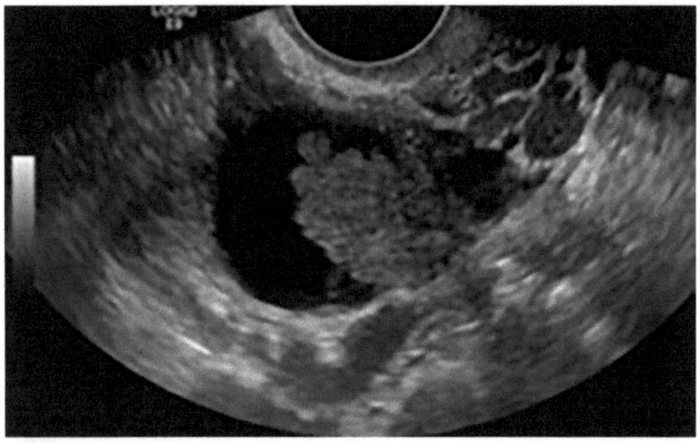

FIGURE 148-151-4. Ultrasound image for the patient described in Scenario 151. (Reprinted from Byron J. A better way to assess ovarian cancer risk. Kaiser Permanente; 2018. Accessed March 17, 2025. https://divisionofresearch.kaiserpermanente.org/a-better-way-to-assess-ovarian-cancer-risk/)

Pelvic masses are commonly encountered in gynecologic clinical practice and have a wide differential diagnosis. Pelvic ultrasonography is the most commonly used first-line imaging technique to evaluate adnexal masses. This allows for assessment of mass characteristics, including size, composition, and the presence or absence of septations, nodules, papillary excrescences, solid components, vascular flow, and free fluid within the pelvis. These findings should guide a clinician's level of concern for malignancy.

Multiple ultrasonography risk stratification systems exist to predict the likelihood of malignancy of an adnexal mass. These can be used alone or in conjunction with tumor markers. CA 125 has been used as a diagnostic biomarker in adnexal masses, but it does not have an acceptable accuracy in population-based screening for ovarian cancer. The CA 125 levels are increased in 50% of early-staged tumors and 92% of advanced-staged disease. Human epididymis protein 4 (HE4) is another tumor marker that has been evaluated in ovarian cancer and has been shown to exhibit higher specificity than CA 125. Biomarker panels and scoring systems involving these markers have been investigated, and the results of these panels, along with menopausal status and imaging findings, can assist with triage to appropriate levels of care in patients with an adnexal mass.

Examples of imaging risk-stratification systems include the Risk of Malignancy Index, the International Ovarian Tumor Analysis (IOTA) group regression model 2, and the Ovarian-Adnexal Reporting and Data System (O-RADS). The Risk of Malignancy Index was the first system developed and combines ultrasonography, menopausal status, and serum CA 125 levels. The IOTA was introduced in the late 1990s in Europe and is still globally used to help the clinician differentiate benign from malignant ovarian masses solely using ultrasonography. The IOTA Logistic Regression model 2 uses the patient's age and five ultrasound findings suggestive of malignancy that are entered into a formula to calculate the probability of malignancy. The O-RADS system was introduced in 2018 by the American College of Radiology. The system stemmed from IOTA but assesses other adnexal pathology, such as tubal disease, and employs MRI imaging in addition to ultrasonography. Multiple validation studies have shown a score of O-RADS US 4 as the appropriate cutoff for suspicion for malignancy (Fig. 148–151-5). Table 148–151-1 demonstrates the components of these risk stratification systems. Although these systems are promising, they are limited by their validation occurring only in research studies with specific ultrasound training (IOTA), or being retrospectively validated (O-RADS), and the suitability for routine clinical use has not been proven. Additionally, there is not one risk stratification system that is endorsed by American College of Obstetricians & Gynecologists. Although scoring criteria vary across the various stratification systems, most assign a low risk score to sonolucent cysts with smooth walls, thin or absent septations, and absence of solid components.

When the likelihood of ovarian cancer is high, referral to a gynecologic oncologist is preferred, as outcomes for patients with ovarian cancer are improved when initial surgical management is undertaken by a gynecologic oncologist. The patient in Scenario 148 is postmenopausal with a complex adnexal mass that demonstrates greater than 80% solid components, shadowing, and internal vascular flow on imaging. Given these findings, in combination with her age and increased CA 125, the concern for malignancy is high, and referral to a gynecologic oncologist is recommended.

If a lesion is classified as intermediate based on a chosen risk-stratification system, additional imaging can provide information about mass characteristics. Magnetic resonance imaging is most useful for solid lesions and cystic lesions with solid components and often is most helpful in establishing the origin of a pelvic mass if it is not clear on ultrasound.

The patient in Scenario 149 has a solid lesion continuous with the uterus and appears consistent with a uterine leiomyoma. Because she is symptomatic with heavy menstrual bleeding and has future fertility desires, an MRI, in this instance, can

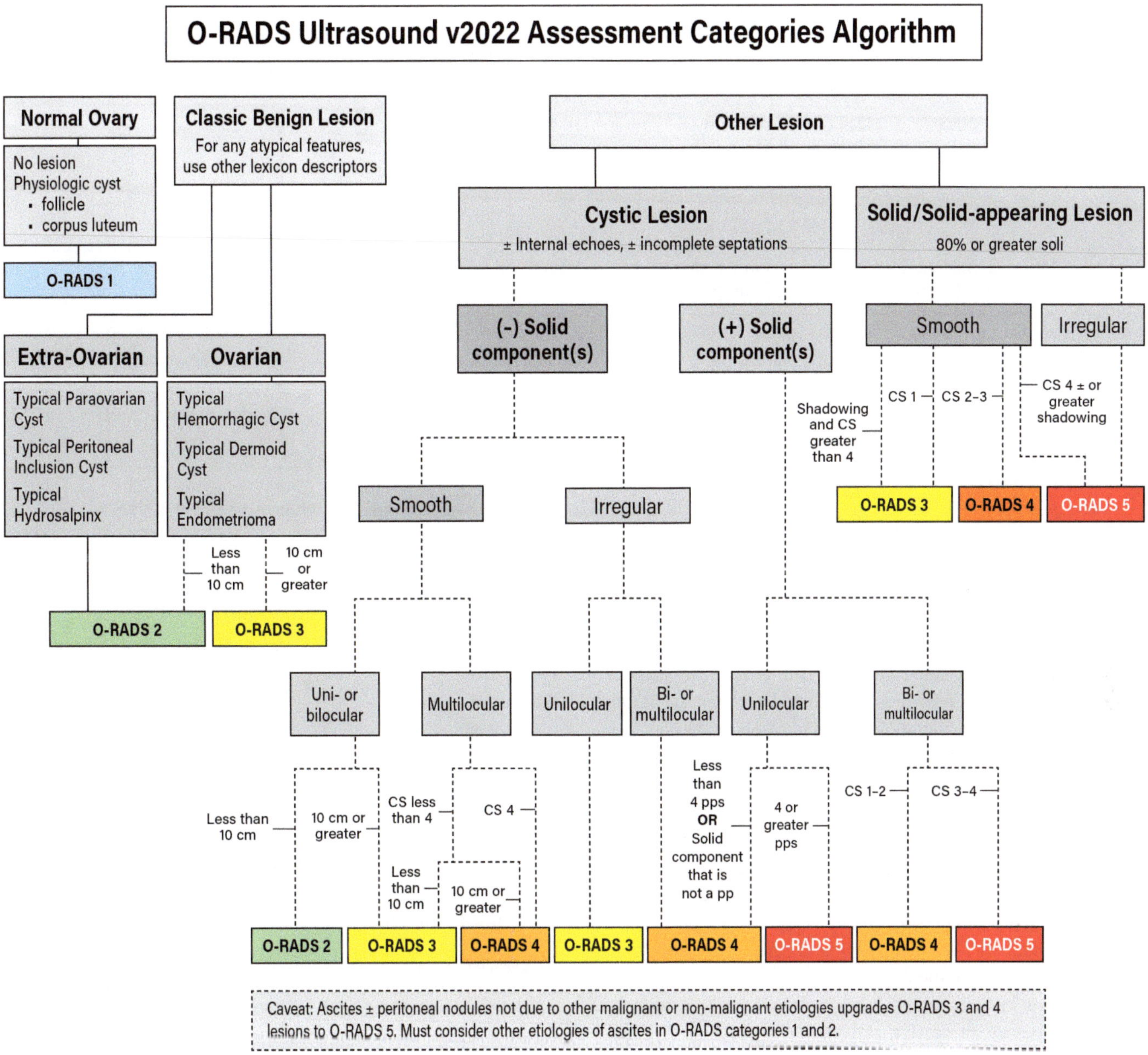

FIGURE 148-151-5. The American College of Radiology Ovarian-Adnexal Reporting and Data System (O-RADS) assessment categories algorithm. (Reprinted from Strachowski LM, Jha P, Phillips CH, Blanchette Porter MM, Froyman W, Glanc P, et al. O-RADS US v2022: an update from the American College of Radiology's Ovarian-Adnexal Reporting and Data System US Committee. Radiology 2023;308:e230685. doi: 10.1148/radiol.230685)

TABLE 148-151-1. Comparison of Ultrasound Risk Stratification Systems

		RISK OF MALIGNANCY	
METHOD	**COMPONENTS**	**HIGH RISK OF MALIGNANCY**	**LOW RISK OF MALIGNANCY**
Risk of malignancy index (RMI)	Calculation of risk by Ultrasound score (U), menopausal status (M), and CA 125 level RMI= U x M x CA 125	RMI 200 or greater	RMI 200 or less
Ovarian-Adnexal Reporting and Data System (O-RADS)	Detailed scoring system based on imaging findings	Score of 4 or 5	1–3
International Ovarian Tumor Analysis (IOTA) group regression model 2	Patient age Menopausal status Symptoms US findings	Mass size greater than 5 cm Cystic vs solid components Presence of septations Papillary projections Vascularity	Size less than 5 cm Simple, unilocular cyst Smooth borders Absence of solid components Low vascularity

Abbreviations: M, menopausal; RMI, Risk of Malignancy Index; U, ultrasound.

Data from Ngu SF, Chai YK, Choi KM, Leung TW, Li J, Kwok GS, et al. Diagnostic performance of Risk of Malignancy Algorithm (ROMA), Risk of Malignancy Index (RMI) and expert ultrasound assessment in a pelvic mass classified as inconclusive by International Ovarian Tumour Analysis (IOTA) simple rules. Cancers (Basel) 2022;14:810. doi: 10.3390/cancers14030810

assist with counseling on management options such as surgical planning for myomectomy.

Unilocular cysts, as noted in the patient in Scenario 150, are almost always benign regardless of age and menopausal status. Findings concerning for malignancy on ultrasonography include larger cyst size (greater than 10 cm), papillary projections or solid components, irregularity or lobular cyst contour, presence of ascites, and high color Doppler flow. Unilocular cysts up to 10 cm in diameter on ultrasonography may be safely monitored using repeat imaging. As the patient in Scenario 150 has a unilocular cyst of less than 10 cm in size without solid components, follow-up with repeat ultrasonography is appropriate and the best step for this patient. The ideal timing and duration for ultrasonography has yet to be defined.

The patient in Scenario 151 has a unilocular cyst with an irregular papillary projection. Given the suspicious findings of a papillary projection in conjunction with her age and an increased CA 125, this mass meets criteria for referral to gynecologic oncology. Biopsy of ovarian masses is not recommended when there is any level of suspicion for cancer as this can induce spillage and seeding of cancer cells into the peritoneal cavity, thereby leading to an increased stage of disease at time of diagnosis. In patients with widespread metastatic disease who may not be optimal primary surgical candidates, the use of infrared fluorescence-guided surgery to obtain a biopsy of a distant metastatic site, such as the omentum, or triage laparoscopy allows for collection of tissue for pathological evaluation.

The use of tumor markers and ultrasound risk-stratifications systems can help triage a patient to appropriate levels of care. Transvaginal ultrasound is the recommended imaging modality for a pelvic mass. Tumor markers can aid in further classification of masses as benign or malignant and tailor a management plan. For masses with concerning features and presence of increased tumor markers, consultation with a gynecologic oncologist is warranted.

Charkhchi P, Cybulski C, Gronwald J, Wong FO, Narod SA, Akbari MR. CA125 and ovarian cancer: a comprehensive review. Cancer (Basel) 2020;12:3730. doi: 10.3390/cancer12123730. doi: 10.3390/cancer12123730

Evaluation and management of adnexal masses. Practice Bulletin No. 174. American College of Obstetricians and Gynecologists. Obstet Gynecol 2016;128:e210–26. doi: 10.1097/AOG.0000000000001768

Strachowski LM, Jha P, Phillips CH, Blanchette Porter MM, Froyman W, Glanc P, et al. O-RADS US v2022: an update from the American College of Radiology's Ovarian-Adnexal Reporting and Data System US Committee. Radiology 2023;308:e230685. doi: 10.1148/radiol.230685

The role of the obstetrician-gynecologist in the early detection of epithelial ovarian cancer in women at average risk. Committee Opinion No. 716. American College of Obstetricians and Gynecologists. Obstet Gynecol 2017;130:e146–9. doi: 10.1097/AOG.0000000000002299

152–155 Survivorship

Choose the most appropriate therapy (A–E) for each clinical scenario (152–155). Each answer may be used more than once.

(A) Combined estrogen and progestin
(B) Gabapentin
(C) Selective serotonin reuptake inhibitor (SSRI)
(D) Transdermal estrogen
(E) Vaginal estrogen

152. E. A 76-year-old reports vaginal dryness with recurrent urinary tract infections. She has a history of stage IA, grade 1, endometrioid endometrial adenocarcinoma and underwent total hysterectomy with bilateral salpingo-oophorectomy at age 55 years. The examination today is consistent with significant vulvovaginal atrophy.

153. A. A 38-year-old who completed primary radiation therapy with chemosensitization for stage IIA2 squamous cell carcinoma of the cervix 6 months ago. She reports hot flushes that occur more than 10 times per day and frequent night sweats that interrupt her sleep. Her examination and imaging indicate a complete response to treatment.

154. A. A 35-year-old *BRCA1* mutation carrier undergoes a laparoscopic risk-reducing bilateral salpingo-oophorectomy. Pathology is negative for carcinoma. She has no personal history of cancer.

155. C. A 45-year-old who underwent a total abdominal hysterectomy with bilateral salpingo-oophorectomy and optimal cytoreduction for stage IIB low-grade serous ovarian adenocarcinoma reports depressive symptoms and diminished quality of life from persistent hot flushes.

Hormone therapy with estrogen with or without progestin is the first-line treatment of vasomotor symptoms, but not all patients are candidates for hormones or need systemic treatment for their specific symptoms (Table 152–155-1).

The patient in the Scenario 152 has a remote history of endometrial cancer and symptomatic vulvovaginal atrophy. Because her endometrial cancer was early-stage disease and treated more than 20 years ago, she could be a candidate for hormonal therapy. Due to her age and specific symptoms of dryness and recurrent urinary tract infections, vaginal estrogen would be the most appropriate treatment. Local estrogen therapy (eg, creams, tablets, rings, or softgel vaginal inserts) is indicated for genitourinary syndrome of menopause. These therapies are preferred over systemic formulations because of their minimal systemic absorption. Systemic hormone therapy initiation after age 60 years, or more than 10 years from menopause onset, has additional risks and does not treat vulvovaginal atrophy as well as topical hormones. Gabapentin or an SSRI would not treat vaginal dryness.

The patient in Scenario 153 has symptomatic premature menopause resulting from chemoradiation for cervical cancer. She is in active surveillance as part of her cancer treatment, having had a complete response to therapy. Due to her young age and severe vasomotor symptoms, she is a candidate for hormonal therapy. This is the standard treatment unless there are contraindications. This patient still has a uterus and needs a combined estrogen and progestin formulation for endometrial protection. Her premature treatment-induced menopause increases her risk of osteoporosis, cardiovascular disease, diabetes mellitus, sexual dysfunction, cognitive and mood changes, and overall mortality. Hormonal therapy will help mitigate these risks and should be continued until she reaches approximately age 52 years (average age of menopause), along with vitamin D, exercise, and screening for comorbidities.

Patients who undergo risk-reducing salpingo-oophorectomy for hereditary breast and ovarian cancer syndromes, such as the patient in Scenario 154, are candidates for hormone therapy if they do not have a personal history of cancer, particularly hormone receptor positive breast cancer. This patient did not have a hysterectomy and would need estrogen and progestin to protect the uterine lining from neoplasia; however, this regimen may increase her risk of breast cancer. A hysterectomy would simplify her hormone management to estrogen alone, which decreases breast cancer incidence, even in high-risk patients (12% versus 22%, Table 152–155-2). The risks of premature menopause and treatment are similar to those in the patient in the second scenario. Hormone replacement therapy is the best option to mitigate her risks.

The patient in Scenario 155 has hormone receptor-positive ovarian cancer, and hormone therapy is contraindicated despite

TABLE 152-155-1. Recommendations for Hormone Therapy in Gynecologic Cancer Survivors

	RECOMMENDATIONS	SELECTED ARTICLES	NOTES
Uterine cancer Early-stage endometrial cancer	HT acceptable	1. Barakat et al JCO 2006 2. Shim et al. European J Cancer 2014	1. 1236 patients, stage I-II EC randomized to HT vs placebo. Closed early due to WHI results. No difference in recurrence rate (2.3% vs 1.9% NS) 2. Meta-analysis—no increased risk of recurrence in EC survivors who receive HT
Advanced-stage endometrial cancer	HT not recommended		
Uterine sarcoma	HT not recommended		
Ovarian cancer High-grade serous ovarian cancer	HT acceptable	1. Guidozzi et al. Cancer 1999 2. Eels et al. JCO 2015	1. RCT; 130 patients less than 59 years ol randomized to HT of placebo, no difference in PFS or OS 2. RCT; 150 patients randomized to HT versus placebo OS improved in patients HT arm (hazard ratio, 0.63; 95% CI, 0.44–0.90; *P*=.011)
Low-grade serous and endometrioid ovarian cancer	HT not recommended		
Cervical cancer	HT acceptable	Polch et al Gynecol Oncol 1987	Prospective study, 120 patients, no difference in recurrence rate with use of HT

Abbreviations: EC, endometrial cancer; HT, hormone therapy; OS, overall survival; PFS, progression-free survival;. RCT, randomized controlled trial.

Reprinted from Sinno AK, Pinkerton J, Febbraro T, Jones N, Khanna N, Temkin S, et al. Hormone therapy (HT) in women with gynecologic cancer and in women at high risk for developing a gynecologic cancer: a Society of Gynecologic Oncology (SGO) clinical practice statement. Gynecol Oncol 2020;157:303-6. doi: 10.1016/j.ygyno.2020.01.035

TABLE 152-155-2. Recommendations for Hormone Therapy in Women at High Risk of Developing Gynecologic Cancer

	RECOMMENDATIONS	SELECTED ARTICLES	NOTES
***BRAC* mutation with no personal history of breast cancer**	HT acceptable	Kotsopolus et al. JAMA Oncol 2018	Prospective cohort 872 *BRCA* mutation carriers post prophylactic oophorectomy. No increased risk of breast cancer with HT use: HR 0.97 (95% CI, 0.62–1.25; *P*=.89). Patients treated with progesterone containing HT had a significantly higher rate of breast cancer versus estrogen only regimens (12% versus 22%; *P*=.04)
***BRCA* mutation with personal history of breast cancer**	HT not recommended	Holmbert et al. JNCI 2008	RCT; 221 women with a personal history of breast cancer. Patients treated with HT had a significantly increased risk of a new breast cancer event: HR 2.4 (95% CI, 1.3–4.2)
Lynch syndrome	HT acceptable	1. Symer et al. Clin Colorectal Cancer 2018 2. Dashati et al. JAMA 2015	1. Prospective cohort of the PLC Reduction in colon cancer risk in general population with HT (0.81; 95% CI, 0.69–0.94; *P*=.005) 2. Women with Lynch syndrome can be counseled similar to the general population regarding the use of HT

Abbreviations: HT, hormone therapy; RCT, randomized controlled trial.

Reprinted from Sinno AK, Pinkerton J, Febbraro T, Jones N, Khanna N, Temkin S, et al. Hormone therapy (HT) in women with gynecologic cancer and in women at high risk for developing a gynecologic cancer: a Society of Gynecologic Oncology (SGO) clinical practice statement. Gynecol Oncol 2020;157:303-6. doi: 10.1016/j.ygyno.2020.01.035

her moderate to severe vasomotor symptoms. The most appropriate treatment for this patient is an SSRI. Additional nonhormonal ways to treat hot flushes and night sweats beside medication (eg, cooling techniques, exercise, weight loss, avoidance of triggers) are understudied, but cognitive behavioral therapy and clinical hypnosis have been shown to reduce vasomotor symptom severity and interference with quality of life. Prescription therapies that address vasomotor symptoms include SSRIs (paroxetine), selective NK3R inhibitors (fezolinetant), serotonin and norepinephrine reuptake inhibitors (SNRIs), gabapentin, and oxybutynin. Paroxetine and fezolinetant are the only formulations that the U.S. Food and Drug Administration has approved for genitourinary syndrome of menopause. Both SSRIs and SNRIs can improve vasomotor symptoms and have the benefit of treating depression as well. Gabapentin is an option for vasomotor symptoms, but would not be the first choice because it would not treat her depression. Patients taking tamoxifen should avoid use of paroxetine or fluoxetine co-administration due to inhibition of CYP2D6. Serotonin and norepinephrine reuptake inhibitors have less effect on this enzyme and are better choices in this circumstance.

Sinno AK, Pinkerton J, Febbraro T, Jones N, Khanna N, Temkin S, et al. Hormone therapy (HT) in women with gynecologic cancer and in women at high risk for developing a gynecologic cancer: a Society of Gynecologic Oncology (SGO) clinical practice statement. Gynecol Oncol 2020;157:303–6. doi: 10.1016/j.ygyno.2020.01.035

The 2022 hormone therapy position statement of The North American Menopause Society. Menopause 2022;29:767–94. doi: 10.1097/GME.0000000000002028

The 2023 nonhormone therapy position statement of The North American Menopause Society. Menopause 2023;30:573–90. doi: 10.1097/GME.0000000000002200

156–159 Management of recurrent cervical cancer

For each clinical scenario 156–159, choose the best next step in treatment (A–E).

(A) Curative radiation
(B) Curative systemic anticancer therapy
(C) Palliative radiation
(D) Palliative systemic anticancer therapy
(E) Pelvic exenteration

156. A. A 42-year-old patient was treated with radical hysterectomy for stage IB2 cervical cancer 18 months ago. Adjuvant therapy was not indicated. She presents now with vaginal bleeding and a 4-cm mass at the vaginal apex. Biopsy confirms recurrent cervical cancer. Imaging demonstrates that the lesion abuts her posterior bladder and rectum without evidence for invasion into either organ. No other regional or distant metastatic disease is present.

157. E. A 55-year-old patient was treated with primary chemoradiotherapy for stage IIB cervical cancer 5 years ago. She now has a 3-cm lesion involving the posterior cervix that extends to the posterior vagina. Imaging demonstrates that the lesion invades the rectum without additional regional or distant metastasis.

158. C. A 78-year-old patient completed primary chemoradiotherapy for stage IIIB cervical cancer 3 months ago. She now presents with debilitating back pain. A physical examination reveals a 3-cm mass at the vaginal apex, and a positron emission tomography (PET) scan shows a 5-cm right para-aortic lymph node invading an adjacent vertebral body.

159. D. A 55-year-old patient who completed primary chemoradiotherapy for stage IIIC1 cervical cancer 3 months ago presents with flank pain. Computed tomography revealed progression of disease with left obturator adenopathy, which is causing hydronephrosis. There is no additional evidence of metastatic disease.

The prognosis and optimal management of recurrent cervical cancer depends on the type of primary treatment received, the anatomic site(s) involved with recurrent cancer, and the characteristics of the individual patient. Only a small percentage of recurrent cervical cancer is amenable to curative intent therapies. When cure is not feasible, noncurative or palliative therapies are an option. The primary goal of palliative cancer treatment is to reduce the burden of cancer in hopes of reducing cancer symptoms and improving quality of life. A secondary goal is the potential to prolong life. When deciding upon palliative cancer therapies, patients, families, and doctors must carefully weigh the probability of achieving a stated palliative goal against the risks of the intervention in terms of toxicity, time, and cost.

Directed cancer therapy at recurrence may consist of surgery, various radiotherapy strategies, systemic therapy, or combined modality therapies. Often, however, there are added limitations at cancer recurrence due to concerns related to treatment tolerance. Prior treatment history can affect available options at recurrence. For example, up to 70% of patients with cervical cancer receive pelvic radiotherapy at some point in their treatment, either as primary chemoradiation or as a component of adjuvant therapy after radical hysterectomy. Due to cumulative radiation dose constraints and the risk of incurring severe organ toxicity, re-irradiation in the pelvis is generally not an option for patients who have had prior pelvic radiation. In addition, cisplatin-associated neuropathy may remain from initial therapies and can limit systemic therapy decisions at recurrence. Finally, depending on their tumor burden, patients diagnosed with cancer recurrence often also experience worsening nutrition and performance status. Such physical decline inevitably reduces their treatment tolerance and may further affect the appropriateness of available palliative treatment options.

Cervical cancer recurrences that have treatment implications can be broadly categorized according to location. Recurrences may be central pelvic, lateral pelvic, or extrapelvic. Central pelvic recurrences may involve the vaginal vault or native cervix and uterus, the parametria, the bladder, or the rectum. Lateral pelvic recurrences occur in pelvic lymph nodes or involve the pelvic side wall and lateral muscles of the pelvic floor. Extrapelvic recurrence includes any metastatic cancer outside of a traditional pelvic radiation field. Metastatic spread can be lymphatic, hematogenous, or peritoneal. Whereas central pelvic recurrences have potential curative options, generally extrapelvic and peritoneal recurrences are not amenable to cure. The response potential of therapies for lateral pelvic recurrences depends greatly on the prior therapies administered at initial treatment.

Scenario 156 describes a patient with a central pelvic cancer recurrence after prior radical hysterectomy. She has never received pelvic radiotherapy, and because there is only a single site of recurrence in the central pelvis, there is potential for cure in this case. Definitive treatment with radiation therapy is the best next step. This would likely include both external beam radiotherapy with concurrent chemotherapy sensitization followed by interstitial brachytherapy. Treatment planning makes careful consideration of radiation dosing to balance effective tumor eradication with the risk of pelvic organ toxicity to the adjacent bladder, small bowel, and rectum. Although surgical excision of this type of recurrence is technically feasible, it would require a pelvic exenteration to obtain adequate surgical margins (Fig. 156–159-1). Compared with chemoradiation

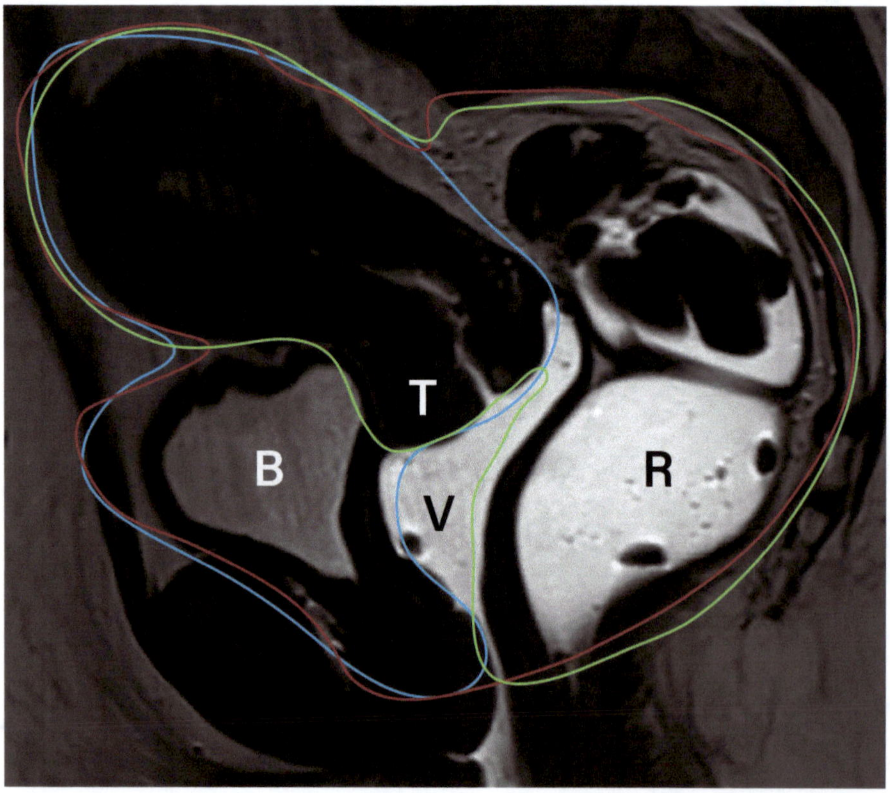

FIGURE 156-159-1. Pelvic exenteration. Pelvic magnetic resonance imaging depicting a centrally recurrent cervical cancer and organ resection targets for anterior, posterior and total pelvic exenteration. (Reprinted from Merz J, Bossart M, Bamberg F, Eisenblaetter M. Revised FIGO staging for cervical cancer a new role for MRI. Rofo 2020;192:937–44. doi: 10.1055/a-1198-5729)

KEY

- total pelvic exenteration
- posterior pelvic exenteration
- anterior pelvic exenteration

B bladder
R rectum
T tumor
V vagina

therapy, exenteration carries an overall greater risk for treatment toxicity and results in poorer overall quality of life and is not the preferred strategy in this setting when radiation has not yet been utilized.

The patient in Scenario 157 has central pelvic recurrence and did receive radiation therapy previously. Treatment in this setting would have potential for cure with second-line therapies, but she is not a candidate for additional radiation therapy. Surgical excision with pelvic exenteration is recommended and offers a potential curative option. Pelvic exenteration has the goal of complete tumor resection with negative margins and can be categorized based on the organs that are removed into anterior, posterior, or total exenteration. Shown in Figure 156–159-1, it consists of the en bloc resection of the uterus, fallopian tubes, ovaries (if these organs are still in situ), and vagina along with the bladder (anterior), rectum (posterior), or both (total). Additional pelvic tissues that are not a part of the pelvic sidewall structures may also be removed. Once en bloc resection has taken place, reconstruction of the intestinal tract, urinary tract, pelvic floor, and vagina may be necessary.

Surgical morbidity and mortality rates after pelvic exenteration have historically been high. Major complication rates reported in the literature have ranged from 25% to 75%, with infectious complications representing a large proportion of this morbidity. A multidisciplinary team is vital to optimizing surgical outcomes in pelvic exenteration. Additionally, careful patient selection also has led to better outcomes. Pretreatment evaluation is critical and often includes PET and computed tomography (CT) to exclude distant metastatic disease, and pelvic MRI for more detailed surgical planning. Given the high risk of physical and psychological morbidity of this procedure, careful patient selection based on age, physical frailty, nutritional status, medical comorbidities, BMI, and psychological readiness is paramount before undertaking this procedure.

The patient in Scenario 158 has manifested new recurrent disease outside of her prior pelvic radiation field as well as persistent disease within her prior radiation field. The new lesion has developed within a very short time after completion of prior therapies. The quick timeline for this symptomatic progression suggests a poor prognosis, and palliative treatment to reduce her debilitating pain is priority. Palliative radiation therapy to her para-aortic nodal recurrence has a high probability of improving pain and reducing vertebral fracture risk, but this targeted radiation will not cure her disease. Additional radiation for the remaining disease within the pelvis is not an option given her prior chemoradiation. Systemic therapies to address this persistent pelvic disease have a slower onset of action and a lower overall probability of treatment response. This strategy is not the preferred initial intervention in the setting of debilitating back pain due to a focal recurrent mass in the vertebrae. The option of systemic therapy after palliative radiotherapy is completed may be appropriate. The decision to proceed, however, would require careful counseling about risks and benefits and depend on patient preferences and goals at that time.

In Scenario 159, the described patient has a lateral pelvic recurrence of cancer in the setting of prior pelvic radiation. The previous pelvic radiation field limits the option of further radiation, making cure unachievable in this setting. Palliative systemic anticancer therapies are available. Due to radiation induced changes in the biology of the tumor and its blood supply, response rates to systemic therapies can be lower when target lesions that are in a prior radiation field. Again, careful counseling regarding risks and benefits in the context of individual patient goals will be essential. Palliative procedures, such as ureteral stenting or nephrostomy, can also be considered and may more directly improve quality of life by relieving pain due to ureteral obstruction.

Treatment selection for recurrent cervical cancer should include factors influencing prognosis, the treatment options available, and the individual patient goals and priorities. Treatment for cure is possible in patients with central pelvic cancer recurrence. Post-recurrence survival in all other settings can be poor, and quality of life often is negatively influenced by pain and organ dysfunction. Balancing trade-offs that consider the probability of clinical benefit with the known toxicities of treatment need to be carefully considered.

National Comprehensive Cancer Network. Cervical cancer. Version 3.2025. NCCN Clinical Practice Guidelines in Oncology [after login]. NCCN; 2025. Accessed February 26, 2025. https://www.nccn.org/guidelines/guidelines-detail?category=1&id=1426

Krakauer EL, Kwete X, Kane K, Afshan G, Bazzett-Matabele L, Bien-Aimé DDR, et al. Cervical cancer-associated suffering: estimating the palliative care needs of a highly vulnerable population. JCO Glob Oncol 2021;7:862–72. doi: 10.1200/GO.21.00025

Ubinha AC, Pedrão PG, Tadini AC, Schmidt RL, Santos MH, Andrade CE, et al. The role of pelvic exenteration in cervical cancer: a review of the literature. Cancer (Basel) 2024;16:817. doi: 10.3390/cancer16040817

160–163 Perioperative venous thromboprophylaxis

Choose the most appropriate prophylaxis (A–D) for venous thromboembolism (VTE) for each of the described patients (160–163).

(A) Mechanical and pharmacologic
(B) Mechanical and pharmacologic with pharmacologic prophylaxis extended 28 or more days
(C) Mechanical alone
(D) Pharmacologic alone

160. A. A 64-year-old patient undergoing robot-assisted total laparoscopic hysterectomy with bilateral salpingo-oophorectomy and sentinel lymph node staging for grade 2 endometrioid endometrial carcinoma.

161. C. A 38-year-old patient undergoing laparoscopic risk-reducing bilateral salpingo-oophorectomy for *BRCA1* mutation.

162. D. A 76-year-old patient with a BMI of 42 undergoing exploratory laparotomy, total abdominal hysterectomy, and unilateral salpingo-oophorectomy for a 12-cm hydrosalpinx and uterine leiomyomas with severe peripheral arterial occlusive disease in the bilateral lower extremities.

163. B. A 61-year-old patient with ovarian cancer on postoperative day 5 from exploratory laparotomy for interval debulking with average risk of postoperative bleeding.

Venous thromboembolism is a significant source of postoperative morbidity and requires risk-based prophylaxis. Prophylaxis must be balanced with the patient's specific clinical risk factors and bleeding risk. The Caprini score is a scoring system that uses the patient's history and physical examination to assign points based on risk factors. The Caprini score has been validated across several surgical disciplines and is a widely accepted tool for risk assessment of VTE in gynecologic surgery.

The points are assigned categories of low to high based on risk of symptomatic VTE. The risk category determines VTE prophylaxis recommendations. Table 160–163-1 lists recommended thromboprophylaxis options and risk of deep vein thrombosis (DVT). Additionally, the risk of postoperative bleeding for the individual patient also needs to be considered when selecting thromboprophylaxis.

Mechanical prophylaxis is recommended for all surgical patients who do not have contraindications. The preferred device is intermittent pneumatic compression, which has been as effective as pharmacologic methods at reducing incidence of DVT in some studies. Graduated compression stockings can be used in addition or as an alternative to intermittent pneumatic compression devices. Although there are few contraindications to either of these options, increased pressure on extremities in patients with peripheral artery occlusive disease could cause a detrimental loss of blood supply, and this is a contraindication to mechanical prophylaxis.

TABLE 160-163-1. Recommended Thromboprophylaxis for Patients at Average Risk of Major Bleeding Complication When Undergoing Gynecologic Surgery

RISK OF SYMPTOMATIC DEEP VEIN THROMBOSIS	CAPRINI SCORE	RECOMMENDED THROMBOPROPHYLAXIS
Low (~1.5%)	1–2	Mechanical prophylaxis*
Moderate (~3.0%)	3–4	Pharmacologic or mechanical
High (~6.0%)	5 or greater	Pharmacologic plus mechanical
High-risk cancer surgery	5 or greater	Pharmacologic plus mechanical and extended duration prophylaxis post discharge

*Mechanical prophylaxis refers to graduated compression stockings or intermittent pneumatic compression devices (preferred). Pharmacologic options include low-dose unfractionated heparin, low-molecular weight heparin, and direct oral anticoagulants.

Modified from Gould MK, Garcia DA, Wren SM, Karanicolas PJ, Arcelus JI, Heit JA, et al. Prevention of VTE in nonorthopedic surgical patients: antithrombotic therapy and prevention of thrombosis, 9th ed: American College of Chest Physicians evidence-based clinical practice guidelines [published erratum appears in Chest. 2012 May;141(5):1369]. Chest 2012;141(2 suppl):e227S–77S. doi: 10.1378/chest.11-2297 https://journal.chestnet.org/article/S0012-3692(12)60125-1/fulltext

Options for pharmacologic prophylaxis include low-dose unfractionated heparin, low-molecular-weight heparin (LMWH), and direct oral anticoagulants. The most extensively studied drug is low-dose unfractionated heparin. This is highly effective for prevention of VTE and can be used safely without dose adjustment in patients with renal disease. Because its half-life is short, and it requires frequent dosing (three times daily), LMWH was developed as an alternative. Low-molecular-weight heparin also is very effective in the prevention of VTE, but it can be cost prohibitive and is not as readily reversed as unfractionated heparin.

Low-molecular-weight heparin must be reduced if a patient's creatinine clearance is less than 30 mL/min. Either of these is an appropriate option for pharmacologic prophylaxis. For patients deemed at highest risk, such as those with malignancy undergoing major open abdominal surgery, extended prophylaxis is recommended. Many guidelines suggest 28 days, but others recommend up to 6 months for patients with cancer.

Direct oral anticoagulants increasingly are being used for thromboprophylaxis. A randomized controlled trial of 400 patients with gynecologic cancer randomized to extended prophylaxis with apixaban versus LMWH showed no difference in risk of bleeding or development of VTE. Additionally, patient satisfaction was significantly improved due to ease of taking the medication and lack of pain associated with injection.

In Scenario 160, the patient has a Caprini score of 6 (2 points each for age 64 years, laparoscopic surgery more than 45 minutes, and malignancy). This puts her in a high-risk category for development of VTE, and mechanical plus pharmacologic prophylaxis during hospitalization is recommended.

The patient in Scenario 161 has a Caprini score of 2 (1 point for age 38 years, 1 point for minor surgery). Her risk of development of VTE is low, and only mechanical prophylaxis is recommended.

The patient in Scenario 162 has a Caprini score of 6 (3 points for age 76, 2 points for major abdominal surgery, 1 point for a BMI greater than 25). Although this puts her into a high-risk category for development of VTE, she has a contraindication to mechanical prophylaxis due to peripheral arterial occlusive disease; therefore, pharmacologic prophylaxis alone is the best option for her. The pathology is benign, and extended prophylaxis is not indicated.

The patient in Scenario 163 has a Caprini score of 6 (2 points each for age 61, major abdominal surgery, and malignancy). Due to high risk of late-onset VTE in this patient in the setting of malignancy, mechanical and extended pharmacologic prophylaxis are indicated.

Gressel GM, Marcus JZ, Mullen MM, Sinno AK. Direct oral anticoagulant use in gynecologic oncology: a Society of Gynecologic Oncology Clinical Practice Statement. Gynecol Oncol 2021;160:312–21. doi: 10.1016/j.ygyno.2020.11.02033257014

Guntupalli SR, Brennecke A, Behbakht K, Tayebnejad A, Breed CA, Babayan LM, et al. Safety and efficacy of apixaban vs enoxaparin for preventing postoperative venous thromboembolism in women undergoing surgery for gynecologic malignant neoplasm: a randomized clinical trial. JAMA Netw Open 2020;3:e207410. doi: 10.1001/jamanetworkopen.2020.7410

Prevention of venous thromboembolism in gynecologic surgery. ACOG Practice Bulletin No. 232. American College of Obstetricians and Gynecologists. Obstet Gynecol 2021;138:e1–15. doi: 10.1097/AOG.0000000000004445

Rabe E, Partsch H, Morrison N, Meissner MH, Mosti G, Lattimer CR, et al. Risks and contraindications of medical compression treatment a critical reappraisal. An international consensus statement. Phlebology 2020;35:447–60. doi: 10.1177/0268355520909066

Wagner BE, Langstraat CL, McGree ME, Weaver AL, Sarangi S, Mokri B, et al. Beyond prophylaxis: extended risk of venous thromboembolism following primary debulking surgery for ovarian cancer. Gynecol Oncol 2019;152:286–92. doi: 10.1016/j.ygyno.2018.11.021

164–167 Treatment approach to cervical cancer

Choose the most appropriate treatment (A–E) for each clinical scenario (164–167).

(A) Cervical conization
(B) Chemoradiation
(C) Extrafascial hysterectomy
(D) Pelvic exenteration
(E) Radical hysterectomy with lymph node assessment

164. A. A 26-year-old nulligravida presents with cervical cytology demonstrating high-grade squamous intraepithelial lesion (HSIL). No gross cervical, vaginal, or parametrial abnormalities are seen on physical examination. Colposcopic biopsies demonstrate cervical intraepithelial neoplasia 3 (CIN 3). An excisional procedure shows the findings listed below:

Loop electrosurgical excision procedure (LEEP) pathology
- Squamous cell carcinoma, depth of stromal invasion: at least 2 mm
- No lymphovascular space involvement
- LEEP margin positive for CIN 3

165. D. A 64-year-old with a history of stage IVA cervical cancer underwent chemoradiation 3 years ago. She presents with vaginal spotting. A pelvic examination demonstrates an endophytic lesion involving the cervix. The parametrium is firm with radiation change, but no obvious tumor involvement is detected. She undergoes further evaluation, which reveals the findings below:

Cervical biopsy
- Squamous cell carcinoma, depth of stromal invasion at least 10 mm
- Lymphovascular space invasion present
- Margins positive for carcinoma

Positron emission tomography (PET) and computed tomography (CT) imaging
- 5-cm hypermetabolic cervical mass extending to the parametria
- No evidence of regional or distant metastasis

166. E. A 32-year-old nulligravida presents with cervical cytology showing atypical glandular cells (AGCs). On examination, there are no gross cervical, vaginal, or parametrial abnormalities. She undergoes further evaluation, which reveals the findings below:

Pathology
- Endocervix curettage demonstrates endocervical adenocarcinoma, usual type
- Endometrial biopsy is unremarkable

PET and MRI
- 2.4-cm cervical lesion, 33% cervical stromal invasion, no regional or distant metastasis

167. B. A 48-year-old presents with worsening abnormal uterine bleeding. A pelvic examination demonstrates a globally enlarged cervix measuring 7 cm that is friable and bleeding. Vaginal fornices are blunted, but there are no obvious parametrial or vaginal abnormalities. She undergoes further evaluation, which reveals the findings below:

Cervical biopsy
- Squamous cell carcinoma, depth of stromal invasion exceeding 10 mm
- Lymphovascular space invasion present
- Margins positive for carcinoma

PET and MRI
- 7-cm cervical mass infiltrating the lower uterine segment
- No evidence of regional or distant metastasis

The treatment options for cervical cancer include surgery, chemoradiation, or both, depending on the clinical scenario. How and when treatment is applied depends on the clinical findings at pretreatment evaluation as well as International Federation of Gynecology and Obstetrics (FIGO) stage and represent a balance between optimizing oncologic outcomes and minimizing treatment associated toxicities. The clinical scenarios above illustrate a spectrum of findings at pretreatment evaluation that determine FIGO 2018 stage and inform subsequent treatment decisions.

The patient in Scenario 164 underwent LEEP for CIN 3 and was found to have early invasive squamous cell carcinoma. Her relevant pathologic findings are as follows: 1) depth of cervical stromal invasion of at least 2 mm; 2) absence of lymphovascular space involvement; and 3) CIN 3 extending to the LEEP specimen margin. This patient has FIGO stage IA1 cervical cancer (Appendix G). Given these findings, the risk for lymphatic spread is considered to be negligible. Cervical conization should be undertaken as the best next step in this patient, with the goals of achieving free surgical margins and further confirming depth of invasion. If no additional invasive cancer were identified on the subsequent surgical specimen, then the FIGO stage remains IA1 and cervical conization is sufficient treatment. Standard post-conization surveillance protocols are then implemented.

The patient in Scenario 165 has locally recurrent cancer of the previously irradiated cervix. Due to cumulative radiation dose constraints and the risk for incurring severe organ toxicity, repeat irradiation in the pelvis is not an option for patients who have had prior pelvic radiation. Findings on examination and imaging demonstrate that this is a central pelvic recurrence without evidence for distant metastases or extension to pelvic sidewall structures. In this case, pelvic exenteration with en bloc removal of the uterus, cervix, parametria, bladder, rectum, and upper vagina offers the potential of cure, and this is the best next step for this patient.

Although radical hysterectomy can theoretically encompass the identified disease by resection of both cervix and parametria, it is not recommended in this setting for several reasons. The probability of achieving curative margins with radical hysterectomy is low for recurrent cervical cancer cases. Additionally, there is parametrial extension of disease and an attempt at radical hysterectomy would likely result in cutting through tumor. Moreover, complications rates with radical hysterectomy are exceedingly high after high-dose radiation. This includes severe complications that would require additional major interventions, such as ureteral injury, vaginal cuff necrosis, and bladder and rectum fistula formation.

The patient in Scenario 166 has stage IB2 adenocarcinoma of the cervix (Appendix G). A standard treatment recommendation for patients with early-stage cervical cancer includes radical hysterectomy with lymph node assessment and has an associated overall 5-year survival rate that ranges between 75% and 95%. Although treatment with chemoradiation is associated with similar oncologic outcomes, surgery allows better preservation of hormonal, sexual, and physical functioning and is the preferred treatment strategy in young patients. Radical hysterectomy with lymph node assessment is the best next step for the patient in this scenario; however, important caveats to this strategy exist and are addressed in the next scenario.

The patient in Scenario 167 has stage IB3 cervical cancer (Appendix G), and chemoradiation is the preferred treatment. Her lesion appears to be confined to the cervix, but it is a large, 7-cm tumor. Radical hysterectomy with surgical lymph node assessment is a treatment option for patients with FIGO stage IB1 to IB3 disease, but primary chemoradiation is preferred for bulky (greater than 4 cm) stage IB tumors. This is mainly due to a high incidence of unfavorable histopathological findings in the radical hysterectomy specimen that would then compel a recommendation for adjuvant pelvic radiotherapy after surgery to reduce risk of recurrent disease. A strategy that combines both radical surgery and adjuvant radiation does not achieve better oncologic outcomes than treatment with primary chemoradiation, but it is associated with significantly higher severe treatment-related toxicity.

Bhatla N, Berek JS, Cuello Fredes M, Denny LA, Grenman S, Karunaratne K, et al. Revised FIGO staging for carcinoma of the cervix uteri [published erratum appears in Int J Gynaecol Obstet 2019;147:279-80]. Int J Gynaecol Obstet 2019;145:129–35. doi: 10.1002/ijgo.12749

Guimarães YM, Godoy LR, Longatto-Filho A, Reis RD. Management of early-stage cervical cancer: a literature review. Cancer (Basel) 2022;14:575. doi: 10.3390/cancer14030575

Landoni F, Maneo A, Colombo A, Placa F, Milani R, Perego P, et al. Randomised study of radical surgery versus radiotherapy for stage IB-IIA cervical cancer. Lancet 1997;350:535–40. doi: 10.1016/S0140-6736(97)02250-2

National Comprehensive Cancer Network. Cervical cancer. Version 3.2025. NCCN Clinical Practice Guidelines in Oncology [after login]. NCCN; 2025. Accessed February 26, 2025. https://www.nccn.org/guidelines/guidelines-detail?category=1&id=1426

Ubinha AC, Pedrão PG, Tadini AC, Schmidt RL, Santos MH, Andrade CE, et al. The role of pelvic exenteration in cervical cancer: a review of the literature. Cancer (Basel) 2024;16:817. doi: 10.3390/cancer16040817

168–171 Preoperative imaging in endometrial cancer

Choose the best imaging study (A–D) for each clinical scenario (168–171).

(A) Chest X-ray
(B) Pelvic ultrasound
(C) Magnetic resonance imaging (MRI)
(D) Computed tomography (CT)

168. A. A woman with newly diagnosed clinical stage I, grade 2, endometrioid endometrial cancer is scheduled to undergo surgical staging. Clinical examination reveals a mobile 6-cm uterus without adnexal mass. She reports having a 3-month history of new cough but has no other symptoms and has not lost weight.

169. C. A 36-year-old asymptomatic woman with grade 1 endometrioid endometrial cancer desires future fertility.

170. D. A 44-year-old woman who underwent hysterectomy for abnormal uterine bleeding has grade 3 endometrioid endometrial cancer with 5% myometrial invasion and no lymphovascular invasion identified at pathology.

171. D. A woman with a history of stage I serous endometrial cancer with vaginal recurrence diagnosed at the time of routine surveillance elects surgical resection.

Clinical scenarios and disease biology drive the appropriate selection of imaging modality in patients with endometrial cancer. Endometrial cancer is usually surgically staged after endometrial sampling shows malignancy. Imaging helps guide decision making about proceeding to surgery and the surgical plan before staging occurs. Routine imaging for low-risk, asymptomatic patients with endometrial cancer is not indicated, given the high rates of stage I disease. Rather, clinicians should evaluate the patient's specific symptoms and physical examination findings to guide the role and type of imaging to order. Routine computed tomography (CT) for high-grade endometrial cancer (ie, poorly differentiated endometrioid, serous, clear cell, carcinosarcoma) is recommended given the higher propensity for metastatic disease at the time of presentation.

Chest imaging X-ray should be performed in patients with pulmonary symptoms who do not require other preoperative imaging. If an abnormality is seen, a non-contrasted chest CT should be performed for further evaluation. The patient in Scenario 168 has stage I low-grade cancer and reports only isolated pulmonary symptoms, and a preoperative chest X-ray would be most appropriate to guide additional imaging as part of her assessment. Pelvic imaging with ultrasonography or MRI is not required because her clinical examination is not concerning for a bulky uterus or local extension given the small, mobile uterus, and plan for surgical staging.

Endometrial cancer may be diagnosed in young women who have not completed childbearing. National Comprehensive Cancer Network guidelines recommend adhering to strict criteria to offer fertility preservation:

- Grade 1 endometrioid adenocarcinoma confirmed on dilation and curettage specimen with expert pathology review
- Disease limited to the endometrium (MRI preferred, but ultrasonography also is acceptable)
- Absence of metastatic disease on imaging
- Lack of contraindications to medical therapy or pregnancy

Patients also should be counseled that fertility preservation is outside of the standard of care and is understudied in this population. The patient in Scenario 169 is asymptomatic with grade 1 endometrial cancer, and an MRI of the pelvis is the most appropriate imaging study to assess for myometrial invasion and to determine if cancer management with fertility preservation is appropriate.

Endometrial cancer may be diagnosed after hysterectomy performed for apparently benign indications. In these scenarios, the role of cross-sectional imaging is guided by uterine pathology (grade, myometrial invasion, and lymphovascular invasion). Patients may be observed without imaging if they are younger than 60 years and if uterine pathology shows stage IA, grade 1–2 cancer and no lymphovascular space invasion, or shows stage IA, grade 3 cancer, no lymphovascular space invasion, and no myometrial invasion. All other patients require cross-sectional imaging, preferably of the chest, abdomen, and pelvis. Cross-sectional CT of the chest, abdomen, and pelvis is recommended for the patient described in Scenario 170, given surgically unstaged myoinvasive grade 3 cancer. Routine positron emission tomography (PET) generally is not recommended unless there are inconclusive findings on CT or an alternative clinical indication for PET, such as contrast allergy or renal dysfunction precluding the use of intravenous contrast.

The role of routine surveillance imaging in endometrial cancer is controversial. No high-quality data support the use of routine imaging for surveillance of endometrial cancer. More than one-half of all recurrences are diagnosed based on symptoms or physical examination findings. In a patient presenting with an examination finding concerning for recurrence, such as that in the patient in Scenario 171, cross-sectional imaging with CT of the chest, abdomen, and pelvis to evaluate the extent of disease and help guide treatment planning is warranted. Unresectable metastatic disease is a contraindication to surgery or local therapy. When isolated disease is identified, MRI may help evaluate the local extent for consideration of surgical resection or radiation. Therefore, for the patient in Scenario 171, performing CT to evaluate for metastatic disease is the best next step, with MRI added secondarily if needed for radiation or surgical planning.

Haldorsen IS, Salvesen HB. What is the best preoperative imaging for endometrial cancer? Curr Oncol Rep 2016;18:25–0. doi: 10.1007/s11912-016-0506-0

National Comprehensive Cancer Network. Uterine neoplasms. Version 2.2025. NCCN Clinical Practice Guidelines in Oncology [after login]. NCCN; 2024. Accessed February 26, 2025. https:// https:// www.nccn.org/guidelines/guidelines-detail?category=1&id=1473

Salani R, Khanna N, Frimer M, Bristow RE, Chen L. An update on post-treatment surveillance and diagnosis of recurrence in women with gynecologic malignancies: Society of Gynecologic Oncology (SGO) recommendations. Gynecol Oncol 2017;146:3–10. doi: 10.1016/j.ygyno.2017.03.022

Zanfagnin V, Ferrero A, Biglia N, Aletti G, Gill SE, Makdisi PB, et al. The role of surgery in recurrent endometrial cancer. Expert Rev Anticancer Ther 2016;16:741–50. doi: 10.1080/14737140.2016.1190650

Appendix A

Normal Values for Laboratory Tests*

ANALYTE	CONVENTIONAL UNITS
Alanine aminotransferase, serum	8–35 units/L
Albumin, serum	3.5–5.5 g/dL
Alkaline phosphatase, serum	15–120 units/L
Amniotic fluid index	3–30 mL
Amylase 20–300 units/L	
Older than 60 years	21–160 units/L
Aspartate aminotransferase, serum	15–30 units/L
Bicarbonate	
Arterial blood	21–27 mEq/L
Venous plasma	23–29 mEq/L
Bilirubin	
Total	0.3–1 mg/dL
Conjugated (direct)	0.1–0.4 mg/dL
Newborn, total	1–10 mg/dL
Blood gases (arterial) and pulmonary function	
Base deficit	Less than 3 mEq/L
Base excess, arterial blood, calculated	−2 mEq/L to +3 mEq/L
Forced expiratory volume (FEV_1)	3.5–5 L
Greater than 80% of predicted value	
Forced vital capacity	3.5–5 L
Oxygen saturation (So_2)	95% or higher
Pao_2	80 mm Hg or more
Pco_2	35–45 mm Hg
Po_2	80–95 mm Hg
Peak expiratory flow rate	Approximately 450 L/min
Pvo_2	30–40 mm Hg
Blood urea nitrogen	
Adult	7–18 mg/dL
Older than 60 years	8–20 mg/dL
CA 19-9	Less than 37 units/mL
CA 125	Less than 34 units/mL
Calcium	
Ionized	4.6–5.3 mg/dL
Serum	8.6–10 mg/dL
Carcinoembryonic antigen (CEA)	Less than 3 ng/mL
Chloride	98–106 mEq/L

(continued)

*Values listed are specific for adults or women, if relevant, unless otherwise differentiated.

Appendix A (continued)

ANALYTE	CONVENTIONAL UNITS
Cholesterol	
Total	
Desirable	140–199 mg/dL
Borderline high	200–239 mg/dL
High	240 mg/dL or more
High-density lipoprotein	40–85 mg/dL
Low-density lipoprotein	
Desirable	Less than 130 mg/dL
Borderline high	140–159 mg/dL
High	Greater than 160 mg/dL
Total cholesterol-to-high-density lipoprotein ratio	
Desirable	Less than 3
Borderline high	3–5
High	Greater than 5
Triglycerides	
20 years and older	Less than 150 mg/dL
Younger than 20 years	35–135 mg/dL
Cortisol, plasma	
8 AM	5–23 micrograms/dL
4 PM	3–15 micrograms/dL
10 PM	Less than 50% of 8 AM value
Creatinine, serum	0.6–1.2 mg/dL
Dehydroepiandrosterone sulfate	60–340 micrograms/dL
Erythrocyte	
Count	3,800,000–5,100,000/mm^3
Distribution width	10 plus or minus 1.5%
Sedimentation rate	
Wintrobe method	0–15 mm/hour
Westergren method	0–20 mm/hour
Estradiol-17β	
Follicular phase	30–100 pg/mL
Ovulatory phase	200–400 pg/mL
Luteal phase	50–140 pg/mL
Child	0.8–56 pg/mL
Ferritin, serum	18–160 micrograms/L
Fibrinogen	150–400 mg/dL
Follicle-stimulating hormone	
Premenopause	2.8–17.2 mIU/mL
Midcycle peak	15–35 mIU/mL
Postmenopause	24–170 mIU/mL
Child	0.1–7 mIU/mL

(continued)

*Values listed are specific for adults or women, if relevant, unless otherwise differentiated.

Appendix A (continued)

ANALYTE	CONVENTIONAL UNITS
Glucose	
Fasting	70–105 mg/dL
2-hour postprandial	Less than 120 mg/dL
Random blood	65–110 mg/dL
Hematocrit	36–48%
Hemoglobin	12–16 g/dL
Fetal	Less than 1% of total
Hemoglobin A_{1c}	
Normal	Less than 5.5–8.5%
Prediabetic	5.7%–6.4%
Human chorionic gonadotropin	0–5 mIU/mL
Pregnant	Greater than 5 mIU/mL
17α-Hydroxyprogesterone	
Adult	50–300 ng/dL
Child	32–63 ng/dL
25-Hydroxyvitamin D	10–55 ng/mL
International Normalized Ratio	Greater than 1
Prothrombin time	10–13 seconds
Iron, serum	65–165 micrograms/dL
Binding capacity total	240–450 micrograms/dL
Lactate dehydrogenase, serum	313–618 units/L
Lactate, serum	Less than 2.0 mmol/L
Leukocytes	
Total	5,000–10,000/cubic microliter
Differential counts	
Basophils	0–1%
Eosinophils	1–3%
Lymphocytes	25–33%
Monocytes	3–7%
Myelocytes	0%
Band neutrophils	3–5%
Segmented neutrophils	54–62%
	1,500–8,000 cells/microliter
Lipase	
60 years or younger	10–140 units/L
Older than 60 years	18–180 units/L
Luteinizing hormone	
Follicular phase	3.6–29.4 mIU/mL
Midcycle peak	58–204 mIU/mL
Postmenopause	35–129 mIU/mL
Child	0.5–10.3 mIU/mL

(continued)

*Values listed are specific for adults or women, if relevant, unless otherwise differentiated.

Appendix A (continued)

ANALYTE	CONVENTIONAL UNITS
Magnesium	
Adult	1.6–2.6 mg/dL
Child	1.7–2.1 mg/dL
Newborn	1.5–2.2 mg/dL
Mean corpuscular	
mCH Hemoglobin	27–33 pg
mCHC Hemoglobin concentration	33–37 g/dL
mCV Volume	80–100 cubic micrometers
Partial thromboplastin time, activated	21–35 seconds
Phosphate, inorganic phosphorus	2.5–4.5 mg/dL
Platelet count	140,000–400,000/mm^3
Potassium	3.5–5.3 mEq/L
Progesterone	
Follicular phase	Less than 3 ng/mL
Luteal phase	2.5–28 ng/mL
On oral contraceptives	0.1–0.3 ng/mL
Secretory phase	5–30 ng/mL
Older than 60 years	0–0.2 ng/mL
First trimester	9–47 ng/mL
Second trimester	16.8–146 ng/mL
Third trimester	55–255 ng/mL
Prolactin	0–17 ng/mL
Pregnant	34–386 ng/mL by third trimester
Prothrombin time	10–13 seconds
Reticulocyte count	Absolute: 25,000–85,000 cubic micrometers 0.5–2.5% of erythrocytes
Semen analysis, spermatozoa	
Antisperm antibody	% of sperm binding by immunobead technique; greater than 20% = decreased fertility
Count	Greater than or equal to 20 million/mL
Motility	Greater than or equal to 50%
Morphology	Greater than or equal to 15% normal forms
Sodium	135–145 mEq/L
Testosterone, female	

(continued)

*Values listed are specific for adults or women, if relevant, unless otherwise differentiated.

Appendix A (continued)

ANALYTE	CONVENTIONAL UNITS
Total	6–86 ng/dL
Pregnant	3–4 × normal
Postmenopause	One half of normal
Free	
20–29 years old	0.9–3.2 pg/mL
30–39 years old	0.8–3 pg/mL
40–49 years old	0.6–2.5 pg/mL
50–59 years old	0.3–2.7 pg/mL
Older than 60 years	0.2–2.2 pg/mL
Thyroid-stimulating hormone	0.2–3 microunits/mL
Thyroxine	
Serum free	0.9–2.3 ng/dL
Triiodothyronine uptake	25–35%
Urea nitrogen, blood	
Adult	7–18 mg/dL
Older than 60 years	8–20 mg/dL
Uric acid, serum	2.6–6 mg/dL
Urinalysis	
Epithelial cells	0–3/HPF
Erythrocytes	0–3/HPF
Leukocytes	0–4/HPF
Protein (albumin)	
Qualitative	None detected
Quantitative	10–100 mg/24 hours
Pregnancy	Less than 300 mg/24 hours
Urine specific gravity	
Normal hydration and volume	1.005–1.03
Concentrated	1.025–1.03
Diluted	1.001–1.01

*Values listed are specific for adults or women, if relevant, unless otherwise differentiated.

Appendix B (18, 90)

TABLE B-1. Derivation of Sensitivity, Specificity, Positive Predictive Value, and Negative Predictive Value of a Screening Test for Ovarian Cancer

	OVARIAN CANCER PRESENT	OVARIAN CANCER ABSENT	FORMULA
TEST POSITIVE	True positive (A)	False positive (B)	PPV=A/(A+B)
TEST NEGATIVE	False negative (C)	True negative (D)	NPV=D/(C+D)
FORMULA	Sensitivity=A/(A+C) ("positive in disease")	Specificity=D/(B+D) ("negative in health")	

Data from Wolford JE, Ferrigni E, Margul D, Herzog TJ. Integrating precision medicine into the contemporary management of gynecologic cancer. Curr Oncol Rep 2022;24:889–904. doi: 10.1007/s11912-021-01163-2

TABLE B-2. Calculation of Positive Predictive Value and Negative Predictive Value for an Ovarian Cancer Screening Test With 90% Sensitivity and 80% Specificity in a Population With 40% Ovarian Cancer Prevalence

	OVARIAN CANCER PRESENT (400)	OVARIAN CANCER ABSENT (600)	FORMULA
TEST POSITIVE	True positive (360)	False positive (120)	PPV=A/A+B =360/360+120=75%
TEST NEGATIVE	False negative (40)	True negative (480)	NPV=D/C+D =480/40+480=92%
FORMULA	Sensitivity=A/A+C =360/400=90%	Specificity=D/B+D =480/600=80%	

Data from Wolford JE, Ferrigni E, Margul D, Herzog TJ. Integrating precision medicine into the contemporary management of gynecologic cancer. Curr Oncol Rep 2022;24:889–904. doi: 10.1007/s11912-021-01163-2

Appendix C (22, 70)

TABLE C-1. Common Molecular Targets in Gynecologic Oncology

	HISTOLOGY	TESTING	TARGETED AGENT
OVARIAN CANCER			
BRCA 1/2 and HRD	High-grade serous	DNA sequencing	PARP-inhibitor (olaparib, niraparib, rucaparib)
Microsatellite instability–high or mismatch repair deficient (MSI-H, dMMR)	High-grade serous, clear cell	IHC, DNA sequencing, PCR	Immunotherapy (pembrolizumab)
ERBB2 or HER2/neu	High-grade serous, low-grade serous, mucinous	IHC, FISH	Monoclonal antibody to HER 2/neu (trastuzumab), antibody–drug conjugate (fam-trastuzumab deruxtecan)
Estrogen/progesterone receptor positive	High-grade serous, low-grade serous	IHC	Endocrine therapy (tamoxifen, raloxifene, medroxyprogesterone acetate, or megestrol acetate)
BRAF	Low-grade serous	IHC, DNA sequencing, PCR	*BRAF* inhibitors (trametininib, vemurafenib, dabrafenib, encorafenib)
ARID1A	Endometrioid, clear cell	DNA sequencing	Enhancer zeste homolog inhibitor, PARPi, immunotherapy
PTEN	Endometrioid, clear cell	DNA sequencing	mTOR inhibitors (temsirolimus, everolimus)
KRAS	Mucinous	DNA sequencing	Monoclonal antibody that targets *KRAS* (adagrasib)
FOLR-α	High-grade serous	IHC	Antibody–drug conjugate (mirvetuximab)
ENDOMETRIAL CANCER			
PTEN	Endometrioid	DNA sequencing	mTOR inhibitors (temsirolimus, everolimus)
MSI-H or dMMR	Endometrioid	IHC, DNA sequencing, PCR	Immunotherapy (pembrolizumab, dostarlimab)
ERBB2 or *HER2/neu*	High-grade serous, clear cell, mucinous	IHC, FISH	Monoclonal antibody to HER 2/neu (trastuzumab), antibody–drug conjugate (fam-trastuzumab deruxtecan)
PTEN	High-grade stromal sarcoma	DNA sequencing	mTOR inhibitors (temsirolimus, everolimus)
CERVICAL CANCER			
PDL-1/2	HPV related	IHC	Immunotherapy (pembrolizumab)
ERBB2 or *HER2/neu*	Squamous cell, adenocarcinoma	IHC	Antibody–drug conjugate (fam-trastuzumab deruxtecan)

Abbreviations: ADL, activity of daily living; BMI, body mass index; BOMC, Blessed Orientation-Memory-Concentration; CARG, Cancer and Aging Research Group; CIRS-G, Cumulative Illness Rating Score-Geriatrics; CRASH, Chemotherapy Risk Assessment Scale for High-Age Patients; ECOG PS, Eastern Cooperative Oncology Group performance status; G8, Geriatric-8; GA, geriatric assessment; GDS, Geriatric Depression Scale; IADL, instrumental activity of daily living; LDH, lactate dehydrogenase; MMSE, Mini-Mental State Examination; MNA, Mini Nutritional Assessment; MOCA, Montreal Cognitive Assessment; OARS, Older Americans Resources and Services; PRO, patient-reported outcome; SPPB, Short Physical Performance Battery; TUG, Timed Up and Go; VES-13, Vulnerable Elders Survey-13.

Data from Wolford JE, Ferrigni E, Margul D, Herzog TJ. Integrating precision medicine into the contemporary management of gynecologic cancer. Curr Oncol Rep 2022;24:889–904. doi: 10.1007/s11912-021-01163-2

Appendix D (23)

TABLE D-1. Recommended Geriatric Oncology Tools

Assessment of the Below GA Domains Recommended for All Patients Aged 65+	Recommended Tool and Score Signifying Impairment	Evidence to Support Recommendation	Administration Characteristics	Considerations and Other Evaluation Options
Function	IADLs: dependence on any task signifies impairment.	Large prospective studies of older patients with cancer show that IADLs predict chemotherapy toxicity, mortality, hospitalizations, and functional decline. Advocated by experts in Delphi consensus panels.	PRO; less than 5 minutes	Consider ADLs. Any ADL deficit is used for characterization of frailty. Consider objective measure of physical performance such as SPPB, TUG, or gait speed.
Falls	Single item: "How many falls have you had over the last 6 months (or since the last visit)?" One or more recent falls.	Falls are common in older adults with cancer and can lead to serious injury. Falls have been associated with chemotherapy toxicity. Assessment for falls is recommended by geriatric oncology expert panels and the American Geriatrics Society for all older adults.	PRO; less than 1 minute	
Comorbidity	Robust review of chronic medical conditions and medications through routine history: three or more chronic health problems or one or more serious health problems.	Comorbidity is associated with poorer survival, chemotherapy toxicity, mortality, and hospitalizations.	Part of routine history	Consider validated tools such as CIRS-G or Charlson. History, CIRS-G, and OARS comorbidity recommended by experts.
Cognition	Mini-Cog: an abnormal test is defined by zero words recalled OR one to two words recalled + abnormal clock-drawing test. This screening test for cognitive impairment and abnormal scores requires further follow-up and decision-making capacity assessment. OR BOMC test: a score of 6 or greater identifies patients who have moderate deficits, and a cut point of 11 or greater identifies patients with severe cognitive impairment.	Growing data show that cognitive impairment is associated with poorer survival in older patients with cancer and increased chemotherapy toxicity risk. Mini-Cog has been shown to have high sensitivity and specificity for identifying cognitive impairment when compared with longer tools. BOMC scale is practical and is included in the cancer-specific GA developed by Hurria et al.	Administered; 5 minutes or less	Multiple tools are available for cognitive assessment. The MMSE has more robust data for prediction of outcomes in older patients with cancer and has been shown to predict chemotherapy toxicity; it is included in the CRASH tool developed by Extermann et al. The MOCA is also used by geriatricians. Both MMSE and MOCA are considerably longer than Mini-Cog and BOMC.

(continued)

Table D-1. Recommended Geriatric Oncology Tools (continued)

Assessment of the Below GA Domains Recommended for All Patients Aged 65+	Recommended Tool and Score Signifying Impairment	Evidence to Support Recommendation	Administration Characteristics	Considerations and Other Evaluation Options
Depression	GDS 15 item: a score of greater than 5 suggests depression and requires follow-up.	Depression has been associated with unexpected hospitalizations, treatment tolerance, mortality, and functional decline in older adults with cancer receiving chemotherapy; these studies primarily assessed depression with the GDS.	PRO; 5 minutes or less	GDS recommended also by ASCO guidelines for depression. The Patient Health Questionnaire-9 is an alternative and is also recommended by ASCO guidelines for depression. The mental health inventory is an option and has been associated with outcomes in older patients with breast cancer.
Nutrition	Unintentional weight loss; greater than 10% weight loss from baseline weight; BMI less than 21 kg/m².	Poor nutrition is associated with mortality in older patients with cancer.	PRO; less than 1 minute	Consider G8 and MNA as alternatives; both are associated with mortality in older patients with cancer.

Tools That Can Provide Estimates of Risk for Chemotherapy Toxicity	Items	Study Population	Administration Characteristics	Considerations
CARG toxicity tool: provides estimates for overall risk of grade 3 to 5 chemotherapy toxicity.	Eleven items; prior falls (one or more v none), hearing problems (deaf to excellent), limitations in walking one block (limited a lot, limited a little, not limited), difficulties with taking medications, interference of social activities by physical health and/or emotional problems (all of the time to none of the time) as well as age, height, weight, gender, cancer type (GI vs genitourinary vs other), dosage (standard vs dose reduced), number of chemotherapy agents (mono vs poly), hemoglobin level, and creatinine clearance.	Patients aged 65+ with a solid tumor malignancy or lymphoma starting a new chemotherapy regimen (any line).	PRO/administered; 5 minutes Available online: www.mycarg.org/Chemo_Toxicity_Calculator	Can ask GA variables as part of history or include as part of PRO assessment.
CRASH tool: provides estimates separately for risk of grade 3 hematologic and grade 3 to 4 nonhematologic toxicity.	Assessment of risk of hematologic toxicity includes diastolic blood pressure (greater than 72 mm Hg), IADL score (less than 26), and LDH (greater than 459 U/L). Assessment of risk of nonhematologic toxicity includes ECOG PS, MMSE (less than 30), and MNA (less than 28). Chemotherapy intensity is assessed with MAX2 index.	Patients aged 70+ years with histologically proven cancer who were starting chemotherapy.	PRO/administered; estimated time to completion is on par with full GA (20–30 minutes). Available online: https://moffitt.org/for-healthcare-providers/clinical-programs-and-services/senior-adult-oncology-program/senior-adult-oncology-program-tools	The CRASH scale includes GA measures known also to predict other adverse outcomes, such as mortality, functional decline, and hospitalizations: IADLs, MMSE, and MNA.

(continued)

Table D-1. Recommended Geriatric Oncology Tools (continued)

Screening Tools That Have Been Independently Associated with Adverse Outcomes in Older Patients with Cancer Receiving Chemotherapy	Items	Study Population and Evidence	Administration Characteristics	Considerations
G8	Eight items covering appetite, weight loss, neuropsychological problems, BMI, number of medications, patient self-rated health, and age. Score of 14 or higher signifies impairment. Derived from the MNA.	Several large studies have been conducted that include patients aged 70+, which included patients with both solid and hematologic malignancies starting a new chemotherapy agent. G8 is independently associated with mortality (1 year and 3 years), even when controlling for ECOG PS and stage of cancer.	Administered; 5–10 minutes	G8 can also be used as a screening tool to identify older patients who need more comprehensive GA.
VES-13	Thirteen items including age, self-rated health, common functional tasks, and ability to complete physical activities. Score of 3 or higher is associated with mortality and chemotherapy toxicity in older patients with cancer. A score of 7 or higher has been shown to be associated with functional decline.	VES-13 score has been shown to be associated with mortality, chemotherapy toxicity, and functional decline.	Administered or PRO (but errors are common with PRO administration); 5–10 minutes	VES-13 can also be used as a screening tool to identify older patients who need more comprehensive GA.

If Resources Available, Consider Assessment of These Domains	Items	Study Population	Administration Characteristics	Considerations
Objective physical performance: SPPB, TUG, or gait speed	SPPB includes three tests (balance, chair stands, and gait speed); a score of less than 9 is associated with increased functional decline, nursing home use, and mortality in community-dwelling older adults. TUG measures the ability of a patient to get out of a chair and walk 3 m or 10 ft and back; a score of greater than 12 s is associated with an increased risk of falling.	Low SPPB score is associated with increased mortality in older women with gynecologic malignancies. TUG and gait speed have been shown to be associated with early mortality (6 months) in older patients with cancer receiving chemotherapy. SPPB and gait speed are associated with functional decline in patients with nonmetastatic breast cancer receiving chemotherapy.	All administered; 1–5 minutes, depending on test	

Abbreviations: ADL, activity of daily living; BMI, body mass index; BOMC, Blessed Orientation-Memory-Concentration; CARG, Cancer and Aging Research Group; CIRS-G, Cumulative Illness Rating Score-Geriatrics; CRASH, Chemotherapy Risk Assessment Scale for High-Age Patients; ECOG PS, Eastern Cooperative Oncology Group performance status; G8, Geriatric-8; GA, geriatric assessment; GDS, Geriatric Depression Scale; IADL, instrumental activity of daily living; LDH, lactate dehydrogenase; MMSE, Mini-Mental State Examination; MNA, Mini Nutritional Assessment; MOCA, Montreal Cognitive Assessment; OARS, Older Americans Resources and Services; PRO, patient-reported outcome; SPPB, Short Physical Performance Battery; TUG, Timed Up and Go; VES-13, Vulnerable Elders Survey-13.

Data from Mohile SG, Dale W, Somerfield MR, Schonberg MA, Boyd CM, Burhenn PS, et al. Practical assessment and management of vulnerabilities in older patients receiving chemotherapy: ASCO Guideline for Geriatric Oncology. J Clin Oncol 2018;36:2326–47. doi: 10.1200/JCO.2018.78.8687

Appendix E (25, 37)

TABLE E-1. The Prospective Trial of Conservative Surgery for Low-Risk Early-Stage Cervical Cancer and Simple Hysterectomy and Pelvic Node Assessment

CONCERV TRIAL
International Federation of Gynecology and Obstetrics (FIGO) 2009 stage IA2–IB1 cervical carcinoma
Squamous cell (any grade) or adenocarcinoma (grade 1 or 2 only) histology
Tumor size of 2 cm or less by physical examination or imaging studies
Stromal invasion of 10 mm or less
No evidence of lymphovascular space invasion
Negative imaging for metastatic disease
Conization margins and endocervical curettage negative for malignancy or high-grade dysplasia
SHAPE TRIAL
FIGO 2009 stage IA2–IB1
Squamous-cell, adenocarcinoma or adenosquamous carcinoma histology, any grade
Tumor size of 2 cm or less
Stromal invasion less than 10 mm on excision specimen or less than 50% stromal invasion on preoperative MRI

Data from Schmeler KM, Pareja R, Lopez Blanco A, Humberto Fregnani J, Lopes A, Perrotta M, et al. ConCerv: a prospective trial of conservative surgery for low-risk early-stage cervical cancer. Int J Gynecol Cancer 2021;31:1317–25. doi: 10.1136/ijgc-2021-002921 *and* Plante M, Kwon JS, Ferguson S, Samouëlian V, Ferron G, Maulard A, et al. Simple versus radical hysterectomy in women with low-risk cervical cancer. CX.5 SHAPE investigators. N Engl J Med 2024;390:819–29. doi: 10.1056/NEJMoa2308900

Appendix F (27, 64)

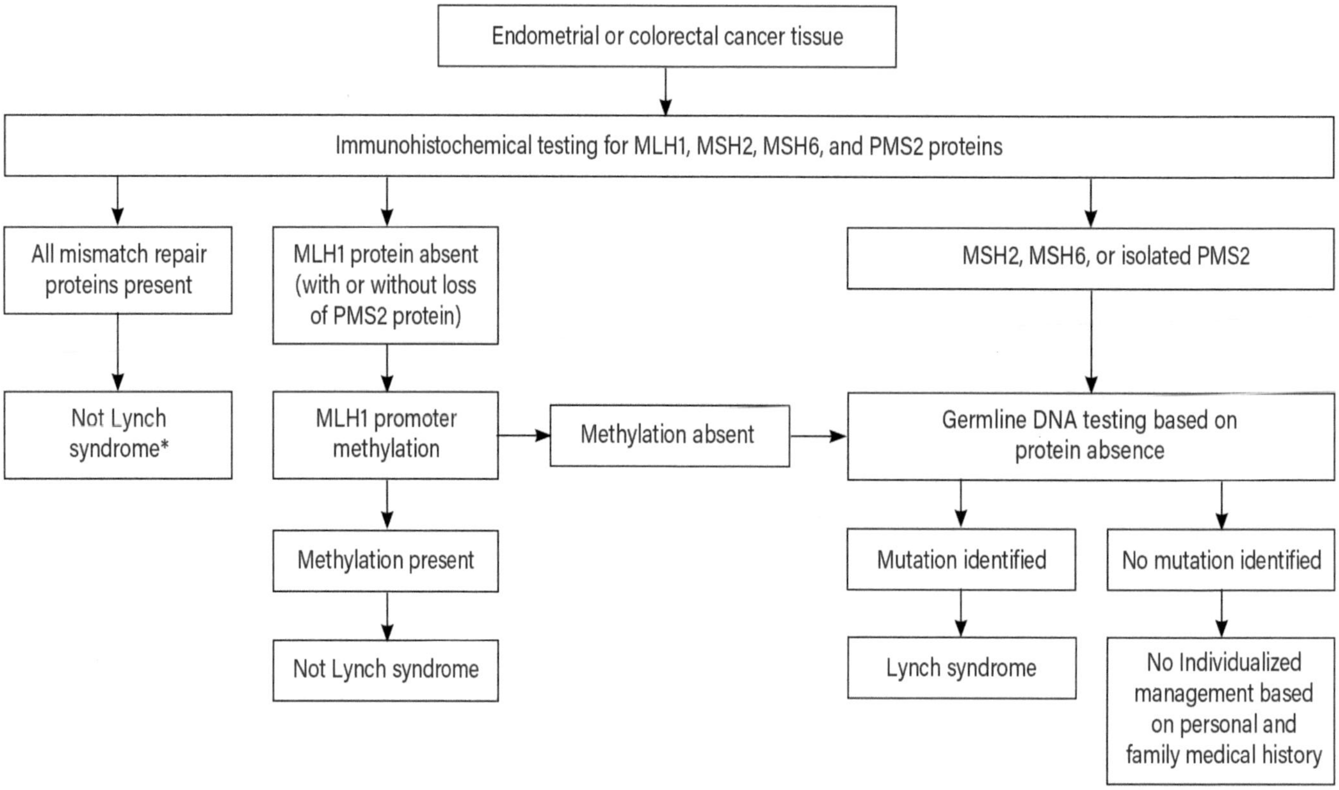

FIGURE F-1. Immunohistochemistry-based endometrial or colorectal tumor testing for mismatch repair gene expression to assess for the possibility of Lynch syndrome. *The scenario in which the presence of all four mismatch repair proteins does not rule out Lynch syndrome is the relatively uncommon situation in which a deleterious mutation allows the production of a full-length but nonfunctional mismatch repair protein. Given this possibility, in the setting of a very high clinical suspicion of Lynch syndrome and normal immunohistochemical testing results, the tumor can be further evaluated by a microsatellite instability testing. (Reprinted from Lynch syndrome. Practice Bulletin No. 147. American College of Obstetricians and Gynecologists [published erratum appears in Obstet Gynecol 2022;139:696]. Obstet Gynecol 2014;124:1042–54. doi: 10.1097/01.AOG.0000456325.50739.72)

Appendix G (28, 104, 164-167)

TABLE G-1. International Federation of Gynecology and Obstetrics (FIGO) Staging System

STAGE	DESCRIPTION
I	Carcinoma is strictly confined to the cervix uteri (extension to the corpus should be disregarded)
IA	Invasive carcinoma that can be diagnosed only by microscopy, with maximum depth of invasion less than 5 mm
IA1	Stromal invasion less than 3 mm in depth
IA2	Stromal invasion 3 mm or greater and less than 5 mm in depth
IB	Invasive carcinoma confined to the uterine cervix, with measured deepest invasion 5 mm or greater
IB1	Tumor measures less than 2 cm in greatest dimension
IB2	Tumor measures 2 cm or greater and less than 4 cm in greatest dimension
IB3	Tumor measures 4 cm or greater in greatest dimension
II	Carcinoma invades beyond the uterus, but has not extended onto the lower third of the vagina or to the pelvic wall
IIA	Limited to the upper two-thirds of the vagina without parametrial involvement
IIA1	Tumor measures less than 4 cm in greatest dimension
IIA2	Tumor measures 4 cm or greater in greatest dimension
IIB	With parametrial involvement but not up to the pelvic wall
III	Carcinoma involves the lower third of the vagina and/or extends to the pelvic wall and/or causes hydronephrosis or nonfunctioning kidney and/or involves pelvic and/or para-aortic lymph nodes
IIIA	Involves the lower third of the vagina, with no extension to the pelvic wall
IIIB	Extension to the pelvic wall and/or hydronephrosis or nonfunctioning kidney from tumor
IIIC	Involvement of pelvic and/or para-aortic lymph nodes, irrespective of tumor size and extent
IIIC1	Pelvic lymph node metastasis only
IIIC2	Para-aortic lymph node metastasis
IV	Carcinoma has extended beyond the true pelvis or has involved (biopsy-proven) the mucosa of the bladder or rectum
IVA	Spread to adjacent pelvic organs
IVB	Spread to distant organs

Reprinted from Bhatla N, Berek JS, Fredes MC, et al. Revised FIGO Staging for carcinoma of the cervix uteri. Int J Gynecol Obstet 2019;145:129-135 and Corrigendum to "Revised FIGO Staging for carcinoma of the cervix uteri" [Int J Gynecol Obstet 2019;145:129-135] Int J Gynecol Obstet 2019;147:279-280.

Appendix H (32, 76, 86, 140-143)

TABLE H-1. International Federation of Gynecology and Obstetrics (FIGO) Staging for Gestational Trophoblastic Neoplasia

FIGO STAGE	DESCRIPTION
I	Gestational trophoblastic tumors strictly confined to the uterine corpus
II	Gestational trophoblastic tumors extending to the adnexa or to the vagina, but limited to genital structures
III	Gestational trophoblastic tumors extending to the lungs, with or without genital tract involvement
IV	All other metastatic sites

Reprinted from Ngan HY, Seckl MJ, Berkowitz RS, Xiang Y, Golfier F, Sekharan PK, et al. Diagnosis and management of gestational trophoblastic disease: 2021 update. Int J Gynaecol Obstet 2021;155(suppl 1):86–93. doi: 10.1002/ijgo.13877

Appendix I (32, 34, 76, 140–143)

TABLE I-1. Modified World Health Organization Prognostic Scoring System

	SCORES			
	0	**1**	**2**	**4**
Age (y)	Less than 40	40 or older	—	
Antecedent pregnancy	Mole	Abortion	Term	
Interval months from index pregnancy	Less than 4	4 to less than 7	7 to less than 13	13 or more
Pretreatment serum hCG (IU/L)	Less than 10^3	10^3 to less than 10^4	10^4 to less than 10^5	Greater than 10^5
Largest tumor size (including uterus)	3 to less than 5 cm	5 cm or greater		
Site of metastases	Lung	Kidney/spleen	Gastrointestinal/liver	Brain
Number of metastases	—	1–4	5–8	Greater than 8
Previous failed chemotherapy	—	—	Single drug	2 or more drugs

Format for reporting to International Federation of Gynecology and Obstetrics Annual Report: In order to stage and allot a risk factor score, a patient's diagnosis is allocated to a stage as represented by a roman number I, II, III, and IV. This is then separated by a colon from the sum of all the actual risk factor scores expressed in Arabic numerals, for example, stage II:4, stage IV:9. This stage and score will be allotted for each patient.

Definition of Risk Categories:

Low Risk – Stage I or Stage II/III with a WHO prognostic score less than 7.

High Risk – Stage IV disease or any stage and WHO score 7 or greater.

Ultra-high Risk – Any stage with WHO score greater than 12.

Reprinted from Horowitz NS, Eskander RN, Adelman MR, Burke W. Epidemiology, diagnosis, and treatment of gestational trophoblastic disease: a Society of Gynecologic Oncology evidenced-based review and recommendation. Gynecol Oncol 2021;163:605–13. doi: 10.1016/j.ygyno.2021.10.003. With permission from Elsevier.

Appendix J **(34, 76)**

TABLE J-1. International Federation of Gynecology and Obstetrics (FIGO) Criteria for Diagnosis of Postmolar Gestational Trophoblastic Neoplasia

1. Plateauing of hCG +/− 10% for four consecutive values over 3 weeks (ie, days 1, 7, 14, 21)
2. A rise in hCG levels of 10% or higher for three values over 2-week period (ie, days 1, 7, 14)
3. Histologic diagnosis of choriocarcinoma or clinical and/or radiologic evidence of metastases
4. Abbreviation: hCG, human chorionic gonadotropin

Appendix K (42, 136–139)

TABLE K-1. Summary of Syndromes With Malignant Manifestations Associated With Breast and Ovarian Cancer

SYNDROME	BREAST CANCER	OVARIAN CANCER	ENDOMETRIAL CANCER	COLON CANCER	OTHER TYPES OF CANCER
Hereditary breast and ovarian cancer	X	X			Pancreatic, prostate, and melanoma
Lynch		X	X	X	Gastric, ureteral, biliary, pancreatic, glioblastoma, renal pelvis
Li-Fraumeni	X			X	Sarcomas, brain, adrenocortical
***PTEN* hamartoma tumor syndrome**†	X		X	X	Benign mucocutaneous lesions, thyroid, gastrointestinal hamartomas
Peutz-Jeghers	X	X		X	Cervical adenoma malignum, gastrointestinal hamartomas, pancreatic, gastric, small bowel
Hereditary diffuse gastric cancer	X				Gastric, colorectal

†Formerly referred to as Cowden syndrome.

Data from National Comprehensive Cancer Network. Breast cancer: NCCN Evidence Blocks. Version 2.2019. NCCN Clinical Practice Guidelines in Oncology [after login]. Fort Washington [PA]: NCCN; 2019 and Hampel H, Bennett RL, Buchanan A, Pearlman R, Wiesner GL. A practice guideline from the American College of Medical Genetics and Genomics and the National Society of Genetic Counselors: referral indications for cancer predisposition assessment. Guideline Development Group, American College of Medical Genetics and Genomics Professional Practice and Guidelines Committee and National Society of Genetic Counselors Practice Guidelines Committee. Genet Med 2015;17:70–87.

TABLE K-2. Hereditary Gynecologic Cancer Syndromes

SYNDROME	GENE	INCIDENCE	CANCER	SCREENING	RISK-REDUCING SURGERY
Lynch syndrome	*MLH1, MSH2, MSH6, PMS2*	1/660–2,000	Colon, uterus, ovary, pancreas, gastrointestinal, kidney	CS – annually after 40 years of age; PE, US, Ca-125 – annually after 30–45 years of age	THBSO after completion of childbearing
HBOCS	*BRCA1, BRCA2*	1/300–600	Breast, ovary, fallopian tube, peritoneum, pancreas, skin (melanoma)	PE, US, Ca-125 – every 6 months at age 35 MRI/mammogram – annually after 25 years of age	RRSO for *BRCA1 1/2 BRCA1*: 35–40 years BRCA2: 40–45 years Or after completion of childbearing; PBM after childbearing
***PTEN* hamartoma tumor syndrome**†	*PTEN*	1/200,000	Breast, uterus, thyroid	MRI/mammography – annually after 30–35 years of age; ES and US after 30–35 years of age	THBSO and PBM after the completion of childbearing
Li-Fraumeni syndrome	*TP53*	1/20,000	Breast, sarcoma, leukemia, adrenal gland, lung, stomach	MRI/mammography after 20 years of age	Discuss PBM

(continued)

TABLE K-2. Hereditary Gynecologic Cancer Syndromes (continued)

SYNDROME	GENE	INCIDENCE	CANCER	SCREENING	RISK-REDUCING SURGERY
Peutz-Jeghers syndrome	*STK11*	1/50,000–200,000	Breast, ovary, gastrointestinal, uterus, uterine cervix, lung, bone, leukemia	PAP smear and PE after 18–20 years of age; MRI/mammography after 30 years of age	Not estimated
Ataxia-telangiectasia	*ATM*	1/40,000–100,000	Leukemia, lymphomas, ovary, breast	Not estimated	Not estimated
DICER1 syndrome	*DICER1*	1/10,600	Lung, kidney, uterine cervix, ovary	Not estimated	Not estimated
Gonadal dysgenesis	46,XY; 45,X; 46,XX	1/4,500–5,000	Ovary	Not estimated	RRSO after 16–16 years of age
Tuberous sclerosis	*TSC1*; *TSC2*	1/6,760–13,520			
MEN Type I	*MEN* I	1/30,000	Parathyroid, pituitary, pancreas, small bowels, ovary	Not estimated	Not estimated
MEN Type II	*RET*	1/30,000	Thyroid, parathyroid, adrenal glands (PHEO) ovary	Not estimated	Not estimated
HSCCOHT, HUUS	*SMARCA4*	Unknown	Ovary, uterus	PE, CA-125, serum calcium level - annually	Not estimated
HDGC	*CDH1*	5/10–100,000	Stomach, breast	CS - 25–30 years; MRI after 30 years of age	PG after 20–30 years of age; PBM - not recommended
MUTYH-associated polyposis	*MUTYH*	0.01–0.04% of the Caucasian population	Colon, rectum, ovary, uterus, breast	Not estimated	RRSO after 45–50 years of age

Abbreviations: CS, colonoscopy; ES, endometrial samplings; HBOCS, hereditary breast-ovarian cancer syndrome; HDGC, hereditary diffuse gastric cancer; HSCCOHT, hereditary small cell carcinoma of the ovary, hypercalcemic type; HUUS, hereditary undifferentiated uterine carcinoma; MEN, multiple endocrine neoplasia; PBM, prophylactic bilateral mastectomy; PE, pelvic examination; PG, prophylactic gastrectomy; PHEO, pheochromocytoma; RRSO, risk-reducing bilateral salpingo-oophorectomy; THBSO, total hysterectomy with bilateral salpingo-oophorectomy; US, ultrasonography.

†Formerly referred to as Cowden syndrome.

Data from Hereditary cancer syndromes and risk assessment. ACOG Committee Opinion No. 793. American College of Obstetricians and Gynecologists. Obstet Gynecol 2019;134:e143–9. doi: 10.1097/AOG.0000000000003562; Kostov S, Watrowski R, Kornovski Y, Dzhenkov D, Slavchev S, Ivanova Y, et al. Hereditary gynecologic cancer syndromes - a narrative review. Onco Targets Ther 2022;15:381–405. doi: 10.2147/OTT.S353054; *and* National Comprehensive Cancer Network. Breast cancer: NCCN Evidence Blocks. Version 6.2024. NCCN Clinical Practice Guidelines in Oncology [after login]. NCCN; 2024. Accessed February 26, 2025.

Index

NOTE: Numbers refer to questions, not pages.

NOTE: Numbers refer to questions, not pages.

NOTE: Numbers refer to questions, not pages.

NOTE: Numbers refer to questions, not pages.

Q

R

S

T

NOTE: Numbers refer to questions, not pages.

NOTE: Numbers refer to questions, not pages.

PROLOG Personal Review of Learning in Obstetrics and Gynecology

Gynecologic Oncology and Critical Care

NINTH EDITION

Assessment Book

ONLINE ASSESSMENT

See instructions on the inside front cover.

ACOG

American College of Obstetricians & Gynecologists

Assessment Instructions

To earn continuing medical education (CME) credits, you need to submit the assessment online. Assessment results must be 80% or higher to achieve a passing score and attain CME credit. Instructions for the electronic submission are included on this page.

The online assessment is included with the price of the print book of this edition of PROLOG. You can retake the online assessment as many times as needed at no cost.

Instructions for Submitting the Electronic Assessment for CME Credit

To complete the online assessment for *Gynecologic Oncology and Critical Care*, Ninth Edition, follow these steps:

1. Go to https://prolog.acog.org.
2. Click "GET STARTED."
3. Log in to your ACOG account.
4. After you are logged in, your browser should redirect you to the PROLOG dashboard.
5. If it does not redirect you, refresh the page or go back to https://prolog.acog.org.
6. Find the assessment for *Gynecologic Oncology and Critical Care*, Ninth Edition, and click "Redeem Code."
7. Enter the key code located inside the red box on the inside cover of the Critique book. Follow the instructions provided and click "Redeem Code."

You will then be taken to the online assessment.

You will receive your test results immediately after submitting the online assessment. With a passing score of 80% or higher, your CME certificate will be available as a PDF within the online assessment. You are able to take the assessment as many times as needed to achieve the passing score for CME credit.

Electronic Assessment for CME Credit

To receive the CME credits for this edition, participants must complete an online assessment. Assessment results must be 80% or higher to achieve a passing score and attain CME credit. To access the online assessment, please visit https://prolog.acog.org. Test results and the CME certificate will be available upon completion of the examination.

If you purchased a print book, use the key code located on the inside front cover of the Critique Book and follow the directions provided. If you purchased an eBook, please follow the instructions online through https://prolog.acog.org to purchase and access the assessment.

DIRECTIONS: Each of the questions or incomplete statements below is followed by suggested answers or completions. On the online assessment select the ONE option that is BEST in each case.

1 Vulvar irritation

A 46-year-old woman presents with new vulvar itching and irritation. Her physical examination is notable for a 2 × 1.5-cm raised gray lesion on the right labium majus. A punch biopsy is performed, and the results are shown in Figure 1-1. The best next step in management is

(A) carbon dioxide laser ablation
(B) cryotherapy ablation
(C) high-potency topical corticosteroid
(D) topical imiquimod
(E) wide local excision

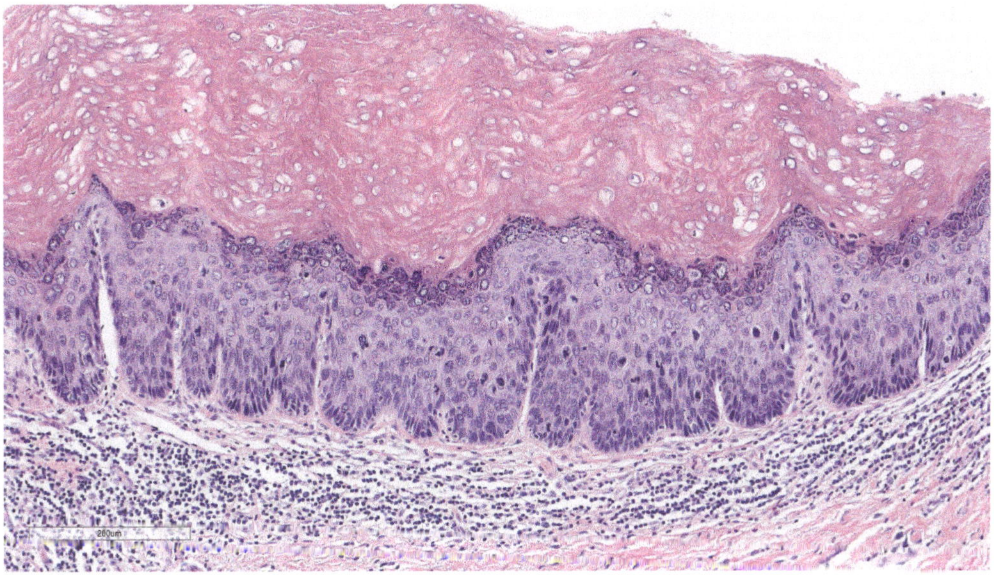

FIGURE 1-1. Vulvar punch biopsy.

2 Cancer-related electrolyte imbalances

A 58-year-old patient with recurrent platinum-resistant high-grade serous ovarian cancer treated with liposomal doxorubicin and bevacizumab presents to the emergency department. She has experienced worsening oral intake, abdominal pain, and nausea and vomiting during the last week. Her partner reports that she seems confused and disoriented. Her vital signs include a temperature of 37.2 °C (99 °F), a blood pressure of 98/60 mm Hg, a heart rate of 112 bpm, and a respiratory rate of 14, and her oxygen saturation is 99% on room air. On examination, she is oriented to self, but not place or time, and has diffuse abdominal tenderness to palpation without rebound or guarding. Serum electrolytes are notable for concentrations of calcium (14.1 mg/dL) and albumin (3 g/dL). An electrocardiogram demonstrates sinus tachycardia with a shortened QT interval. The best next step in treatment is the administration of

(A) calcitonin
(B) furosemide
(C) normal saline
(D) prednisone
(E) zoledronic acid

3 Laparoscopic complications

A 61-year-old woman with serous endometrial cancer presents for surgical staging. Her history is remarkable for a BMI of 41 and prior colonic resection due to a perforated diverticulitis and subsequent hernia repair with mesh. During laparoscopic entry with an open technique at the umbilicus, the small bowel is encountered during sharp dissection. After additional trocar placement and lysis of adhesions, an 8-mm enterotomy is identified in the ileum. No through and through defect is identified. The best next step is

(A) bowel diversion
(B) omental patch
(C) placement of enteral stent
(D) primary repair
(E) resection with anastomosis

4 Atypical glandular cells on cervical cytology

A 45-year-old woman presents for evaluation of cervical cytology showing atypical glandular cells (AGCs). She has no concerns at today's visit and no prior history of abnormal cervical cytology. She is not taking hormonal contraception and notes regular menstrual cycles. In addition to colposcopy and endocervical curettage, the best next step is

(A) cervical excisional procedure
(B) endometrial sampling
(C) human papillomavirus (HPV) testing
(D) pelvic ultrasonography
(E) repeat cervical cytology

5 Massive transfusion protocol

A patient with a grade 3C placenta accreta spectrum disorder with extension into the parametria has a postcesarean hysterectomy hemorrhage with an estimated blood loss exceeding 5 L. The institutional massive transfusion protocol (MTP) is activated. In an MTP, the best ratio of units of packed red blood cells (PRBCs) to units of fresh frozen plasma (FFP) to six packs of platelets is

(A) 4:2:1
(B) 2:1:1
(C) 1:1:1
(D) 3:1:2

6 Neurologic symptoms

A 68-year-old woman with a history of advanced-stage endometrial cancer presents to the emergency department after a fall. Her history is notable for weakness and headaches during the last several weeks. She also notes nausea and vomiting. A neurologic examination is notable for gait disturbance. Her vital signs are within normal limits, and the laboratory workup is unremarkable. There was no evidence of hemorrhage, hydrocephalus, or mass effect on a noncontrast head computed tomography (CT). The best next step in her evaluation is

(A) contrast-enhanced CT
(B) electroencephalogram (EEG)
(C) lumbar puncture
(D) MRI
(E) positron emission tomography (PET)

7 Postoperative nutrition

A 51-year-old woman with epithelial ovarian cancer underwent a total abdominal hysterectomy, bilateral salpingo-oophorectomy, omentectomy, peritoneal stripping, extensive lysis of adhesion requiring oversewing of the bowel, and optimal debulking. She is otherwise healthy. In the immediate postoperative period, the best next step for nutrition management is

(A) bowel rest until flatus
(B) clear liquid diet
(C) immunonutrient supplementation
(D) regular diet
(E) total parenteral nutrition

8 Soft tissue infections

A 54-year-old woman presents to the emergency department with a 2-day history of worsening vulvar swelling and pain. Her medical history is notable for a BMI of 42, hypertension, and type 2 diabetes (her recent outpatient hemoglobin A_{1C} was 10.4). Her vital signs are significant for a temperature of 38.1 °C (100.5 °F), a pulse of 110 bpm, and a blood pressure of 95/60 mm Hg. Her glucose today is 289 mg/dL. On physical examination, there is erythema and edema of the right vulva with central bulla and severe pain with palpation. Blood cultures were obtained, and the emergency department has initiated fluid resuscitation, broad-spectrum antibiotics, and insulin. The best next step in management is

(A) await blood culture results
(B) obtain computed tomography (CT)
(C) perform serial vulvar examinations
(D) perform surgical debridement
(E) perform vulvar biopsy

9 Nosocomial pneumonia

A 73-year-old patient develops a fever (38.5 °C [101.3 °F]) and shortness of breath 7 days after exploratory laparotomy, total hysterectomy, bilateral salpingo-oophorectomy, and complete cytoreduction for ovarian cancer. Her physical examination is notable for decreased breath sounds on the left and oxygen saturation of 93% on 4 L of O_2 by nasal cannula. Her laboratory test results are notable for a white blood cell count of 16.8×10^3/microliter with 98% neutrophils and a serum creatinine level of 1.74 mg/dL. A chest X-ray demonstrates a left lower lobe infiltrate. The patient has a history of treatment with intravenous antibiotics 4 weeks ago for lower leg cellulitis. In addition to piperacillin-tazobactam, the best antibiotic agent to add to this patient's therapy is

(A) cefazolin
(B) gentamycin
(C) linezolid
(D) oxacillin
(E) vancomycin

10 Placental site trophoblastic tumor

A 39-year-old gravida 1, para 1, had a hysterectomy for a 10-cm myomatous uterus and abnormal uterine bleeding. She had a molar pregnancy 5 years ago. Her preoperative urine test for human chorionic gonadotropin (hCG) was negative. Final pathology showed a vascular myometrial mass invading greater than 50% of the uterine wall. The photomicrographs below show a hematoxylin-eosin–stained section (Fig. 10-1A) and an immunohistochemical stain for Ki-67 (Fig. 10-1B). In this patient, the factor most consistently associated with an unfavorable prognosis is

(A) age less than 40 years
(B) deep myometrial invasion
(C) long interval from index pregnancy
(D) low hCG
(E) uterine size

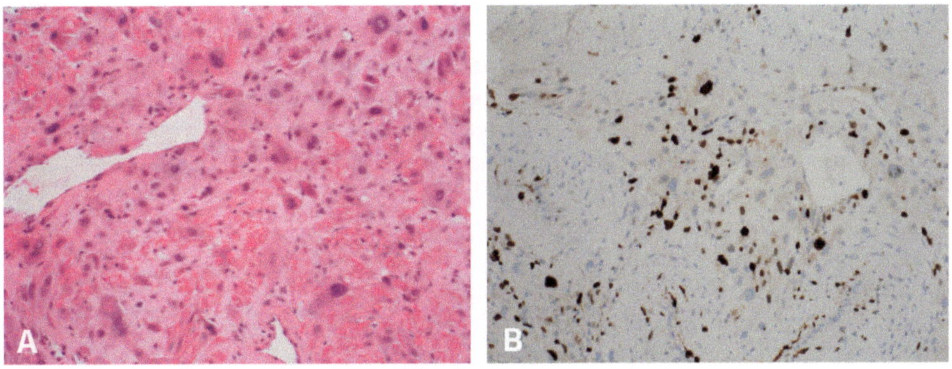

FIGURE 10-1. A. Highly atypical trophoblasts (hematoxylin-eosin). B. Immunohistochemical stain for Ki-67 shows a proliferation index of about 30%, supporting placental site trophoblastic tumor. (Reprinted from Polnaszek B, Mullen M, Bligard K, Raghuraman N, Massad LS. Term pregnancy after complete response of placental site trophoblastic tumor to immunotherapy. Obstet Gynecol 2021;138:115–8. doi: 10.1097/AOG.0000000000004434)

11 Bariatric surgery

A 32-year-old with a BMI of 45 and type 2 diabetes undergoes a sleeve gastrectomy. Weight loss is likely to most effectively reduce her risk for cancer of the

(A) breast
(B) colon
(C) endometrium
(D) pancreas
(E) stomach

12 Surveillance after borderline tumor

A 28-year-old underwent a left oophorectomy for a 12-cm adnexal mass, which was found to be a serous borderline tumor. No other disease was seen at the time of surgery. Her medical history and family history are unremarkable. She has not completed childbearing and asks about surveillance. You inform her that the best test to detect a recurrence is

(A) CA 125 level
(B) computed tomography (CT) of the abdomen and pelvis
(C) human epididymis protein 4 level
(D) MRI
(E) pelvic ultrasonography

13 Bowel preparation

A 65-year-old woman presents with new-onset abdominal pain and bloating. Her past medical history is notable for hypertension, which is well-controlled on medications. The physical examination demonstrates a mobile, 12-cm mass. Computed tomography (CT) demonstrates a 12-cm complex adnexal mass, ascites, and an omental cake without bowel involvement, and the patient is scheduled for an exploratory laparotomy and tumor debulking. Preoperatively, the best gastrointestinal intervention to optimize surgical outcomes is to

(A) avoid oral intake after midnight
(B) begin treatment with oral antibiotics
(C) have a carbohydrate drink 2 hours before surgery
(D) initiate probiotic therapy immediately
(E) undergo a mechanical bowel preparation

14 Depression

A 67-year-old presents for a surveillance visit after treatment for stage IIIC serous ovarian carcinoma. She has undergone surgical debulking and completed six cycles of carboplatin-paclitaxel chemotherapy 6 months ago. She is accompanied by her daughter, who expresses concern about the patient's mood, noting increasing irritability, decreased appetite and energy, and insomnia, all of which are interfering with her ability to participate in her daily activities. Her Patient Health Questionnaire 9 (PHQ-9) score is 21. The best next step is to recommend

(A) behavioral activation
(B) cognitive behavioral therapy
(C) electroconvulsive therapy (ECT)
(D) selective serotonin reuptake inhibitor (SSRI)
(E) tricyclic antidepressant

15 Endometrial cancer

A 31-year-old gravida 1, para 1, with abnormal uterine bleeding receives a diagnosis of grade 1 endometrioid endometrial adenocarcinoma after hysteroscopy with directed sampling. She desires future fertility. You counsel her that imaging is needed to assess her candidacy for fertility-sparing treatment. The best imaging test to assess her fertility status is

(A) computed tomography (CT)
(B) lymphoscintigraphy
(C) MRI
(D) positron emission tomography (PET)
(E) ultrasonography

16 Minimally invasive surgery for endometrial cancer

A 75-year-old woman with a diagnosis of International Federation of Gynecology and Obstetrics (FIGO) grade 3 endometrial cancer is undergoing surgical staging. A sentinel lymph node (SLN) protocol with indocyanine green tracer injected into the cervix is performed during the operation. A right SLN was detected in the obturator space and was excised. A left SLN was not identified. The best next operative step to evaluate for lymph node metastases is to

(A) inject intrauterine indocyanine green tracer
(B) inject the cervix with isosulfan blue dye
(C) obtain frozen section of the right sentinel node
(D) perform left-sided lymphadenectomy

17 Mortality risk factors

A 56-year-old woman with a BMI of 45 presents for an annual visit. Five years ago, she underwent a hysterectomy and bilateral salpingo-oophorectomy to treat abnormal uterine bleeding caused by the pathology shown in Figure 17-1. She is concerned about her mortality risk, and you counsel her that her highest risk of mortality is from

(A) cardiovascular disease
(B) colon cancer
(C) diabetes mellitus
(D) endometrial cancer
(E) fatty liver

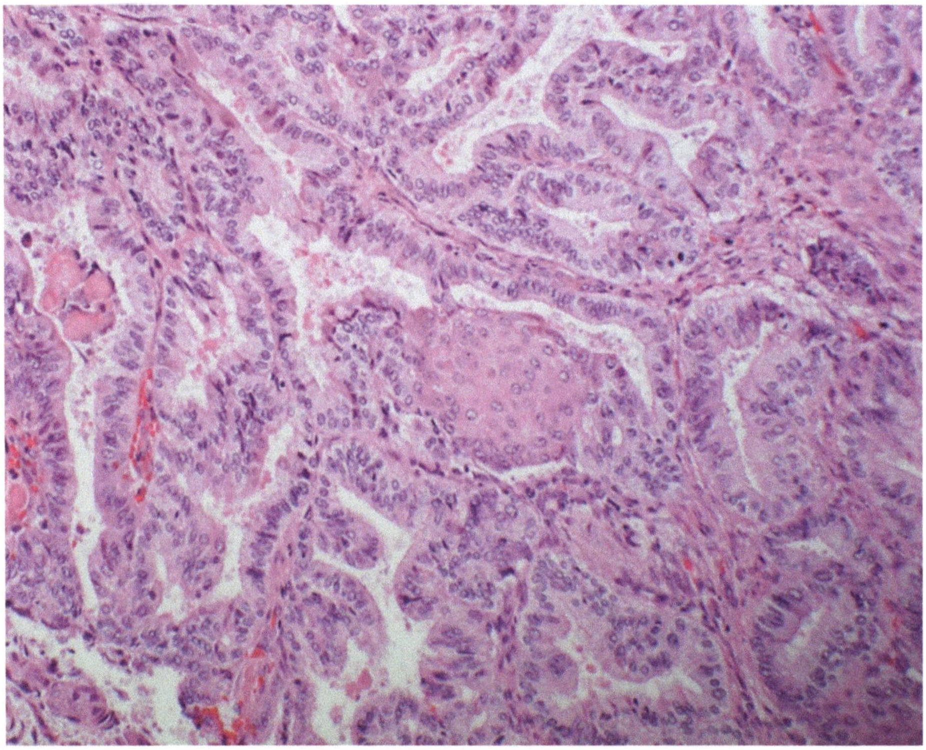

FIGURE 17-1. High-power image with crowded back-to-back glands with nuclear rounding, vesicular nuclei, small nucleoli, and squamous metaplasia. (Courtesy of Dr. Christine Bookhout, Department of Pathology, University of North Carolina.)

18 Statistical measures in antibiotic choice

A 52-year-old woman with endometrial adenocarcinoma is scheduled for hysterectomy and surgical staging. Her surgical history includes an appendectomy complicated by a methicillin-resistant *Staphylococcus aureus* wound infection. Considering her potential risk of antibiotic resistance, the most important statistical measure in prophylactic antibiotic selection for this patient is

(A) negative predictive value
(B) positive predictive value
(C) sensitivity
(D) specificity

19 Surgical site infection prevention

A 54-year-old patient with ovarian cancer undergoes interval debulking surgery with exploratory laparotomy, total abdominal hysterectomy, bilateral salpingo-oophorectomy, and omentectomy. She has a history of diabetes mellitus, and her hemoglobin A_{1C} is 9.5%. Her BMI is 29. She received cefazolin 30 minutes before incision, and her skin and vagina were prepped with chlorhexidine–alcohol skin preparation before surgery. Her midline incision is closed with a series of interrupted subcuticular monocryl sutures. There are no complications during surgery. On postoperative day 5, she develops a wound infection that requires opening the incision and packing. The factor that increased her risk of surgical site infection (SSI) the most is

(A) antibiotic selection
(B) BMI
(C) chlorhexidine–alcohol skin preparation
(D) diabetes
(E) skin closure method

20 Palpable breast mass

A 42-year-old gravida 3, para 3003, presents for her annual well-woman examination. She is currently using a levonorgestrel-releasing intrauterine device for contraception. Her baseline mammogram at age 40 was negative. Her family history includes a grandmother with breast cancer diagnosed when she was 64 years old. On physical examination, the patient is afebrile. She has a 2-cm nontender, firm, mobile mass just lateral to the left nipple with no skin changes. The best next step to evaluate the mass is

(A) core needle biopsy
(B) diagnostic digital breast tomosynthesis
(C) examination in 2 months
(D) fine needle aspiration
(E) MRI

21 Vulvar cancer micrometastasis

A 75-year-old patient underwent a partial radical vulvectomy with ipsilateral inguinal sentinel lymph node biopsy for squamous cell carcinoma of the vulva. Final pathology reveals negative surgical margins and a 1-mm metastasis in the sentinel lymph node with no extracapsular spread. The best next step to treat this cancer is

(A) external beam radiotherapy
(B) full inguinal-femoral lymphadenectomy
(C) immune checkpoint inhibitor
(D) lymph node assessment in 3 months
(E) systemic chemotherapy

22 Molecular testing

A 60-year-old patient with a history of stage IA, grade 3, endometrioid adenocarcinoma of the uterus presents for routine surveillance. Her cancer was initially managed with surgery and observation. She has been doing well without evidence of disease for 2 years. She now reports new-onset abdominal bloating and early satiety. A physical examination is notable for mild abdominal distension but is otherwise unremarkable. Imaging of the chest, abdomen, and pelvis reveals multifocal peritoneal implants. A biopsy of a peritoneal nodule confirms recurrent endometrioid adenocarcinoma. When considering options for initial systemic therapy, the best initial tumor test is

(A) folate receptor α (FOLR-α)
(B) homologous recombination deficiency (HRD)
(C) human epidermal growth factor receptor 2 (*HER2*)
(D) mismatch repair (MMR)
(E) phosphatase and tensin analog (*PTEN*)

23 Geriatric oncology

An 89-year-old patient with newly diagnosed metastatic ovarian cancer presents to the office to discuss treatment recommendations. Her BMI is 24. She has chronic obstructive pulmonary disease, arthritis, and hypertension. On examination, you note a fixed right adnexal mass with impingement on the rectum, a distended abdomen, and decreased breath sounds at the bases. Computed tomography (CT) reveals omental caking, ascites, pleural effusions, and a large adnexal mass. A CT-guided biopsy of the omentum indicates high-grade serous ovarian cancer. You discuss the standard treatment of metastatic ovarian cancer and explain that she may not be able to tolerate systemic therapy due to her age, comorbidities, and cancer burden. The best surrogate to assess her tolerance for chemotherapy is her

(A) BMI calculation
(B) Charlson Comorbidity Index score
(C) instrumental activities of daily living (IADL) score
(D) nutritional status
(E) performance status assessment

24 Familial cancer

A 29-year-old gravida 2, para 2, presents for her routine gynecologic examination. Her history is significant for two cesarean deliveries and a tubal ligation. Her family history is notable for epithelial ovarian cancer in her mother (now deceased) at age 54 years. The patient is using combined oral contraceptives (COCs) for cycle control. During your interview, she informs you that her 43-year-old sister received a diagnosis of breast cancer earlier this year and did not have a *BRCA* mutation. Her clinical breast examination is unremarkable. The best next step is to recommend

(A) bilateral salpingo-oophorectomy
(B) cessation of COCs
(C) genetic testing
(D) pelvic ultrasonography
(E) screening mammography

25 Fertility-sparing management of cervical cancer

A 36-year-old nulligravida who is interested in fertility preservation presents for follow-up after cervical conization for cervical intraepithelial neoplasia 3 (CIN 3). The final pathology from the cone reveals invasive squamous cell carcinoma with a depth of invasion of 6 mm, no lymphovascular space invasion (LVSI), and negative margins. The endocervical curettage also is negative for invasive carcinoma and high-grade dysplasia. Magnetic resonance imaging of the pelvis is normal. The best next step for this patient is

(A) colposcopy and high-risk human papillomavirus (HPV)-based testing at 6 months
(B) pelvic lymph node sampling
(C) radical hysterectomy
(D) radical trachelectomy
(E) simple hysterectomy

26 Endometrial sampling

A 33-year-old nulligravida presents to your office after hysteroscopy with dilation and curettage. Her biopsy result is shown in Figure 26-1. She desires future fertility. She has a history of polycystic ovary syndrome, a BMI of 38, and factor V Leiden heterozygous status with previous femoral vein thromboembolism. The best next step for the management of this pathology is to

(A) initiate oral contraceptive pills
(B) insert a levonorgestrel-releasing intrauterine device (LNG-IUD)
(C) perform endometrial ablation
(D) perform a hysterectomy
(E) perform hysteroscopic resection

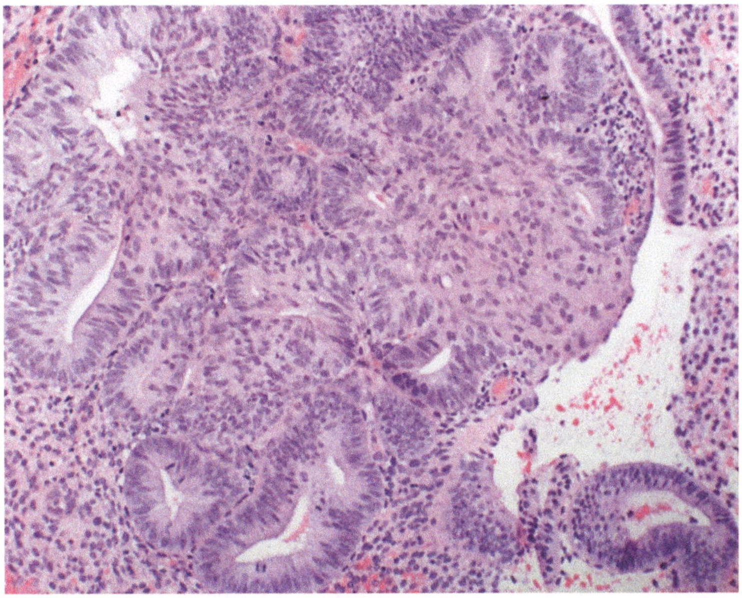

FIGURE 26-1. Glandular crowding and complexity as well as altered cytology characterized by nuclear rounding, vesicular nuclei, small nucleoli, and squamous metaplasia distinct from the surrounding endometrium.

27 Endometrial cancer evaluation

A 61-year-old receives a diagnosis of grade 2 endometrioid endometrial adenocarcinoma after hysteroscopic biopsy for postmenopausal bleeding. Mismatch repair testing is performed with immunohistochemistry on her tumor specimen with the following results: MSH6 intact, MSH2 intact, PMS2 absent, and MLH1 absent. The best next step in evaluation is to test for

(A) germline mutation
(B) homologous recombination deficiency
(C) microsatellite instability
(D) promoter methylation

28 Treatment of cervical cancer

A 59-year-old woman recently received a diagnosis of cervical cancer. Her pelvic examination reveals a 2-cm cervical lesion. Positron emission tomography/computed tomography (PET/CT) demonstrated a single 3-cm fluorodeoxyglucose-avid right pelvic lymph node. Image-guided biopsy of this node indicates squamous cell carcinoma. The best treatment for her cancer is

(A) pelvic radiotherapy
(B) pelvic radiotherapy with adjuvant chemotherapy
(C) pelvic radiotherapy with concurrent chemotherapy
(D) radical hysterectomy
(E) radical hysterectomy with pelvic lymphadenectomy

29 Adnexal mass in a pregnant patient

A 37-year-old at 11 2/7 weeks of gestation with an intrauterine spontaneous singleton pregnancy is incidentally found to have a 6-cm unilocular adnexal mass on her first-trimester ultrasound (Fig. 29-1). She is asymptomatic, and her physical examination is normal. Her family history is unremarkable. She has had no previous surgery. The best next step in management is

(A) CA 125 testing
(B) human epididymis protein 4 (HE4)
(C) pelvic MRI
(D) repeat ultrasonography in 4–6 weeks
(E) surgical resection

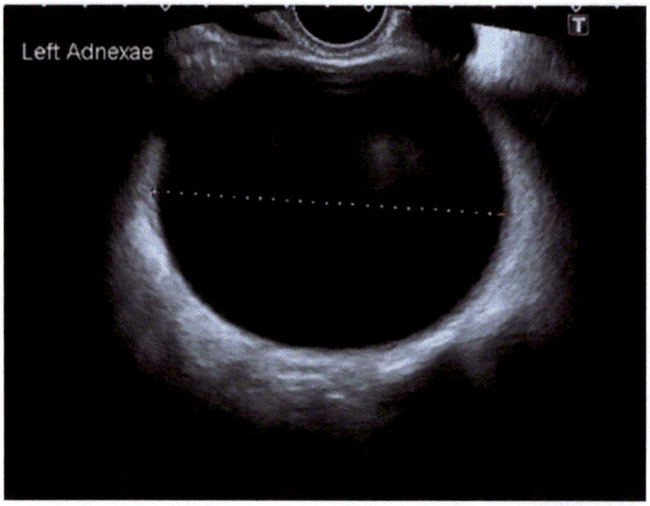

FIGURE 29-1. Ultrasonography showing an adnexal mass. (Reprinted from Puri S. Sonographic assessment of ovarian cysts and masses. In: Jayaprakasan K, Polanski L, Ojha K, editors. Gynaecological ultrasound scanning: tips and tricks. Cambridge University Press; 2020. p. 100–20. Accessed March 17, 2025.)

30 Treatment planning in cervical cancer

A 42-year-old patient has been experiencing vaginal bleeding for the last 8 months. On examination, her cervix is firm and nodular and measures 7 × 7 cm and extends to the vagina. There is no obvious parametrial involvement on rectovaginal examination. A biopsy of her cervical mass demonstrates invasive squamous cell carcinoma. To determine a treatment plan, the preferred imaging modality is

(A) combined transvaginal and transrectal ultrasonography
(B) intravenous pyelogram
(C) MRI
(D) positron emission tomography/computed tomography (PET/CT)

31 Antibody–drug conjugates

A 32-year-old with stage IVB cervical cancer has completed six cycles of chemotherapy with cisplatin, paclitaxel, bevacizumab, and pembrolizumab, and her fifth cycle of maintenance bevacizumab and pembrolizumab is planned. Today, she presents with new-onset pelvic pain and shortness of breath. Positron emission tomography with computed tomography (PET/CT) shows a progression of the disease. After explaining these results, you recommend discontinuing her current treatment and initiating the antibody–drug conjugate tisotumab vedotin. You discuss the potential adverse events and toxicities of tisotumab vedotin use and recommend pre-infusion management to prevent

(A) alopecia
(B) blurred vision
(C) fatigue
(D) hypertension
(E) neuropathy

32 Initial management of high-risk gestational trophoblastic neoplasia

A 36-year-old gravida 2, para 2, presents with amenorrhea for 2 months followed by irregular vaginal bleeding for the last month. Her most recent pregnancy was a full-term vaginal delivery 2 years ago. Her physical examination is notable for an enlarged 12-week-sized uterus. Her β-human chorionic gonadotropin (β-hCG) concentration is 84,500 mIU/mL, and pelvic ultrasonography shows a 3-cm echogenic mass within the uterine cavity. She undergoes dilation and curettage, and pathology reveals an invasive molar pregnancy. Chest computed tomography (CT) is notable for three lung nodules, and a brain MRI is negative. The best next step is

(A) immunotherapy
(B) single-agent chemotherapy
(C) radiotherapy
(D) multi-agent chemotherapy
(E) surgical resection

33 Basal cell carcinoma of the vulva

A 72-year-old patient presents to your clinic with a 3-month history of increasing vulvar pruritus. On examination, there is a 3-cm papular lesion with central ulceration on the right labium majus that is tender to palpation (Fig. 33-1). A punch biopsy of the lesion reveals nodular-type basal cell carcinoma. The best next step in treatment is

(A) carbon dioxide (CO_2) laser ablation
(B) topical imiquimod
(C) total superficial vulvectomy
(D) vulvar radiotherapy
(E) wide local excision

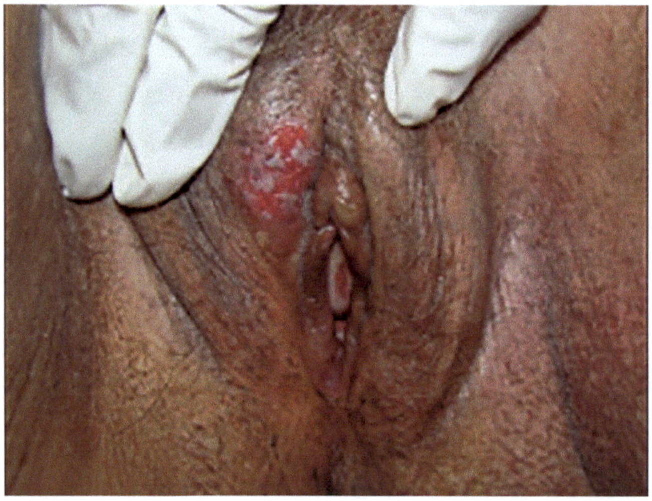

FIGURE 33-1. Vulvar basal cell carcinoma. (Reprinted from Rodríguez VG, De la Fuente García A, Torres MA, Flores MG, Moreno GJ, Candiani JO. Could cryosurgery be an alternative treatment for basal cell carcinoma of the vulva? [published correction appears in Indian Dermatol Online J. 2015 Jul-Aug;6(4):314. doi: 10.4103/2229-5178.160308]. Indian Dermatol Online J. 2014;5(2):160–163. doi:10.4103/2229-5178.131089)

34 Molar pregnancy

A 39-year-old gravida 3, para 0020, at 8 weeks of gestation undergoes an ultrasound-guided uterine aspiration and intrauterine device insertion for management of early pregnancy loss. Her preoperative β-human chorionic gonadotropin (β-hCG) concentration is 75,150 mIU/mL. Pathology demonstrates diffusely enlarged hydropic villi without fetal tissue and the presence of cisterns. Genetic testing of the surgical specimen reveals a 46,XX karyotype, and p57 staining is negative. The best next step is to

(A) determine maternal karyotype
(B) follow β-hCG levels until negative
(C) initiate chemotherapy
(D) remove the intrauterine device

35 Complications of chemotherapy

A 76-year-old patient with metastatic, recurrent ovarian cancer presents to the clinic, reporting weight loss and fatigue. She started her third cycle of weekly paclitaxel with bevacizumab 2 weeks ago. She has nausea but can eat three small meals a day. She had a bowel movement 1 day ago. Her vital signs are unremarkable except for the loss of 2% of her weight since her assessment (before cycle 3). Her BMI today is 17. On examination, her abdomen is distended but nontender. Bimanual examination reveals no palpable pelvic and rectal masses. Computed tomography is ordered, and the results indicate that her pretreatment abdominal tumors have shrunk. The best next step to address her symptoms is to

(A) initiate an appetite stimulant
(B) place an enteral feeding tube
(C) refer her to a dietitian
(D) start parenteral nutrition

36 Postoperative altered mental status

An 82-year-old woman is evaluated on postoperative day 1 after ovarian cancer debulking surgery. The surgery included extensive pelvic dissection and required 5 hours of operative time. She was given intravenous fluids at a rate of 100 mL/h upon transfer from her post-anesthesia care unit. The next morning, she is lethargic and confused. Her vital signs and laboratory values are noted below in Table 36-1. She weighs 176 lb (80 kg). A physical examination and symptom assessment are otherwise noncontributory. The best next step to evaluate the patient's condition is to obtain

(A) blood cultures
(B) head computed tomography
(C) kidney ultrasound
(D) serial basic metabolic profile
(E) urine electrolytes

TABLE 36-1. The Described Patient's Vital Signs and Laboratory Study Results

	6 PM	MIDNIGHT	6 AM
Pain Score	8	6	2
Temperature (°C [°F])	37.5 (99.5)	37.1 (98.8)	36.9 (98.4)
Blood pressure	110/75	101/60	98/68
Pulse	101	92	115
Respiratory rate	22	16	18
Oxygen saturation (%)	97	96	98
Urine output (mL/h)	40	16	8
White blood cell count (per mm^3)	12,000	—	8,000
Hemoglobin (g/dL)	9	—	9
Creatinine (mg/dL)	0.9	—	2.9
Sodium	137	—	140
Chloride	102	—	101
Bicarbonate	26	—	27
Potassium	4	—	4.1

37 Early-stage cervical cancer

A 43-year-old gravida 3, para 3, presents with 2 months of postcoital bleeding and dyspareunia. Her surgical history is significant for bilateral tubal ligation. Her physical examination is notable for a 2.5-cm friable mass limited to the posterior lip of the cervix. A biopsy of the mass confirms invasive squamous cell carcinoma. Positron emission tomography with computed tomography is negative for metastatic disease. In addition to pelvic lymph node assessment, the best next step is

(A) cold knife cone
(B) simple trachelectomy
(C) radical trachelectomy
(D) simple hysterectomy
(E) radical hysterectomy

38 Diagnostic tools to evaluate postmenopausal bleeding

A 56-year-old woman presents for follow-up of postmenopausal vaginal bleeding. She experienced menopause when she was 49 years old. Three months ago, she presented to the office with an episode of vaginal spotting. Transvaginal ultrasonography at that time revealed a normal-appearing uterus with an endometrial thickness that measured 1.1 mm. Since that visit, she has had an additional episode of vaginal bleeding. Her pelvic examination reveals vaginal atrophy and is otherwise normal. Her cervical cancer screening is negative from her annual examination 6 months ago. The best next step is

(A) endometrial sampling
(B) repeat transvaginal ultrasound
(C) systemic hormonal therapy
(D) tranexamic acid
(E) vaginal estrogen

39 Deep vein thrombosis

A 58-year-old patient with a history of ovarian cancer presents to the clinic for a surveillance visit. She is taking a poly(ADP-ribose) polymerase (PARP) inhibitor after completion of primary taxane and platinum-based chemotherapy. She reports left calf pain that started a few days ago. On examination, her vital signs are within normal limits. Her physical examination is notable for an enlarged left calf that is tender to palpation. Bilateral venous Doppler ultrasonography shows a deep vein thrombosis (DVT). The best next step in treatment is

(A) direct oral anticoagulant (DOAC)
(B) inferior vena cava filter placement
(C) low-molecular-weight heparin (LMWH)
(D) unfractionated heparin
(E) warfarin

40 Opioids in cancer-related pain

A 58-year-old patient with platinum-refractory ovarian cancer recently discontinued cancer-directed therapy. She has been seen in the clinic during the last several months with increasing pain due to progressive disease. She is eating and drinking without nausea or vomiting and is having regular bowel movements. For the last several weeks, she has been taking 15 mg of immediate-release oxycodone every 4 hours day and night in addition to over-the-counter pain medications. Her vital signs are normal, and her physical examination is notable for palpable abdominal masses with generalized tenderness but no rebound or guarding. The best next step in this patient's opioid treatment is to

(A) change to a different immediate-release opioid
(B) decrease the oxycodone dosing interval
(C) increase the oxycodone dose
(D) initiate intravenous opioids
(E) initiate an extended-release opioid

41 Risk reduction for recurrent cervical dysplasia

A 31-year-old gravida 1, para 1, presents for follow-up after a loop electrosurgical excision procedure (LEEP) treatment for cervical intraepithelial neoplasia 3 (CIN 3). Her medical history is significant for obesity, with a BMI of 31. A physical examination reveals a well-healed cervical bed with no apparent lesions. Final pathology reveals cervical high-grade squamous intraepithelial lesion (HSIL [CIN 3]) with negative margins and negative endocervical curettings. She has a desire for future fertility but is not actively trying to get pregnant. She does not use tobacco and is in a monogamous, stable relationship. She asks how to decrease her risk of cervical dysplasia in the future. The best next step to reduce her risk of recurrence is

(A) dietary modifications
(B) herbal supplementation
(C) human papillomavirus (HPV) vaccination
(D) repeat excisional procedure
(E) topical imiquimod

42 Identifying hereditary cancer syndromes

A 28-year-old woman presents for a well-woman examination. Her family history is significant for endometrial cancer in her mother, breast cancer in her maternal aunt, and colon cancer in her maternal grandfather. Her physical examination is notable for several cutaneous findings (Fig. 42-1). The patient's most likely gene mutation is

(A) *BRIP1*
(B) *MSH6*
(C) *PTEN*
(D) *STK11*
(E) *TP53*

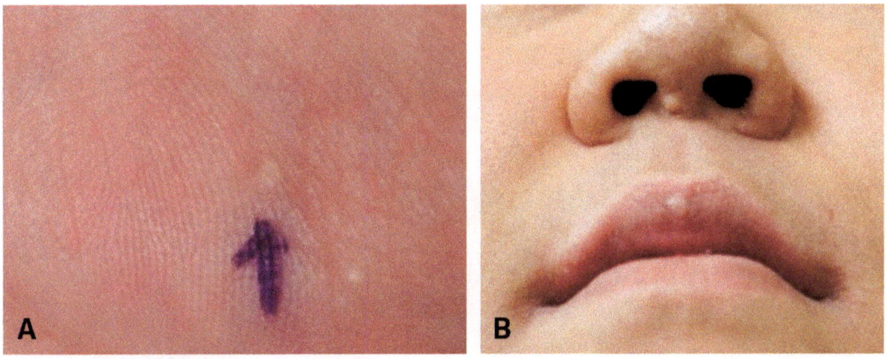

FIGURE 42-1. Patient's palm (A) and face (B). (Reprinted from Lee J, Shin DM, Oh SJ, Park J, Lee D. Ann Dermatol 2023;35:146–50. doi: 10.5021/ad.20.265)

43 Abdominal wall hematoma

A 52-year-old patient presents to the emergency department for the abrupt onset of abdominal pain on her left side 3 days after a laparoscopic hysterectomy and bilateral salpingo-oophorectomy. Her medical history is notable for recurrent venous thromboembolism, and she resumed chronic anticoagulation with apixaban 24 hours after her surgery. On examination, the anterior abdominal wall surrounding the left laparoscopic port site is firm. The incision has opened, and there is scant dark red bleeding. She is tachycardic with a heart rate of 115 beats per minute. Her temperature and blood pressure are within normal limits. Her preoperative hemoglobin was 12 mg/dL, and a repeat hemoglobin in the emergency department is 9.5 mg/dL. Computed tomography (CT) with contrast is notable for a hematoma within the left rectus muscle with active extravasation. There is a small amount of complex fluid within the pelvis. She is given intravenous fluid resuscitation with a plan to hold anticoagulation. The best management of the abdominal wall hematoma is

(A) bedside closure of the port site
(B) endovascular arterial embolization
(C) placement of percutaneous drain
(D) placement of a pressure dressing
(E) surgical exploration and evacuation

44 Recurrent vulvar pruritus

An 88-year-old woman presents with vulvar pruritus. She has multiple medical comorbidities, including congestive heart failure and chronic obstructive pulmonary disease (COPD). Her examination findings are shown in Figure 44-1A and -1B. Five years ago, she underwent an excision of a similar right vulvar lesion. Vulvar and perineal biopsies are obtained at her current visit (Fig. 44-2A and -2B) and are consistent with pathology from her previous excision 5 years ago. The best next step is

(A) topical imiquimod
(B) Mohs micrographic surgical excision
(C) simple vulvectomy
(D) radical vulvectomy
(E) external beam radiotherapy

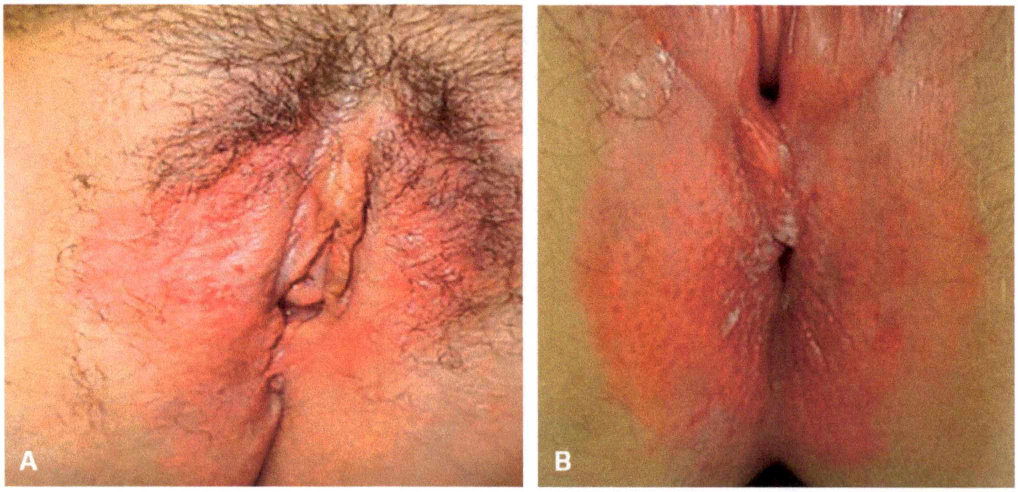

FIGURE 44-1. A. Vulvar examination findings. (Reprinted from Mayo-Martínez F, Moro R, Millán-Esteban D, Ríos-Viñuela E, Bautista IJ, Nagore E, et al. Topical imiquimod in primary cutaneous extramammary Paget's disease: a systematic review. Cancers (Basel) 2023;15:5665. doi: 10.3390/cancers15235665). B. Perineal and perianal examination findings. (Reprinted from Santos MD, Soares F, Presa-Fernandes JM, Silva DS. Perianal Paget disease: different entities with the same name. Cureus 2021;13:e15161. doi: 10.7759/cureus.15161)

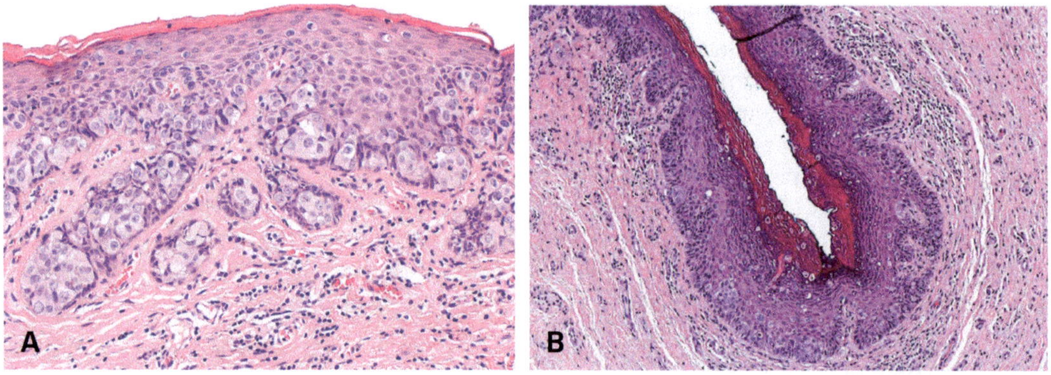

FIGURE 44-2. A. Representative vulvar biopsy: low-power magnification. (Reprinted from Mayo-Martínez F, Moro R, Millán-Esteban D, Ríos-Viñuela E, Bautista IJ, Nagore E, et al. Topical imiquimod a primary cutaneous extramammary Paget's disease: a systematic review. Cancers (Basel) 2023;15:5665. doi: 10.3390/cancers15235665). B. Representative vulvar biopsy with high-power magnification. (Reprinted from Salari E, Ma L. Vulva and vagina: other carcinomas, Paget disease. Pathology Outlines; 2024. Accessed March 17, 2025. https://www.pathologyoutlines.com/topic/vulvapagetsdisease.html. Courtesy of PathologyOutlines.com, contributed by Priya Nagarajan, MD, PhD)

45 Malignant ovarian germ cell tumor

A 33-year-old gravida 2, para 2, presents with a 4-month history of right lower quadrant pain, bloating, and constipation. She has no medical comorbidities and has completed childbearing. Her physical examination is significant for an enlarged right ovary, and ultrasonography reveals a 12-cm complex cyst with a hyperechoic solid nodule. She undergoes a laparoscopic right salpingo-oophorectomy, and an intraoperative frozen section reveals an immature teratoma. A total hysterectomy, left salpingo-oophorectomy, lymphadenectomy, and peritoneal biopsies are performed for surgical staging. The final pathology confirms an immature teratoma with high-grade neural elements confined to the right ovary. The best treatment to prevent disease recurrence is

(A) bleomycin, etoposide, and cisplatin (BEP)
(B) carboplatin and paclitaxel
(C) external beam radiotherapy
(D) megestrol acetate
(E) pembrolizumab

46 Surgical management of borderline tumor

A 37-year-old underwent a right ovarian cystectomy for a 12-cm complex left adnexal mass. The contralateral ovary was normal appearing, and no extraovarian disease was noted. Intraoperative rupture of the mass occurred. Pathology demonstrated a serous borderline tumor with micropapillary features. Her risk of recurrence is increased most by

(A) her age
(B) intraoperative rupture
(C) micropapillary architecture
(D) ovarian cystectomy
(E) size of mass

47 Diarrhea

A 67-year-old patient with ovarian cancer presents with worsening diarrhea 14 days after cytoreductive surgery. She reports 2 days of watery diarrhea with associated abdominal cramping. In the office, she has normal vital signs with mild abdominal tenderness and no rebound or guarding. Her serum laboratory values are within normal limits, her computed tomography result is unremarkable, and her stool cultures reveal a gram-positive, spore-forming anaerobic bacterium. The best management for this condition is to administer

(A) bezlotoxumab
(B) fidaxomicin
(C) metronidazole
(D) tigecycline
(E) vancomycin

48 Cervical cancer recurrence

A 42-year-old patient with a history of stage IB2 squamous cell carcinoma of the cervix who underwent chemoradiation therapy with cisplatin 4 years ago presents for a follow-up visit. She reports an unintentional 30-lb weight loss and new left leg swelling. Positron emission tomography shows a new fluorodeoxyglucose F 18 (FDG)-avid pelvic mass concerning for rectal invasion and multiple FDG-avid liver lesions. Tumor testing is positive for programmed death-ligand 1 (PD-L1). The best next step in treatment is chemotherapy combined with

(A) bevacizumab
(B) gemcitabine
(C) pembrolizumab
(D) tisotumab vedotin
(E) topotecan

49 Complications of an epidural after surgery

Recent literature has suggested that epidural anesthesia for postoperative pain relief may not be the best option for patients undergoing gynecologic surgery. In addition to the risks of urinary retention and difficulty ambulating, the main reason for the decrease in the use of epidural anesthesia is

(A) anesthesia failure
(B) cardiac arrest
(C) epidural abscess
(D) neuraxial hematoma

50 Chemotherapy for recurrent ovarian cancer

A 62-year-old patient presents to the emergency department reporting shortness of breath, nausea and vomiting, and a swollen abdomen. She finished six cycles of chemotherapy for stage IIIC ovarian cancer 3 months ago. Tumor testing is notable for homologous recombination proficiency and low folate receptor α expression. She has persistent neuropathy from her previous treatments, which limits her daily activities. On examination, her blood pressure is 110/60 mm Hg. Her lungs have decreased breath sounds at the bases bilaterally, and her abdomen is distended. Her white blood cell count is 10×10^9/L, and her creatinine level is 0.9 mg/dL. Computed tomography results show bilateral pleural effusions and peritoneal carcinomatosis. Computed tomography-guided peritoneal biopsy confirms recurrent ovarian cancer. The best next step is chemotherapy with

(A) carboplatin, paclitaxel, and bevacizumab
(B) mirvetuximab soravtansine
(C) pegylated liposomal doxorubicin with bevacizumab
(D) topotecan

51 Acupuncture in cancer

A 76-year-old patient is undergoing chemotherapy for the treatment of advanced ovarian cancer. She is experiencing many bothersome symptoms related to her treatment and is interested in pursuing acupuncture. The best use of acupuncture in cancer patients is to

(A) decrease symptoms of depression
(B) enhance pain management
(C) improve chemotherapy effectiveness
(D) increase the immune response
(E) prevent nausea

52 Cervical cancer screening in a low-resource setting

A 41-year-old woman presents to a health clinic where you often volunteer in Uganda. Her sister was recently treated for cervical cancer, which prompted the patient to seek cervical cancer screening. The patient's community clinic does not have the resources to provide this screening, and because she does not have reliable transportation, she has never been screened. No laboratory services are available to you in the location. On examination during her clinic visit today, her cervix is grossly normal. She wants to know if anything can be done at this visit. You inform her that the best next step is

(A) cryotherapy
(B) excisional procedure
(C) random cervical biopsy
(D) visual inspection with acetic acid

53 Endometrial intraepithelial neoplasia

A 35-year-old, otherwise healthy woman receives a diagnosis of endometrial intraepithelial neoplasia (EIN) on dilation and curettage. The most appropriate surgical procedure to manage EIN is

(A) hysteroscopic endometrial resection
(B) radiofrequency endometrial ablation
(C) supracervical hysterectomy
(D) total hysterectomy

54 Rare ovarian tumors

A 53-year-old woman underwent surgical exploration for an 8-cm complex adnexal mass with corpuscular fluid and vascular solid components. The result from intraoperative frozen section is shown in Figure 54-1. You perform comprehensive surgical staging that ultimately reveals stage IC2 cancer. You recommend primary chemotherapy followed by

(A) endocrine therapy
(B) evaluation in 3 months
(C) poly(ADP-ribose) polymerase (PARP) inhibitor
(D) programmed cell death protein 1 (PD-1) inhibitor
(E) vascular endothelial growth factor inhibitor

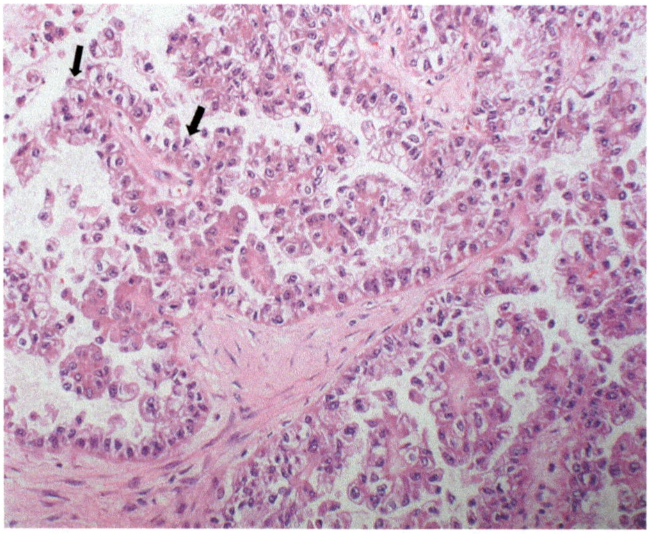

FIGURE 54-1. High-grade nuclei with prominent nucleoli, nuclear hobnailing (arrows), and distinct clear to eosinophilic cytoplasm with hyalinized core. (Courtesy of Dr. Christine Bookhout, Department of Pathology, University of North Carolina.)

55 Recurrent metastatic cancer

A 73-year-old patient with recurrent platinum-resistant metastatic ovarian cancer, who was previously treated with three lines of chemotherapy, is brought to the emergency department by her family due to abdominal pain, bloating, nausea, and vomiting. She is currently enrolled in a clinical trial. On evaluation in the emergency department, her vital signs reveal a temperature of 36.3 °C (97.3 °F), blood pressure of 90/60 mm Hg, heart rate of 120 beats per minute, a respiratory rate of 20 breaths per minute, and oxygen saturation of 90% on room air. Her examination is notable for abdominal bloating with a palpable fluid wave, and computed tomography (CT) reveals progressive disease with moderate volume ascites and metastatic implants of the liver and spleen. Her family reports she has had increasing difficulty with activities of daily living and now spends most of her days in bed. In addition to hospital admission, the best next step for her cancer care is to

(A) change the chemotherapy regimen
(B) consult hospice for enrollment
(C) continue clinical trial treatment
(D) perform a goals-of-care assessment

56 Radiation proctitis

A 48-year-old patient with stage IIIA squamous cell carcinoma of the cervix presents for routine surveillance. She completed chemoradiation 12 months ago. Her medical history is notable for hypertension and a 10-pack-year smoking history. She reports recent-onset fecal urgency, bloody diarrhea, and periodic stool incontinence. On physical examination, there is no evidence of recurrent disease; however, a rectal examination is painful and blood is noted. She undergoes a diagnostic sigmoidoscopy, which confirms the diagnosis of radiation proctitis. Subsequent management with sucralfate retention enemas does not relieve her symptoms. The best next treatment to address her symptoms is

(A) corticosteroid suppositories
(B) mesalamine
(C) ozone therapy
(D) pentoxifylline and vitamin E
(E) rectal formalin application

57 Endometrial cancer surveillance

A 64-year-old patient presents for a surveillance visit 3 months after robot-assisted laparoscopic hysterectomy, bilateral salpingo-oophorectomy, and pelvic lymph node dissection for a stage IA, grade 2, endometrioid endometrial adenocarcinoma. She reports no changes to her health, no new bladder or bowel symptoms, and no bleeding. The best way to assess for cancer recurrence is to perform

(A) CA 125 tumor marker testing
(B) computed tomography (CT) of the abdomen and pelvis
(C) pelvic examination
(D) positron emission tomography combined with computed tomography (PET/CT)
(E) vaginal cytology

58 Febrile neutropenia

A 55-year-old patient with recurrent, metastatic cervical cancer is receiving chemotherapy with cisplatin, paclitaxel, bevacizumab, and pembrolizumab. She presents during cycle 1, day 7, with an at-home temperature of 38.2 °C (100.8 °F) and poor intake. Her vital signs on arrival are blood pressure of 88/50 mm Hg, heart rate of 110 beats per minute, temperature of 38 °C (100.4 °F), a respiratory rate of 18 breaths per minute, and oxygen saturation of 94% on room air. Her physical examination is notable for abdominal pain to palpation without rebound or guarding. Her white blood cell count is 1.2×10^3/L with an absolute neutrophil count of 400 per microliter, and her serum creatinine concentration is 1.3 mg/dL. Computed tomography is negative (no bowel wall thickening and no radiographic source of infection). Intravenous hydration is started, and urine and blood cultures are pending. She has a prior documented allergic reaction to penicillin and cephalosporins. The best initial antibiotic regimen is

(A) ciprofloxacin
(B) levofloxacin
(C) meropenem
(D) vancomycin

59 Kaplan-Meier method

A study of a new treatment is underway. The primary outcome is overall survival, and you want to analyze the study's data with the Kaplan–Meier method. The probability calculation for Kaplan–Meier at each time interval is represented by

(A) change in percent death/change in time
(B) number of deaths/patients enrolled
(C) number of disease-free survivors/number of patients at risk
(D) number of survivors/number of patients at risk

60 Initial management of ovarian cancer

A 57-year-old woman is referred to you after reporting 6 months of pelvic pain, bloating, and early satiety. Her past medical history is notable for hypertension and poorly controlled diabetes mellitus, with a hemoglobin A_{1C} (Hb A_{1C}) of 9.2 mg/dL. The physical examination is notable for a moderately distended abdomen and palpable masses to the level of the umbilicus with fluid wave. Her CA 125 is 432 U/mL. Computed tomography (CT) of her chest, abdomen, and pelvis reveals bilateral adnexal masses, moderate ascites, omental nodularity to the greater curvature of the stomach, mesenteric lymphadenopathy, and a 4-cm liver mass near the portal vein. A CT-guided biopsy of the omentum shows high-grade serous carcinoma of müllerian origin. The best next step in treatment is

(A) chemoradiation
(B) hospice referral
(C) neoadjuvant chemotherapy
(D) primary cytoreductive surgery

61 First-line chemotherapy in ovarian cancer

A 56-year-old patient with stage IVA ovarian cancer with preoperative pleural effusions presents for postoperative follow-up 2 weeks after an exploratory laparotomy, total abdominal hysterectomy, omentectomy, and tumor debulking. She had unresectable disease in the lesser sac and small bowel mesentery. She has no other medical problems. On examination, her midline incision is well healed. In addition to carboplatin, the best chemotherapy regimen for this patient is

(A) gemcitabine and bevacizumab
(B) paclitaxel alone
(C) paclitaxel and bevacizumab
(D) pegylated liposomal doxorubicin

62 Fertility-sparing treatment of endometrial cancer

A 38-year-old nulligravida with a history of polycystic ovary syndrome undergoes hysteroscopy with dilation and curettage for abnormal uterine bleeding. The pathology demonstrates grade 1 endometrioid endometrial adenocarcinoma that is ERPR+. Magnetic resonance imaging of the pelvis shows normal-appearing ovaries, no evidence of residual endometrial mass or myometrial invasion, and no pelvic lymphadenopathy. She strongly desires fertility-sparing treatment. The factor that best predicts this patient's response to treatment is

(A) absence of lymphadenopathy
(B) absence of myometrial invasion
(C) absence of ovarian involvement
(D) her age
(E) progesterone receptor status

63 Somatic testing in ovarian cancer

A 46-year-old patient received a new diagnosis of stage IIIC ovarian cancer and presented for follow-up after cycle 3 of adjuvant therapy with carboplatin and paclitaxel. Her germline genetic testing showed a *BRCA* wild type with a variant of unknown significance in *BRIP1*. She is curious about what maintenance therapy may be advised after her sixth cycle of chemotherapy. You inform her that, in addition to germline testing, the best next step to determine her maintenance plan is to test the tumor for

(A) *BRIP1* mutation
(B) homologous recombination deficiency (HRD)
(C) programmed death-ligand 1 (PD-L1) immunohistochemistry
(D) vascular endothelial growth factor immunohistochemistry

64 Testing for hereditary cancer syndromes in endometrial cancer

A 57-year-old gravida 4, para 4, receives a diagnosis of stage IA, grade 1, endometrioid endometrial adenocarcinoma after hysterectomy and surgical staging. There is no myometrial invasion or lymphovascular space invasion, and pelvic washings are negative. Her brother has a history of colon cancer at age 55 years. The best next somatic test to assess her risk of genetic cancer is

(A) CpG island hypermethylation
(B) homologous recombination deficiency
(C) mismatch repair (MMR) protein expression
(D) *p53* overexpression

65 Management of recurrent malignant ascites

A 68-year-old patient presents with abdominal distension, shortness of breath, and unintentional weight loss. She is being treated for recurrent platinum-resistant ovarian cancer and started chemotherapy 2 weeks ago. She has had four recent paracenteses for ascites, most recently 1 week ago, and she desires more long-term relief of her symptoms. On examination, she has a distended abdomen with a notable fluid wave. Computed tomography demonstrates large ascites, peritoneal carcinomatosis, and enlarged pelvic and periaortic lymph nodes. Her CA 125 concentration is 1,258 U/mL, and her creatinine level is 1.4 mg/dL. The best next step to achieve long-term relief for her symptoms is to

(A) administer albumin
(B) administer a diuretic
(C) perform cytoreductive surgery
(D) perform an ultrasound-guided paracentesis
(E) place an indwelling peritoneal catheter

66 Electrolyte abnormalities in advanced cervical cancer

A 49-year-old woman presents to the emergency department with vaginal bleeding and pelvic and low back pain. Vital signs include a temperature of 37.1 °C (98.7 °F), blood pressure of 112/70 mm Hg, heart rate of 95 beats per minute, respiratory rate of 16 breaths per minute, and oxygen saturation of 98% on room air. She has tenderness to palpation in the bilateral lower abdominal quadrants without rebound or guarding. Speculum examination reveals a fungating cervical mass encompassing the cervix and extending into the upper vagina. On bimanual examination, an 8-cm mass is palpable, and bilateral parametrial invasion is suspected. Computed tomography (CT) confirms the presence of a tumor, with bilateral hydronephrosis noted. Serum testing is notable for potassium of 6.45 mEq/L. Her electrocardiogram (ECG) result is shown in Figure 66-1. The best next treatment is to initiate

(A) calcium gluconate
(B) dialysis
(C) furosemide
(D) insulin
(E) patiromer

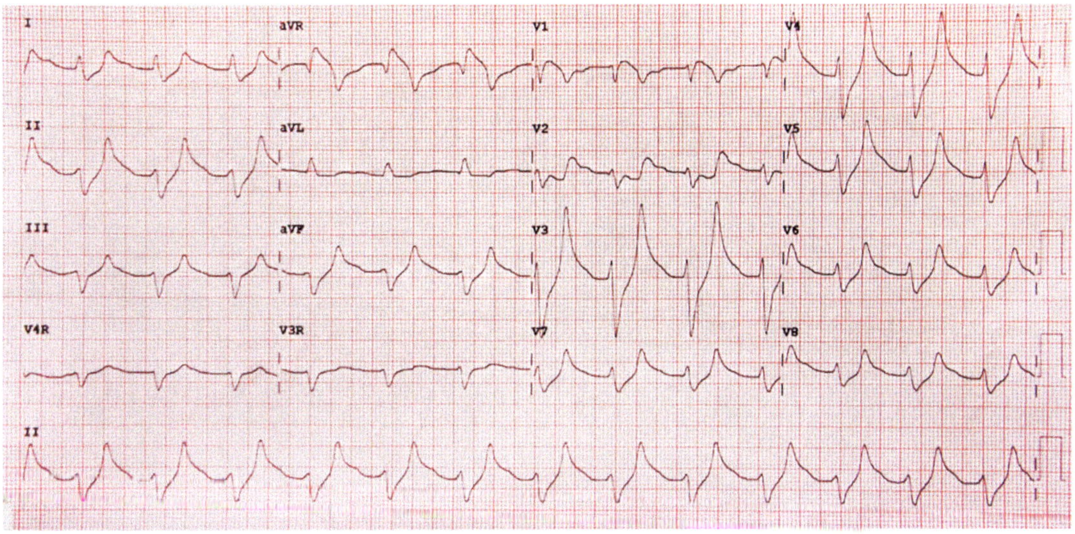

FIGURE 66-1. Normal electrocardiogram. (Reprinted from Hicks B. Hyperkalemia on ECG. J Educ Teach Emerg Med 2016;1:V7-8.)

67 Worsening pelvic pain

A 65-year-old woman presents to the emergency department with pelvic pain that has been present for 2 months and has worsened to a pain score of 10 out of 10 today. Oxycodone has previously been prescribed for pain management. Her past medical history is notable for hypertension, depression managed with cognitive behavioral therapy, liver cirrhosis, and endometrial cancer. She has a firm, immobile pelvic mass on examination. Selected laboratory study results are shown in Table 67-1. The factor that puts this patient at greatest risk for opioid-induced respiratory depression is

(A) altered kidney function
(B) depression
(C) endometrial cancer
(D) hypertension
(E) liver cirrhosis

TABLE 67-1. The Described Patient's Laboratory Study Results

LABORATORY STUDY	VALUE
Alanine aminotransferase	17 units/L
Aspartate aminotransferase	16 units/L
Creatinine	2.1 mg/dL

68 Postoperative complications in an unstable patient

A 63-year-old woman presents to the emergency department with abdominal pain 12 days after a debulking procedure with hysterectomy, bilateral salpingo-oophorectomy, rectosigmoid resection with anastomosis, and omentectomy. Vital signs include a temperature of 38.1 °C (100.5 °F) and a heart rate of 120 beats per minute. Intravenous fluids and broad-spectrum antibiotics are started, and laboratory values are pending. Computed tomography (CT) results are shown in Figures 68-1 and 68-2. The best next step in management is

(A) serial abdominal examinations
(B) Gastrografin study
(C) nasogastric decompression
(D) interventional radiology consultation
(E) surgical exploration

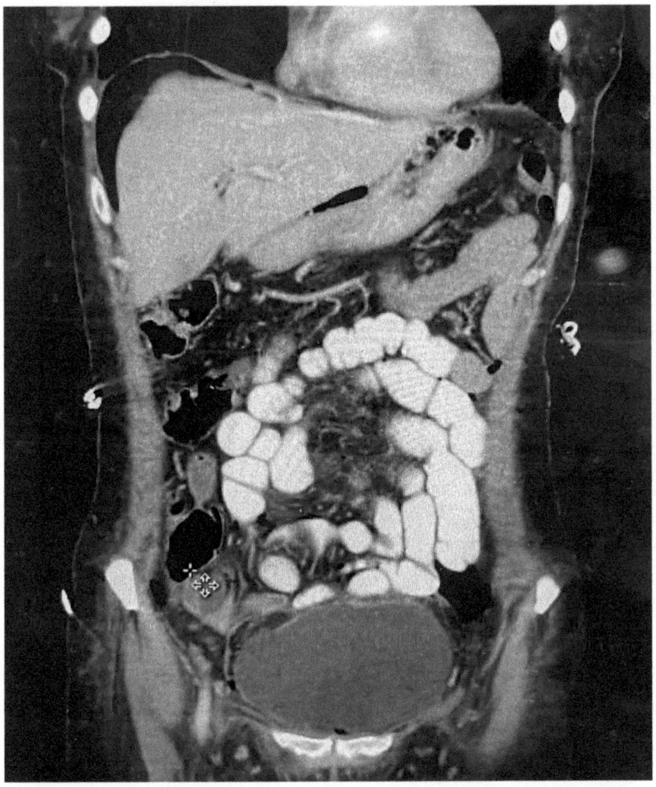

FIGURE 68-1. Computed tomography of the described patient, coronal view.

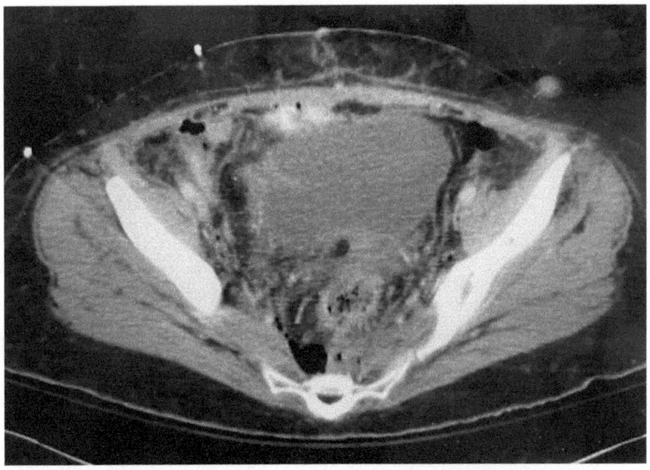

FIGURE 68-2. Computed tomography of the described patient, axial view of the pelvis.

69 Pain management for laparotomy

A 43-year-old patient presents for a preoperative evaluation before total abdominal hysterectomy for chronic pelvic pain and abnormal uterine bleeding due to multiple uterine leiomyomas. Her uterine size is approximately 28 weeks on physical examination, and you plan to perform a midline vertical incision. She expresses concern regarding anticipated pain after surgery and would like to minimize her need for opioid medications. You discuss a multimodal pain regimen with her, including acetaminophen, gabapentin, and celecoxib, to decrease opioid use. The best time to initiate this regimen is

(A) the day before surgery
(B) preoperatively on the day of surgery
(C) in the post-anesthesia care unit
(D) at discharge from the hospital

70 Precision medicine

A 55-year-old patient with stage IIIC high-grade serous ovarian cancer undergoes adjuvant chemotherapy after primary debulking surgery. She has no evidence of disease after platinum-based chemotherapy. Her germline testing for heritable genetic syndromes was negative for known mutations. The best biomarker to determine the efficacy of maintenance therapy is

(A) folate receptor α (FOLR1)
(B) homologous recombination deficiency (HRD)
(C) human epidermal growth factor receptor-2 (HER2)
(D) programmed death-ligand 1 (PD-L1)
(E) tumor mutational burden (TMB)

71 Evaluation of hematuria

A 64-year-old gravida 5, para 5, completed chemoradiation for stage IIA2 squamous cell carcinoma of the cervix 7 years ago. She has a 60-pack-year smoking history and past medical history of chronic obstructive pulmonary disease and coronary artery disease. She now presents to the emergency department with intermittent severe pelvic pain. She also reports worsening urinary incontinence, urinary frequency, and intermittent hematuria over the past 2 years. Her pelvic examination demonstrates vaginal agglutination, and the apex of the vagina and cervix cannot be evaluated. A urine sample demonstrates gross hematuria with associated small clots. Computed tomography demonstrates diffuse bladder wall hypertrophy, with muscosal irregularity and intraluminal debris. The best next step in evaluation is

(A) cystoscopy
(B) positron emission tomography (PET)
(C) tampon test
(D) urine cytology
(E) urodynamic testing

72 Receiver operator characteristic curve

The receiver operator characteristic (ROC) curve is one way to evaluate how well a test performs. A new cancer screening test is developed, and ROC curve is drawn to help select the optimal cut-point. The x and y axes represent

(A) false-positive rate and true-positive rate
(B) prevalence and positive predictive value
(C) sensitivity and negative predictive value
(D) true negative rate and specificity

73 Squamous dysplasia during pregnancy

A 34-year-old gravida 2, para 1, at 28 weeks of gestation undergoes colposcopy for high-grade squamous epithelial lesion (HSIL) cytology, human papillomavirus (HPV) type 16 positive. A colposcopic examination demonstrates dense acetowhite epithelium with coarse mosaicism at the 12:00 position of the cervix, and the lesion does not look concerning for invasion. The biopsy pathology shows cervical intraepithelial neoplasia 3 (CIN 3). The best next step in management is

(A) endocervical curettage
(B) excisional procedure
(C) HPV vaccine series
(D) postpartum colposcopy

74 Risk factors for patients on aromatase inhibitors

A 42-year-old surgically postmenopausal patient with recurrent low-grade serous ovarian cancer is initiating treatment with an aromatase inhibitor. She is taking no other medications, and her medical history is otherwise unremarkable. Before initiation of the aromatase inhibitor, the most appropriate baseline test for this patient is a (an)

(A) bone mineral density scan
(B) echocardiogram
(C) estrogen level
(D) lipid panel
(E) liver function panel

75 Types of clinical studies

A new drug is developed that targets a molecular abnormality occurring in many types of cancer. The most suitable study design to assess the activity of this drug in patients whose tumors have a mutation, irrespective of the primary tumor site, is

(A) basket
(B) noninferiority
(C) phase IV
(D) umbrella

76 Postmolar gestational trophoblastic neoplasia

A 21-year-old received a diagnosis of complete hydatidiform mole during a desired pregnancy and underwent a dilation and curettage. During the third month of post-procedure surveillance, the patient's quantitative serum human chorionic gonadotropin (hCG) values rose to 85,000, which represented an increase of greater than 10% in 2 weeks (measured over three tests). Her pelvic ultrasound is shown in Figure 76-1. Computed tomography (CT) of the patient's chest, abdomen, and pelvis is normal. The best next step in treatment is

(A) chemotherapy
(B) dilation and curettage
(C) hysterectomy
(D) hysteroscopic resection
(E) pelvic radiotherapy

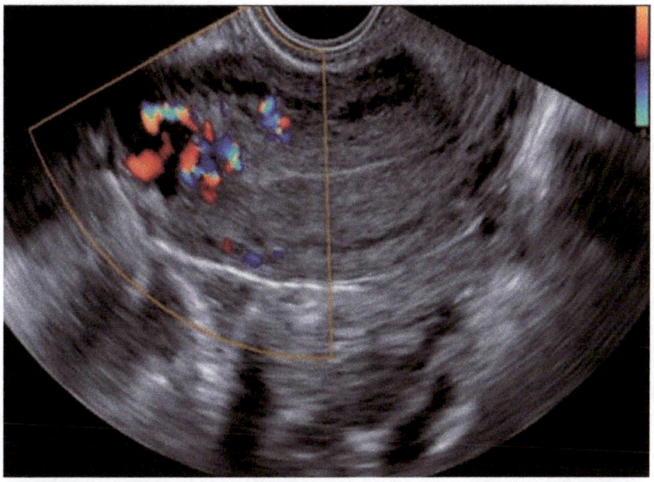

FIGURE 76-1. Three-centimeter mass extending to the uterine myometrium. (Reprinted from Lima LL, Parente RC, Maestá I, Amim Junior J, de Rezende Filho JF, Montenegro CA, Braga A. Clinical and radiological correlations in patients with gestational trophoblastic disease. Radiol Bras. 2016 Jul-Aug;49(4):241–250. doi: 10.1590/0100-3984.2015.0073)

77 Pulmonary evaluation

A 55-year-old underwent a hysterectomy and bilateral salpingectomy for symptomatic uterine fibroids 6 weeks ago. She now presents to the emergency department reporting 3 days of pleuritic chest pain, dyspnea, and cough. Her children are at home with upper respiratory infections. She takes no medications, reports an allergy to intravenous contrast, and has no other significant medical history. She felt fine, and was normally active, prior to the onset of symptoms. On physical examination, her temperature is 37.2 °C (99 °F), her heart rate is 90 beats per minute, her blood pressure is 130/80 mm Hg, and her oxygen saturation is 98% on room air. The remainder of her physical examination yields normal results. In addition to a respiratory panel, the best next step in evaluation is

(A) brain natriuretic peptide (BNP)
(B) chest radiograph
(C) computed tomography–pulmonary angiogram (CTPA)
(D) serum D-dimer
(E) a ventilation perfusion (VQ) scan

78 HER2+ serous endometrial cancer

A 72-year-old patient presents for her postoperative follow-up after a robot-assisted total hysterectomy with bilateral salpingo-oophorectomy, partial omentectomy, and bilateral pelvic sentinel node mapping and biopsy. Her pathology shows a 4-cm serous adenocarcinoma of the endometrium with invasion into the myometrium and two positive lymph nodes. Today's testing reveals that her tumor is human epidermal growth factor 2 positive (HER2+). In addition to treatment with carboplatin and paclitaxel, the best next step is to administer

(A) doxorubicin
(B) external beam radiation therapy (EBRT)
(C) pembrolizumab
(D) trastuzumab

79 Postoperative complications

A 65-year-old woman, postoperative day 13 from an exploratory laparotomy, total abdominal hysterectomy, bilateral salpingo-oophorectomy, and tumor debulking, presents to the emergency department with a 2-day history of increasing intermittent abdominal pain, nausea, and vomiting. Her physical examination is notable for blood pressure of 90/52 mm Hg, heart rate of 123 beats per minute, abdominal distension, and decreased bowel sounds. Her abdominal radiograph is shown in Figure 79-1. The patient is transferred to the intensive care unit, a nasogastric tube is placed, and fluid resuscitation is initiated. Once the patient is stabilized, the best next step in evaluation is

(A) computed tomography (CT)
(B) Gastrografin challenge
(C) MRI
(D) repeat radiograph
(E) ultrasonography

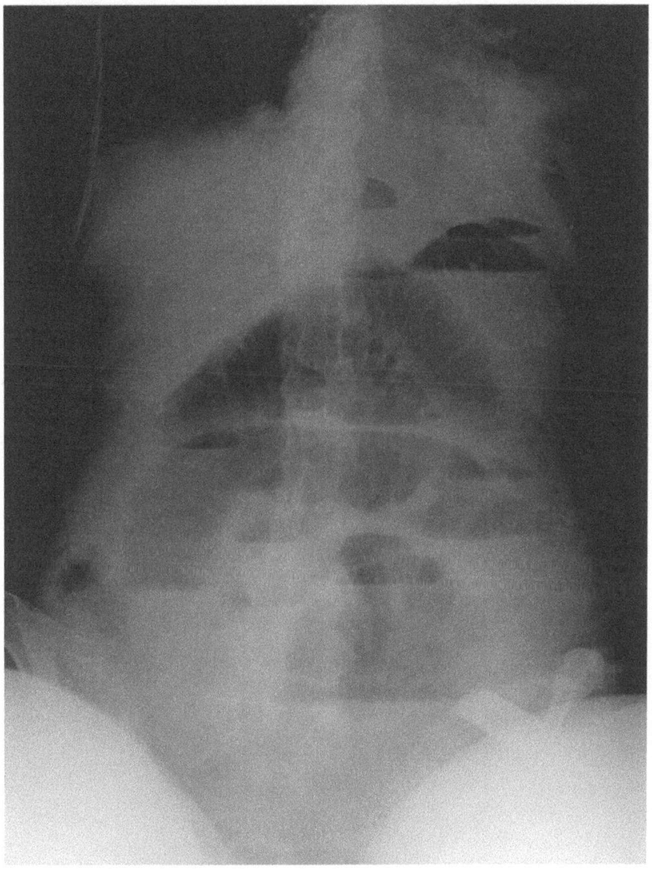

FIGURE 79-1. Abdominal radiograph.

80 Vaginal intraepithelial neoplasia

A 52-year-old patient presents for an annual well-woman examination. She reports having undergone a total hysterectomy at age 40 for management of cervical intraepithelial neoplasia 3. Vaginal cytology reveals high-grade squamous intraepithelial lesion (HSIL) with positive testing for high-risk human papillomavirus (HPV). The best next step is

(A) carbon dioxide laser ablation
(B) partial vaginectomy
(C) repeat cytology in 12 months
(D) topical 5% imiquimod therapy
(E) vaginal colposcopy

81 Nutritional intake after surgery

A 55-year-old woman is admitted to the hospital after undergoing optimal cytoreductive surgery for advanced ovarian cancer. Her body mass index is 27, and her past medical history is significant only for hypertension. On postoperative day 2, she develops nausea, an episode of emesis, decreased appetite, and bloating without passage of flatus or a bowel movement. Examination reveals abdominal distension and absent bowel sounds. Intravenous fluids are administered. The best management of her nutritional intake at this time is

(A) a clear liquid diet
(B) nothing by mouth (NPO)
(C) placement of a feeding tube
(D) total parenteral nutrition (TPN)

82 Back pain

A 54-year-old patient presents with acute onset of fecal incontinence and bilateral lower extremity weakness. She describes progressive lower back pain and a sharp shooting pain down both legs for the last 2 months. She has a history of endometrial cancer treated with chemotherapy 2 years ago and was last seen 6 months ago. Her physical examination is remarkable for point tenderness in the lumbar spine and a score of 3 out of 5 for strength in bilateral lower extremities. Laboratory studies are unremarkable. Magnetic resonance imaging of the lumbar spine is shown in Figure 82-1. You consult with a neurosurgeon and a radiation oncologist and determine that the best next step in treatment is to administer

(A) acetazolamide
(B) dexamethasone
(C) gabapentin
(D) ketorolac
(E) morphine

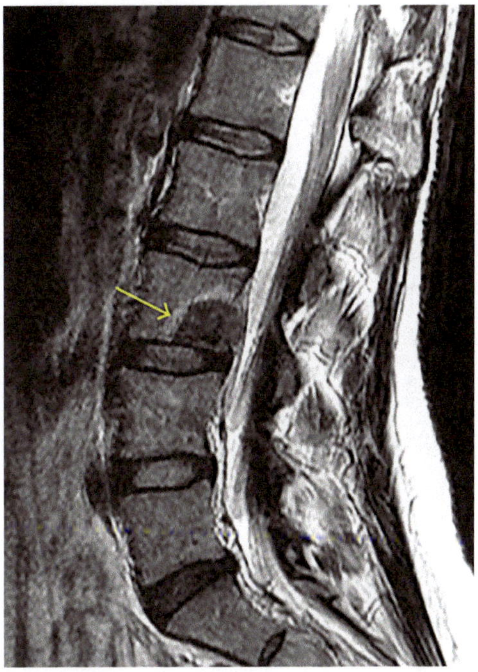

FIGURE 82-1. Magnetic resonance imaging of the lumbar spine. (Reprinted from Shah LM, Salzman KL. Imaging of spinal metastatic disease. Int J Surg Oncol 2011;2011:769753. doi: 10.1155/2011/769753)

83 Regional anesthesia

A 54-year-old patient presents for an exploratory laparotomy for ascites, a large pelvic mass, and an increased CA 125 level. She has no allergies and has not had previous surgery. She is concerned about postoperative adverse effects and pain control. The best perioperative pain management strategy is

(A) erector spinae muscle block
(B) incisional infiltration of bupivacaine
(C) intrathecal morphine injection
(D) thoracic epidural analgesia
(E) transversus abdominis plane (TAP) block

84 Vulvar cancer lymph node evaluation

A 68-year-old with a history of lichen sclerosus presents to the clinic with worsening vulvar pruritus. On examination, there is a 1-cm lesion on the posterior left vulva crossing the midline (Fig. 84-1). A biopsy is performed and confirms invasive squamous cell carcinoma of the vulva with 1.5 mm of invasion. She is referred to a high-volume regional cancer center for disease management. Inguinal lymph nodes are normal to palpation bilaterally, and a radical vulvectomy is recommended. At the time of that procedure, the best recommendation regarding the inguinal-femoral lymph nodes is

(A) bilateral inguinal-femoral lymphadenectomy
(B) bilateral sentinel lymph node biopsy
(C) ipsilateral inguinal-femoral lymphadenectomy
(D) ipsilateral sentinel lymph node biopsy
(E) no lymph node dissection

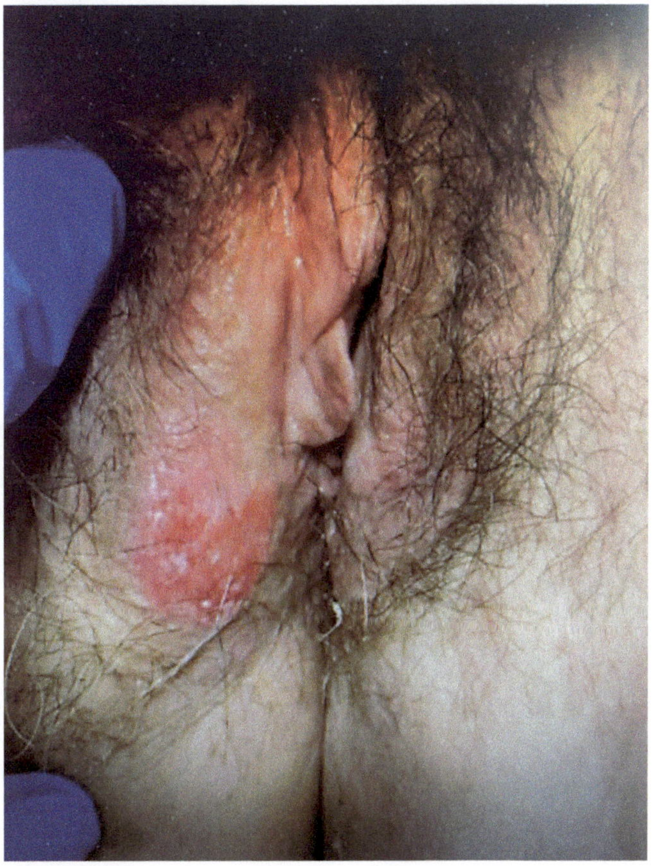

FIGURE 84-1. Vulvar lesion.

85 Hypoxia

A 72-year-old woman with platinum-resistant ovarian cancer presents with shortness of breath. Her physical examination reveals decreased breath sounds in the right lung. Her oxygen saturation is 94% at rest. Her chest X-ray is shown in Figure 85-1. The best next step to manage this condition is to

(A) administer antibiotics
(B) administer diuretics
(C) perform pleurodesis
(D) perform thoracentesis
(E) provide oxygen supplementation

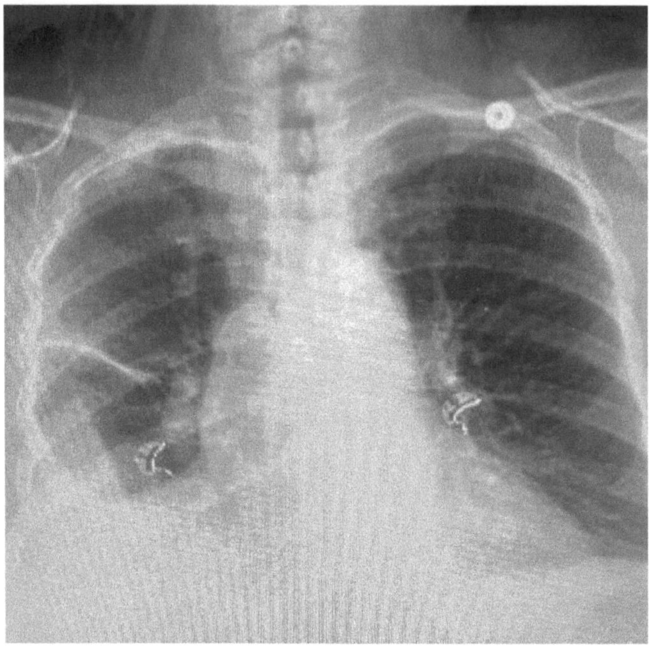

FIGURE 85-1. Patient's chest X-ray with blunting of the costophrenic angle with dependent opacity.

86 Ovarian cancer

A 71-year-old woman presents for evaluation of abdominal distention, bloating, and early satiety. Abdomen and pelvic computed tomography reveal a left ovarian mass invading the rectosigmoid, large-volume ascites, and a tumor replacing the omentum and involving the splenic hilum and the small bowel mesentery. Her serum CA 125 concentration is 6,500 IU/mL. A biopsy of the omental mass confirms high-grade serous cancer consistent with a gynecologic primary. You recommend neoadjuvant platinum-based chemotherapy. The disease factor that best predicts the inability of complete primary tumor resection is

(A) ascites
(B) CA 125 concentration
(C) mesenteric involvement
(D) rectosigmoid involvement
(E) splenic hilum involvement

87 Malignant ascites

A 58-year-old woman with a history of ovarian cancer presents for a surveillance visit with concerns of abdominal swelling, nausea, and bloating. Her last chemotherapy cycle with platinum and taxane was completed 4 months ago. Her examination is notable for a distended abdomen with a fluid wave. Computed tomography of her abdomen and pelvis is consistent with recurrence, revealing large-volume ascites and peritoneal carcinomatosis. In addition to taxol and carboplatin, the most effective therapeutic agent to improve her symptoms is

(A) acetazolamide
(B) albumin
(C) bevacizumab
(D) furosemide
(E) spironolactone

88 Postoperative fever

A 49-year-old woman presents to the emergency department 5 days after an uncomplicated total laparoscopic hysterectomy and bilateral salpingo-oophorectomy. She reports 2 days of fever, diffuse abdominal pain, and generalized malaise. Her medical history includes obesity, hypertension, and type 2 diabetes mellitus. On examination, her vital signs include a temperature of 38.8 °C (101.9 °F), a blood pressure of 91/47 mm Hg, a heart rate of 123 beats per minute, a respiratory rate of 18 breaths per minute, and oxygen saturation 95% on room air. She appears uncomfortable and has diffuse abdominal tenderness. A genitourinary examination demonstrates purulent drainage from the vaginal cuff and a fluctuant mass palpable superior to the vaginal cuff. Laboratory values are shown in Table 88-1. In addition to starting antibiotics, the best next step is

(A) computed tomography
(B) fluid resusitation
(C) subcutaneous insulin
(D) surgical exploration
(E) vasopressors

TABLE 88-1. The Described Patient's Laboratory Study Results

TEST	RESULT
White blood cell count	18,000 micrograms/L
Hemoglobin	12.3 g/dL
Platelets	216,000/microliter
Glucose	237 mg/dL
Creatinine	1.1 mg/dL
Lactate	1.7 mmol/L

89 Vulvar dermatoses

A 65-year-old patient presents with concerns of persistent, generalized vulvar itching during the last 6 months. Her physical examination findings are noted in Figure 89-1, and the vulvar biopsy result is shown in Figure 89-2. The best next step in treatment is topical

(A) antifungal
(B) corticosteroid
(C) estrogen
(D) petroleum jelly
(E) tacrolimus

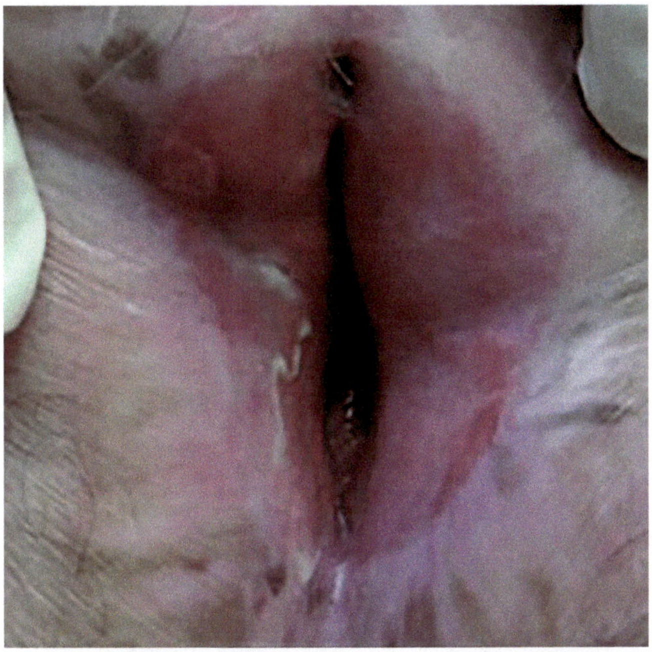

FIGURE 89-1. Physical examination findings. (Reprinted from Howard M, Hall A. Vulval lichen planus–lichen sclerosus overlap. Int J STD AIDS 2018;29:1017–23. doi: 10.1177/0956462418758777)

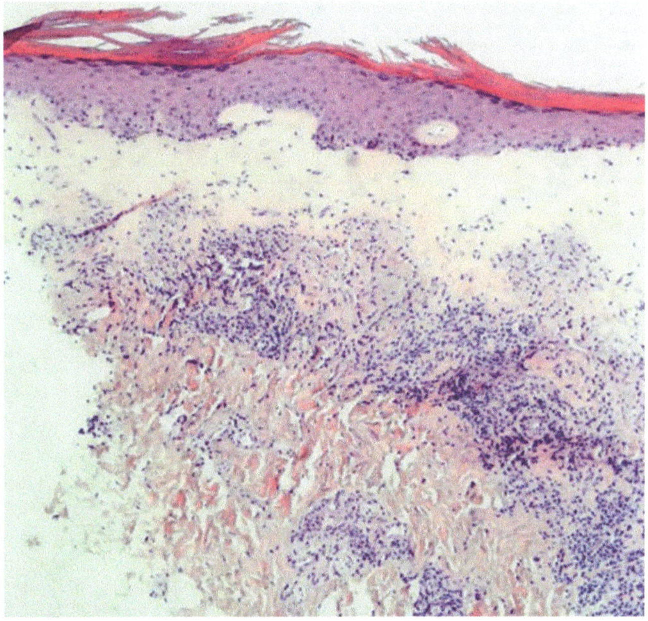

FIGURE 89-2. Patient's vulvar biopsy. (Reprinted from Huvila J, Gilks CB. Lichen sclerosus. PathologyOutlines.com. Accessed July 11, 2025. https://www.pathologyoutlines.com/topic/vulva-lichensclerosus.html)

90 Positive and negative predictive values

A direct-to-consumer marketed blood test is advertised as a screening test for ovarian cancer for women aged 50 and older in the United States and reportedly has 90% sensitivity and 80% specificity. If this test is adopted for screening, and the test result is positive, what are the chances that the patient actually has ovarian cancer? The information you need to answer this question is

(A) false-negative rate
(B) false-positive rate
(C) incidence
(D) population size
(E) prevalence

91 Cancer diagnosis

A 37-year-old patient presents with several months of worsening abdominal distension and discomfort. Computed tomography is shown in Figure 91-1. Her CA 125 level is 108 U/mL, her carcinoembryonic antigen (CEA) level is 20.7 ng/mL, and CA 19-9 level is 195 U/mL. Based on these findings, the most likely primary site of disease is the

(A) appendix
(B) breast
(C) ovary
(D) pancreas
(E) uterus

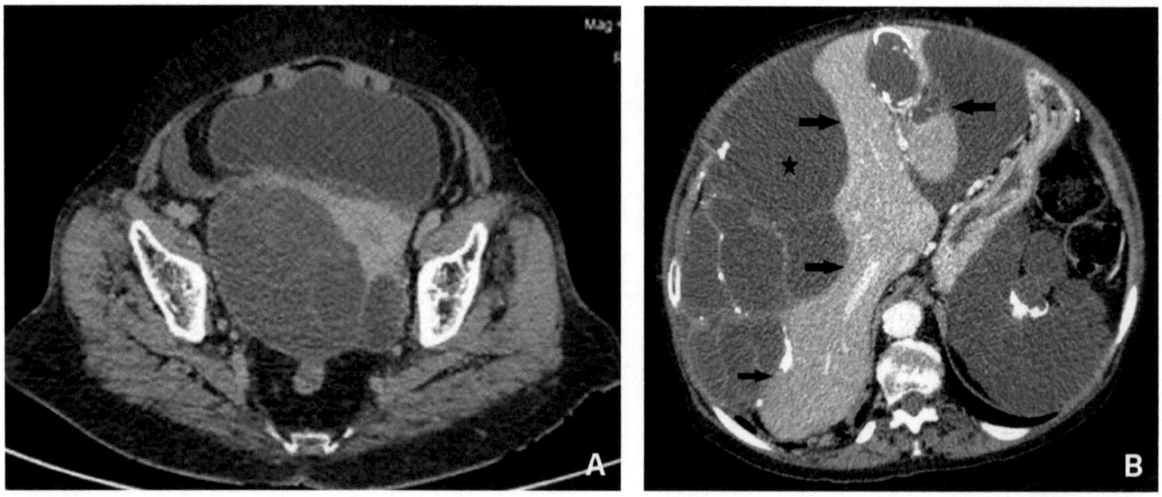

FIGURE 91-1. A. Computed tomography of the pelvis (Reprinted from Joseph R, Sathiamoorthy R, Gnanasekaran R, Gunasekaran L, Ilangovan G. A case report of pseudomyxoma peritonei arising from primary mucinous ovarian neoplasms. Cureus 2022;14:e29309. doi: 10.7759/cureus.29309). B. Upper abdomen showing liver scalloping characteristic of pseudomyxoma peritonei. (Reprinted from Allart K, Sabbagh C, Regimbeau J. Liver scalloping: pseudomyxoma peritonei liver compression. J Visc Surg 2019;156:75–6. doi: 10.1016/j.jviscsurg.2018.09.001)

92 Ovarian cancer screening

A 57-year-old patient presents for her annual examination. She is asymptomatic and has a past medical history remarkable for hypertension. She reports a family history of colon cancer in a paternal aunt. She requests ovarian cancer screening because she is anxious after her older sister received a diagnosis of ovarian cancer. Compared with no screening, available screening strategies for ovarian cancer are associated with

(A) increased likelihood of unnecessary surgery
(B) lower ovarian cancer mortality
(C) reduced patient anxiety
(D) similar stage at diagnosis

93 Clinical findings and associated hereditary cancer syndromes

A 38-year-old patient presents for her annual examination. The physical examination is remarkable for macrocephaly. Mucosal findings (Fig. 93-1) and skin findings (Fig. 93-2) also are appreciated with an otherwise unremarkable examination. After confirmatory genetic testing, the patient undergoes screening for cancer genetically linked with her condition. The screening test most likely to detect an associated cancer is a(n)

(A) colonoscopy
(B) endometrial biopsy
(C) mammogram
(D) renal ultrasonography
(E) thyroid ultrasonography

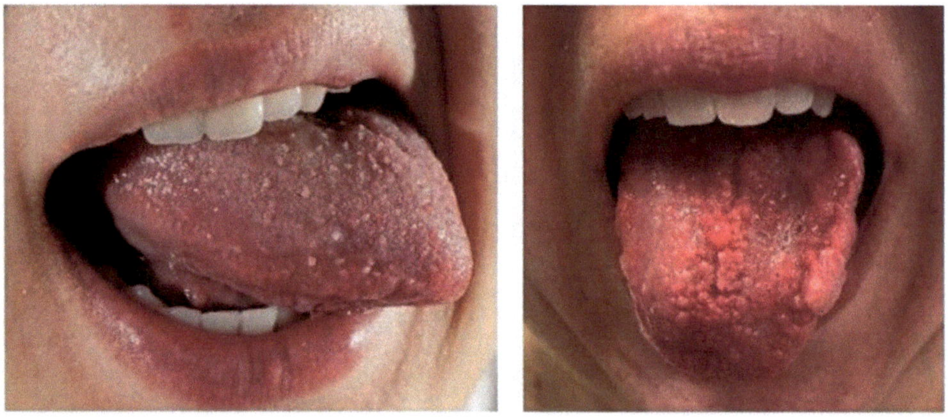

FIGURE 93-1. Extensive oral papillomas resulting in cobblestone appearance of tongue. (Reprinted from National Cancer Institute. Oral papilloma. In: NCI dictionary of genetics terms. Accessed June 3, 2025. https://www.cancer.gov/publications/dictionaries/genetics-dictionary/def/oral-papilloma)

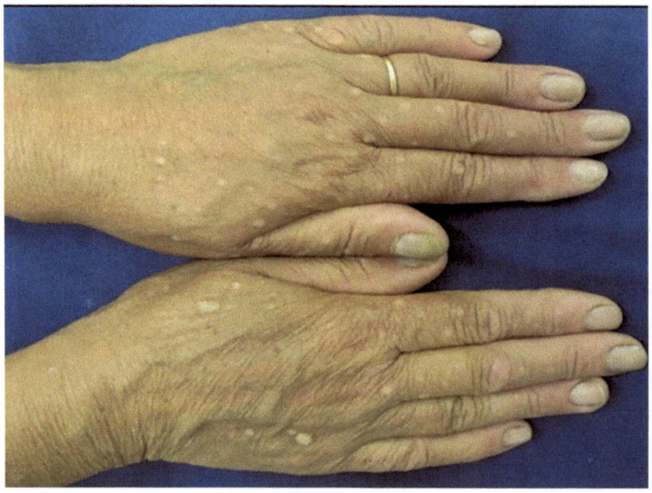

FIGURE 93-2. Warty appearing acral keratosis on the hands. (Reprinted from Flores IL, Romo SA, Tejeda Nava FJ, Roger dos Santos Silva A, Vargas PA, Paes de Almeida O, et al. Oral Surg Oral Med Oral Pathol Oral Radiol 2014;117:E301-10. doi: 10.1016/j.oooo.2014.01.015)

94 Pulmonary complications after surgery

A 64-year-old with no significant cardiac or pulmonary history undergoes an abdominal hysterectomy for symptomatic benign leiomyoma. In the recovery room, she had several episodes of vomiting immediately after surgery. On postoperative day 2, she develops a fever of 38.6 °C (101.4 °F) and worsening shortness of breath. On examination, her heart rate is 100 beats per minute, her blood pressure is 110/60 mm Hg, crackles are present at both lung bases, and her respiratory rate is 32 breaths per minute. Her oxygen saturation is 88% on 6 L of high-flow oxygen by nasal cannula. An electrocardiogram shows sinus tachycardia but no other abnormalities, and a chest X-ray (Fig. 94-1) is performed. You initiate broad-spectrum antibiotics. The best next step is

(A) high-dose corticosteroids
(B) incentive spirometry
(C) mechanical ventilation
(D) nebulizer treatment
(E) thrombolytic therapy

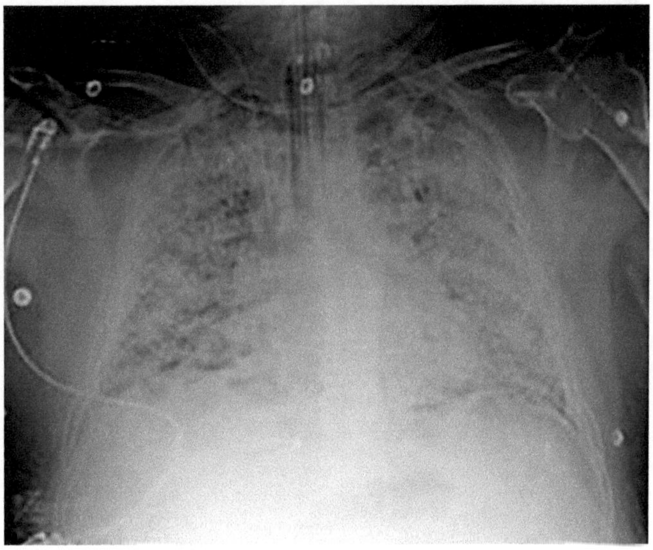

FIGURE 94-1. Chest X-ray.

95 Hemodynamic monitoring

A patient with a diagnosis of advanced-stage ovarian cancer is admitted to the intensive care unit in septic shock. A pulmonary artery catheter is placed and initial values of systemic vascular resistance (SVR), pulmonary vascular resistance (PVR), cardiac index (CI), and pulmonary capillary wedge pressure (PCWP) are obtained. The combination of hemodynamic parameters that is most consistent with septic shock is

(A) increased SVR, normal PVR, decreased CI, increased PCWP
(B) decreased SVR, normal PVR, increased CI, normal PCWP
(C) increased SVR, normal PVR, decreased CI, decreased PCWP
(D) normal SVR, increased PVR, decreased CI, normal PCWP

96 Surgery for leiomyosarcoma

A 40-year-old is scheduled for a total laparoscopic hysterectomy for a uterine mass. Pelvic ultrasonography confirms that the mass has increased in size from 8 to 12 cm during the last 6 months. The growing mass is increasing the patient's symptoms of pelvic pressure and abdominal discomfort. Due to the rapid increase in size, there is concern about the possibility of leiomyosarcoma. During the hysterectomy, it is noted that the uterus is enlarged with no disease outside of the uterus. Leiomyosarcoma is confirmed intraoperatively. The best next step in surgical management is

(A) bilateral salpingectomy
(B) bilateral salpingo-oophorectomy
(C) omentectomy
(D) pelvic lymphadenectomy
(E) peritoneal biopsies

97 Obstipation

A 68-year-old woman with recurrent high-grade serous ovarian cancer presents to the emergency room with severe abdominal pain, nausea, vomiting, and obstipation. She received cycle 2 of carboplatin and paclitaxel 7 days ago. She has otherwise tolerated her treatment and has an Eastern Cooperative Oncology Group performance status of 1. Her vital signs are listed in Table 97-1. A physical examination is notable for moderate abdominal distention, hyperactive bowel sounds, tympany to percussion, and tenderness to palpation in the bilateral lower quadrants. Computed tomography (CT) is shown in Figure 97-1. The best next step in management is a (an)

(A) cecostomy tube
(B) endoscopic stent
(C) enema
(D) nasogastric tube
(E) surgical diversion

TABLE 97-1. The Described Patient's Vital Signs

Temperature	37.3 °C (99.3 °F)
Heart rate	110 beats per minute
Blood pressure	110/70 mm Hg
Respiratory rate	16 breaths per minute
Oxygen saturation on room air	97%

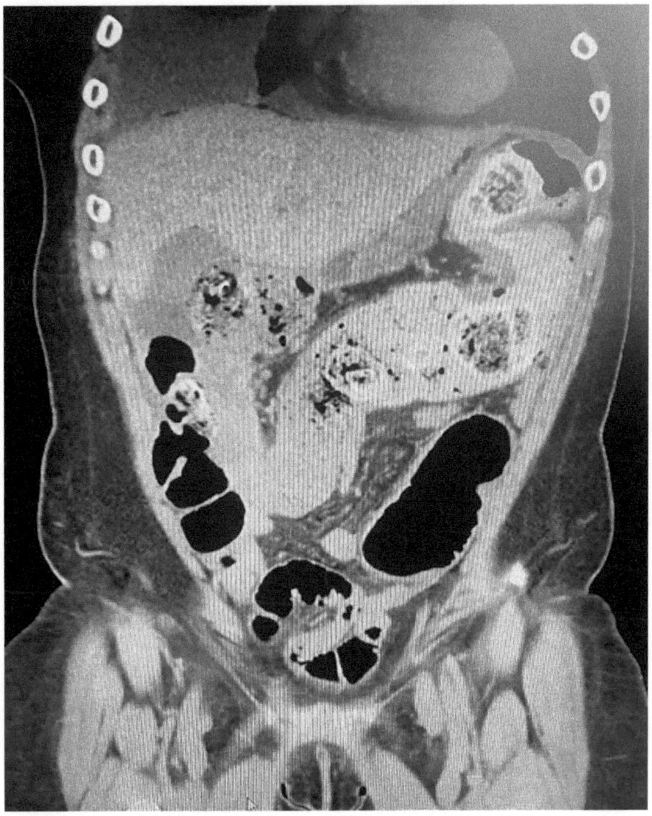

FIGURE 97-1. Patient's computed tomography.

98 Ovarian vein thrombosis

A 63-year-old with advanced ovarian cancer underwent complete cytoreductive surgery followed by six cycles of chemotherapy with carboplatin and paclitaxel. She presents to your office after completing chemotherapy for post-therapy computed tomography (CT). She has no bothersome symptoms, and her physical examination is unremarkable. The CT is notable for a left ovarian vein thrombosis that does not extend into the renal vein. There are no other findings and no evidence of residual malignancy. The best next step in management is

(A) antibiotics
(B) low-dose aspirin
(C) routine ovarian cancer surveillance
(D) therapeutic anticoagulation
(E) thrombectomy

99 Uterine bleeding in patients receiving cancer treatment

A 15-year-old adolescent with Hodgkin lymphoma who is undergoing chemotherapy presents to the emergency department with acute-onset heavy vaginal bleeding. She has a history of a deep venous thrombosis while using the birth control patch last year and is not on anticoagulation currently. On examination, her blood pressure is 100/60 mm Hg, and her pulse is 102 beats per minute. She is pale but otherwise in no acute distress. A pelvic examination is notable for active bleeding from the cervical os. Her hemoglobin is 6.8 g/dL, and a urine pregnancy test is negative. In addition to intravenous (IV) fluid resuscitation and blood transfusion, the best next step in treatment is

(A) depot leuprolide acetate
(B) dilation and curettage
(C) intravenous estrogen
(D) levonorgestrel-releasing intrauterine device (LNG-IUD)
(E) oral progestin

100 Vaginal dysplasia

A 46-year-old gravida 4, para 4, underwent a total laparoscopic hysterectomy for abnormal uterine bleeding. Pathology was notable for benign uterine fibroids. Her cervical cancer screening was up to date at the time of surgery, and she does not have a history of cervical dysplasia. Two years after the hysterectomy, her primary care doctor performs cervical cytology with human papillomavirus (HPV) testing. The results indicate low-grade squamous intraepithelial lesion (LSIL) and return positive for high-risk HPV type. Her pelvic examination reveals a normal-appearing, well-healed vaginal cuff. The best next step in management is

(A) HPV vaccination
(B) laser ablation of vaginal cuff
(C) repeat vaginal cytology and HPV co-testing in 1 year
(D) vaginal colposcopy

101 Cervical cancer screening

A 40-year-old patient has a history of a loop electrosurgical excision procedure (LEEP) performed 8 years ago for the treatment of cervical intraepithelial neoplasia 2-3 (CIN 2-3). Cervical cytology 5 years ago showed atypical squamous cells of undetermined significance (ASC-US), and she has had no testing since then. Her physical examination is notable for vaginal candidiasis, but the cervix appears grossly normal. The best next step for cervical cancer screening is

(A) colposcopy
(B) cytology
(C) endocervical curettage (ECC)
(D) high-risk human papillomavirus (HPV)-based testing

102 Low-grade serous ovarian cancer

A 23-year-old underwent a diagnostic laparoscopy with unilateral salpingo-oophorectomy, omentectomy, and drainage of ascites. Her final pathology was notable for stage IIIC low-grade serous ovarian cancer. Next-generation sequencing is notable for a *BRAF* v600e mutation. Postoperatively, she received chemotherapy with carboplatin and paclitaxel. Before cycle 4 of chemotherapy, she presented with worsening abdominal distension and decreased breath sounds bilaterally. Computed tomography of the chest, abdomen, and pelvis demonstrated bilateral pleural effusions, ascites, and multiple peritoneal implants. The best next step in her treatment is to

(A) add bevacizumab to chemotherapy
(B) begin an aromatase inhibitor
(C) continue paclitaxel and carboplatin
(D) initiate molecular targeted therapy
(E) perform secondary cytoreduction

103 Maintenance therapy in ovarian cancer

A 55-year-old patient underwent a genomic evaluation that revealed a somatic *BRCA2*. After primary optimal debulking surgery for stage IIIC high-grade serous ovarian cancer, she completed six cycles of carboplatin and paclitaxel chemotherapy. Computed tomography after cycle 6 revealed no evidence of disease. The best agent for maintenance therapy is

(A) bevacizumab
(B) mirvetuximab
(C) olaparib
(D) pazopanib
(E) pembrolizumab

104 Microinvasive cervical cancer

A 28-year-old nulligravida receives a diagnosis of cervical adenocarcinoma on biopsy during colposcopy. There is no visible lesion on her physical examination. Cervical cold knife conization is performed, and the result is notable for a 4-mm grade 1 cervical adenocarcinoma with 4-mm depth of invasion, negative lymphovascular space invasion (LVSI), 2-mm negative surgical margins, and benign endocervical curettage. Computed tomography and surgical lymph node assessment are negative for metastatic disease. The patient was undergoing a fertility evaluation before her colposcopy, and she wants to retain her ability to have children. The best next step in management is

(A) cervical cancer surveillance
(B) radical trachelectomy
(C) repeat cold knife conization
(D) total hysterectomy

105 Ovarian cancer risk reduction

A 47-year-old patient presents to the office for a preoperative visit before planned total laparoscopic hysterectomy for abnormal uterine bleeding secondary to fibroids. Her history is notable for well-controlled hypertension and a cesarean delivery. She shares that her friend's mother recently received a diagnosis of ovarian cancer and asks if there is anything that can reduce her own risk. The best next step is to recommend a (an)

(A) aromatase inhibitor
(B) bilateral salpingectomy
(C) bilateral salpingo-oophorectomy
(D) combined oral contraceptive pill
(E) selective estrogen receptor modulator (SERM)

106 Posttreatment surveillance of cervical cancer

A 56-year-old woman who recently completed primary chemoradiotherapy treatment for stage IIIC1 squamous cell carcinoma of the cervix presents for post-therapy follow-up care. You discuss the signs and symptoms of cervical cancer recurrence and the potential benefits of surveillance strategies. The most effective modality for local cancer recurrence detection is

(A) cervical biopsy
(B) cervical cytology
(C) colposcopy
(D) high-risk human papillomavirus (HPV) testing
(E) pelvic examination

107 Respiratory distress

A 78-year-old patient with a medical history of hypertension underwent her first cycle of neoadjuvant chemotherapy for stage IV ovarian cancer. Two days later, she presented to the emergency department with shortness of breath, cough, and heart palpitations. Relevant vital signs and laboratory findings are listed in Table 107-1. An electrocardiogram demonstrates right bundle branch block and sinus tachycardia. Chest computed tomography (CT) is depicted in Figure 107-1. In addition to supplemental oxygen, the best next step is

(A) antibiotics
(B) anticoagulation
(C) diuretics
(D) granulocyte colony-stimulating factor (G-CSF)
(E) thoracentesis

TABLE 107-1. The Described Patient's Vital Signs and Laboratory Study Results

Temperature	37.8 °C (100.04 °F)
Blood pressure	92/60 mm Hg
Heart rate	130 bpm
Oxygen saturation	88%
Hemoglobin	8.2 mg/dL
Absolute neutrophil count	2.0 (x 10^9/L)

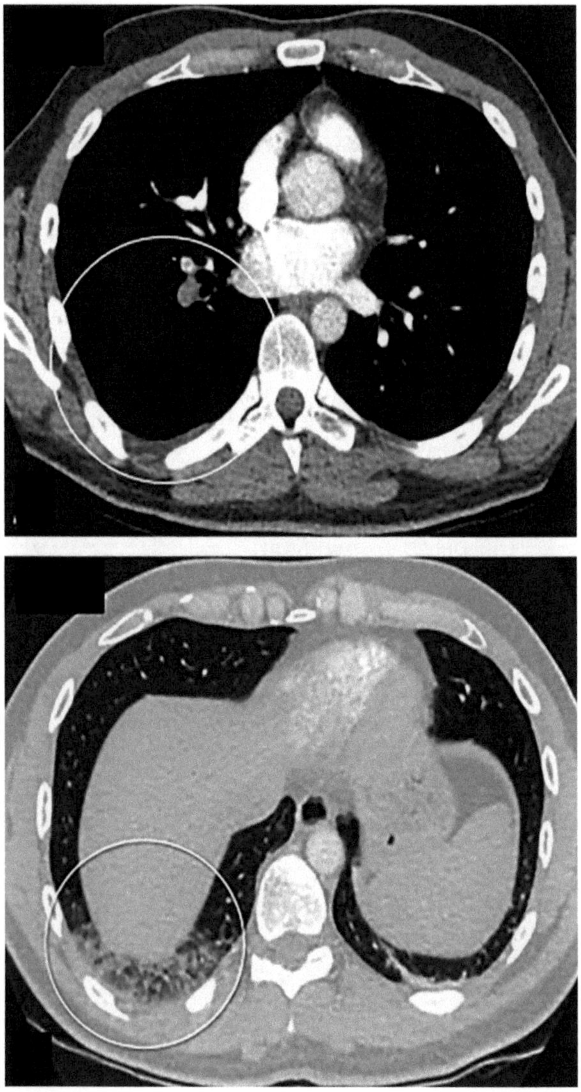

FIGURE 107-1. Chest CT depicting both soft tissue and lung windows. The circles represent the area of interest.

108 Timing of delivery in pregnancies affected by cervical cancer

A 38-year-old gravida 1 at 28 weeks of gestation presents with new vaginal spotting. Her physical examination reveals a 1-cm irregular mass on the cervix with smooth parametria and a normal rectovaginal septum. Biopsy of the mass reveals invasive squamous cell carcinoma. She elects to delay cancer treatment for pregnancy continuation. Her pelvic MRI is notable for the known cervical tumor and otherwise negative. The most appropriate delivery plan is

(A) preterm cesarean
(B) preterm vaginal
(C) term cesarean
(D) term vaginal

109 Database research

The Surveillance, Epidemiology, and End Results (SEER) Program provides cancer statistics in an effort to reduce the cancer burden in the U.S. population. The linked SEER Medicare Cancer database includes data pertaining to the clinical setting, incidence, and survival information from cancer registries that cover a substantial proportion of the U.S. population and links the data to Medicare claims data. A study that analyzed information in this data file reported that women with ovarian cancer who were prescribed metformin do not have improved survival compared with women with ovarian cancer who were not prescribed metformin. The inherent design limitation of this study is that it is

(A) inaccurate
(B) incomplete
(C) not generalizable
(D) subject to information bias

110 Vulvar cancer

An 82-year-old patient with hypertension presents to the office with vaginal bleeding and vulvar pain. She reports that she has never had surgery and walks 2 miles every day. She has had vulvar pain for 6 months, and she noticed an ulcer 3 months ago. Her physical examination is notable for a 1.5-cm ulcerative lesion on the left labium majus approximately 1 cm from the clitoris. There are no palpable inguinal lymph nodes. Biopsy results indicate squamous cell carcinoma of the vulva with 4 mm of invasion. The best next step in cancer treatment is

(A) complete radical vulvectomy with bilateral inguinal lymphadenectomy
(B) neoadjuvant chemotherapy with cisplatin and paclitaxel
(C) radiation therapy with concurrent cisplatin
(D) radical local excision with bilateral sentinel inguinal lymph node biopsies
(E) radical vulvectomy with postoperative radiation therapy

111 Endometriosis-associated ovarian cancer

A 47-year-old patient with a history of biopsy-proven endometriosis was noted 1 year ago to have a 4-cm left adnexal mass. Ultrasound imaging of the mass at that time is shown in Figure 111-1A, and her current ultrasound is shown in Figure 111-1B. She now reports pelvic pain, and her CA 125 level, which was previously in the normal range, is 362 U/mL. Other than endometrioid adenocarcinoma, the most likely cancer histology of this mass is

(A) carcinosarcoma
(B) clear cell
(C) high-grade serous
(D) low-grade serous
(E) mucinous

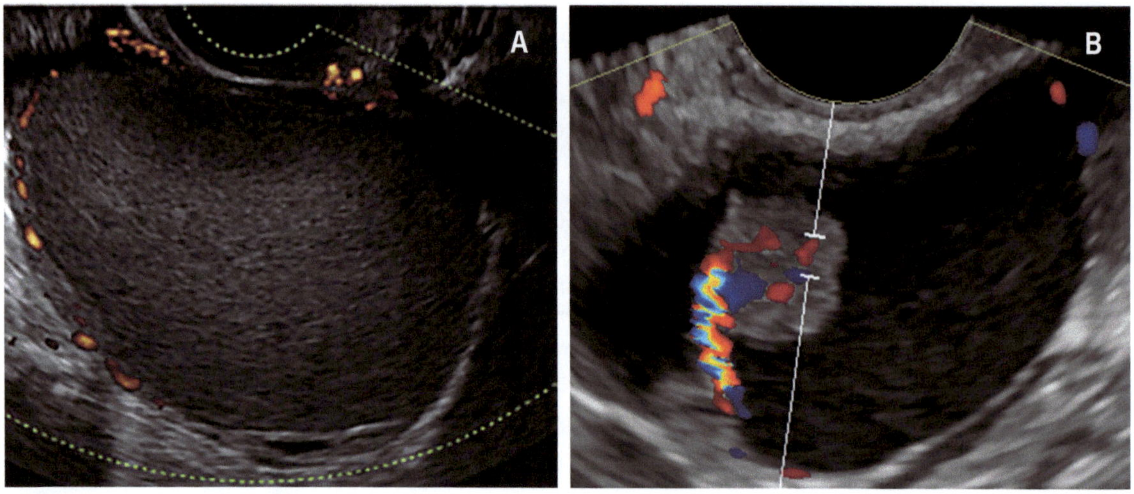

FIGURE 111-1. A and B. Past and current ultrasound images of left adnexal mass. (Figure 111-1A reprinted from Exacoustos C, Manganaro L, Zupi E. Imaging for the evaluation of endometriosis and adenomyosis. Best Pract Res Clin Obstet Gynaecol. 2014 Jul;28(5):655-81. doi: 10.1016/j.bpobgyn.2014.04.010.)

112 Tumor markers

A 59-year-old presents with a 2- to 3-month history of persistent lower abdominal pain, hematochezia, and nausea. She is afebrile with normal vital signs, and her abdominal examination is notable for mild tenderness to deep palpation across the lower abdomen. Laboratory test results are listed in Table 112-1. Imaging of the abdomen and pelvis with computed tomography (CT) is obtained (Fig. 112-1A and -1B). To determine a diagnosis, the best additional tumor marker to evaluate is

(A) α-fetoprotein (AFP)
(B) CA 15-3
(C) carcinoembryonic antigen (CEA)
(D) human chorionic gonadotropin (hCG)
(E) human epididymis protein 4 (HE4)

TABLE 112-1. The Described Patient's Laboratory Study Results

White blood cell count	7,200/microliter
Hematocrit	28.6%
Blood urea nitrogen	10 mg/dL
Creatinine	0.9 mg/dL
CA 125	142 U/mL
CA 19-9	34 U/mL

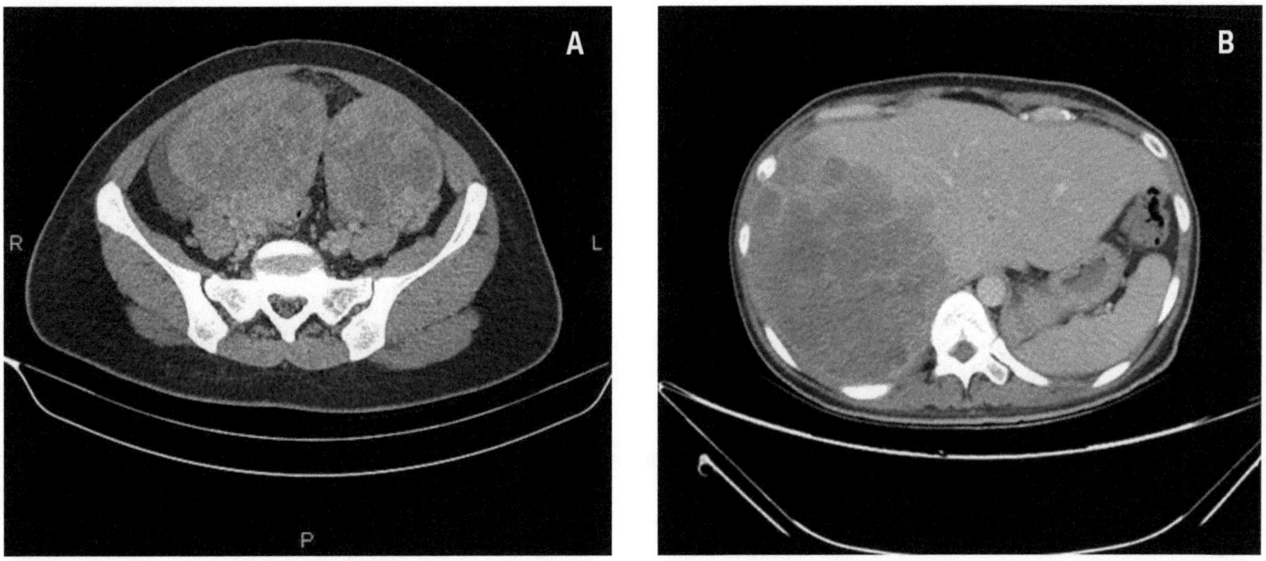

FIGURE 112-1. A and B. Described patient's computed tomography results. (A. Reprinted from Molinari A. Krukenberg tumor. Radiopaedia. Accessed June 3, 2025. https://radiopaedia.org/articles/krukenberg-tumor-2. B. Reprinted from Wang W, Lin CC, Liang WY, Chang SC, Jiang JK. Adenocarcinoma of sigmoid colon with metastasis to an ovarian mature teratoma: A case report. World J Clin Cases. 2024 Feb 6;12(4):853–858. doi: 10.12998/wjcc.v12.i4.853)

113 Hospice

A 68-year-old woman with recurrent ovarian cancer is undergoing fourth-line chemotherapy. At the time of her scheduled follow-up, she reports mild fatigue and intermittent nausea that has been well managed with palliative care. She states that she is able to garden daily, enjoys walks with her spouse, and likes to cook family dinners. The most recent imaging studies reveal progression of the disease. She explains that she would like to continue to feel well and does not want to continue cytotoxic treatment. For this patient, the best type of institution for hospice referral is

(A) assisted-living facility
(B) patient's home
(C) inpatient facility
(D) long-term nursing facility

114–117 Checkpoint inhibitor toxicity

Choose the most appropriate intervention (A–D) in the setting of toxicity caused by checkpoint inhibitor therapy for the described patient (114–117).

(A) Administer intravenous (IV) corticosteroids
(B) Permanently discontinue checkpoint inhibitor therapy
(C) Administer oral corticosteroids
(D) Proceed with next cycle

114. A 55-year-old presents for cycle 2 of maintenance therapy with a checkpoint inhibitor. She reports 10 non-bloody stools a day for the past week.

115. A 62-year-old presents for cycle 4 of platinum, taxane, and a checkpoint inhibitor. She reports that since cycle 3 she has experienced joint pain that limits her ability to dress herself.

116. A 45-year-old presents for cycle 6 of maintenance therapy with a checkpoint inhibitor. She was recently treated and discharged from the hospital for a diagnosis of grade 4 checkpoint inhibitor hepatitis.

117. A 70-year-old presents for cycle 4 of maintenance checkpoint inhibitor therapy. Her pretreatment thyroid-stimulating hormone (TSH) concentration is 5.6 micro-international units/mL but her T_4 level is within normal range.

118–121 Granulosa cell ovarian tumor

Match the correct management (A–F) of the granulosa cell tumor with each patient scenario (118–121).

(A) Aromatase inhibitor
(B) Bleomycin, etoposide, and cisplatin
(C) Endometrial sampling and surgical staging
(D) Hysterectomy with oophorectomy and surgical staging
(E) Paclitaxel and carboplatin
(F) Surveillance examinations and serum inhibin B

118. A 56-year-old patient underwent a robot-assisted laparoscopic hysterectomy with bilateral salpingo-oophorectomy and surgical staging for a 4-cm solid mass of the ovary. The ovary was intact, cytology was negative for malignant cells, and there was no other evidence of disease.

119. A 42-year-old gravida 3, para 3, with a past surgical history of bilateral tubal ligation underwent an oophorectomy with bilateral salpingectomy for ovarian torsion. The 12-cm ovarian mass was removed intact.

120. A 28-year-old nulligravida undergoes surgery for a 6-cm cystic and solid adnexal mass found during infertility evaluation. No other visible disease is present. She undergoes a unilateral oophorectomy with a frozen section, which confirms a sex cord-stromal tumor.

121. A 61-year-old with stage IIIC disease undergoes a hysterectomy and bilateral salpingo-oophorectomy with suboptimal tumor debulking.

122–127 Genitourinary injury

Match the appropriate surgical intervention (A–F) to each ureteral injury (122–127) and the corresponding site indicated in Figure 122–127-1.

(A) Cystoscopy with ureteral stent placement
(B) Percutaneous nephrostomy tube placement with delayed ureteroneocystostomy
(C) Ureteroneocystostomy
(D) Ureteroneocystostomy with psoas hitch
(E) Ureteroneocystostomy with Boari flap
(F) Uretero-ureteral anastomosis

122. Ureter transected with scissors during mobilization of the peritoneum in attempt to remove para-aortic lymph nodes (location 1)

123. Extensive thermal injury during dissection for endometriosis (location 2)

124. Ureter transected using electrosurgery taking down the posterior peritoneum during surgery for leiomyoma (location 3)

125. Ureter clamped in attempt to control bleeding at uterine vessels, recognized, and released before suture, with no devascularization noted (location 4)

126. Ureter incorporated into suture for hemostasis after sacrificing the uterine vessels with devascularization noted (location 4)

127. Worsening flank pain 3 weeks after laparoscopic hysterectomy with a computed tomography urogram showing left hydroureteronephrosis and a contrast defect (near location 3).

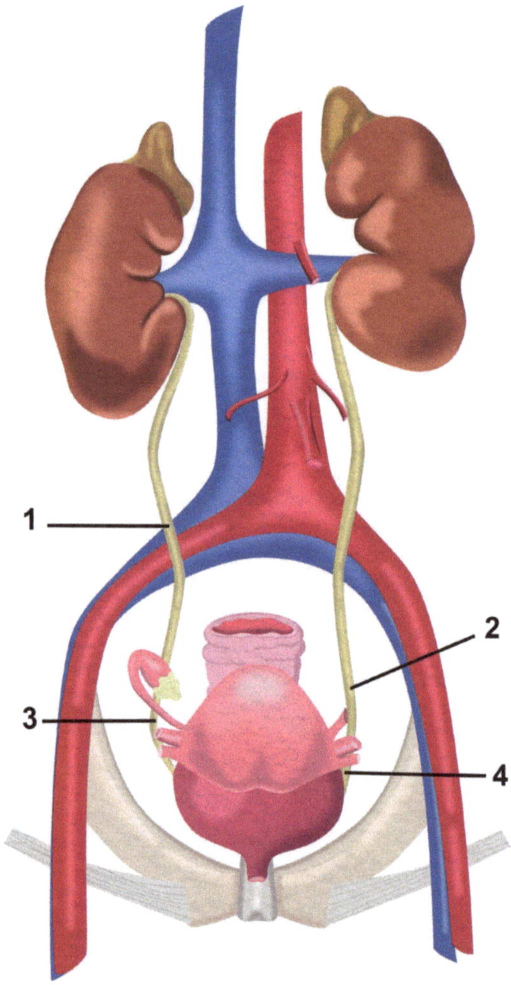

FIGURE 122–127-1. Female pelvic organs. Used with permission from Keytha Collins.

128–132 Cervical cancer screening in patients with human immunodeficiency virus/immunocompromised status

Choose the best testing (A–E) option for each clinical scenario (128–132).

(A) Cervical cytology with human papillomavirus (HPV) testing now
(B) Cervical cytology with HPV testing in 12 months
(C) Cervical cytology with HPV testing in 3 years
(D) Cervical cytology with HPV testing in 5 years
(E) Colposcopy now with endocervical curettage

128. A 35-year-old woman presents for a well-woman examination after a new diagnosis of HIV. Her last cervical cytology was 2 years ago and was negative for intraepithelial lesion or malignancy (NILM).

129. A 45-year-old woman with HIV presents to follow up on cervical cytology results. She has had two prior screenings that returned normal cytology with negative HPV testing. Her most recent result is NILM cytology, HPV negative.

130. A 32-year-old women diagnosed with HIV 1 year ago, with normal cervical cytology and HPV testing at that time, has a repeat screening that indicates NILM cytology, HPV negative.

131. A 55-year-old woman living with HIV presents to discuss the results of her recent cervical cancer screening, which indicated atypical squamous cells of undetermined significance (ASC-US) cytology and non-HPV 16/18 positive status. One year ago, her screening results were NILM cytology and HPV negative status.

132. An 18-year-old woman with newly diagnosed HIV presents for a routine gynecology appointment and has no prior cervical cancer screening. She is not currently sexually active.

133–135 Postoperative treatment of ovarian cancer

Choose the most appropriate treatment (A–C) for each of the patients (133–135) with high-grade epithelial ovarian cancer and Eastern Cooperative Oncology Group (ECOG) performance status of 0.

(A) Paclitaxel and carboplatin
(B) Liposomal doxorubicin
(C) Gemcitabine, carboplatin, and bevacizumab

133. A 60-year-old-presents with stage III disease. She is chemotherapy naive and has undergone optimal primary cytoreduction. She has hypertension and nephrotic syndrome.

134. A 62-year old with recurrent disease who progressed on her most recent treatment with platinum-based chemotherapy has undergone an end sigmoid colostomy for malignant sigmoid obstruction. She has no medical comorbidities.

135. A 63-year old with recurrent disease had complete response to her last course of carboplatin and paclitaxel. She has had optimal secondary cytoreduction. Today she presents with grade III chemotherapy-induced peripheral neuropathy.

136–139 Cancer syndromes

Choose the most likely germline mutation (A–F) for each clinical scenario (136–139).

(A) *BRCA1*
(B) *DICER1*
(C) *MSH6*
(D) *PTEN*
(E) *STK11*
(F) *TP53*

136. A 21-year-old nulligravida receives a diagnosis of cervical adenocarcinoma on biopsy. She has areas of increased pigmentation on their fingers, toes, and inside the mouth.

137. A 35-year-old gravida 2, para 2, undergoes a bilateral salpingectomy for sterilization. Final pathology reveals serous tubal intraepithelial carcinoma (STIC). The patient reports that her mother has a history of triple-negative breast cancer at age 42 years.

138. A 28-year-old gravida 1, para 1, has a history of childhood soft tissue sarcoma and receives a diagnosis of breast cancer on biopsy.

139. A 15-year-old nulligravida presents with clitoromegaly, voice deepening, male-pattern baldness, and amenorrhea. Her pelvic ultrasonography demonstrates a complex mass on the right ovary.

140–143 High-risk gestational trophoblastic neoplasia

Choose the most appropriate treatment (A–D) for each of the patients with gestational trophoblastic neoplasia (GTN) (140–143).

(A) Hysterectomy
(B) Reduced-dose induction multiagent chemotherapy
(C) Immunotherapy
(D) Single-agent chemotherapy

140. A 39-year-old woman had evacuation of a hydatidiform mole 4 months ago. Her human chorionic gonadotropin (hCG) concentration is 1,100,000 mIU/mL. She has nine metastases to the liver, spleen, and peritoneum, the largest of which is 10 cm. She has had no prior chemotherapy.

141. A 25-year-old woman had evacuation of a hydatiform mole 20 months ago. Her hCG is 200,000 mIU/mL. She has seven lung metastases, the largest of which is 2 cm. She declines cytotoxic chemotherapy.

142. A 50-year-old woman had evacuation of a hydatidiform mole 14 months ago and subsequent treatment with single-agent methotrexate followed by single-agent actinomycin-D. The hCG plateaued at 900 (units). Repeat computed tomography shows a mass in the uterus and no evidence of metastatic disease.

143. A 37-year-old woman with low-risk (stage I) GTN is undergoing treatment with actinomycin D. Her β-hCG nadir was 60 mIU/mL and subsequent values plateaued over 3 weeks. She is asymptomatic. Imaging reveals disease confined to the uterus. During counseling, she reports completed childbearing, and she chooses to undergo a hysterectomy and bilateral salpingectomy.

144–147 Optimal modality of breast imaging

Choose the correct breast imaging modality (A–D) for each clinical scenario (144–147).

(A) Mammography
(B) Mammography and ultrasonography
(C) Ultrasonography
(D) Magnetic resonance imaging with contrast

144. A 25-year-old woman presents with a new breast lump that has been present for 4 months. Her maternal grandmother had breast cancer at age 67 years.

145. A 51-year-old asymptomatic patient presents for her annual examination. She is adopted and does not know her family history.

146. A 47-year-old woman has a new breast lump that is palpable on clinical breast examination. She has no family history of breast or ovarian cancer.

147. A 27-year-old asymptomatic woman presents for her annual examination. She is a *BRCA1* mutation carrier.

148–151 Adnexal masses

For each clinical scenario and image (148–151), choose the best next step (A–D):

(A) Gynecologic oncology referral
(B) Interval pelvic ultrasound (US)
(C) Image-guided (RI) biopsy of mass
(D) Magnetic resonance imaging (MRI)

148. A 66-year-old woman presents with 3 months of bloating and lower abdominal pain. Her pelvic examination is significant for a right adnexal mass that is solid and fixed. Her CA 125 concentration is 120 U/mL. Pelvic ultrasonography is performed, and the result is shown in Figure 148–151-1.

149. A 38-year-old woman presents with heavy menstrual bleeding and a firm palpable mass on bimanual examination. She has future fertility desires. Ultrasound imaging is shown in Figure 148–151-2. A urine human chorionic gonadotropin test is negative.

150. A 50-year-old patient presents with recent imaging demonstrating an 8-cm adnexal mass. Her CA 125 concentration is 28 U/mL. Ultrasound imaging is shown in Figure 148–151-3.

151. A 45-year-old patient undergoes pelvic ultrasonography because of heavy menses and right-sided pelvic pain for the past 6 months. Her urine pregnancy test is negative and her CA 125 concentration is 200 U/mL. Imaging of the ovary is shown in Figure 148–151-4.

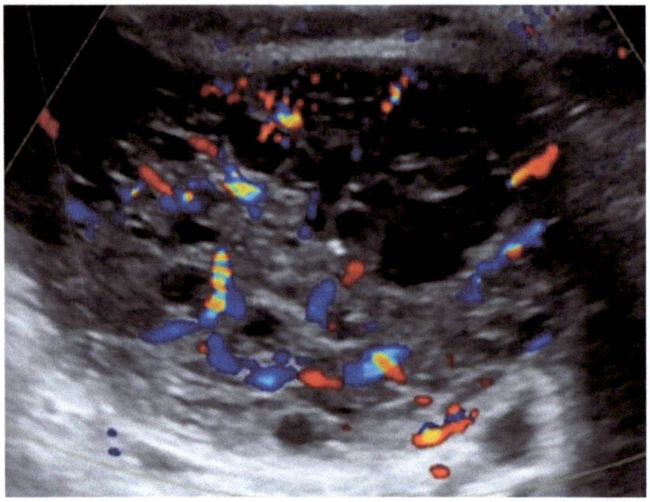

FIGURE 148–151-1. Ultrasonography showing an adnexal mass. (Reprinted from Strachowski LM, Jha P, Phillips CH, Blanchette Porter MM, Froyman W, Glanc P, et al. O-RADS US v2022: an update from the American College of Radiology's Ovarian-Adnexal Reporting and Data System US Committee. Radiology 2023;308:e230685. doi: 10.1148/radiol.230685)

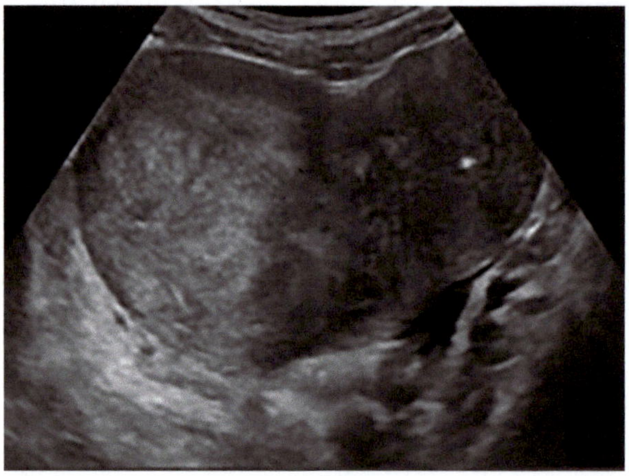

FIGURE 148–151-2. Pelvic ultrasound image for the patient in Scenario 149. (Reprinted from Geertsma T. Uterine fibroids leiomyomas. Ultrasound Cases. Accessed March 17, 2025. https://www.ultrasoundcases.info/uterine-fibroids---leiomyomas-6697/)

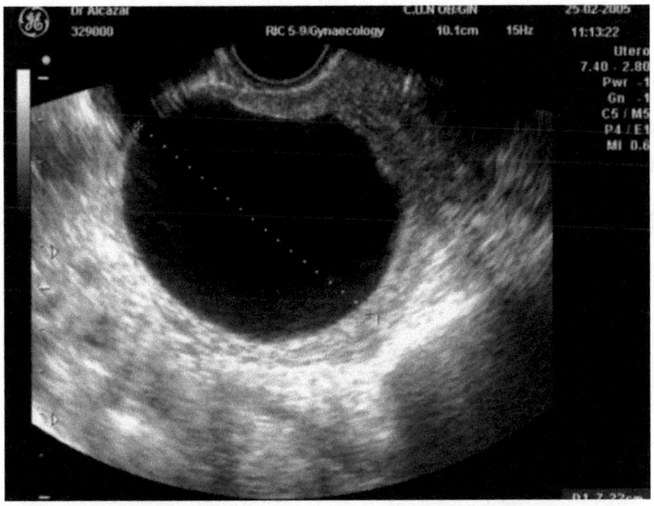

FIGURE 148-151-3. Ultrasound image for the patient in Scenario 150 showing an 8-cm ovarian cyst. (Reprinted from Alcazar JL, Martinez N, Juez L, Caparros M, Salas A, Errasti T. Ovarian simple cysts in asymptomatic postmenopausal women detected at transvaginal ultrasound: A review of literature. World J Obstet Gynecol 2015; 4(4): 108-112 [DOI: 10.5317/wjog.v4.i4.108])

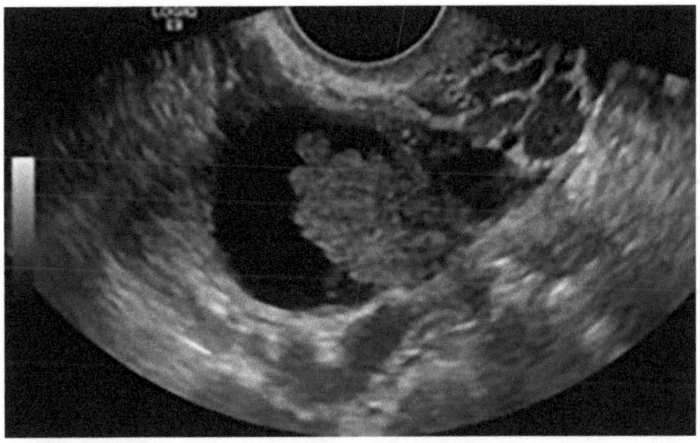

FIGURE 148-151-4. Ultrasound image for the patient described in Scenario 151. (Reprinted from Byron J. A better way to assess ovarian cancer risk. Kaiser Permanente; 2018. Accessed March 17, 2025. https://divisionofresearch.kaiserpermanente.org/a-better-way-to-assess-ovarian-cancer-risk/)

152–155 Survivorship

Choose the most appropriate therapy (A–E) for each clinical scenario (152–155). Each answer may be used more than once.

(A) Combined estrogen and progestin
(B) Gabapentin
(C) Selective serotonin reuptake inhibitor (SSRI)
(D) Transdermal estrogen
(E) Vaginal estrogen

152. A 76-year-old reports vaginal dryness with recurrent urinary tract infections. She has a history of stage IA, grade 1, endometrioid endometrial adenocarcinoma and underwent total hysterectomy with bilateral salpingo-oophorectomy at age 55 years. The examination today is consistent with significant vulvovaginal atrophy.

153. A 38-year-old who completed primary radiation therapy with chemosensitization for stage IIA2 squamous cell carcinoma of the cervix 6 months ago. She reports hot flushes that occur more than 10 times per day and frequent night sweats that interrupt her sleep. Her examination and imaging indicate a complete response to treatment.

154. A 35-year-old *BRCA1* mutation carrier undergoes a laparoscopic risk-reducing bilateral salpingo-oophorectomy. Pathology is negative for carcinoma. She has no personal history of cancer.

155. A 45-year-old who underwent a total abdominal hysterectomy with bilateral salpingo-oophorectomy and optimal cytoreduction for stage IIB low-grade serous ovarian adenocarcinoma reports depressive symptoms and diminished quality of life from persistent hot flushes.

156–159 Management of recurrent cervical cancer

For each clinical scenario 156–159, choose the best next step in treatment (A–E).

(A) Curative radiation
(B) Curative systemic anticancer therapy
(C) Palliative radiation
(D) Palliative systemic anticancer therapy
(E) Pelvic exenteration

156. A 42-year-old patient was treated with radical hysterectomy for stage IB2 cervical cancer 18 months ago. Adjuvant therapy was not indicated. She presents now with vaginal bleeding and a 4-cm mass at the vaginal apex. Biopsy confirms recurrent cervical cancer. Imaging demonstrates that the lesion abuts her posterior bladder and rectum without evidence for invasion into either organ. No other regional or distant metastatic disease is present.

157. A 55-year-old patient was treated with primary chemoradiotherapy for stage IIB cervical cancer 5 years ago. She now has a 3-cm lesion involving the posterior cervix that extends to the posterior vagina. Imaging demonstrates that the lesion invades the rectum without additional regional or distant metastasis.

158. A 78-year-old patient completed primary chemoradiotherapy for stage IIIB cervical cancer 3 months ago. She now presents with debilitating back pain. A physical examination reveals a 3-cm mass at the vaginal apex, and a positron emission tomography (PET) scan shows a 5-cm right para-aortic lymph node invading an adjacent vertebral body.

159. A 55-year-old patient who completed primary chemoradiotherapy for stage IIIC1 cervical cancer 3 months ago presents with flank pain. Computed tomography revealed progression of disease with left obturator adenopathy, which is causing hydronephrosis. There is no additional evidence of metastatic disease.

160–163 Perioperative venous thromboprophylaxis

Choose the most appropriate prophylaxis (A–D) for venous thromboembolism (VTE) for each of the described patients (160–163).

(A) Mechanical and pharmacologic
(B) Mechanical and pharmacologic with pharmacologic prophylaxis extended 28 or more days
(C) Mechanical alone
(D) Pharmacologic alone

160. A 64-year-old patient undergoing robot-assisted total laparoscopic hysterectomy with bilateral salpingo-oophorectomy and sentinel lymph node staging for grade 2 endometrioid endometrial carcinoma.

161. A 38-year-old patient undergoing laparoscopic risk-reducing bilateral salpingo-oophorectomy for *BRCA1* mutation.

162. A 76-year-old patient with a BMI of 42 undergoing exploratory laparotomy, total abdominal hysterectomy, and unilateral salpingo-oophorectomy for a 12-cm hydrosalpinx and uterine leiomyomas with severe peripheral arterial occlusive disease in the bilateral lower extremities.

163. A 61-year-old patient with ovarian cancer on postoperative day 5 from exploratory laparotomy for interval debulking with average risk of postoperative bleeding.

164–167 Treatment approach to cervical cancer

Choose the most appropriate treatment (A–E) for each clinical scenario (164–167).

(A) Cervical conization
(B) Chemoradiation
(C) Extrafascial hysterectomy
(D) Pelvic exenteration
(E) Radical hysterectomy with lymph node assessment

164. A 26-year-old nulligravida presents with cervical cytology demonstrating high-grade squamous intraepithelial lesion (HSIL). No gross cervical, vaginal, or parametrial abnormalities are seen on physical examination. Colposcopic biopsies demonstrate cervical intraepithelial neoplasia 3 (CIN 3). An excisional procedure shows the findings listed below:

Loop electrosurgical excision procedure (LEEP) pathology
- Squamous cell carcinoma, depth of stromal invasion: at least 2 mm
- No lymphovascular space involvement
- LEEP margin positive for CIN 3

165. A 64-year-old with a history of stage IVA cervical cancer underwent chemoradiation 3 years ago. She presents with vaginal spotting. A pelvic examination demonstrates an endophytic lesion involving the cervix. The parametrium is firm with radiation change, but no obvious tumor involvement is detected. She undergoes further evaluation, which reveals the findings below:

Cervical biopsy
- Squamous cell carcinoma, depth of stromal invasion at least 10 mm
- Lymphovascular space invasion present
- Margins positive for carcinoma

Positron emission tomography (PET) and computed tomography (CT) imaging
- 5-cm hypermetabolic cervical mass extending to the parametria
- No evidence of regional or distant metastasis

166. A 32-year-old nulligravida presents with cervical cytology showing atypical glandular cells (AGCs). On examination, there are no gross cervical, vaginal, or parametrial abnormalities. She undergoes further evaluation, which reveals the findings below:

Pathology
- Endocervix curettage demonstrates endocervical adenocarcinoma, usual type
- Endometrial biopsy is unremarkable

PET and MRI
- 2.4-cm cervical lesion, 33% cervical stromal invasion, no regional or distant metastasis

167. A 48-year-old presents with worsening abnormal uterine bleeding. A pelvic examination demonstrates a globally enlarged cervix measuring 7 cm that is friable and bleeding. Vaginal fornices are blunted, but there are no obvious parametrial or vaginal abnormalities. She undergoes further evaluation, which reveals the findings below:

Cervical biopsy
- Squamous cell carcinoma, depth of stromal invasion exceeding 10 mm
- Lymphovascular space invasion present
- Margins positive for carcinoma

PET and MRI
- 7-cm cervical mass infiltrating the lower uterine segment
- No evidence of regional or distant metastasis

168–171 Preoperative imaging in endometrial cancer

Choose the best imaging study (A–D) for each clinical scenario (168–171).

(A) Chest X-ray
(B) Pelvic ultrasound
(C) Magnetic resonance imaging (MRI)
(D) Computed tomography (CT)

168. A woman with newly diagnosed clinical stage I, grade 2, endometrioid endometrial cancer is scheduled to undergo surgical staging. Clinical examination reveals a mobile 6-cm uterus without adnexal mass. She reports having a 3-month history of new cough but has no other symptoms and has not lost weight.

169. A 36-year-old asymptomatic woman with grade 1 endometrioid endometrial cancer desires future fertility.

170. A 44-year-old woman who underwent hysterectomy for abnormal uterine bleeding has grade 3 endometrioid endometrial cancer with 5% myometrial invasion and no lymphovascular invasion identified at pathology.

171. A woman with a history of stage I serous endometrial cancer with vaginal recurrence diagnosed at the time of routine surveillance elects surgical resection.